National Diet and Nutrition Survey:

children aged 1½ to 4½ years

Volume 1: Report of the diet and nutrition survey

A survey carried out in Great Britain on behalf of the Ministry of Agriculture, Fisheries and Food and the Departments of Health by the Social Survey Division of the Office of Population Censuses and Surveys and the Medical Research Council Dunn Nutrition Unit

Janet R Gregory, Office of Population Censuses and Surveys

Deborah L Collins, Office of Population Censuses and Surveys

Peter S W Davies, MRC Dunn Nutrition Unit

Joyce M Hughes, Ministry of Agriculture, Fisheries and Food

Petronella C Clarke, Department of Health

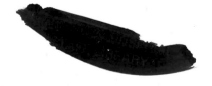

London: HMSO

ISBN 0 11 691611 7

Contents

11 Anthropometric measurements: results

Appendices

Foreword

This Report is the outcome of a successful collaboration between the Ministry of Agriculture, Fisheries and Food and the Department of Health with the Office of Population Censuses and Surveys, and the Medical Research Council Dunn Nutrition Unit.

The survey, of a nationally representative sample of children aged 1½ to 4½ years, is one of a programme of national diet and nutrition surveys aimed at gathering information about the dietary habits and nutritional status of the British population. There is also a related survey of the dental health of the same group of preschool children.

Diet and nutrition have a key role in achieving the targets for reducing the number of deaths from coronary heart disease and stroke set out in the Health of The Nation. The dietary behaviour established in children's early years is not only fundamentally important for their growth and development, but also lays the foundations for later life. The results from this survey will therefore provide a sound basis for understanding the current dietary habits of young children, and for developing future food and health policy to enable today's youngsters to enjoy a longer and healthier life.

We warmly welcome this Report in the National Diet and Nutrition Survey programme and express our thanks to all the respondents who took part.

BARONESS CUMBERLEGE
Parliamentary Secretary
Department of Health

ANGELA BROWNING
Parliamentary Secretary
Ministry of Agriculture,
Fisheries and Food

Authors' acknowledgements

We would like to thank everyone who contributed to the survey and the production of this Report. We were supported by specialist staff in the Social Survey Division of the Office of Population Censuses and Surveys who carried out the sampling, fieldwork, coding and editing stages. Particular thanks are due to the nutritionists at OPCS, Rosaline Ajiboye, Vasant Gorsia and Ceri Lowe, and to the interviewers who showed such commitment and enthusiasm to a survey which placed considerable demands on their skills.

We would also like to record our gratitude to the following people for their support, technical advice and assistance at various stages of the survey:

– the professional staff at the Ministry of Agriculture, Fisheries and Food and the Department of Health, in particular Alison Mills, Gillian Smithers, Michael Day (MAFF), Cecilia McGrath, Gordon Farquharson (formerly of MAFF) and Bob Wenlock (Department of Health);

– staff at the Medical Research Council Dunn Nutrition Unit, particularly Dr T J Cole, Dr A Lucas, Miss A Jennings and Mr K C Day, and at the Hospital for Sick Children, particularly Dr I Hann;

– Dr Elaine Gunter, Chief, NHANES Laboratory, Centers for Disease Control and Prevention, Atlanta, USA, for an independent review of the methodology for the laboratory analyses;

– the phlebotomists and the personnel recruited to collect and process the specimens of blood;

– members of the Panel on Child Nutrition of the Committee on Medical Aspects of Food Policy, for their advice to the Department of Health on the development of the protocol;

– members of the Steering Group on Chemical Aspects of Food Surveillance's Working Party on Dietary Surveys for their advice to the Ministry of Agriculture, Fisheries and Food on the development of the protocol and the analyses of the data.

Most importantly, we would like to thank all the parents and children who participated in the survey, and without whose co-operation it would not have been possible.

Notes

1 Tables showing percentages

In general, percentages are shown if the base is 30 or more. Where a base number is less than 30, actual numbers are shown within square brackets.

The row or column percentages may add to 99% or 101% because of rounding.

The varying positions of the percentage signs and bases in the tables denote the presentation of different types of information. Where there is a percentage sign at the head of a column and the base at the foot, the whole distribution is presented and the individual percentages add to between 99% and 101%. Where there is no percentage sign in the table and a note above the figures, the figures refer to the proportion of children who had the attribute being discussed, and the complementary proportion, to add to 100%, is not shown in the table.

In tables showing cumulative percentages the row labelled 'All' is always shown as 100%. The proportion of cases falling above the upper limit of the previous band can be calculated by subtracting from 100 the proportion in the previous band. Actual maximum values are not shown in tables of cumulative percentages, since they could vary for different subgroups being considered within the same table.

2 Conventions

The following conventions have been used within tables:
  – no cases
    0 values less than 0.5%
    the numbers inside the square brackets are the actual number of observations when the total number of cases, that is the base, is fewer than 30.

3 Tables showing descriptive statistics—mean, percentiles, standard error of the mean, standard deviation

These are shown in tables to an appropriate number of decimal places.

4 Significant differences

Differences commented on in the text are shown as being significant at the 99% or 95% confidence levels ($p < 0.01$ and $p < 0.05$). Throughout the Report the terms 'significant' and 'statistically significant' are used interchangeably. Where differences are shown or described as being 'not statistically significant' or 'NS' this indicates that $p > 0.05$.

Where the differences between subgroups are compared for a number of variables, for example, differences between children living in different regions in their consumption of sugar confectionery, chocolate confectionery and preserves, the significance level shown ($p < 0.01$ or $p > 0.05$) applies to *all* comparisons unless otherwise stated.

5 Standard errors for estimates for simple random sample are calculated as follows:

for a proportion (p) of a sample of n cases the standard error is given by:

$$se(p) = \sqrt{p(1-p)/n}$$

Standard errors for estimates of mean values are shown in the tables.

The standard error of the difference between two proportions or mean (a and b) for different subgroups of the sample is given by:

$$se(a\text{-}b) = \sqrt{[se(a)]^2 + [se(b)]^2}$$

In testing for the significance of the difference between two sample estimates, proportions or means, the sampling error calculated as for a simple random design was multiplied by an assumed design factor of 1.5 to allow for the complex sample design. The reader is referred to Appendix D for a description of the method of calculating true standard errors and for tables of design factors for the main variables and subgroups used throughout this Report. In general design factors were below 1.5 and therefore there will be some differences in sample proportions and means not commented on in the text which are significantly different at least at the $p < 0.05$ level.

6 Age groups

For the purpose of analysis and reporting children have been grouped in three age bands, described in the text and tables as:
  'aged 1½ to 2½ years'—that is, all children aged under 30 months;
  'aged 2½ to 3½ years'—that is, all children aged 30 months to under 42 months;
  'aged 3½ to 4½ years'—that is, all children aged 42 months and over.

For information on the derivation of age see:
  Chapter 3 and Appendix C: age at the time the dietary record was kept;
  Chapter 10: age at the time the blood sample was taken;
  Chapter 11: age at the time the anthropometric measurements were made.

The derivation of age at the time of the dental examination is described in Chapter 1 of *Volume 2: Report of the Dental Survey*.

Summary

Introduction

This Report presents the findings of a survey of the diet and nutrition of British children aged 1½ to 4½ years carried out between July 1992 and June 1993. The survey forms part of the National Diet and Nutrition Survey programme which was set up jointly by the Ministry of Agriculture, Fisheries and Food and the Department of Health in 1992 following the successful Dietary and Nutritional Survey of British Adults[1]. This cross-sectional study of children aged 1½ to 4½ years is part of a planned programme of surveys covering representative samples of defined age groups of the population. Other groups to follow will be older adults aged 65 years or over and school children aged 5 to 15 years, before returning to adults aged 16 to 64 years. Preschool children were chosen as the first of the new groups because no nationally representative survey had been undertaken since the Government survey by the Health Departments in 1967/8[2].

The children in the survey

A nationally representative sample of 2101 children aged 1½ to 4½ years was identified from a postal sift of addresses selected from the Postcode Address File. Only children living in private households were eligible to be included and only one child per household was selected. The interview, which was the first stage of the full survey protocol, was completed for 1859 children (88% of the identified sample). These 1859 children are referred to as the interview sample. The numbers of children in the interview sample were 648 aged 1½ to 2½ years, 668 aged 2½ to 3½ years and 543 aged 3½ to 4½ years. The survey fieldwork covered 12 months to take account of possible seasonal variation in eating habits.

(Chapters 1 and 3 and Appendix C).

The interview sample of children was found to be representative of the population in terms of social and demographic characteristics as assessed by reference to the 1992 General Household Survey[3] and mid year population estimates[4]. *(Chapter 3).*

The survey design included an interview, generally with the child's mother, to provide information about sociodemographic circumstances of the child's household, medication and eating and drinking habits; a weighed dietary record of all food and drink consumed over four consecutive days (including a Saturday and Sunday); a record of bowel movements for the same four days; physical measurements of the child (weight, standing height, mid upper-arm and head circumferences, and supine length for children under 2 years of age); a request for a sample of blood; and a dental examination.

Records of weighed dietary intake were obtained for 1675 children, that is 90% of those completing the interview and 80% of those identified by the sift. Physical measurements were obtained for over 90% of the interview sample. Consent to the request for a blood sample was given for 1157 children (63% of the interview sample) and blood was obtained from 1003 children (54%). The final element in the survey was an assessment of dental health by questionnaire and examination. An examination and/or dental interview was achieved for 1658 children, that is 89% of the children for whom a dietary interview had been obtained. This final element in the survey took place at the end of each of the four 3-month dietary survey fieldwork periods. A full Report of this dental survey is published separately as Volume 2[5]. A summary of the dental survey is at Appendix Q.

The foods and drinks consumed

The proportion of children consuming the various foods was based on the numbers of consumers during the four-day period of recording, which would not necessarily be the same as the proportion of these same children consuming these foods over any longer period. An explanation of the method used to re-weight the food intake data and estimate the average daily intake of nutrients is provided in Appendix J. The following foods and drinks were consumed by more than 70% of the children during the four-day recording period; biscuits; white bread; non-diet soft drinks; whole milk; savoury snacks (includes both potato crisps and cereal-based snacks); boiled, mashed or jacket potatoes; chocolate confectionery and chips. Coated or fried white fish had been eaten by 38%, but white fish cooked by methods other than frying by only 10%, and oily fish by 16% of children. Fifty nine percent of the children had eaten some cheese but the amounts were small, 40% of children had eaten yogurt and 46% eggs. Of fats and oils, polyunsaturated margarine was consumed by the largest proportion of children (36%) and butter by 30%. Sausages, chicken and turkey, and beef and beef dishes were eaten by about half of the children. Peas and carrots were the only cooked vegetables, excluding potatoes, to be eaten by more than half the children (carrots, 54% and peas 53%). Of any vegetable, baked beans were consumed in the greatest quantities and were eaten by 49% of all children in the survey. Leafy green vegetables were eaten by only 39% and in fairly small quantities. Raw vegetables and salad were eaten by less than 24% of children during the four-day period. The most popular fruits were apples and pears, then bananas. Chocolate confectionery was more commonly eaten than sugar confectionery, by 74% and 58% of children respectively.

(Chapter 4)

In the interview mothers reported that whole milk was given as a drink to 68% of children while 19% usually had semi-skimmed and 1% skimmed milk to drink. In all, 8% of the children were reported as having no milk to drink although some of these had it mixed with food, for example, on cereals and in milk puddings. Soft drinks were consumed by the majority of children. Half of those drinking non-diet soft drinks were estimated to be consuming about 1.5 litres a week and half of those who drank diet soft drinks were consuming about 1 litre per week. Fruit juice and tea were each consumed by about one third of children but in smaller quantities.

(Chapter 4)

Twenty one percent of children were reported in the interview to be taking dietary supplements and information from the dietary records showed that 19% of the children had taken dietary supplements during the four days (11% as tablets, 3% as syrups and 5% as drops). Children who were reported as taking dietary supplements generally had higher intakes of vitamins from food than children who did not take supplements.

(Chapter 8)

When the successive age groups were compared, trends in eating patterns with age were identified. More of the youngest children ate bananas, commercial infant and toddlers' foods, fish which was neither coated or fried, yogurt and whole milk, while more of the older children ate white bread, buns, cakes and pastries, ice cream, sugar confectionery, meat products, chips and savoury snacks. The quantity of food consumed generally increased with age including the amounts of sugar and chocolate confectionery. However the mean consumption of whole milk decreased by almost one third from the youngest to the oldest age groups. There were small differences in the amounts of foods consumed by girls and by boys in the older age group. *(Chapter 4)*

Energy consumption

The mean daily energy intakes for children aged 1½ to 2½ years were 4393kJ (1045kcal), for those aged 2½ to 3½ years 4882kJ (1160kcal), and for the oldest group of girls intake was 4976kJ (1183kcal) compared with the oldest group of boys intake of 5356kJ (1273kcal).

(Chapter 5)

For each age/sex group the mean energy intakes were below the Estimated Average Requirements (EARs)[6]. It was considered unlikely that these recorded low levels of energy intakes were due to poor dietary recording methodology following the validation of the method using a doubly-labelled water technique in the feasibility study[7]. Values for EAR for energy for infants set in 1979[8] were revised and lowered in 1991[6]. EAR values for older pre-school children were also slightly revised in 1991, but may still be set too high. The mean energy intakes of subjects in this study probably do not reflect inadequate amounts for the maintenance of health and growth. When compared with the children examined in the Government survey of 1967/8[2], children of the same age in 1992/3 were on average significantly taller *(Fig 11.2)*.

At all ages cereals and cereal products made the largest contribution to energy intake (overall 30%), and this was closely followed by milk and milk products (overall 20%), then vegetables, potatoes and savoury snacks (overall 12%) *(Table 5.7b and Fig 5.6)*. The proportion of energy from milk and milk products reduced from 26% for the youngest age group to 16% for the oldest children whereas the proportion of energy from cereals and cereal products increased from 27% for the youngest group to 32% for the oldest group of children *(Fig 5.6)*. On average children in the sample derived about one fifth of their mean energy intake from foods eaten away from home. The amount of energy derived from each of the macronutrients, protein, carbohydrate and fat for each of the three age groups and for boys and girls is shown in the table below and in *Figure 6.3*.

Macronutrient contribution to food energy intake by age and sex of child

| | Age and sex of child | | | | | | |
| | All aged 1½–2½ years | All aged 2½–3½ years | All aged 3½–4½ years | | All boys | All girls | All |
			Boys	Girls			
Average daily intake:							
Total food energy (kcal)	1045	1160	1273	1181	1172	1108	1141
Total food energy (kJ)	4393	4882	5356	4976	4930	4663	4798
Protein (g)	35.4	36.8	39.4	37.7	37.4	36.2	36.8
Carbohydrate (g)	139	159	177	162	160	150	155
Total fat (g)	42.5	46.3	50.1	47.2	46.7	44.6	45.7
Percentage food energy from:							
Protein (%)	13.6	12.7	12.4	12.7	12.8	13.1	13.0
Carbohydrate (%)	49.9	51.5	52.3	51.7	51.4	50.8	51.1
Fat (%)	36.4	35.8	35.3	35.5	35.7	36.1	35.9

The nutrients: protein

The mean protein intake for all children was 36.8g which contributed about 13% of the total food energy. Children aged 1½ to 2½ years obtained a slightly higher proportion of their energy from protein than older children. Mean intakes of protein for each group defined by age and sex, in all cases, considerably exceeded the Reference Nutrient Intake (RNI)[6]. Milk and milk products (overall 33%), then cereals and cereal products (overall 23%) and meat and meat products (overall 22%) all made major contributions to protein intake.

(Chapter 6)

The nutrients: carbohydrates including non-starch polysaccharides (dietary fibre)

The mean daily carbohydrate intake (excluding non-starch polysaccharides) for all children was 155g which contributed about 51% of the total food energy. The average daily intake of total sugars for all children was 87g which contributed 29% of the total food energy and that of starch was 68g which contributed 22% of total food energy. Total sugars have been further subdivided into non-milk extrinsic sugars and intrinsic and milk sugars. Non-milk extrinsic sugars provided on average about 19% of total food energy. The main dietary sources of non-milk extrinsic sugars were soft drinks, which contributed a third of the total, followed by confectionery which contributed about one fifth. Other major contributors were biscuits (7%) and fruit juices (6%).

(Chapter 6)

Of the starch in the diets of these children two thirds was obtained from cereals and cereal products and about a quarter was obtained from vegetables, potatoes and savoury snacks. The intakes of total starch increased with age and also provided an increasing proportion of energy intake with increasing age of the child. When intrinsic and milk sugars were added to starch they contributed overall 32% of the total food energy.

(Chapter 6)

The average daily intake of non-starch polysaccharides (NSP) was 6.1g. However intakes increased with age with the youngest children having an average daily intake of 5.5g and the oldest boys 6.8g (oldest girls 6.4g) *(Table 6.20)*. The main dietary sources of NSP were vegetables (excluding potatoes) (17%), potatoes including fried potatoes (13%), high fibre and whole grain breakfast cereals (12%) and fruit (11%) with a smaller contribution from bread (white 7% and wholemeal 6%) *(Table 6.21b)*. There was a positive correlation between increasing levels of NSP intake and numbers of bowel movements daily.

(Chapter 6)

Dietary fats and blood lipids

The average daily total fat intake for all children was 45.7g which contributed 35.9% of total food energy. Saturated fatty acids contributed an average of 16.2% of total food energy. The proportion of energy from total fat and saturated fatty acids tended to decline with increasing age, from 36.4% and 16.9% respectively for the youngest age group to 35.3% from total fat and 15.4% from saturated fatty acids for boys in the oldest age group and 35.5% from total fat and 15.5% from saturated fatty acids for girls in the oldest age group. The main food sources of total fat were milk and milk products (35% at 1½ to 2½ years; 26% at 2½ to 3½ years and 22% for both boys and girls in the oldest age group). Cereals and cereal products contributed one fifth of the total fat and meat and meat products contributed one sixth overall. Milk, meat, savoury snacks and biscuits were major contributors of saturated fatty acids in the diet.

(Chapter 7)

Trans fatty acids provided about 1.7% of total food energy from an average daily intake of between 2.0 to 2.4g. Most *trans* fatty acids were derived from cows' milk (21%), fat spreads (14%), biscuits (13%), buns, cakes and pastries (8%) *(Table 7.18a and b)*.

Cis-monounsaturated fatty acids provided about 11% of food energy. These were mainly derived from meat and meat products (20%), cows' milk (17%), savoury snacks (8%), fat spreads (8%), biscuits (6%) and fried potatoes (6%). The average intake of *cis* polyunsaturated fatty acids of the n-3 series contributed less than 1% of food energy which came in small amounts from fried potatoes, fish, meat, milk and cereal products. *Cis* n-6 polyunsaturated fatty acids contributed about 4% of total food energy, the main sources in the children's diets being polyunsaturated fat spreads, fried potatoes, meat and meat products, cereals and cereal products and milk.

Blood lipid results are reported for plasma total cholesterol, high density lipoprotein (HDL) cholesterol and for plasma triglycerides. The blood was not taken with the child fasting and therefore the values relating to triglyceride levels must be interpreted with caution. Plasma levels of both total and HDL cholesterol generally correlated positively (blood levels increasing as dietary intakes increased) with intakes of total fat, saturated, *trans* and *cis* monounsaturated fatty acids and with dietary cholesterol. However these relationships were generally weak, particularly with respect to levels of plasma total cholesterol. There was no consistent association between plasma total cholesterol and HDL cholesterol levels and intakes of *cis* n-3 and *cis* n-6 polyunsaturated fatty acids. *(Table 10.43)*.

(Chapter 10)

The nutrients: vitamins

Vitamin A intakes were derived from an assessment of daily retinol intakes with a contribution from carotenoid precursors of vitamin A combined as 'retinol equivalent'. The mean daily intake from food and dietary supplements for the whole group of children was 578μg. The skewed distribution of intakes of vitamin A (retinol equivalents) resulted in the median intake being lower than the mean intake, 428μg daily. About half of the children had average daily intakes of vitamin A which fell below the RNI value of 400μg. Eight percent of children aged under 4 years and 7% of children aged 4 years and over had intakes of vitamin A below the lower reference nutrient intake (LRNI) level. The food sources of vitamin A were mainly milk and vegetables. Overall liver provided about one sixth of total intake although only 4% of children had eaten it in the four-day recording period. Dietary supplements containing vitamin A contributed substantial amounts but they tended to be taken by children who were already towards the upper end of the range of intake levels.   *(Chapter 8)*

Blood was analysed for retinol and several carotenoids. There were no clear associations between plasma retinol levels and dietary intakes of pre-formed retinol and total carotene.   *(Chapter 10)*

On average the mean daily intakes for thiamin, riboflavin, niacin, vitamin B_6, vitamin B_{12} and folate were well above the RNI values. The average daily intakes for all children from both food sources and dietary supplements (that is, all sources) were for thiamin 0.8mg, for riboflavin 1.2mg, for niacin 16.3mg, for vitamin B_6 1.2mg, for vitamin B_{12} 2.8µg and for folate 132µg. None of the children aged under 4 years had intakes below the LRNI for niacin and vitamin B_{12} and only 1% or less had intakes below the LRNI for thiamin, riboflavin, vitamin B_6 and folate. Similarly none of the children aged 4 years and over had intakes below the LRNI for niacin and vitamin B_{12} and only 1% had intakes below the LRNI for thiamin, riboflavin and folate and 5% below that for vitamin B_6. The mean intakes of riboflavin per kilogram body weight declined from 0.1mg/kg to 0.07mg/kg with increasing age and this can be accounted for by the declining consumption of milk with increasing age. The range of intakes of vitamin C was wide and the distribution of intakes was skewed, with some children having intakes many times the RNI value. The mean daily intake from all sources was 51.8mg which was well above the RNI for vitamin C (30mg). Dietary supplements contributed 7% but none of the children in the bottom 2.5 percentile of intake took vitamin C supplements during the four days. Only 1% of all children had intake levels below the LRNI.   *(Chapter 8)*

Results for blood analyses of the erythrocyte glutathione reductase activation coefficient (EGRAC), a measure of riboflavin status, and of vitamin B_{12}, red blood cell folate, plasma folate and vitamin C are reported. The data from this survey reflect, for the first time, levels of these analytes for the national population of children aged 1½ to 4½ years in Great Britain and thus provide population standards. The mean values for the blood samples provided by the children were for the EGRAC 1.24, for vitamin B_{12} 636pmol/l, for red cell folate 914nmol/l, and for plasma folate 21.1nmol/l *(Tables 10.17 to 10.21)*. Overall the mean level of plasma vitamin C was 67.6µmol/l, with a wide range between the lower and upper 2.5 percentiles (8.8µmol/l to 124.5 mol/l) *(Table 10.22 and Fig 10.4)*. There was almost no variation in plasma vitamin C by age but boys had significantly lower levels than girls. Dietary intakes of riboflavin for each age/sex cohort were significantly negatively correlated with the EGRAC. Red cell folate correlated positively with dietary intakes of folate and plasma levels of vitamin C with dietary intakes of vitamin C.   *(Chapter 10)*

Average daily intakes of vitamin D from foods were low, 1.2µg in both the youngest and middle age groups and very slightly higher in the 3½ to 4½ years group (boys 1.4µg, girls 1.3µg). Dietary supplements resulted in an increase in total intakes to 1.8µg for both the youngest and middle groups and 2.0µg for the boys, 1.9µg for the girls in the 3½ to 4½ years group. The RNI at age 1 to 3 years is 7µg, a level met by only 5% of children aged under 4 years. No DRVs are set for vitamin D for children aged 4 years or over because most of the body's requirement for vitamin D in this age group can be synthesised by the skin if they are sufficiently exposed to sunlight. Children in the youngest age group, 1½ to 2½ years, were obtaining about one sixth of their mean daily intake of vitamin D from milk products, mainly infant formula, whereas boys in the oldest age group were obtaining only 5% and girls 2% from this food source. The other main food sources for all the children were breakfast cereals and fat spreads, many of which are fortified with vitamin D.   *(Chapter 8)*

Blood levels of plasma 25-hydroxyvitamin D were determined and a mean value of 68.1nmol/l *(Table 10.34 and Fig 10.6)* was reported. There was no apparent association between the mean values and either the age or the sex of the child. However plasma vitamin D levels varied by season, with mean levels being highest in July to September and lowest in January to March *(Figure 10.7)*. In addition plasma levels correlated significantly with dietary intakes of vitamin D, plasma levels rising with increasing intakes.   *(Chapter 10)*

The mean daily intake of vitamin E was 4.4mg for all children and there was a small increase with age from 3.9mg for the youngest age group to 5.1mg for boys and 4.6mg for girls in the oldest age group. Dietary supplements contributed only 2% to the intake of this vitamin.   *(Chapter 8)*

Plasma α-and γ-tocopherols concentrations were measured. The mean plasma α-tocopherol level was 18.8µmol/l and the mean γ-tocopherol level was 1.6µmol/l. Levels of both tended to increase with age. Overall plasma α-tocopherol levels were positively correlated with total intakes of vitamin E.   *(Chapter 10)*

The nutrients: minerals

Iron was the only mineral to which dietary supplements made a substantive contribution. Iron in the children's diet was assessed as haem iron (mainly found in meat) and non-haem iron. The average daily intake of total iron from food was 5.4mg, of which haem iron contributed only 4%. Dietary supplements increased the total iron intake by only 2% to 5.5mg daily. The average daily intakes were well below the RNI for iron, with 84% of those under 4 years of age and 57% of those aged 4 years and over having intakes below the RNI. Sixteen percent of those under 4 years of age had intakes from all sources below the LRNI which increased to 24% in those aged 1½ to 2½ years. The LRNI value for children aged 4 years and over is lower than for younger children and only 4% had intakes below the LRNI. The main food sources of iron were cereal products, many of which are fortified, vegetables, potatoes and savoury snacks and meat and meat products. *(Chapter 9)*

The mean haemoglobin concentration in samples from the children as a whole group was 12.2g/dl. Average values were lowest for the youngest group at 12.0g/dl and highest for boys aged 3½ to 4½ years at 12.4g/dl. Haemoglobin concentrations below 11.0g/dl were defined as an indication of anaemia[9]. One in eight in the youngest group were anaemic and one in 12 of all children were anaemic using this definition. Low ferritin levels also implied that a proportion of the children had poor iron status, with 20% of all children having ferritin levels below 10μg/l, and 5% having levels below 5μg/l. The ferritin levels matched the haemoglobin levels in that there was a higher proportion of children with low levels in the youngest age group. Other haematological measurements such as mean corpuscular volume (MCV), haematocrit, mean cell haemoglobin (MCH), and mean cell haemoglobin concentration (MCHC) as well as zinc protoporphyrin (ZPP) results all supported the haemoglobin and ferritin results to confirm that iron deficiency occurred commonly and that it was more prevalent in the youngest age group. Generally the correlations between haemoglobin, ferritin and ZPP and dietary intakes were weak. Only haemoglobin showed any significant correlation with intakes of total, haem and non-haem iron. *(Chapter 10)*

The mean daily intake for all children of calcium was 637mg, of phosphorus was 742mg and of magnesium was 136mg which for each of these minerals was well above the RNI values. The range of intakes of both calcium and phosphorus was large but for calcium only 1% of children under the age of 4 years and 2% of those aged 4 years and over had intakes below the LRNI. Likewise the proportions with intakes below the LRNI for magnesium were small, less than 1% of children aged under 4 years and 2% of those aged 4 years and over. The main source of calcium was milk and milk products which provided 64% of the mean intake. Average calcium intakes decreased markedly with age which reflects the decrease in milk consumption. Fortified cereals and cereal products are the second main source and the contribution from this source increased with age.

Sodium and chloride intakes (which do not include additions during cooking or at the table) were both, on average, more than twice the RNI values. For all children the estimated average daily intake of sodium was 1506mg and for chloride 2261mg. The mean daily intakes of potassium were 1476mg for children aged 1½ to 2½ years, 1513mg for those aged 2½ to 3½ years and 1501mg for girls in the oldest age group and 1573mg for boys in the oldest group. Average daily intakes were well in excess of the RNI values and only 1% or less of all children had intakes below the LRNI values.

Zinc intakes were generally below reference values. The average daily intake for children aged 1½ to 2½ years was 4.3mg and similar average intake was recorded for the middle age group. In the 3½ to 4½ years age group, the average intake for boys was 4.6mg and for girls 4.4mg. Seventy two percent of those aged under 4 years had intakes less than 5.0mg (the RNI value for this age

group) and 14% had mean intakes below 3.0mg (the LRNI value). A greater proportion of children aged 4 years and over had intakes below the RNI (89%) and LRNI (37%) values. The average intake of copper for children in the survey was 0.5mg. Thirty six percent of children aged under 4 years and 68% of those aged 4 years and over had intakes below the RNI. Average daily iodine intakes were above the RNI values, and only 3% of children aged under 4 years and 5% of those 4 years and over had intakes below the LRNIs. Intakes of manganese increased with age with a mean daily intake of 1.2mg for all children aged 1½ to 4½ years. *(Chapter 9)*

Blood samples were analysed for plasma zinc, which showed very little variation with either age or sex; the overall mean level was 13.0μmol/l. *(Chapter 10)*

Anthropometric measurements

The average weight of girls and boys aged 1½ to 2½ years was 11.9kg and 12.6kg respectively, of those 2½ to 3½ years group 14.3kg and 14.9kg and at age 3½ to 4½ years the average weights were 16.4kg and 16.6kg for girls and boys. The average standing heights were 86.9cm for boys and 85.3cm for girls in the youngest group, 95.6cm for boys and 94.7cm for girls in the middle age group and 102.1cm for boys and 101.3cm for girls in the 3½ to 4½ year age group. In addition, supine length was measured for children under 2 years of age. For boys supine length was on average 1.60cm greater than standing height; for girls the difference was 1.63cm. On average, the head circumferences of girls were smaller than those of boys. In the youngest age group the mean head circumference was 50.1cm for boys and 48.8cm for girls, and in the oldest age group the average measurements were 51.9cm for boys and 51.0cm for girls. Only in the youngest age group was there a significant difference in the mid upper-arm circumference between boys, 16.5cm and girls, 16.2cm. At 2½ to 3½ years arm circumferences were 17.0cm for both boys and girls and at 3½ to 4½ years arm circumferences were 17.5cm and 17.6cm respectively. When these measurements were compared with the results from the 1967/8 survey of children of a similar age, children today in the youngest age group were slightly lighter, boys aged 2½ to 4½ years were about the same average weight and girls aged 2½ to 4½ years were slightly heavier. There had been estimated increases in average heights between the two surveys of up to 3.5cm.

The body mass index (BMI) of children aged 3½ to 4½ years was the same for both sexes, 15.9. At younger ages boys had BMIs greater than girls. As was reported for the 1967/8 survey food energy intakes were correlated positively with BMI and arm circumference. *(Chapter 11)*

Unwell children

Twenty seven percent of the children were reported as being unwell at some time during the dietary recording period, and for 16% mothers reported that being unwell had affected their eating. For this latter group being unwell resulted in a mean energy intake about 13% lower than the mean intake for children who were well. For those for whom it had been reported that being unwell had not affected their eating habits mean energy intake was about 6% lower than that for children who were well *(Table 5.3a)*.

The children who were reported as being unwell during the dietary recording period had lower average intakes of protein, all carbohydrates, total fat and fatty acids, most vitamins and minerals than other children; this generally applied whether or not their eating was reported to have been affected by their illness. Most differences were associated with differences in energy intake between well and unwell children and not to the nutrient density of their diet.

Region

The nationally representative sample of children was subdivided into four regions for purposes of analyses based on where the child was living at the time of interview (see *Fig 3.1*).

There were differences in the proportions of children eating the various foods between the regions but patterns of eating behaviour associated with region were not always distinct. However, children in the Northern region were the most likely, and children in the London and the South East the least likely to be eating meat pies and products, baked beans and boiled, mashed and jacket potatoes and to be drinking coffee. In contrast children in the Northern region were least likely to be eating rice, coated chicken, raw and salad vegetables (not tomatoes or carrots). Children in Scotland were most likely to be eating chips, beef and beef products, canned fruit in syrup and drinking soft drinks and were least likely to be eating cheese, most types of vegetables and drinking fruit juice. *(Chapter 4)*

The differences in foods eaten were not reflected in differences in average daily energy intake since there were no significant differences in energy intake according to region. *(Chapter 5)*

There was almost no variation between children living in different regions in the proportion of energy they derived from protein, total carbohydrate and total fat. Only intakes of NSP and starch varied significantly by region, intakes of starch being lowest for children living in London and the South East and highest among those from the Central, South West and Wales region. Intakes of NSP were also highest for children in the Central, South West and Wales region, but were lowest among children in Scotland. There were very few differences in average intake of fatty acids between children living in different parts of Great Britain. Any differences were associated with the small differences in energy intake. *(Chapters 6 and 7)*

There were regional variations in the vitamin intakes of children. Children in Scotland had the lowest intakes of vitamin C and total carotene. Children in London and the South East together with children living in the Northern region of England had the lowest intakes of folate. In most cases these differences were still apparent after adjusting for any differences in energy intake. *(Chapter 8)*

Children living in London and the South East tended to have the highest intakes of minerals except that their intakes of sodium, chloride and iodine were on average among the lowest. In Scotland, the position was reversed. Even after adjusting for the small differences in energy intakes, the intakes of several minerals by children living in Scotland tended to be lower than in children living elsewhere. *(Chapter 9)*

There were no marked associations between the results for the blood haematology and region. However there were differences in the results from the water soluble vitamins measured in blood (apart from the EGRAC), with children from the Northern region having generally lower values than for children living elsewhere in Great Britain. *(Chapter 10)*

Boys living in Scotland and the Northern region of England had a BMI above the average but there was no significant difference in BMI for girls in the different regions. *(Chapter 11)*

Socio-economic characteristics

Children were classified according to the social class of head of household (based on their occupation), which for reporting was described as manual and non-manual backgrounds. Other measures of socio-economic status were based on the employment status of head of household, whether the household was receiving Family Credit and/or Income Support, and the mother's highest educational qualification level.

There were several differences in the consumption of foods between children from manual and non-manual backgrounds. Children from non-manual home backgrounds were more likely to have eaten rice, wholemeal bread, wholegrain and high-fibre breakfast cereals, and buns, cakes and pastries than were children from a manual home background although the average amounts eaten did not differ greatly. However children from a manual home background were more likely to have eaten white bread and non-wholegrain and high fibre breakfast cereals and in significantly greater amounts. There was a marked difference in consumption of fruit juice which was twice as likely in the non-manual group when compared with the manual group of children, while significantly more children from manual home backgrounds consumed tea. Children from non-manual homes were significantly more likely to be taking dietary supplements than children from manual homes. *(Chapter 4)*

Although there were differences in food consumption patterns, there were no significant differences in mean energy intake for children from manual and non-manual home backgrounds (manual 4830kJ/1148kcal, non-manual 4767kJ/1132kcal). Nor were there any significant differences related to the other indicators of socio-economic status. *(Chapter 5)*

Girls from a non-manual home background and with mothers with no formal educational qualifications tended to have a lower than average BMI but there was no significant difference between boys from different socio-economic backgrounds. *(Chapter 11)*

When carbohydrate intakes were related to indicators of socio-economic status, there was a significant trend for children from households of lower economic status to have lower average intakes of total sugars but higher starch intakes than other children. This relationship was consistent for measures based on mothers' educational qualifications, the employment status of the head of household, and social class. There was also a tendency for children from a manual social class background to have lower intakes of protein and higher absolute intakes of total fat and certain fatty acids (especially *cis* monounsaturated fatty acids). However the percentage energy from total fat was not significantly different for children from less economically advantaged backgrounds (with the exception of the group whose mothers had no formal educational qualifications where the contribution from fat was higher) than other children. *(Chapters 6 and 7)*

Lower intakes of most vitamins were recorded for children from manual home backgrounds. When the intakes were adjusted for differences between the groups in energy intake, the diets of children from manual backgrounds were found to have proportionately lower amounts of total carotene, niacin, vitamin B_{12}, vitamin C and E. Within the range of values recorded for blood levels of vitamins, there were associations with all vitamin status levels recorded (except the EGRAC) and socio-economic characteristics. Thus, except for the EGRAC, lowest values tended to be recorded in children from manual homes or where the head of household was not working, where parents were receiving Income Support and/or Family Credit or where the mother had a low level of educational qualifications. *(Chapters 8 and 10)*

Children from non-manual home backgrounds tended to have higher average intakes of most minerals except sodium and chloride for which higher average intakes were recorded in the diets of children from manual home backgrounds. Furthermore, children from manual home backgrounds had lower intakes than other children of many minerals even after adjusting for differences in energy intakes. *(Chapter 9)*

Most haematological analytes showed no variation by social class, employment status or receipt of benefits but there was an observed difference in mean levels of ferritin between samples from children whose head of household was working (24μg/l) and those from children where the head was economically inactive (21μg/l). *(Chapter 10)*

Family type

Children in the survey were ascribed to one of four family types for reporting purposes: married or cohabiting couple with one child; married or cohabiting couple with more than one child; lone parent with one child; lone parent with more than one child. Eighty two percent of the children were living with married or cohabiting adults (two-parent families) and only 18% were living with one parent (lone-parent families). A higher proportion of two-parent families had two or more children compared with lone-parent families, 73% compared with 60%. *(Chapter 3)*

There were no significant differences in mean energy intake according to family type, although the data suggest that intakes of children in lone-parent families tended to be higher than for children in two-parent families. Average daily energy intake for one child living in a two-parent family was 4680kJ (1112kcal), for a child that had siblings living in a two-parent family 4802kJ (1141kcal), for one child living in a lone-parent family 4959kJ (1181kcal) and for a child with siblings living in a one-parent family 4911kJ (1169kcal). The range of energy intakes for children in lone-parent families, particularly where there was only one child, was large; 2560kJ (610kcal) to 8341kJ (1986kcal) between the lower and upper 2.5 percentiles. *(Chapter 5)*

Differences in body weight, height and BMI between children from different family types were not statistically significant although single children (boys and girls) and girls with siblings in lone-parent families were slightly heavier than the average weight for all children and both boys and girls in two-parent families were slightly lighter. Children from lone-parent families were slightly taller than other children and single children (boys and girls) and girls with siblings in lone-parent families had slightly greater BMIs than the mean for all children. *(Chapter 11)*

Overall there was no significant variation in the average daily intake of carbohydrates and protein associated with family type nor did the proportion of energy derived from carbohydrates vary significantly. However children from lone-parent families where there was more than one child in the family had significantly higher intakes of starch than other children, but lower intakes of total sugars and non-milk extrinsic sugars (as compared with children from two-parent families with more than one child) *(Table 6.30)*. The mean daily intake of total sugars for children (single and with siblings) living in two-parent families was 88g, for one child living with one parent, 86g and for a child with siblings living with one parent, 81g. *(Chapter 6)*

There was a pattern of higher intakes of total fat and fatty acids by children in one-parent families compared with children in two-parent families, and a general tendency for children with siblings to have somewhat higher intakes than children with no siblings. Some differences in the percentage of energy derived from total fat and fatty acids between the groups were evident but they were small. For example, the mean percentage of food energy derived from total fat for one child in a two-parent family was 35.9%, for a child with siblings in a two-parent family 35.8%, for a single child in a one-parent family 36.1% and for a child with siblings in a one-parent family 36.5% *(Table 7.28).* *(Chapter 7)*

Children in one-parent families with more than one child had the lowest absolute intakes of both total carotene and vitamin C. After adjusting for variation in energy intakes vitamin C levels for these children were still lower than for other children. Children who had brothers or sisters, both in one-parent and two-parent families, had lower intakes of most vitamins than other children *(Table 8.52).* *(Chapter 8)*

Average intake of most minerals varied little according to family type. However there was a tendency for absolute intakes of calcium, phosphorus and potassium to be lower and intakes of sodium and chloride to be higher in children from one-parent families with brothers and sisters than those of other children. Those differences remained even after allowing for differences in energy intake. *(Chapter 9)*

There were no clear associations between mean levels of the haematological analytes and family type, nor with whether the child was an only child, or had siblings. Levels of water soluble vitamins assayed (except the EGRAC) were generally lower for children from one-parent families compared with those for other children. The variation was not generally as marked as for the other socio-economic characteristics, but levels of vitamin C showed the largest relative differences, for example comparing two-parent families with one child and lone-parent families with more than one child the vitamin C levels for the children in the survey were 75.2μmol/l and 58.4μmol/l respectively. *(Chapter 10)*

References

1 Gregory J, Foster K, Tyler H, Wiseman M. *The Dietary and Nutritional Survey of British Adults.* HMSO (London, 1990).
2 Department of Health and Social Security. Report on Health and Social Subjects: 10. *A Nutrition Survey of Pre-school Children 1967–68.* HMSO (London, 1975).
3 Thomas M, Goddard E, Hickman M, and Hunter P. *1992 General Household Survey.* HMSO (London, 1994).
4 Population Estimates Unit, OPCS, Crown Copyright (unpublished data). In mid-1992 the number of children born in 1988, 1989, 1990 and 1991 and living in Great Britain was estimated to be 3,019,644. Of these children 25% were born in each of the four years showing an equal distribution in the population from which the survey sample was drawn.
5 Hinds K, Gregory J. *The National Diet and Nutrition Survey: Children aged 1½ to 4½ years. Volume 2. Report of the Dental Survey.* HMSO (London, 1995).
6 Department of Health. Report on Health and Social Subjects: 41. *Dietary Reference Values for Food Energy and Nutrients for the United Kingdom.* HMSO (London, 1991).
7 White A, Davies PSW. *Feasibility Study for the National Diet and Nutrition Survey of Children aged 1½ to 4½ years.* OPCS (1994) (NM22).
8 Department of Health and Social Security. Report on Health and Social Subjects: 15. *Recommended Daily Amounts of Food Energy and Nutrients for Groups of People in the United Kingdom.* HMSO (London, 1979).
9 World Health Organisation. WHO Technical Report Series No: 503 *Nutritional Anaemias.* WHO (Geneva, 1972).

1 Background, purpose and research design

This chapter describes the background to the survey, its main aims and the overall research design and methodologies. Subsequent chapters and appendices give more detailed accounts of the methodologies used in the various components which together make up the National Diet and Nutrition Survey of children aged 1½ to 4½ years.

1.1 The National Diet and Nutrition Survey Programme

The National Diet and Nutrition Survey programme (NDNS) is a joint initiative, established in 1992, between the Ministry of Agriculture, Fisheries and Food and the Department of Health.

The NDNS programme aims to provide a comprehensive cross-sectional picture of the dietary habits and nutritional status of the population of Great Britain. It will also contribute to the health monitoring programme set out in the Government's Health of the Nation White Paper[1].

The programme aims to:

- provide detailed quantitative information on the food and nutrient intakes, sources of nutrients, and nutritional status of various subgroups in the population to inform Government policy;

- describe the characteristics of those with intakes of specific nutrients above and below the national average;

- provide a database which could be used to estimate dietary intakes of natural toxicants, contaminants and additives for risk assessment;

- measure haematological, biochemical and other indices that give evidence of nutritional status and relate these to dietary, physiological and social data;

- provide height, weight and other measurements of body size and examine their relationship to social, dietary and other data, including data from blood analyses;

- monitor the diet of the population to establish the extent to which it is nutritionally adequate and varied;

- monitor the extent to which quantitative dietary targets set by Government are being met; and

- help determine possible relationships between morbidity, cause of death and diet.

The NDNS programme builds on the experience gained from the earlier Dietary and Nutritional Survey of British Adults[2]. Because different methodologies may be appropriate for different age groups, the programme is separately considering different age groups in the population; children aged 1½ to 4½ years, school children aged 5 to 15 years, adults aged 16 to 64 years, and older adults aged 65 years and over. It is expected that it will take two to three years to carry out a survey for each age group, hence it is intended that the whole population will have been studied in an eight to ten-year period.

1.2 The need for the survey

Preschool children were chosen as a priority group for study because of the paucity of up-to-date information at a national level on their diets and nutritional status. Data on the diets of British school children[3], on infant feeding practices[4,5] and on the diets of British adults[2] have been collected since 1985 but no data on those aged 1½ to 4½ years have been collected since 1968.[6] Appendix P summarises the main findings of the 1967/68 preschool children's nutrition survey.

The 1988 Third Report on Present Day Practice in Infant Feeding recommended that 'the diets of British preschool children should be surveyed so as to provide quantitative analyses of the nutrients consumed by children between 2 and 5 years.'[7]

Preschool children are identified in the Government's White Paper *The Health of the Nation* as a key group. It notes that '...the adoption of healthy lifestyles during childhood encourages optimum growth and resistance to ill health, both emotional and physical. There is increasing evidence to suggest that there is a relationship between growth and development starting from before birth and during childhood, and risk in later life of coronary heart disease, raised blood pressure and other risk factors'.[1]

These considerations led the Ministry of Agriculture, Fisheries and Food and the Department of Health to commission the Social Survey Division of the Office of Population Censuses and Surveys (OPCS) and the Medical Research Council (MRC) Dunn Nutrition Unit at Cambridge to carry out this survey.

1.3 The aims of the survey

The survey is designed to meet the aims of the NDNS programme in providing detailed information on the current dietary behaviour and nutritional status of preschool children living in private households in Great Britain.

Additionally this survey will:

(i) provide data to assist with the development of dietary guidelines for preschool children;

(ii) characterise the socio-demographic and domestic circumstances which may affect how young children are fed;

(iii) determine the pattern of stool frequency in this age group;

(iv) provide baseline data for some anthropometric and biochemical indices in this age group; and

(v) provide information on the dental habits and dental condition of preschool children.[8,9]

To meet these aims it was necessary to design a survey capable of collecting detailed information about the quantities of foods and nutrients consumed by preschool children. The survey also had to include anthropometric measurements and measurements of blood indices, and collect information on household circumstances and stool frequency.

1.4 The sample design and selection

A nationally representative sample of preschool children living in private households in Great Britain was required. It was estimated that an achieved sample of about 1500 children was needed for analysis, ideally evenly distributed across the three age groups 1½ to 2½, 2½ to 3½ and 3½ to 4½ years and covering all months of the year to represent any seasonality in eating behaviour.

The study focused on one eligible child per selected household to reduce clustering of similar dietary patterns within households, and also to reduce the burden on informants, which might have affected co-operation rates and the quality of the data. A more detailed explanation is given in Appendix C.

The sample was selected using a multi-stage random probability design, with postal sectors as first stage units. The small users' Postcode Address File (PAF) was used as the sampling frame. The frame was stratified by region, and by 1981 Census variables.

A total of 100 postal sectors was selected as first stage units, with probability proportional to the number of postal delivery points; from each sector 280 addresses were randomly selected. To identify households which contained an eligible child, each address was sent a sift form which asked for details of the sex and date of birth of every person living in the household. Non- responding addresses were called on by an interviewer who attempted to collect the same information as on the sift form. Copies of the sift forms are reproduced in Appendix A. From the returns households containing an eligible child were identified. A child's eligibility, being aged between 1½ and 4½ years, was determined by taking the mid point of the fieldwork period as the reference date for defining

eligible dates of birth. As each wave of fieldwork covered a three month period, eligible children, at the time of interview, could have been slightly under 1½ years or slightly over 4½ years. For further details on eligibility refer to Appendix C.

One eligible child was randomly selected from each household. Interviewers were told which child had been selected before they started the fieldwork.

Since the requirement was for a sample of children living in private households, institutions were excluded at the sample selection stage wherever possible; institutions identified at the fieldwork stage were excluded from the interview sample.

To allow for seasonality in eating behaviour, fieldwork was distributed over four waves, each of three month's duration. The four fieldwork waves were:

Wave 1: July to September 1992
Wave 2: October to December 1992
Wave 3: January to March 1993
Wave 4: April to June 1993

At the selection of the first stage units, that is the 100 postal sectors, 25 sectors were allocated to each of the four fieldwork waves. The allocation took account of the need to aim to have equal numbers of households in each wave of fieldwork, and for each wave to be nationally representative.

A letter was sent to each eligible household in advance of the interviewer calling, telling them about the survey. Given the age group and the sensitivity of some of the subject matter letters were sent to Chief Constables of Police, Directors of Public Health and Directors of Social Services with responsibility for one or more of the selected postal sectors, informing them of when and where the survey would be taking place, giving them information about the survey and asking them to notify the appropriate people at a more local level as required. These letters are reproduced in Appendix B.

A more detailed account of the sampling procedures and response to the postal sift is given in Appendix C. Appendix D gives true standard errors and design factors for the main classificatory variables and for selected nutrients and energy intakes, anthropometric measurements and blood analytes.

1.5 The elements of the survey

To meet the aims of the research it was necessary to design a study which would incorporate both dietary and physical measurements.

This was achieved by asking the parent(s) or guardian(s) of the child to:

– answer an interview questionnaire, giving information about themselves and their household, and general information on the child's dietary habits;

– keep a four-day weighed intake record of all food and drink consumed by the child, both in and out of the home;

- keep a record of the number of bowel movements the child had over the dietary recording period;
- provide information on the use of dietary supplements, for example, vitamin tablets, and on all prescribed medicines being taken by the child;
- agree to the following measurements being taken—height, supine length (for those children aged under 2 years on the day the measurement was taken), weight, mid upper-arm circumference and head circumference;
- give written consent to a sample of the child's blood being taken;
- agree to answer a short questionnaire covering the child's dental habits and history and to the child having a dental examination. (The methodology and results of this dental survey are covered in a separate report.[9])

To assist the survey nutritionists in evaluating the quality of recording in the food diary, the parent or guardian was also asked to answer a short interview questionnaire after the recording period had finished, concerning any difficulties or problems in keeping the dietary record, and about any circumstance which may have affected the child's eating habits during the recording period, such as illness.

Copies of the fieldwork documents are provided in Appendix A.

As a token of appreciation, £10 was paid to the parent or guardian who kept the diary for four days. The child was given a height chart as thanks for their co-operation with the anthropometric measurements.

Feasibility work carried out by the Social Survey Division of OPCS and the MRC Dunn Nutrition Unit in 1989 tested the questionnaire and dietary methodology and developed protocols for the taking of anthropometric measurements. The validity of the dietary data was tested using the doubly-labelled water technique to assess energy expenditure against reported energy intake[10]. The results of this study showed that the methodologies proposed were feasible, that the accuracy and validity of the dietary data were acceptable and that the survey protocol was acceptable to informants.

The main purpose of pilot work which was carried out in 1991 was to test sampling procedures and develop the protocol for taking blood. Further details of these development stages are documented in Appendix E and in the Feasibility Study for the National Diet and Nutrition Survey of Children aged 1½ to 4½ years report.[11]

1.6 Fieldwork

All interviewers working on the survey had been fully trained by the Social Survey Division of OPCS and were experienced, having worked on other surveys. In addition each interviewer attended a personal briefing over five days conducted by research and professional staff from Social Survey Division including three nutritionists who were recruited to work on the survey, staff from the two client departments, and from the Dunn Nutrition Unit, who were responsible for gaining ethical approval to take blood and the recruitment of the blood takers. Prior to the briefing interviewers were asked to keep their own three-day weighed intake record and to code a day from a preschool child's diary[12]. At the residential briefings interviewers received feedback on their record keeping and coding from the nutritionists and were trained in all aspects of the survey including how to complete the weighed intake record, techniques for checking and detailed probing of the dietary record and training on how to code the entries in the diaries. Interviewers were also trained to take the anthropometric measurements, and instructed in the procedures for obtaining parental consent to the blood sample being taken and results being reported back to the parents and the child's GP. These procedures are discussed in detail in Chapter 2 and Appendices L and O. Emphasis was placed on the need for accuracy in the recording and coding of the dietary information and the measurement techniques.

In addition to the personal briefings written instructions were provided for interviewers and for those taking blood samples. Interviewers working on more than one fieldwork wave were recalled for a one-day refresher briefing between waves to maintain the accuracy of the diary coding and anthropometric measurements.

1.7 Plan of the report

Chapter 2 and its associated appendices describe the methodology of the four-day weighed intake record, anthropometry and blood sampling. The reasons for the choice of a four-day weighed intake methodology for obtaining the dietary information are discussed. Full details of the recording and weighing procedures for foods eaten in and out of the home, food and brand coding and editing procedures carried out on the completed dietary records are given. The purpose and choice of the anthropometric measurements made and the techniques and instruments used are reported in detail. The chapter also explains the purpose of obtaining the blood sample, the techniques and equipment used, and the analyses carried out on the samples. Appendix N gives an account of the procedures used by the laboratories for analysing the samples and quality control data.

Chapter 3 gives details on response to the different elements of the survey and on the characteristics of the responding samples.

Some informants chose not to co-operate with all elements of the survey, and the data in the subsequent chapters are based on those co-operating with that element, rather than on those who completed all elements of the survey package.

Chapters 4 to 11 report the substantive results of the survey. Chapters 4 to 9 are devoted to results based on the data collected in the dietary records. They cover quantities of food consumed (*Chapter 4*) and energy and nutrient intakes (*Chapters 5 to 9*). Chapter 10 reports on the blood analyses and Chapter 11 the anthropometric data.

The report is largely concerned with providing basic descriptive statistics for the variables measured and information on their association with demographic, social and behavioural characteristics of the sample population. One of the aims of the analysis was to relate the dietary and biological data and some results from these analyses are presented in Chapters 10 and 11. Where appropriate, data from this survey have been compared to other similar dietary surveys which used the weighed intake methodology, particularly the 1967–68 preschool children's survey.[6]

A copy of the survey database containing the full dataset, including results not presented in this initial Report, will be deposited with the ESRC Data Archive at the University of Essex following publication of this Report. Independent researchers who wish to carry out their own analyses should apply to the Archive for access.[13]

References and notes

1 Department of Health. *The Health of the Nation: a strategy for health in England.* HMSO (London, 1992).

2 Gregory J, Foster K, Tyler H, Wiseman M. *The Dietary and Nutritional Survey of British Adults.* HMSO (London, 1990).

3 Department of Health. Report on Health and Social Subjects: 36. *The Diets of British School children.* HMSO (London, 1989).

4 White A, Freeth S, O'Brien M. *Infant Feeding 1990.* HMSO (London, 1992).

5 Mills A, Tyler H. *Food and Nutrient Intakes of British Infants aged 6 to 12 months.* HMSO (London, 1992).

6 Department of Health and Social Security. Report on Health and Social Subjects: 10. *A Nutrition Survey of Preschool Children, 1967–68.* HMSO (London, 1975).

7 Department of Health and Social Security. Report on Health and Social Subjects: 32. *Present Day Practice in Infant Feeding: Third Report.* HMSO (London, 1988).

8 Parents who had taken part in the dietary survey were asked to agree to an OPCS interviewer calling back with a dentist seconded from the Community Dental Service of the NHS, to carry out an examination of the child's teeth. Parents were asked about the child's dental health and habits without the dentist present. Results of this survey are presented in a separate report.

9 Hinds K, Gregory J. *National Diet and Nutrition Survey of children aged 1½ to 4½ years. Volume 2: Report of the Dental Survey.* HMSO (London, 1995).

10 Davies PSW, Coward WA, Gregory J, White A, Mills A. Total energy expenditure and energy intake in the preschool child: a comparison. *Brit J Nutr.* 1994; 72:1:13-20.

11 White A, Davies PSW. *Feasibility Study for the National Diet and Nutrition Survey of Children aged 1½ to 4½ years.* OPCS (London, 1994) (NM22).

12 The coding exercise given to interviewers before attending the residential briefing was based on weighed intake records collected at the pilot stage. It was designed to give interviewers an idea of the kinds of foods preschool children were eating, and practice in coding them.

13 For further information about archived data please contact:
      Ms Kathy Sayer
      ESRC Data Archive
      University of Essex
      Wivenhoe Park
      Colchester
      Essex CO4 3SQ
      Great Britain
      Tel: [UK] 01206 872323
      Fax: [UK] 01206 872003
      EMAIL: SAYEK @:ESSEX.AC.UK

2 Dietary, anthropometry and blood sampling methodologies and procedures

2.1 The choice of dietary methodology

The survey used a weighed intake methodology since the study's main aims are to provide detailed information on the range and distribution of intakes of foods and nutrients for children aged 1½ to 4½ years in Great Britain, and to investigate relationships between intakes of selected nutrients and various health measures.

The advantages and disadvantages of this method and the factors affecting the choice are discussed in Appendix F.

Feasibility work was conducted to determine whether the weighed intake methodology was suitable for use with children aged 1½ to 4½ years, and to provide information on an appropriate length of recording period (see *Appendices E and J*)[1]. In particular the feasibility study was designed to test whether accurate information could be obtained on the amount of food consumed by children in this age group, given that losses from the weights of foods served were expected to be high, and possibly unmeasurable, because of spillage or rejection. Estimates of energy expenditure, derived from measurements of the excretion of water labelled with stable isotopes, doubly-labelled water, were compared with energy intake, estimated from the weighed intake record. The results showed a high level of agreement for the three one-year age cohorts in the feasibility sample, indicating that the methodology would provide sufficiently accurate estimates of intakes[2].

2.2 Choice of number and pattern of recording days

In deciding to use a weighed intake methodology, the period over which to collect information for an individual needed to be considered. Ideally it needed to be long enough to give reliable information on usual food consumption, but this had to be balanced against the likelihood of poor compliance if the recording period was lengthy.

Analysis of the feasibility study data, carried out by MAFF, also showed that among children in this age group, intakes of certain nutrients and energy varied according to the day of the week. Intakes of energy, carbohydrate, starch, sugar, and iron were significantly different when weekdays were compared with weekend days, and protein intakes were significantly different when data for Saturdays and Sundays were compared. In respect of the nutrients and energy intakes examined, there appeared to be no significant differences in intakes between different weekdays (see *Appendix J*).

The feasibility report concluded that four days was likely to be the maximum period acceptable to respondents if a high level of co-operation was to be obtained; financial constraints also meant that this was the maximum period that could be covered for the required sample size in the main survey[1].

In the light of findings from further analysis of the energy and nutrient data collected in the feasibility survey it was decided that, at the main stage, a four-day weighed intake record should be sought, and each record should include both weekend days. A placement pattern was determined, such that within four consecutive days, Mondays, Tuesdays, Thursdays and Fridays would be equally represented. At the analysis stage information for the two weekdays has been weighted to five days, before adding it to the data for the two weekend days and subsequently calculating average daily intakes[3].

2.3 The questionnaire

Before starting the dietary record mothers were asked to agree to an interview to provide background information about the household and their child's usual dietary behaviour[4]. Information was also collected on the child's consumption of artificial sweeteners, herbal teas and herbal infant drinks; the age at which different types of milk were introduced into the child's diet; the use of fluoride preparations and dietary supplements, and information on the child's health status. The interview questionnaire is reproduced in Appendix A.

Information was also collected which was of use to the interviewer when checking the dietary record. If, for example, the mother worked, whether the child was looked after by anyone else; whether the child attended a nursery or playgroup where food was provided; and whether the child was allergic to, or not given, particular foods. A record was also made of the child's usual eating pattern on weekdays and at weekends.

When the interviewer called back on the household at the end of the four dietary recording days the main diary keeper was asked if there had been any special circumstances which may have affected the child's eating behaviour during the period, such as going to a party. Other questions provided information on any problems the informant had with weighing and recording. Information was also collected on any illness the child had during the recording period and any prescribed medication taken.

2.4 The dietary record

The parent or carer of the child was asked to keep a weighed record of all food and drink consumed by the child, both in and out of the home, over four consecutive days including a Saturday and Sunday.

Parents were issued with a set of accurately calibrated Soehnle Quanta digital food scales. Two recording documents were also given to the parent; the 'home record' diary for use when it was possible for foods to be weighed, generally foods eaten in the home, and a smaller 'eating out' diary for use when foods could not be weighed—generally foods eaten away from home. The instruction and recording pages from these documents are included in Appendix A.

The parent or carer was shown by the interviewer how to use the scales to weigh food and drinks, including how to zero the scales after each item was weighed so that a series of items put on to the same plate could be weighed separately. Instructions were also given on how to weigh and record leftovers, and how to record any food that was spilt or not eaten which could not be re-weighed.

The 'home record' diary was the main recording and coding document. For each item consumed over the four days a description of the item was recorded, including the brand name of the product, and where appropriate the method of preparation. Also recorded was the weight served and the weight of any leftovers, the time food was served, whether it was eaten at home or away from home, and for fruit and vegetables, whether the item was home grown, defined as being grown in the household's own garden or allotment.

2.4.1 The recording procedure

Recording what the child consumed in the diaries started from the time the interviewer left the home; the interviewer called back approximately 24 hours after placing the diary in order to check that the parent or carer was recording items correctly, to give encouragement and to re-motivate where appropriate. Entries made up to midnight on the day the interviewer left the diary were discarded at the analysis stage as the dietary recording period started at midnight.

Everything consumed by the child had to be recorded, including medicines, vitamin and mineral supplements and drinks of water. Where a served item could not be weighed, the parent or carer was asked to record a description of the portion size, using standard household measures, such as teaspoons, or to describe the size of the item.

Each separate item of food in a served portion needed to be weighed separately in order that the nutrient composition of each food item could be calculated. For example, for a sandwich the bread, spread and filling(s) all needed to be weighed and recorded separately.

The amount of salt used either at the table or in cooking was not recorded as it would have been very difficult to weigh accurately. However questions on the use of salt in the cooking of the child's food and the child's use of salt at the table were asked at the interview. All other sauces, pickles and dressings were recorded. Vitamin and mineral supplements and artificial sweeteners were recorded as units consumed, for example, one teaspoon of Canderel Spoonful.

A large amount of detail needed to be recorded in the dietary record to enable similar foods prepared and cooked by different methods to be coded correctly, as such foods will have different nutrient compositions. For example, the nutrient composition of crinkle cut chips made from new potatoes and fried in a polyunsaturated oil is different from the same chips fried in lard. Therefore, depending on the food item, information could be needed on cooking method, preparation and packaging as well as an exact description of the product before it could accurately be coded.

Interviewers were responsible for coding the food diaries so they could readily identify the level of detail needed for different food items, and probe for missing detail at later visits to the household. In addition, recipes for all homemade dishes were collected.

Parents and carers were encouraged to record details in the diary, including weight information if at all possible, of any leftovers or food that was spilt or dropped. Further details on the recording of leftovers and spillages are given in Appendix F.

The eating out diary was intended to be used only when it was not possible to weigh the food items. In such cases, record keepers were asked to write down as much information as possible about the food item consumed, particularly the portion size. To encourage this the diary had a centimetre rule printed on the bottom of each page. Prices, descriptions, brand names, place of purchase and where the food was consumed were all recorded; duplicate items were bought and weighed by the interviewer where possible.

Further information on recording procedures is provided in Appendix F.

2.4.2 Coding the food record

Interviewers were trained in recognising the detail required for coding foods of different types at the briefing and by exercises they had completed before the briefing.

A food code list giving code numbers for about 3000 items and a full description of each item was prepared by nutritionists at MAFF for use by the interviewers. The list was organised into sections by food type, for example milk and cream, soft drinks, breakfast cereals, fruit, vegetables and different types of meat. Interviewers were also provided with an alphabetical index to help them find particular foods in the code list. Additional check lists were provided to assist the interviewers when coding fats and soft drinks.

As fieldwork progressed, further codes were added to the food code list for recipes and new products found in the dietary records; by the end of fieldwork there were approximately 3600 separate food codes. A page from the food code list is reproduced in Appendix G.

Brand information was collected for all food items bought pre-wrapped, as some items, such as biscuits and breakfast cereals could not be easily food coded unless the brand was known. However brand information has been coded for only artificial sweeteners, mineral waters, herbal teas and herbal infant drinks and soft drinks, to ensure adequate differentiation of these items.

After the interviewers had coded the entries in the dietary records, the documents were checked by OPCS headquarters coding staff. OPCS and MAFF nutritionists dealt with specific queries from interviewers and coding staff, and advised on and checked the quality of coding. They were also responsible for converting descriptions of portion sizes to weights, and checking that the appropriate codes for recipes and new products had been used. The first diary returned by each interviewer received a 100% coding check; feedback was given on the quality of their coding and probing. Coding of certain items was checked on all diaries, for example, vitamin and mineral supplements.

2.4.3 Editing the dietary information

Computer checks for completeness and consistency of information were run on the dietary and questionnaire data. At this stage the weight of each food item consumed was calculated by subtracting the weight of any leftovers from the weight of food served; where a combined weight was given for a number of leftover items the total weight of leftovers was divided among the food items indicated as being leftover, usually in proportion to the served weights of those items. Computer checks were run to identify cases where the weight of food consumed was outside a specified range; such cases were individually checked and any errors corrected.

Following completion of these checks and calculations the information from the dietary record was linked to the nutrient databank and nutrient intakes were thereby calculated from quantities of food consumed. This nutrient databank, which was compiled by MAFF, holds information on 54 nutrients for each of the food codes. Further details of the nutrient databank are described in Appendix H.

Checks were run to identify cases where the intake of any nutrient was outside the expected range for normal intakes, although in most cases only a maximum value could be specified; again such cases were individually checked and errors corrected. MAFF supplied range information for both food weights and nutrient intakes.

Most of the dietary analysis presented in this Report is based on average daily intakes of nutrients from all sources, either including or excluding dietary supplements. Each food code used was, however, also allocated to one of 54 main food types which were further divided into a number of subgroups (*Appendix I*). Information on the quantity of food consumed from each subgroup is tabulated in Chapter 4, and data on the contribution of the main food groups to intakes of energy and specific nutrients are included in Chapters 5 to 9.

2.5 Anthropometry

One of the main aims of this survey was to provide anthropometric data on a representative sample of children, which could be related to socio-demographic and dietary data.

Anthropometry, the measurement of body size, weight and proportions, is an intrinsic part of any nutritional survey and can be an indicator of health, development and growth. Derived indices, for instance to assess the proportion of body weight that is fat, provide additional information.

2.5.1 Choice of anthropometric measurements

In deciding which measurements should be taken a number of factors needed to be considered; these included the acceptability of the measurement to the child and parent, whether equipment suitable for use in the home was available, and whether interviewers could be trained to take the measurements accurately.

Measurements of standing height, weight, mid upper-arm circumference and head circumference were required for all children. Additionally supine length was measured for children who were under two years of age, because growth standards for this age group are based on supine length rather than height. The measurement of both height and supine length for these children has also enabled comparisons to be made between the two.

Height and weight can also be used to calculate the Quetelet or Body Mass Index (weight[kg]/height[m]^2) or other indices which control for variations in body weight associated with height. Mid upper-arm circumference was measured to give information on body size, and head circumference is a standard measure of development and growth.

Measures of skinfold thickness were not included in the anthropometric measurements as it was felt that inter-observer variability would be too great for the measures to be reliable and there were concerns regarding the extent to which children would tolerate such measurements being attempted. The feasibility study had found it extremely difficult to achieve consistent measures of waist and hip circumferences, and thus these measures were not included in the main stage of this survey (see *Appendix E*)[1].

2.5.2 Techniques and instruments used

OPCS interviewers have experience of taking height and weight measurements on surveys of adults[5,6]. However it was recognised that children were likely to be more difficult to measure accurately; deciding on appropriate equipment, techniques and training was therefore a requirement of the feasibility and pilot studies (see *Appendix E*)[1].

At the main stage all interviewers were trained in accurate measurement techniques at personal briefings. Once trained, any interviewer working on a subsequent wave of fieldwork attended a one-day refresher briefing where the techniques were checked. Interviewers were able to practice the measurement techniques on young children at the briefings.

Interviewers were allowed to take the measurements at any point after the initial questionnaire had been completed; it was thought that specifying a particular time to take the measurements could affect response, as gaining the co-operation of young children might be problematic and more than one attempt might be needed. Detailed descriptions of the techniques used to take the measurements are given in Appendix O.

Interviewers recorded the measurement, the date on which it was taken, how many attempts were made and if there were any special circumstances which might have affected the accuracy of the measurement. The Department of Health advised on circumstances which were likely to affect the accuracy to such an extent that the measurement should be excluded from the analysis; these included wearing a wet nappy when the child was being weighed, and the child being unable to keep the correct posture when standing height or supine length were being measured.

Standing height: the measurement was taken using a portable, digital, telescopic stadiometer, modified to OPCS specification from a building surveyor's measuring device. Measurements were taken to the nearest millimetre.

The measurement was taken with the child wearing only vest and pants. The child's head was positioned such that the Frankfort plane was horizontal, and while maintaining this position, gentle traction was applied to attain the maximum unsupported height. For further details on the equipment used and the Frankfort plane see *Appendix O*.

As the stadiometer had a fixed minimum height of 0.75m any child less than 0.75m tall could not be measured; four children could not be measured for this reason.

Supine length: the techniques and instruments used were the same as for standing height except the child laid on his or her back on a hard, flat surface. The head was positioned so that the Frankfort plane was vertical, and while maintaining this position, gentle traction was applied to achieve maximum length.

If the child was less than 0.75m tall a metal spacer block 10cm square, was placed at the feet. The measurement was then taken and 10cm deducted before recording. Use of the spacer block was recorded on the questionnaire. Only two children needed the spacer block for their length to be measured.

Weight: Soehnle Quantratronic digital personal weighing scales, calibrated in kilogram and 100 gram units were used, and placed on a hard level surface for taking the measurement. Where no hard level surface was available the interviewer made a note on the questionnaire. All the scales were checked for accuracy prior to each fieldwork wave before being issued to interviewers.

Children were asked to undress to vest and pants. The measurement was not taken at a standard time of day.

Mid upper-arm circumference: for consistency of technique this measurement was taken from the left side of the child's body. If for any reason the interviewer was unable to take the measurement on the left side, then the measurement was taken on the right and a note made on the questionnaire.

Mid upper-arm circumference was measured in two stages using a standard tape to identify the mid-point of the upper arm, and an insertion tape to measure the circumference.

Interviewers were instructed to take the measurement on bare skin with the child in a vest. Where the child was unable or unwilling to comply with this request the measurement was not taken.

The position of the child's arm was standardised for each stage of the measurement. The mid-point of the upper arm was identified as halfway between the inferior border of the acromion process and the tip of the olecranon process. In taking the circumference measurement care was taken to ensure that the tape was horizontal and that the tissues of the upper arm were not compressed. Circumference measurements were taken to the nearest millimetre.

Head circumference: this was taken using an insertion tape. The tape was placed around the child's head just above the brow ridges, at the point of maximum circumference. The measurement was taken over the child's hair, under slight tension. Head circumference was not measured for children whose hair was dressed in a 'permanent' hairstyle which would affect the measurement. The measurement was recorded to the nearest millimetre.

As a token of thanks, children were given a height chart for co-operating with the measurements.

2.6 Purpose of obtaining a sample of venous blood

One of the main aims of the NDNS programme is to measure haematological and other blood indices which give evidence of nutritional status and to relate these to dietary and social data. In the preschool children's survey a main concern was to measure haemoglobin concentrations and other indicators of iron status, since iron deficiency is common among this age group in Britain[7].

Blood concentrations of other nutrients and analytes would give valuable information about the nutrient status of preschool children, and in many cases establish normative ranges for a healthy preschool population of children in Great Britain. To measure haematological status, a venous blood sample is preferred to a capillary sample and it is widely accepted that venepuncture is usually less painful and a more managed technique for obtaining a blood sample than fingerprick techniques.

Approval from National Health Service (NHS) Local Research Ethics Committees for blood sampling was subject to a maximum volume of 4ml blood being taken and thus the number of analyses which could be carried out was restricted. Therefore analytes were prioritised according to nutritional interest for analysis dependent on the volume of blood obtained. The order was as follows[8]:

> measures of iron status; haemoglobin and other haematological indices;
> measures of vitamin status; water and fat soluble vitamins including retinol and vitamin D;
> levels of blood lipids, including high density lipoproteins, plasma total cholesterol and triglycerides;
> acute phase proteins;
> red cell folate and plasma ascorbate;
> markers of immune function; IgA, IgM, IgG.

It was hoped that any residual plasma left after the haematological analyses could be used to measure levels of a number of trace elements of toxicological interest. However the level of incidental contamination of the sample was too great to give reliable results (see *Chapter 10*).

Approval was obtained from the NHS Local Research Ethics Committees for any unused sample remaining after the above analyses to be stored, subject to parental consent, and an undertaking was given that neither the original sample nor any stored sample would be tested for HIV.

2.7 Procedures for obtaining the blood sample

All procedures associated with obtaining and analysing the blood samples were contracted to the Medical Research Council Dunn Nutrition Unit in Cambridge whose staff worked closely with OPCS throughout all stages of the survey.

All the procedures were tested prior to the main stage survey to ensure that they were safe and acceptable to children, to their parents, to those taking the blood samples and to the medical profession[9].

2.7.1 Ethical approval

The Dunn Nutrition Unit sought ethical approval for the study from the NHS Local Research Ethics Committees covering each of the 100 sampled areas; one area failed to give consent in sufficient time for work to begin, all other Committees gave their approval. The Ethical Committees of the British Medical Association and of the British Paediatric Association were informed about the survey. Information about the survey was also sent to Directors of Public Health, Chief Constables of Police and Directors of Social Services with responsibility for the areas of residence of participant children; they were asked to inform appropriate local staff[10].

2.7.2 Training and recruitment of the blood takers

As taking blood from small children is more difficult than bleeding adult subjects it was decided that those recruited to take the blood samples should have recent paediatric experience of taking blood. Thus the majority of those recruited by the Dunn Nutrition Unit were phlebotomists working with infants and young children; the remainder were paediatricians or GPs. A total of 80 suitably qualified personnel was recruited; some worked on more than one wave of fieldwork, some in more than one area, and some worked in pairs. All received written instructions and attended for a half day during the five-day interviewer briefing sessions where they had the opportunity to meet the interviewer with whom they would be working, and were given training in the protocols for obtaining the sample, despatching part of it and processing and storing the remainder. Emphasis was placed on the need to standardise procedures and adhere strictly to the protocol that had been presented to and agreed by the NHS Local Research Ethics Committees. Further details of the recruitment of blood takers are described in Appendix L.

2.7.3 Outline consent procedures

Explicit formal consent was required for taking the blood sample from the child. Interviewers were required to tell parents at the time they conducted the questionnaire interview that their consent to a blood sample being taken would be sought, to avoid the possibility that having built a rapport with the interviewer, parents might have felt obliged to consent to this procedure against their true wishes.

Parents received a written statement of the purpose and procedures involved in taking the blood sample and were given time to discuss this with others, for example their child's family doctor, and with the blood taker. Written, witnessed consent for the procedure was sought, as well as consent for OPCS to waive the confidentiality pledge in respect of informing the Dunn Nutrition Unit of the child's name and address and the name of the child's GP (General Practitioner). This was needed in order that parents could be routinely informed of the result of the haemoglobin analysis and that, with consent, the child's GP could be told of any abnormal result for certain specified analytes, such as low iron status or high lipid levels.

It should be noted that agreement to this aspect of the survey was independent of agreement to other elements in the survey, the payment of £10 for completing the dietary record, and the gift to the child for co-operating with the anthropometric measurements.

Parents were informed that consent to the procedure could be withdrawn at any time, even after written consent had been given, and blood takers were instructed that they should stop the procedure at any point if they felt the child or family became unduly distressed.

A copy of the consent forms used and information sheet handed to parents is given in Appendix M.

2.7.4 Outline venepuncture procedure

Blood was taken in the child's home with the OPCS interviewer present.

Parents were advised that a venepuncture procedure would be less painful for their child than a finger prick; nevertheless if they requested a finger prick then this was complied with. Topical anaesthetic cream (Emla cream) was only used for children in areas where NHS Local Research Ethics Committee approval was conditional on its use.

The approved protocol allowed for a maximum of two attempts at bleeding and for a maximum of 4ml of blood to be obtained by venepuncture or 1ml by finger prick. The preferred site for the venepuncture was the antecubital fossa, although some phlebotomists opted for the back of the hand.

It was not felt appropriate in the context of a voluntary survey of small children to require a fasting sample nor was the time at which the sample was taken standardised, although it was acknowledged that these arrangements might compromise the accuracy of results of the triglyceride assay. Details of the procedures for taking blood samples and the processing procedures are described in Appendices L and N.

2.8 Procedures for reporting results to parents and General Practitioners

Subject to parental consent, GPs were notified of the child's participation in the survey and they and the parents were informed of the results of the haemoglobin analysis.

As noted earlier, for many analytes this survey is intended to establish baseline normative values for preschool children; for such analytes it was not possible to identify 'abnormal' results nor could General Practitioners be advised on the clinical significance of any particular result.

In respect of haemoglobin, ferritin, zinc protoporphyrin, retinol, vitamin D and lipids, ranges for preschool children were defined and any result outside the range was sent to the child's parents and, subject to parental consent, to the child's GP. Parents were advised to arrange for their child to see his or her GP[11].

References and notes

1 White A, Davies PSW. *Feasibility Study for the National Diet and Nutrition Survey of Children aged 1½ to 4½ years.* Crown Copyright. OPCS (1994) (NM22).
2 Davies PSW, Coward WA, Gregory J, White A, Mills A. Total energy expenditure and energy intake in the preschool child: a comparison. *Brit J Nutr.* 1994; 72; 1: 13–20.
3 See Chapter 4 and Appendix J for notes on the effects of re-weighting data on four-days' intakes.
4 The child's mother or female parent-figure was interviewed if she was in the household as certain questions, such as whether the child was ever put to the breast, could best be asked of her. The questionnaire is reproduced in Appendix A. In the few cases where there was no mother or female parent-figure in the household the father was interviewed. Some interviews were with both parents.
5 Knight I. *The Heights and Weights of Adults in Great Britain.* HMSO (London, 1984).
6 Gregory J, Foster K, Tyler H, Wiseman M. *The Dietary and Nutritional Survey of British Adults.* HMSO (London, 1990).
7 Department of Health. Report on Health and Social Subjects: 45. *Weaning and the Weaning Diet.* HMSO (London, 1994).
8 For a full list of analytes see Appendix K.
9 See Appendix E for a report on the pilot study.
10 Copies of these letters are given in Appendix B.
11 Results were reported to the GP as follows:
   Haemoglobin: less than 11g/dl
   Ferritin: This value is age related and varies between 12μg/l at age 1½ years to about 18μg/l at age 4½ years.
   Zinc protoporphyrin (ZPP): values are increased due to iron deficiency, lead toxicity and inflammatory disease. This value is aged related and, for this study, ZPP levels at or above the 90th centile of data from a study carried out at the Hospital for Sick Children, Great Ormond Street in 1992 were reported to the GP.
   The values are:
   age 1½ to under 2 years 75μmol/mol haem
   age 2 to under 3 years   113μmol/mol haem
   age 3 to under 4 years   80μmol/mol haem
   age 4 to under 5 years   78μmol/mol haem
   Retinol: less than 0.3 μmol/l
   25-hydroxyvitamin D: less than 12.5nmol/l
   Lipids: For all cases where plasma total cholesterol was greater than 5.5mmol/l full lipid results were scrutinised for clinical significance before referral.

3 Response to the survey and characteristics of the co-operating sample

This chapter reports on the response achieved for different components of the survey package and describes the characteristics of the responding sample, that is those who co-operated with the interview.

As a large part of the survey analysis presented in this Report is based on those who completed a four-day diary, which covered both weekend days, a more detailed description of the characteristics of this 'diary' sample is also shown.

To make some assessment of the representativeness of the sample comparisons have been made between responding and non-responding households and, for some of the main socio-demographic characteristics, between the responding sample and a subsample from the 1992 General Household Survey (GHS). The GHS subsample used for comparison is of private households containing at least one child under the age of five years. Although not an exact match, it is the only data source readily available, and it is unlikely there are any major differences between the characteristics of households containing a child under 5 years and those containing a child aged 1½ to 4½ years.

In this chapter some classificatory variables are tabulated with each other to point the reader to possible interactions which may aid interpretation of results presented later in the analysis chapters, where data are tabulated by the classificatory variables independently.

Not all tables in this chapter are commented on.

3.1 Response to the various components of the survey

As described previously, the sample for this survey was selected from the small users' file of the Postcode Address File by means of a postal sift and interviewer follow up of non-responders and of those who returned their sift form indicating that more than one household lived at the selected address. Further details on the sample design and response to the sift stages are given in Appendix C.

Of the 2101 eligible households identified by the sift stages, 88% co-operated with the interview, and 81% completed a four-day diary. Only 1% of those who gave an interview started to keep a diary but gave up part way through the record-keeping period. About 6% of the eligible sample (6% of those interviewed) refused to keep the diary. There were no significant differences between the different waves of fieldwork in co-operation with the interview and diary. *(Table 3.1)*

A small number of diaries, about 1%, were excluded from the analysis at the coding or editing stages either because the diary was not thought to be an accurate record of the child's diet or because the child's diet was affected by a serious medical condition. The decision to exclude a diary was based on information recorded by the interviewer during the diary keeping period and in the post-diary questionnaire, on the advice of the OPCS and MAFF nutritionists who checked all the diaries.

Analysis of the feasibility survey data by MAFF had indicated significant differences in certain nutrient intakes between weekdays and weekend days, and between Saturdays and Sundays, but no significant differences between weekdays (see *Appendix J*). Therefore parents were asked to keep the diary over four consecutive days which, if at all possible, should include both a Saturday and a Sunday. Only 2% of four-day diaries, 1% of cases overall, did not cover both weekend days. Thus it was decided that partial and four-day diaries not covering both weekend days would be excluded from the analysis. Analyses of the dietary data are therefore based on the 1675 diaries which contained both weekend days.

3.1.1 Co-operation with the anthropometric measurements

A number of anthropometric measurements were attempted; weight, standing height, mid upper-arm and head circumferences, and, for children under 2 years of age on the day the measurement was taken, supine length.

With the exception of supine length, over 90% of the responding sample, that is those children whose parents were interviewed, had each measurement taken.

Co-operation rates with taking supine length were lower; the measurement was taken for only 73% of children aged under 2 years. This was partly because the technique for measuring supine length is more difficult, and because the very youngest children were more likely to be unco-operative.

Of the other measurements standing height was the most difficult to obtain; it was taken for 92% of children. Weight was obtained for 96%, mid upper-arm circumference was taken for 95%, and head circumference for 96% of children.

There was little variability in co-operation with each measurement by wave of fieldwork. *(Table 3.2)*

There were no differences in co-operation with each of the measurements between boys and girls. Height was the only measurement where co-operation varied significantly by age, being lower for the youngest age group than for the middle and oldest age groups, 86% compared with 95% (p<0.01).

Co-operation with each measurement was somewhat higher for children from a non-manual compared with a manual home background. However weight was the only measurement where these differences reached statistical significance, 98% compared with 94% (p<0.01).

(Tables 3.3 to 3.5)

3.1.2 Co-operation with the blood sample

Parents were asked for their written consent to a sample of blood (maximum 4ml) being taken for analysis. Parents or the child could withdraw their co-operation at any stage. Consent to an attempt being made was obtained from 63% of the responding sample.

However, in 5% of cases where consent had been obtained an attempt was not made. This was usually because blood takers were not available at a time convenient to the parents or in the blood taker's opinion an attempt should not be made because, for example, the child was distressed.

Moreover not all attempts to take a sample were successful as young children can be difficult to bleed; there is often difficulty in finding a suitable vein, and on puncturing, the vein of a very young child is more likely to collapse than that of an older child or adult. Thus in a further 9% of cases where consent had been given the attempt to take blood was not successful. Overall samples were obtained for 54% of children in the responding sample. Although a high proportion of the responding sample refused consent to the blood sample, of those who gave their consent to the sample being taken the success rate was high; a blood sample was obtained for 87% of the consenting sample. The results of a separate follow-up study which asked parents about their reactions to the blood taking part of the survey will be reported elsewhere[1]. *(Table 3.6)*

There were no significant differences in the proportions consenting to a blood sample being taken between boys and girls, different age groups or children from different social class backgrounds. *(Tables 3.7 to 3.9)*

3.2 Characteristics of the sample

A comparison with mid-1992 population estimates[2] suggests that the responding sample may slightly under-represent the oldest group of children and slightly over-represent children in the middle age cohort, although the differences are not statistically significant. It is likely that differences result from random variations in the distribution of children in these age groups in the 100 postal sectors, which formed the primary sampling units, particularly as there was no significant difference between responding and non-responding households in household composition or the ages of eligible children.

(Tables 3.10 and 3.11)

Table 3.12 shows that the age and sex distributions of the responding and diary samples were virtually identical.

A map showing the four regions used for analysis purposes and a list of the counties they contain is shown in Figure 3.1.

Comparison of the regional distribution between the responding and diary samples and 1992 GHS data show no regional bias. *(Table 3.13)*

Tables 3.14 and 3.15 show some differences in the distribution of children by sex and age group within the broad regions used for analysis in this Report. In particular, the proportion of girls and children aged 3½ to 4½ years in Scotland is higher than in other regions. In the Northern region there is a higher proportion of children in the middle age cohort than elsewhere. These differences were not statistically significant.

Social class of head of household
Social class was derived for both the head of household, usually the child's father, and for the child's mother, from information about their occupation. For fathers, this information related to their current or most recent job. For mothers, information to derive social class was collected about their main life job. This was decided on the basis of evidence from the feasibility and pilot studies which found that mothers who had left the labour market to have children had often either taken a lower grade occupation on their return to work or had gone back to their old job but at a lower level. Thus their current job might not adequately reflect their education, training or social status.

Throughout this Report analysis using social class information is based on that of the head of household as it is available for the largest number of cases and readily allows comparisons to be made with other data sources.[3] In 16% of cases the mother was the head of household.

Social class could not be derived for 4% of cases where the head of household's occupation was inadequately described, or he or she was a member of the Armed Forces, or was economically inactive and had never worked.

Table 3.16 shows no difference between the responding and diary samples in the distribution of social class of head of household for boys and girls.

In order to provide adequate numbers for analysis in this Report the six social class categories have been collapsed into two groups as follows:

Non-manual Social Classes I and II — professional, managerial and technical occupations, and Social Class IIInm — skilled non-manual occupations.

Manual Social Class IIIm — skilled manual occupations, and Social Classes IV and V — unskilled occupations.

There were virtually no differences between the responding and diary samples and the 1992 GHS data in

Figure 3.1 Standard Regions of England, Scotland and Wales and aggregated regions for analysis

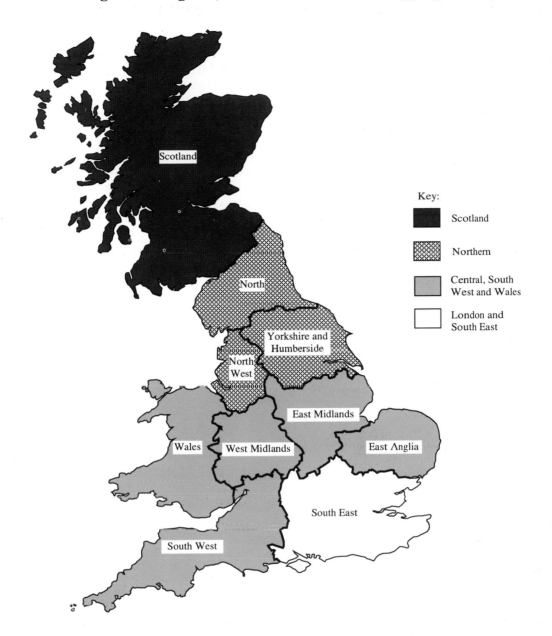

North
Tyne and Wear Metropolitan County
Cleveland
Cumbria
Durham
Northumberland

Yorkshire and Humberside
South Yorkshire Metropolitan County
West Yorkshire Metropolitan County
Humberside
North Yorkshire

East Midlands
Derbyshire
Leicestershire
Lincolnshire
Northamptonshire
Nottinghamshire

East Anglia
Cambridgeshire
Norfolk
Suffolk

South East
Greater London
Bedfordshire
Berkshire
Buckinghamshire
East Sussex
Essex
Hampshire
Hertfordshire
Isle of Wight
Kent
Oxfordshire
Surrey
West Sussex

South West
Avon
Cornwall and Isles of Scilly
Devon
Dorset
Gloucestershire
Somerset
Wiltshire

West Midlands
West Midlands Metropolitan County
Hereford and Worcester
Shropshire
Staffordshire
Warwickshire

North West
Greater Manchester Metropolitan County
Merseyside Metropolitan County
Cheshire
Lancashire

the social class distribution. In each of the three age groups of children social class distribution was similar.

(Tables 3.17 and 3.18)

As would be expected children living in London and the South East were more likely to come from a non-manual home background than children living elsewhere. Thus in London and the South East 55% of heads of household were in the non-manual group, compared with 37% in the Northern region and Scotland ($p < 0.01$), and 43% in the Central and South West regions of England and Wales ($p < 0.05$). *(Table 3.19)*

Employment status of head of household
Information was collected from the head of household, usually the child's father, and from the child's mother to establish their employment status, although in the analyses presented in this Report employment status of the head of the household has been used.

Respondents were asked whether they were working full time or part time during the week prior to the interview. Those not in paid employment were asked further questions and their responses categorised to identify those who were unemployed and those who were economically inactive.

Unemployed was defined as being out of work during the previous week and either:

– waiting to take up a job, or
– looking for work, or
– prevented from working by temporary sickness.

Informants classified as economically inactive were those unemployed or not working, such as full-time students, the retired, those keeping house and those permanently unable to work due to ill health or disability.

The responding and diary samples contained similar proportions of heads of households who were working, unemployed and economically inactive. *(Table 3.20)*

There were no significant differences between the three age groups in the proportion of heads of household in different employment status groups. *(Table 3.21)*

London and the South East had the highest proportion of heads of household in work. *(Table 3.22)*

Heads of household who were classified as being in the manual social classes were more likely than those in the non-manual group to be unemployed, 16% compared with 3% ($p < 0.01$). *(Table 3.23)*

Receipt of benefits
As an indicator of relative economic deprivation, information was collected on parents' receipt of certain state benefits, Income Support and Family Credit, and this has been used as a classificatory variable throughout this Report.

Levels of disposable income might be expected to affect the choice of diet, particularly where resources are limited. However, detailed information on income was not collected because it might have jeopardised co-operation with other parts of the survey.

Table 3.24 shows that there were no differences between boys and girls in the responding and diary samples in the proportion of parents receiving these benefits. Six per cent of the diary sample were in receipt of Family Credit while 27% were receiving Income Support. Overall, nearly a third of parents were receiving one or other of these benefits. These proportions correspond closely to figures supplied by the Department of Social Security for households containing at least one child under 5 years old[4].

Children living in London and the South East were the least likely to have parents receiving these benefits; 23% of parents in London and the South East were receiving benefits compared with 35% in the Northern region ($p < 0.05$), and 36% in both Central and South West regions of England and Wales ($p < 0.01$) and Scotland (NS). *(Table 3.26)*

Those households whose head worked in a manual occupation were more likely to be receiving benefit than those in non-manual occupations, 42% compared with 18% ($p < 0.01$). *(Table 3.27)*

Household composition and family type
Details were recorded of the number of adults and children living in the household at the time of interview and their relationship to the sampled child and each other. From this, classificatory variables describing the household composition, which allowed comparison with 1992 GHS data, and family type, which is used in this Report, were derived.

There were no significant differences between the responding and diary samples in household composition or family type. However comparison with 1992 GHS data indicates that households containing two adults with children were over-represented in this survey, 79% compared with 75% ($p < 0.05$), and that households containing three or more adults with children were under-represented in this survey, 6% compared with 12% ($p < 0.01$). *(Tables 3.28 and 3.34)*

Almost half the respondents had two children under the age of 16 in their household, and one third had two children under the age of five. In 63% of households the sampled child was the only child under the age of 5, with no difference between the responding and diary samples. *(Table 3.33)*

Just under a fifth of respondents were lone parents. A higher proportion of married and cohabiting couples had two or more children compared with lone parents, 73% compared with 60% ($p < 0.01$).[5]

(Tables 3.35 and 3.36)

In London and the South East there was a smaller proportion of lone parents than elsewhere in the country, although the only statistically significant regional difference was between London and the South East and Central and South West England and Wales, 12% compared with 20% ($p < 0.05$). *(Table 3.37)*

Table 3.38 shows that lone parent heads of household were more likely to be economically inactive than their married or cohabiting counterparts, for example, for those with one child 62% of lone parents were economically inactive compared with 3% of married or cohabiting parents (p<0.01). There were no differences between different family types in their social class composition. *(Table 3.39)*

Lone parents were much more likely to be in receipt of benefits than their married or cohabiting counterparts, for example 84% of lone parents with one child were receiving either Income Support or Family Credit compared with 14% of married or cohabiting couples with one child (p<0.01). However married or cohabiting couples with two or more children were more likely to be receiving Income Support or Family Credit than those with one child, 22% compared with 14% (p<0.05). *(Table 3.40)*

Mother's highest educational qualification
The mother's education might affect the type of diet she gives her child and other aspects of the child's nutrition and behaviour. For example the duration of breast feeding is positively associated with the mother's educational attainment[6]. Information was therefore collected on the highest educational qualification achieved by the child's mother. There was no difference between the responding and diary samples by sex of the child in the proportions of mothers with different qualifications. About one in three mothers had obtained GCE 'A' level or equivalent qualifications or higher, for a similar proportion their highest qualification was at GCE 'O' level or equivalent. One in seven mothers achieved one or more CSE passes or equivalents and one in five had no educational qualification. *(Tables 3.41 and 3.42)*

Mothers in London and the South East were more likely to have obtained qualifications above GCE 'A' level than those in the Northern region, 24% compared with 16% (p<0.05) or in the Central and South West regions of England and Wales, 24% compared with 14% (p<0.01). Scotland had the highest proportion of mothers with no qualifications, 30% compared with 17% in London and the South East (p<0.05). *(Table 3.43)*

Table 3.44 shows the distribution of mother's highest educational qualification by social class of head of household. Mothers from a non-manual household were more likely to hold a qualification above GCE 'A' level than those from manual households, 34% compared with 5% (p<0.01). Conversely mothers from a manual household were more likely to have no qualifications than those from non-manual households, 30% compared with 10% (p<0.01).

3.3 Childcare

Forty one per cent of the children in the sample had a working mother, a very similar proportion as in the 1992 GHS, where 43% of women with a youngest child aged under 5 years were working[7]. Five per cent of children were primarily cared for by a paid childminder, and 6% mainly attended a nursery while the mother was at work. *(Table 3.45)*

Two thirds of all children in this survey attended a nursery, playgroup, mother and toddler group, or childminder for part of each week, rising from 45% of those aged 1½ to 2½, to 87% of 3½ to 4½ year olds.[8] Almost half had a meal while there, and a further 16% had a snack. Food and drink consumed outside the home during the

survey diary period was recorded either by the child's mother, or by the carer. *(Table 3.46)*

3.4 Illness, the use of dietary supplements and prescribed medicines

Parents were asked a number of questions about their child's health and use of dietary supplements and prescribed medicines during the interview, to help with the interpretation and analysis of both the dietary and blood data. In particular, parents who kept the dietary record were asked whether their child had been teething, had diarrhoea, been sick or vomited, or been unwell in any other way during the record-keeping period, and if so, whether this had affected the child's eating habits.

Unwell children
Twenty seven per cent of children were reported as being unwell during the diary recording period, but eating habits had only been affected in 16% of cases. No significant differences were found between boys and girls in rates of reported illness. As would be expected, a greater proportion of children were reported as being unwell during the winter months which covered Waves 2 and 3, than the summer months, covered by Waves 1 and 4, but these differences were not statistically significant. *(Tables 3.47 and 3.48)*

Children in the youngest age group were more likely to have been unwell than those in the oldest age group, 35% compared with 20% (p<0.01). *(Table 3.49)*

Dietary supplements
Overall 21% of children were taking dietary supplements. Although not reaching statistical significance, a higher proportion of children were taking dietary supplements during the winter than the summer. *(Table 3.50)*

There was little difference in the proportions of children taking supplements by either sex or age. However children from a non-manual home background were more likely to be taking dietary supplements than those from a manual home background, 28% compared with 16% (p<0.01). *(Tables 3.51 to 3.53)*

Details of the type of dietary supplement the child was taking were recorded in the diary and on the questionnaire; nine discrete groups of dietary supplement were defined and these are shown in Table 3.54. Vitamins A, C and D which include Department of Health Children's Vitamin Drops, and multivitamins were the most commonly taken, accounting for just over three quarters of all supplements being taken.

Prescribed medicines
It was important to identify children taking prescribed medicines which might affect the levels of the blood analytes being measured. Therefore details of any prescribed medicines the child was taking were recorded in the questionnaire; these were later classified into groups using the British National Formulary[9]. For further details of interactions between blood analytes and prescribed medicines see Chapter 10.

Table 3.55 shows that one in ten children were taking at least one prescribed medicine at the time of interview.

Although not reaching statistical significance, a higher proportion of children were taking prescribed medicines during the winter than the summer, and the proportion of children taking prescribed medicines was higher in the youngest age group reflecting trends observed earlier in the rates of reported illness. *(Table 3.57)*

The two types of prescribed medication most commonly taken by children in this survey were antibacterial medication, classified as drugs for the treatment of infections, such as Amoxycillin, and bronchodilatory drugs for the treatment of asthma, such as Ventolin. These groups of medicines accounted for just under half of all prescribed drugs being taken. *(Table 3.58)*

References and notes

1 Davies PSW, Collins DL, and Clarke PC. *Reactions to Venepuncture in Children aged 1½ to 4½ years*. In preparation.
2 Population Estimates Unit, OPCS, Crown Copyright (unpublished data). In mid-1992 the number of children born in 1988, 1989, 1990 and 1991 and living in Great Britain was estimated to be 3,019,644. Of these children 25% were born in each of the four years showing an equal distribution in the population from which the survey sample was drawn.
3 Information on the social class of the head of household and the mother is included on the copy of the Survey database held at the University of Essex Data Archive (see *Reference 13 to Chapter 1* for details of obtaining a copy or subset of the data).
4 Department of Social Security, Crown Copyright, unpublished data. As at May 1993, 31% of households containing a child under 5 years were receiving Income Support and 7% were receiving Family Credit.
5 Bridgwood A, Savage D. *1991 General Household Survey*. HMSO (London, 1993). GHS reported that among married and cohabiting couples the average number of dependent children was 1.9 compared with an average of 1.7 children among lone parents.
6 White A, Freeth S, O'Brien M. *Infant Feeding 1990*. HMSO (London, 1992).
7 Thomas M, Goddard E, Hickman M, Hunter P. *1992 General Household Survey* HMSO (London, 1994).
8 Information on the use of day care services by parents of children aged under 8 years old in England has been published in Meltzer H. *Day care services for children*. HMSO (London, 1994). Data from this dietary survey and from the survey of day care services are not comparable.
9 *British National Formulary*. Number 23 (March 1992). British Medical Association and the Royal Pharmaceutical Society of Great Britain (London, 1992).

Table 3.1 Response to interview and diary by wave of fieldwork*

Response	Wave of fieldwork									
	Wave 1		Wave 2		Wave 3		Wave 4		All	
	No.	%	No.	%	No.	%	No.	%	No.	%
Eligible sample=100%	**474**	*100*	**544**	*100*	**559**	*100*	**524**	*100*	**2101**	*100*
Non-contacts	1	*0*	6	*1*	5	*1*	–	–	12	*1*
Movers	14	*3*	25	*5*	13	*2*	24	*5*	76	*4*
Refusals	33	*7*	41	*7*	38	*7*	42	*8*	154	*7*
Co-operation with:										
interview	426	*90*	472	*87*	503	*90*	458	*87*	1859	*88*
four-day diary, both weekend days	374	*79*	431	*79*	462	*83*	408	*78*	1675	*80*
other four-day diaries	8	*2*	6	*1*	4	*1*	13	*2*	31	*1*
partial diaries	4	*1*	4	*1*	1	*0*	2	*0*	11	*0*
rejected diaries	8	*2*	6	*1*	4	*1*	5	*1*	23	*1*
Refused diary	32	*7*	25	*5*	32	*6*	30	*6*	119	*6*

*Wave 1: July–September 1992, Wave 2: October–December 1992, Wave 3: January–March 1993, Wave 4: April–June 1993.

Table 3.2 Co-operation with anthropometric measurements by wave of fieldwork*

Anthropometric measurement	Wave of fieldwork				
	Wave 1	Wave 2	Wave 3	Wave 4	All
Weight:					
Measurements made	**409**	**451**	**484**	**437**	**1781**
as % of eligible sample	86%	83%	87%	83%	85%
as % of responding sample	96%	96%	96%	95%	96%
Standing height:					
Measurements made	**389**	**424**	**473**	**423**	**1709**
as % of eligible sample	82%	78%	85%	81%	81%
as % of responding sample	91%	90%	94%	92%	92%
Mid upper-arm circumference:					
Measurements made	**404**	**443**	**481**	**432**	**1760**
as % of eligible sample	85%	81%	86%	82%	84%
as % of responding sample	95%	94%	96%	94%	95%
Head circumference:					
Measurements made	**408**	**447**	**486**	**435**	**1776**
as % of eligible sample	86%	82%	87%	83%	84%
as % of responding sample	96%	95%	97%	95%	96%
Supine length:					
Measurements made	**60**	**58**	**52**	**56**	**226**
as % of eligible sample**	73%	70%	76%	74%	73%

*Wave 1: July–September 1992, Wave 2: October–December 1992, Wave 3: January–March 1993, Wave 4: April–June 1993.
**Only children aged under two years of age on the day the measurement was taken were eligible to be measured.

Table 3.3 Co-operation with anthropometric measurements by sex of child for responding sample

Anthropometric measurements	Sex of child		
	Boys	Girls	All
Weight	95%	96%	96%
Standing height	92%	92%	92%
Mid upper-arm circumference	94%	95%	95%
Head circumference	95%	96%	96%
Base	*943*	*916*	*1859*

Table 3.4 Co-operation with anthropometric measurements by age of child for responding sample

Anthropometric measurements	Age of child (in years)			
	1½–2½	2½–3½	3½–4½	All
Weight	94%	97%	96%	96%
Standing height	86%	95%	95%	92%
Mid upper-arm circumference	92%	96%	96%	95%
Head circumference	94%	97%	96%	96%
Base	*648*	*668*	*543*	*1859*

Table 3.5 Co-operation with anthropometric measurements by social class of head of household for responding sample

Anthropometric measurements	Social class of head of household		
	Non-manual	Manual	All*
Weight	98%	94%	96%
Standing height	94%	91%	92%
Mid upper-arm circumference	96%	94%	95%
Head circumference	97%	94%	96%
Base	*818*	*972*	*1859*

*Total includes those heads of household who were not allocated a social class because their job was either inadequately described, they were a member of the Armed Forces, or had never worked.

Table 3.6 Response to the request for a blood sample by wave of fieldwork*

Response to the request for a blood sample	Wave of fieldwork				
	Wave 1	Wave 2	Wave 3	Wave 4**	All
Consented to blood sample	**251**	**316**	**310**	**280**	**1157**
as % of eligible sample	53%	58%	55%	55%	56%
as % of responding sample	59%	67%	62%	64%	63%
Attempted blood sample	**235**	**306**	**295**	**266**	**1102**
as % of eligible sample	50%	56%	53%	53%	53%
as % of responding sample	55%	65%	59%	60%	60%
as % of consenting sample	94%	97%	95%	95%	95%
Obtained blood sample	**215**	**279**	**261**	**248**	**1003**
as % of eligible sample	45%	51%	47%	49%	48%
as % of responding sample	50%	59%	52%	56%	54%
as % of consenting sample	86%	88%	84%	89%	87%

*Wave 1: July–September 1992
Wave 2: October–December 1992
Wave 3: January–March 1993
Wave 4: April–June 1993
**One NHS Local Ethical Committee failed to give ethical clearance in time for fieldwork to begin in one area in Wave 4. Figures for the eligible and responding sample have been adjusted to exclude this area.

Table 3.7 Response to the request for a blood sample by sex of child

Response to the request for a blood sample	Sex of child		
	Boys	Girls	All
	%	%	%
Consent refused	38	36	37
Consent given:			
blood obtained	54	55	54
attempt unsuccessful	5	5	5
no attempt	3	3	3
*Base=100%**	*934*	*907*	*1841*

*Excludes one area where the Local NHS Ethical Committee failed to give ethical clearance in time for fieldwork to begin.

Table 3.8 Response to the request for a blood sample by age of child

Response to the request for a blood sample	Age of child (in years)			
	1½–2½	2½–3½	3½–4½	All
	%	%	%	%
Consent refused	39	37	36	37
Consent given:				
blood obtained	53	55	56	54
attempt unsuccessful	6	6	4	5
no attempt	2	3	5	3
*Base=100%**	*640*	*660*	*541*	*1841*

*Excludes one area where the Local NHS Ethical Committee failed to give ethical clearance in time for fieldwork to begin.

Table 3.9 Response to the request for a blood sample by social class of head of household

Response to the request for a blood sample	Social class of head of household		
	Non-manual	Manual	All*
	%	%	%
Consent refused	34	39	37
Consent given:			
blood obtained	58	51	54
attempt unsuccessful	5	6	5
no attempt	3	3	3
Base=100%**	810	963	1841

*Total includes those who could not be ascribed a social class either because their job was inadequately described, they were a member of the Armed Forces or had never worked.

**Excludes one area where the Local NHS Ethical Committee failed to give ethical clearance in time for fieldwork to begin.

Table 3.10 Comparison of household composition for responding and non-responding households

Household composition	Non-responding eligible households		Responding sample	
	No.	%	No.	%
1 adult with child(ren)	53	19	280	15
2 adults with child(ren)	211	74	1453	78
3 or more adults with child(ren)	20	7	126	7
Base=100%	284	100	1859	100

Table 3.11 Comparison of age of sampled child for responding and non-responding households

Age of child	Non-responding eligible households		Responding sample	
	No.	%	No.	%
1½–2½ years	98	36	648	35
2½–3½ years	86	31	668	36
3½–4½ years	92	33	543	29
Base=100%	276	100	1859	100

Table 3.12 Age and sex of child for responding and diary samples

Age of child	Responding sample			Diary sample*		
	Boys	Girls	All	Boys	Girls	All
	%	%	%	%	%	%
1½–2½ years	36	34	35	35	34	34
2½–3½ years	35	37	36	35	37	36
3½–4½ years	29	29	29	30	29	29
Base = 100%	943	916	1859	848	827	1675
	(51%)	(49%)		(51%)	(49%)	

*Diary sample refers only to those diaries reported on, that is those including two weekdays and both weekend days.

Table 3.13 Regional distribution of responding and diary samples

Region	Responding sample	Dairy sample	1992 GHS sample*
	%	%	%
Scotland	**10**	**10**	**9**
North	5	6	6
Yorkshire and Humberside	9	9	9
North West	11	11	12
Northern	**25**	**26**	**27**
East Midlands	8	8	6
East Anglia	4	4	3
West Midlands	9	9	10
South West	7	8	8
Wales	6	5	5
Central, South West and Wales	**34**	**34**	**32**
London and South East	**31**	**31**	**31**
Base = 100%	1859	1675	5264

*1992 GHS subsample of households containing at least one child aged under 5 years.

Table 3.14 Sex of child by region
Diary sample

Sex of child	Region				
	Scotland	Northern	Central, South West and Wales	London and South East	All
	%	%	%	%	%
Boys	45	51	51	52	51
Girls	55	49	49	48	49
Base = 100%	*165*	*427*	*563*	*520*	*1675*

Table 3.15 Age of child by region
Diary sample

Age of child	Region				
	Scotland	Northern	Central, South West and Wales	London and South East	All
	%	%	%	%	%
1½–2½ years	33	33	35	35	34
2½–3½ years	34	40	36	34	36
3½–4½ years	33	27	29	31	29
Base = 100%	*165*	*427*	*563*	*520*	*1675*

Table 3.16 Social class of head of household by sex of child for responding and diary samples

Social class of head of household	Responding sample			Diary sample		
	Boys	Girls	All	Boys	Girls	All
	%	%	%	%	%	%
I and II	32	31	32	32	32	32
IIInm	11	14	12	11	14	12
IIIm	33	31	32	32	30	31
IV and V	21	20	20	21	20	20
Unclassified*	3	4	4	3	4	4
Base = 100%	*943*	*916*	*1859*	*848*	*827*	*1675*

*Includes those who were not allocated a social class either because their job was inadequately described, they were a member of the Armed Forces or had never worked.

Table 3.17 Social class of head of household for responding and diary samples compared with 1992 GHS data

Social class of head of household	Responding sample	Diary sample	1992 GHS sample**
	%	%	%
Non-manual	44	45	44
Manual	52	52	51
Unclassified*	4	4	5
Base = 100%	*1859*	*1675*	*5264*

*Includes those who were not allocated a social class either because their job was inadequately described, they were a member of the Armed Forces or had never worked.
**1992 GHS subsample of households containing at least one child aged under 5 years.

Table 3.18 Social class of head of household by age of child
Diary sample

Social class of head of household	Age of child (in years)			
	1½–2½	2½–3½	3½–4½	All
	%	%	%	%
Non-manual	45	46	43	45
Manual	50	51	54	52
Unclassified*	4	3	3	4
Base = 100%	*576*	*606*	*493*	*1675*

*Includes those who were not allocated a social class either because their job was inadequately described, they were a member of the Armed Forces or had never worked.

Table 3.19 Social class of head of household by region
Diary sample

Social class of head of household	Region				
	Scotland	Northern	Central, South West and Wales	London and South East	All
	%	%	%	%	%
Non-manual	37	37	43	55	45
Manual	58	59	54	41	52
Unclassified*	5	3	2	4	4
Base = 100%	*165*	*427*	*563*	*520*	*1675*

*Includes those who could not be allocated a social class either because their job was inadequately described, they were a member of the Armed Forces or had never worked.

Table 3.20 Employment status of head of household by sex of child for responding and diary samples

Employment status of head of household	Responding sample			Diary sample		
	Boys	Girls	All	Boys	Girls	All
	%	%	%	%	%	%
Working	75	74	74	75	74	75
Unemployed	9	10	10	9	10	10
Economically inactive	16	16	16	16	15	15
Base = 100%	*943*	*916*	*1859*	*848*	*827*	*1675*

Table 3.21 Employment status of head of household by age of child
Diary sample

Employment status of head of household	Age of child (in years)			
	1½–2½	2½–3½	3½–4½	All
	%	%	%	%
Working	72	77	75	75
Unemployed	11	9	10	10
Economically inactive	16	15	15	15
Base = 100%	*576*	*606*	*493*	*1675*

Table 3.22 Employment status of head of household by region
Diary sample

Employment status of head of household	Region				
	Scotland	Northern	Central, South West and Wales	London and South East	All
	%	%	%	%	%
Working	71	72	73	79	75
Unemployed	7	10	11	10	10
Economically inactive	22	18	16	11	15
Base = 100%	*165*	*427*	*563*	*520*	*1675*

Table 3.23 Employment status of head of household by social class of head of household
Diary sample

Employment status of head of household	Social class of head of household		
	Non-manual	Manual	All*
	%	%	%
Working	84	68	75
Unemployed	3	16	10
Economically inactive	12	16	15
Base = 100%	*748*	*867*	*1675*

*Includes those who were not allocated a social class either because their job was inadequately described, they were members of the Armed Forces or had never worked.

Table 3.24 Child's parents in receipt of Income Support or Family Credit for responding and diary samples by sex of child

Type of benefit	Percentage in receipt of named benefit					
	Responding sample			Diary sample		
	Boys	Girls	All	Boys	Girls	All
Family Credit	5	7	6	5	7	6
Income Support	28	28	28	27	27	27
One or both of the above	32	33	32	31	33	32
*Base**	*943*	*916*	*1859*	*848*	*827*	*1675*

*Includes those not answering.

Table 3.25 Child's parents in receipt of Income Support or Family Credit by age of child

Diary sample

Age of child	Receiving benefit(s)	Base
1½–2½ years	34%	576
2½–3½ years	30%	606
3½–4½ years	32%	493
All ages	32%	1675

Table 3.26 Child's parents in receipt of Income Support or Family Credit by region

Diary sample

Region	Receiving benefit(s)	Base
Scotland	36%	165
Northern	35%	427
Central, South West and Wales	36%	563
London and South East	23%	520
All regions	32%	1675

Table 3.27 Child's parents in receipt of Income Support or Family Credit by social class of head of household

Diary sample

Social class of head of household	Receiving benefit(s)	Base
Non-manual	18%	748
Manual	42%	867
Unclassified*	60%	60
All cases	32%	1675

*Includes those who were not allocated a social class either because their job was inadequately described, they were a member of the Armed Forces or had never worked.

Table 3.28 Household composition by sex of child for responding and diary samples compared with 1992 GHS data

Household composition	Responding sample			Diary sample			1992 GHS*
	Boys	Girls	All	Boys	Girls	All	All
	%	%	%	%	%	%	%
1 adult and child(ren)	15	15	15	15	15	15	13
2 adults and child(ren)	78	79	78	79	79	79	75
3 or more adults and child(ren)	7	7	7	6	6	6	12
Base = 100%	943	916	1859	848	827	1675	5264

*1992 GHS subsample of households containing at least one child aged under 5 years.

Table 3.29 Household composition by sex of child

Diary sample

Household composition	Sex of child		
	Boys	Girls	All
	%	%	%
1 adult with:			
1 child	5	5	5
2 children	6	6	6
3 or more children	3	3	3
2 adults with:			
1 child	20	23	21
2 children	39	37	38
3 or more children	20	19	20
3 or more adults with:			
1 child	2	2	2
2 children	2	3	2
3 or more children	2	2	2
Base = 100%	848	827	1675

Table 3.30 Household composition by age of child

Diary sample

Household composition	Age of child (in years)			
	1½–2½	2½–3½	3½–4½	All
	%	%	%	%
1 adult and child(ren)	15	14	16	15
2 adults and child(ren)	80	79	78	79
3 or more adults with child(ren)	5	7	6	6
Base = 100%	576	606	493	1675

Table 3.31 Household composition by region

Diary sample

Household composition	Region				
	Scotland	Northern	Central, South West and Wales	London and South East	All
	%	%	%	%	%
1 adult and child(ren)	19	15	17	11	15
2 adults and child(ren)	74	75	79	83	79
3 or more adults and child(ren)	6	10	4	6	6
Base = 100%	165	427	563	520	1675

Table 3.32 Household composition by social class of head of household
Diary sample

Household composition	Social class of head of household		
	Non-manual	Manual	All*
	%	%	%
1 adult and child(ren)	14	13	15
2 adults and child(ren)	80	80	79
3 or more adults with child(ren)	5	6	6
Base = 100%	748	867	1675

*Includes those who were not allocated a social class either because their job was inadequately described, they were a member of the Armed Forces or had never worked.

Table 3.33 Number of children in the household under 5 and 16 years of age for the responding and diary samples

No. of children in the household	Responding sample	Diary sample
	%	%
aged under 5 years		
1 child	63	63
2 children	33	33
3 or more children	4	4
Base = 100%	1859	1675
aged under 16 years		
1 child	29	28
2 children	47	47
3 children	17	18
4 or more children	7	8
Base = 100%	1859	1675

Table 3.34 Child's family type for responding and diary samples

Family type	Responding sample	Diary sample
	%	%
Married or cohabiting couple with:		
one child	22	22
more than one child	60	60
Lone parent* with:		
one child	7	7
more than one child	11	11
Base = 100%	1859**	1675

 *Includes four lone fathers.
**Includes one case where child was a foster child.

Table 3.35 Child's family type by sex of child
Diary sample

Family type	Sex of child		
	Boys	Girls	All
	%	%	%
Married or cohabiting couple with:			
one child	21	23	22
more than one child	62	59	60
Lone parent* with:			
one child	7	7	7
more than one child	10	11	11
Base = 100%	848	827	1675

*Includes four lone fathers.

Table 3.36 Child's family type by age of child
Diary sample

Family type	Age of child (in years)			
	1½–2½	2½–3½	3½–4½	All
	%	%	%	%
Married or cohabiting couple with:				
one child	31	18	15	22
more than one child	52	65	65	60
Lone parent* with:				
one child	7	7	8	7
more than one child	10	10	12	11
Base = 100%	576	606	493	1675

*Includes four lone fathers.

Table 3.37 Child's family type by region
Diary sample

Family type	Region				
	Scotland	Northern	Central, South West and Wales	London and South East	All
	%	%	%	%	%
Married or cohabiting couple with:					
one child	18	19	21	26	22
more than one child	59	61	59	62	60
Lone parent* with:					
one child	8	10	7	5	7
more than one child	14	10	13	7	11
Base = 100%	165	427	563	520	1675

*Includes four lone fathers.

Table 3.38 Child's family type by employment status of head of household
Diary sample

Employment status of head of household	Family type				All
	Married or cohabiting couple with:		Lone parent* with:		
	one child	more than one child	one child	more than one child	
	%	%	%	%	%
Working	88	84	33	22	75
Unemployed	10	12	5	2	10
Economically inactive	3	4	62	76	16
Base = 100%	366	1011	121	177	1675

*Includes four lone fathers.

Table 3.39 Child's family type by social class of head of household
Diary sample

Family type	Social class of head of household		
	Non-manual	Manual	All**
	%	%	%
Married or cohabiting couple with:			
one child	23	21	22
more than one child	61	62	60
Lone parent* with:			
one child	6	7	7
more than one child	10	11	11
Base = 100%	748	867	1675

*Includes four lone fathers.
**Includes those not allocated a social class either because their job was inadequately described, they were a member of the Armed Forces or had never worked.

Table 3.40 Child's family type by whether parents in receipt of Income Support or Family Credit
Diary sample

Family type	Receiving benefit(s)	Base
Married or cohabiting couple with:		
one child	14%	366
more than one child	22%	1011
Lone parent* with:		
one child	84%	121
more than one child	90%	177
All families	32%	1675

*Includes four lone fathers.

Table 3.41 Mother's highest educational qualification for responding and diary samples by sex of child

Mother's highest educational qualification	Responding sample			Diary sample		
	Boys	Girls	All	Boys	Girls	All
	%	%	%	%	%	%
Above GCE 'A' level	18	17	18	19	18	18
GCE 'A' level and equivalents	9	12	11	10	12	11
GCE 'O' level and equivalents	35	33	34	36	34	35
CSE and equivalents*	14	16	15	13	15	14
None	24	22	23	22	20	21
Base = 100%**	943	916	1859	848	827	1675

*Includes 'other' qualifications.
**Includes those not answering and two cases where there was no mother living in the household.

Table 3.42 Mother's highest educational qualification by age of child
Diary sample

Mother's highest educational qualification	Age of child (in years)			
	1½–2½	2½–3½	3½–4½	All
	%	%	%	%
Above GCE 'A' level	19	19	16	18
GCE 'A' level and equivalents	11	12	9	11
GCE 'O' level and equivalents	38	32	36	35
CSE and equivalents*	13	14	15	14
None	19	22	24	21
Base = 100%**	576	606	493	1675

*Includes 'other' qualifications.
**Includes those not answering and two cases where there was no mother living in the household.

Table 3.43 Mother's highest educational qualification by region
Diary sample

Mother's highest educational qualification	Region				
	Scotland	Northern	Central, South West and Wales	London and South East	All
	%	%	%	%	%
Above GCE 'A' level	21	16	14	24	18
GCE 'A' level and equivalents	12	9	11	12	11
GCE 'O' level and equivalents	30	34	37	36	35
CSE and equivalents*	8	16	18	11	14
None	30	25	20	17	21
Base = 100%**	165	427	563	520	1675

*Includes 'other' qualifications.
**Includes those not answering and two cases where there was no mother living in the household.

Table 3.44 Mother's highest educational qualification by social class of head of household
Diary sample

Mother's highest educational qualification	Social class of head of household		
	Non-manual	Manual	All†
	%	%	%
Above GCE 'A' level	34	5	18
GCE 'A' level and equivalents	14	8	11
GCE 'O' level and equivalents	33	38	35
CSE and equivalents*	10	18	14
None	10	30	21
Base = 100%**	748	867	1675

*Includes 'other' qualifications.
**Includes those not answering and two cases where there was no mother living in the household.
†Includes those who were not allocated a social class either because their job was inadequately described, they were a member of the Armed Forces or had never worked.

Table 3.45 Main carer of the child whilst the mother was at work by age of child

Main carer of the child whilst mother was at work	Age of child (in years)			
	1½–2½	2½–3½	3½–4½	All
	%	%	%	%
Mother not working	62	57	57	59
Mother working, child looked after by:				
father	12	16	13	14
other relative*	12	11	14	12
paid childminder**	5 }38	5 }42	4 }43	5 }41
nursery†	3	6	8	6
child stays with mother	5	4	4	4
Base = 100%††	648	668	543	1859

*Includes friends and neighbours.
**Includes nannies.
†Includes schools, day nurseries, creches, playgroups and other arrangements.
††Includes those not answering.

Table 3.46 Whether the child attends playgroup, nursery or childminder and has anything to eat by age and sex of child

Whether child attends playgroup, nursery or childminder and eats there	Sex of child		Age of child (in years)			All
	Boys	Girls	1½–2½	2½–3½	3½–4½	
	%	%	%	%	%	%
Does not attend	32	35	55	29	13	33
Attends and has:						
only a snack	16	15	12	17	18	16
a meal*	49 }68	48 }65	31 }45	53 }71	65 }87	49 }67
nothing to eat	3	2	2	1	4	2
Base = 100%**	943	916	648	668	543	1859

*Includes children who had both a meal and a snack and those having only a meal.
**Includes those not answering.

Table 3.47 Whether child was reported as being unwell during the four-day recording period by wave of fieldwork

Whether child was reported as being unwell	Wave of fieldwork*				
	Wave 1	Wave 2	Wave 3	Wave 4	All
	%	%	%	%	%
Unwell during four-day recording period and:					
eating affected	13	17	19	14	16
eating not affected	11	14	11	10	11
Not unwell during recording period	76	70	70	76	73
Base = 100%	374	431	462	408	1675

*Wave 1: July to September 1992.
Wave 2: October to December 1992.
Wave 3: January to March 1993.
Wave 4: April to June 1993.

Table 3.48 Whether child was reported as being unwell during the four-day recording period by sex of child

Diary sample

Whether child was reported as being unwell	Sex of child		
	Boys	Girls	All
	%	%	%
Unwell during four-day recording period and:			
eating affected	16	16	16
eating not affected	10	13	11
Not unwell during recording period	74	71	73
Base = 100%	*848*	*827*	*1675*

Table 3.49 Whether child was reported as being unwell during four-day recording period by age of child

Diary sample

Whether child was reported as being unwell	Age of child (in years)			
	1½–2½	2½–3½	3½–4½	All
	%	%	%	%
Unwell during four-day recording period and:				
eating affected	20	15	12	16
eating not affected	15	11	8	11
Not unwell during recording period	66	74	80	73
Base = 100%	*576*	*606*	*493*	*1675*

Table 3.50 Percentage of children who were taking dietary supplements by wave of fieldwork*

Diary sample

Wave of fieldwork	Percentage taking dietary supplements	
		*Base***
Wave 1	21	*374*
Wave 2	24	*431*
Wave 3	23	*462*
Wave 4	18	*408*
All children	*21*	*1675*

*Wave 1: July to September 1992.
Wave 2: October to December 1992.
Wave 3: January to March 1993.
Wave 4: April to June 1993.
**Includes those not answering.

Table 3.51 Percentage of children who were taking dietary supplements by sex of child

Diary sample

Sex of child	Percentage taking dietary supplements	
		*Base**
Boys	20	*848*
Girls	23	*827*
All children	*21*	*1675*

*Includes those not answering.

Table 3.52 Percentage of children who were taking dietary supplements by age of child

Diary sample

Age of child	Percentage taking dietary supplements	
		*Base**
1½–2½ years	19	*576*
2½–3½ years	22	*606*
3½–4½ years	23	*493*
All children	*21*	*1675*

*Includes those not answering.

Table 3.53 Percentage of children who were taking dietary supplements by social class of head of household

Diary sample

Social class of head of household	Percentage taking dietary supplements	
		*Base**
Non-manual	28	*748*
Manual	16	*867*
Unclassified**	18	*60*
All children	*21*	*1675*

*Includes those not answering.
**Includes those who were not allocated a social class either because their job was inadequately described, they were a member of the Armed Forces or had never worked.

Table 3.54 Dietary supplements being taken by children

Diary sample

Type of dietary supplement	Proportion of total supplements being taken
	%
Cod liver oil based supplements	6
Single vitamin supplements	2
Vitamins A, C & D only	39
Multivitamins	36
Vitamins with iron	5
Multivitamins and multiminerals	8
Minerals only	1
Other/don't know/no answer	4
Total number of supplements being taken = 100%	*381*

Table 3.55 Percentage of children who were taking prescribed medicines by wave of fieldwork*

Responding sample

Wave of fieldwork	Percentage taking prescribed medicines	
		*Base***
Wave 1	9	*426*
Wave 2	10	*472*
Wave 3	13	*503*
Wave 4	11	*458*
All children	*11*	*1859*

*Wave 1: July to September 1992.
Wave 2: October to December 1992.
Wave 3: January to March 1993.
Wave 4: April to June 1993.
**Includes those not answering.

Table 3.56 Percentage of children who were taking prescribed medicines by sex of child
Responding sample

Sex of child	Percentage taking prescribed medicines	Base*
Boys	11	943
Girls	10	916
All children	*10*	*1859*

*Includes those not answering.

Table 3.57 Percentage of children who were taking prescribed medicines by age of child
Responding sample

Age of child	Percentage taking prescribed medicines	Base*
1½–2½ years	12	648
2½–3½ years	11	668
3½–4½ years	8	543
All children	*10*	*1859*

*Includes those not answering.

Table 3.58 Type of prescribed medicine being taken
Responding sample

Type of prescribed medicine	Proportion of total prescribed medicines being taken
	%
Drugs for diseases of:	
gastro-intestinal system*	4
respiratory system	41
of which:	
—bronchodilators	*20*
—corticosteroids	*7*
central nervous system	16
of which:	
—analgesics	*14*
infections**	27
skin	3
Other†	7
All medicines being taken = 100%	*275*

*All drugs in this category were laxatives.
**All drugs in this category were antibacterial.
†Includes unknown drugs and drugs for treatment of diseases of the endocrine system; urinary-tract disorders; nutrition and blood disorders; eyes, ear, nose and oropharynx; and vaccines.

26

4 Quantities of foods consumed

4.1 Introduction

The main part of this chapter reports on the proportions of children who were consuming different foods and the amounts they were consuming; this information is derived from the four-day weighed intake dietary records. The chapter also includes related information from the interview with the child's mother which preceded her keeping the dietary record, including data on the child's consumption of different types of milk and the age at which the child was first given cows' milk as a drink.

The great majority of children in the survey were living in households where facilities and appliances for storing and cooking food were available. All the children were living in households with a kitchen — defined as a separate room for cooking, and almost all households owned or at least had the use of a refrigerator (96%), and a separate freezer (95%); in 72% of households there was a microwave oven. More than three quarters of the households owned or had the use of a car, 28% having more than one car or van. The proportions owning or with the use of these various domestic appliances correspond closely to the data on consumer durables and cars for small and large families in the 1992 General Household Survey[1]. *(Table 4.1)*

Most households also had a range of food items in the house at the time of interview, which, had an emergency arisen, would have provided some food and drink for the child, at least in the short term. From a list of seven prompted items — breakfast cereal, bread, milk (including infant formula), tinned baked beans or spaghetti, eggs, any kind of biscuits, and potatoes, all households had at least two items in the house and over 70% reported having all seven in the house at the time of the interview. *(Table 4.2)*

4.2 Foods consumed

4.2.1 Deriving food consumption data from the four-day weighed intake dietary records

Every item of food consumed by the child was weighed and recorded in the dietary record and subsequently allocated an individual food code. It is therefore possible to analyse the data on food consumption at an individual food code level. However patterns of consumption and differences are more easily identified if the individual food codes are grouped into larger subgroups.

Each food code was allocated by MAFF to one of 99 *food subgroups;* these food subgroups can be collapsed into 54 *food groups*, which in turn can be grouped into 12 *food types*. The complete list of food types, groups and subgroups, with examples of the types of foods included in the food groups, is given in Appendices I(i) and I(ii).

For each child for whom a four-day dietary record was obtained, the gram quantity of each food item consumed during the four-day period was calculated; food item data were then grouped to food subgroup level and the gram quantities weighted to provide an estimate of the total amount consumed over a seven-day period. Thus the total consumption of an item recorded for the two weekdays was multiplied by $5 \div 2$ and then added to the total consumption of the item recorded for Saturday and Sunday.

For items such as beverages and fruit squashes which were recorded in the diary either as 'dry weight', for example instant coffee, or as the weight of a concentrate, for example orange squash, the weight was multiplied by a dilution factor to convert to a 'made-up weight'. This has resulted in fluid consumption being overestimated, as the water used to dilute a concentrate or dry weight was also recorded in the diary. The tables should therefore not be used to estimate the fluid consumption of children in the survey.

NOTE

The proportion of children consuming the various foods, as shown in the tables, represents *consumers over a four-day period*, and is, of course, likely to be lower than the proportion of the same sample of children who would be consumers of the same item over a seven-day, or any other longer recording period. The mean and median amounts of food items consumed over seven days, as shown in the tables, have however been estimated from the four-days' information and the possible effects of this on the estimated amounts reported need to be borne in mind. The weighting applied to the data assumes that the consumption pattern on the three (non-recording) weekdays will be the same as on the two (recording) weekdays; information for the two weekend days is not subject to any re-weighting. Thus a child recorded as eating a large quantity of an item on two weekdays will be assumed to have eaten a similarly (proportionate) large amount on the three non-recording weekdays; conversely the child recorded as consuming very little of an item on two weekdays will be assumed to have had the same low consumption pattern on the other three weekdays for which no information was recorded; at an individual level such consistency in consumption is unlikely. However in order to produce information on intakes that would allow, as far as possible, comparisons to be made with other dietary survey data, which are conventionally expressed as seven-day intakes, it was decided that quantities and intakes *estimated for seven days based on four-days' data*, should be calculated and presented in this Report, with this caveat[2].

Table 4.3 shows the mean and median quantity of each food subgroup consumed for the total sample of boys and girls and for consumers only (that is, those eating the item during the recording period)[3]. In the text that follows references to amounts of foods and drinks are for consumers, unless otherwise stated. *(Table 4.3)*

Although consumption of artificial sweeteners and dietary supplements was recorded in the dietary record, presenting information for these items showing gram quantities consumed is not appropriate and hence these items have been excluded from the main food consumption tables in this chapter. Information taken from the diaries on the proportion of children consuming these items is given in Section 4.7 below together with additional information about the use of artificial sweeteners and dietary supplements taken from the interview questionnaire.

The foods consumed by the largest proportions of children were biscuits (88%), white bread (86%), non-diet soft drinks (86%), whole milk (83%), savoury snacks (78%), other potatoes (77%), that is boiled, mashed and jacket potatoes, and chocolate confectionery (74%). Boys and girls were equally likely to have eaten these foods. Consumption of milk is discussed separately in Section 4.2.2 below.

During the dietary recording period more than half the children in the sample had not eaten eggs in any form (54%), any coated or fried white fish (62%) or fish in dishes or cooked any other way (90%)[4], any leafy green vegetables such as cabbage, greens, or broccoli (61%) or drunk fruit juice (64%).

In Section 4.2.3 below reasons why some children avoided or did not eat particular foods are briefly discussed, with reference to information collected during the interview.

There were very few differences between boys and girls in the foods eaten. Boys were more likely than girls to have eaten preserves ($p<0.01$) and 'other' bread ($p<0.05$) which includes brown and granary breads. Girls were more likely than boys to have eaten salad and raw vegetables ($p<0.01$), raw tomatoes, bacon and ham, and to have drunk tea ($p<0.05$).

Overall, the data showed very few significant differences between boys and girls in the total quantities of the different foods consumed. Among consumers, boys ate greater amounts than girls of wholegrain and high fibre breakfast cereals, and biscuits, and drank greater amounts of diet soft drinks ($p<0.05$, $p<0.01$ and $p<0.05$ respectively) while girls on average ate greater amounts of green beans ($p<0.05$).

The majority of children ate some form of bread and consumed breakfast cereals. Among both boys and girls white bread was eaten by a greater proportion of children and in greater amounts than wholemeal, soft grain or any other type of bread ($p<0.01$). High fibre and wholegrain breakfast cereals were consumed by a smaller proportion of children than consumed other types, by

61% of children compared with 66% ($p<0.05$), but the mean amount of high fibre and wholegrain breakfast cereals eaten by consumers was significantly greater than the mean amount consumed of other types of breakfast cereal ($p<0.01$).

Over half the children in the sample had eaten some cheese (other than cottage cheese) during the recording period (59%), but the median amount consumed was quite small (52 grams). Forty per cent of children had eaten yogurt; fromage frais was less popular, eaten by 26% of children ($p<0.01$).

Of the types of fats and oils identified, 'polyunsaturated' margarine was consumed by the largest proportion of children, 36%, with butter the next most popular but consumed by a smaller proportion of children, 30% ($p<0.01$). Relatively small proportions of children were eating low or reduced fat spreads and only 1% of children were consuming hard 'block' margarine.

Of the types of meat and meat dishes separately identified, sausages, chicken and turkey, and beef and veal (and dishes made with them) were eaten by the largest proportions of children, in each case by about half the children. Less than 20% of children ate pork, lamb, or chicken coated in egg and crumb or in batter, and only 4% of children had liver in any form during the dietary recording period.

Coated white fish and fried white fish were eaten by 38% of children[5]; 16% of children had eaten some form of oily fish, which includes sardines, pilchards and tuna.

Raw vegetables and salad were eaten by relatively small proportions of children in relatively small quantities; for example only 10% of children had eaten raw carrots and 17% raw tomatoes. Of cooked vegetables, peas and carrots were eaten by more than half the children; 49% had eaten baked beans. The median consumption of baked beans (125 grams) was significantly greater than that of either peas or carrots (40 grams each).

The majority of children had eaten potato chips (71%) and savoury snacks (78%), which includes both potato crisps and cereal-based snacks. Over a third (37%) had eaten roast or other fried potatoes. Potato chips, boiled, mashed and jacket potatoes and savoury snacks were consumed in relatively large amounts; among consumers, 50% ate more than 147 grams of chips, 150 grams of boiled, mashed or jacket potatoes, and 70 grams (about three packets) of savoury snacks.

Half the children in the sample had eaten apples or pears and 46% had eaten bananas, but citrus fruits, such as oranges and satsumas, were only eaten by about one quarter of the children, despite fieldwork for the survey covering all four seasons. Just under half the children eating bananas were consuming more than 200 grams; the median amounts of apples and pears, and of citrus fruits consumed, were somewhat smaller, 157 and 144 grams respectively (NS). Less than 10% of children had eaten fruit canned in juice or in syrup.

Over half the children had consumed table sugar and over a third had eaten preserves such as jam or marmalade during the dietary recording period. Table sugar is defined as sugar that was weighed and recorded as a separate item in the food diary; thus it includes sugar added 'at the table', for example, to beverages, breakfast cereals, and fruit, but excludes the sugar included in composite or recipe items (unless recorded separately in the diary), and excludes the sugar in processed foods. For consumers, the median amount of table sugar estimated as consumed over seven days was 18 grams, equivalent to about 4½ level teaspoons, but some children consumed much larger quantities, giving a mean amount of nearly twice the median—33 grams. Chocolate confectionery was more commonly eaten than sugar confectionery, by 74% and 58% of children respectively (p<0.01), but the median amounts consumed were very similar, about 80 grams.

Most children had consumed non-diet soft drinks during the recording period (86%) and nearly half had drunk diet drinks (49%). The amounts of soft drinks consumed were quite large; across the total sample, consumers and non-consumers, the median quantity of non-diet soft drinks consumed was 1295 grams. Among consumers, half of those drinking non-diet soft drinks were estimated as having more than 1635 grams per week; the median quantity of diet soft drinks consumed was somewhat smaller, 1160 grams. This represents about 1.5 litres of non-diet and about 1 litre of diet soft drinks per week.

Only about one third of children had fruit juice and a very small proportion (4%) had mineral water. During the recording period over one third of children had drunk tea (37%), but only 7% had drunk coffee. The estimated median amounts of tea and coffee consumed were 463 and 327 grams respectively, the equivalent of about 2½ cups of tea and 1½ cups of coffee over seven days.

Although commercial infant food and drinks are classified to the same food subgroup, they were separately identified at the food code level and have been shown separately in the tables in this Chapter. Overall 4% of children were eating commercially prepared infant foods and 2% were having drinks specially formulated for infants and young children.

4.2.2 Current milk consumption and infant feeding practices

As noted earlier, information in the dietary records showed that most children (83%) were having whole milk, either as a drink or in some other way, but nearly one third were having semi-skimmed milk (32%) and 4% of children were consuming some skimmed milk, although the median amount of skimmed milk for consumers was relatively small (425 grams). Fifty per cent of children who had whole milk consumed more than 1500 grams over seven days.

In the interview with the child's mother which preceded her keeping the dietary record, more information was collected about the child's consumption of milk, including the age at which cows' milk had been introduced and on the types of milk given to a child as a drink and used in cooking; these data are shown in Tables 4.4 to 4.12.

As can be seen from Table 4.4 only 5% of children were reported never to have had cows' milk as a drink and a further 8%, although they had in the past done so, were no longer drinking cows' milk[6].

Semi-skimmed and skimmed milks, as a consequence of their lower fat content, have a lower energy value and lower levels of fat soluble vitamins than whole milk. Their consumption has been recommended for adults who wish to reduce their fat intake, but for young children who have high energy requirements, fat reduced milks, particularly as a drink, are not generally recommended. Fully skimmed milk should not generally be given before 5 years of age[7].

In the interview, 68% of children were reported as usually having whole milk as a drink; 19% usually had semi-skimmed and 1% skimmed milk to drink. The proportions of children having either semi- or skimmed milk as a drink increased with age.

A distinction was made in the interview between milk given to the child 'as a drink' and milk used on breakfast cereal or in cooking, and as Table 4.6 shows semi-skimmed milk was more likely to be used for cooking and on cereal than as a drink for the child; over one quarter of all children were having semi-skimmed milk in cooked dishes or on breakfast cereal and again the proportions increased as the children got older.

The introduction of cows' milk as a drink during infancy is not recommended, partly because it offers a poor source of iron. An infant who is not yet consuming a diverse diet may not be getting an adequate iron intake[7] and the manufactured products, infant formula or follow-on formula provide iron fortified drinks[8].

Table 4.7 shows 3% of children had started having cows' milk as a drink before they were six months old; by the age of nine months nearly one third of children had cows' milk to drink and 57% of children had been given cows' milk before reaching their first birthday. Semi-skimmed milk as a drink had been given to 2% of children before they were 9 months old; and 4% had semi-skimmed milk to drink before they were 12 months old

In the interview mothers were asked whether they had ever breast-fed their child, and ever used infant formula or follow-on milk; how long each feeding practice was continued was also recorded although it should be noted, particularly for the mothers of the oldest group of children, that the information may be subject to inaccuracies of memory.

It was reported that 59% of the survey children had been put to the breast at birth, but 8% of the mothers had stopped breast-feeding in the first week. By six weeks 38% were still breast-feeding but by six months this had fallen to only 18%; 10% of mothers were still breast-feeding their child, at least once a day, nine months after the birth. These percentages are slightly lower than those reported in the last national survey of infant feeding practices carried out in 1990 where 63% of mothers reported putting their child to the breast at birth; at six weeks, six months and nine months the proportions still breast-feeding were 39%, 21% and 11% respectively[9].

Only 12% of children in this survey had never had either infant formula or follow-on milk and as Table 4.10 shows over a third of children in the sample were having a formula feed or follow-on milk at least once a day at the age of 12 months. Between the ages of 12 and 18 months however most children gave up formula and follow-on milk, with only 7% continuing beyond age 18 months.

Table 4.11 shows the age of the child when cows' milk was introduced as a drink according to the age the child was when she or he stopped having formula feeds (including having follow-on milk). As both pieces of information were collected and recorded in age bands, it is not possible to identify precisely the children who were no longer having any formula feeds when they started having cows' milk as a drink; however the boxed area on the table provides a minimum estimate of the likely percentage. Table 4.12 presents similar information in relation to the age of the child when breast-feeding stopped. Again, as the information on the age of the child was collected in age bands, only estimates can be made of the percentage of children who were no longer being breast-fed when cows' milk as a drink was introduced. It should also be remembered that some children will have been both formula and breast-fed, and they may not have both been stopped at the same time.

(Tables 4.4 to 4.12)

4.2.3 Reasons for not eating certain foods

The reasons for avoidance of particular foods are various and, apart from personal preference, may include medical or health reasons, and religious or other reasons of personal principle, including vegetarianism.

It was noted above, for example, that over half the children had not eaten any eggs during the recording period. For 51 children—3% (30 boys and 21 girls)—there were no entries in the food diaries for any meat or meat product. From the information collected during the interview only 35 of these children 2%—(19 boys and 16 girls)—were reported as never eating any meat; the remaining 16 children may not have been vegetarians but simply happened not to have eaten meat on any of the recording days.

Although in the interview information was collected on the foods avoided or not given to the children and the reasons, this information was intended to assist the interviewer in checking the dietary record, particularly for what might be omissions in recording; hence the various foods not given to children were not coded and the information was not analysed. Informants were asked however whether certain foods were avoided because their child was, or was thought to be, allergic to them; 14% said they avoided giving certain foods for this reason including 5% who said the allergy had been diagnosed by a doctor. Hyperactivity and behavioural problems were the most frequent type of allergic reaction, reported as experienced by 6% of all children; 3% were reported to suffer from rashes or blotches if certain foods were given and 2% had an allergic eczema; 2% of children had gastrointestinal problems, such as diarrhoea, vomiting or stomach upsets if given certain foods[10].

(Table 4.13)

4.3 Variation by age group in the foods eaten

The proportion of children in each of the three age groups who had eaten foods of various types, and the mean and median amounts eaten by consumers are shown in Table 4.14.

(Table 4.14)

The general pattern was for the proportion of children eating the various foods to increase with age. There were however a few exceptions. Not surprisingly the youngest children, those aged 1½ to 2½ years, were more likely than other children to have consumed commercially prepared infant or toddlers' foods and drinks (p<0.01); they were also more likely to have eaten bananas (p<0.01) and, compared with those aged 3½ to 4½ years, were more likely to have consumed yogurt, whole milk, wholegrain and high fibre breakfast cereals and peas (p<0.05). They were also more likely than children aged 2½ to 3½ years to have eaten fish which was neither fried nor coated (p<0.05).

The proportion of children consuming white bread, other breakfast cereals, buns, cakes and pastries, ice cream, semi-skimmed milk, bacon and ham, other meat products, raw carrots, chips, savoury snacks, sugar confectionery and non-diet soft drinks increased significantly with age (for oldest and youngest groups compared, p<0.05 for white bread, other breakfast cereals, other meat products, raw carrots and savoury snacks; for other foods p<0.01). The proportion of children eating coated chicken significantly increased after age 3½ years from 16% to 24% (p<0.05), and after the age of 2½ years significantly more children drank diet soft drinks, 52% compared with 41% (p<0.01).

The average quantities of the various foods consumed (by consumers) also generally increased with age, but with some notable exceptions. For example, there was no significant difference in the mean amount of high fibre and wholegrain breakfast cereals consumed by the youngest and oldest age groups, although for other types of breakfast cereal there was such an increase (p<0.05). Similarly there was no significant difference in the mean consumption of wholemeal bread associated with age, but consumption of white bread did increase with age (p<0.01).

Children under 2½ years were not only more likely to be drinking whole milk than older children, but, on average, they were having significantly larger quantities, a mean of 2233 grams (about 4 pints) compared with 1543 grams (about 2¾ pints) by those aged 3½ to 4½ years (p<0.01), but their consumption of reduced fat types of milk was not significantly different from that of older children. The mean amounts of fruit juice, diet and non-diet soft drinks, tea and coffee consumed did not vary significantly with age. There was also no significant difference in the average amounts of fruit or table sugar being eaten by the youngest and oldest groups of children, but the oldest children had eaten, on average, about one third more confectionery than the youngest group (p<0.01).

Among the youngest children, aged between 1½ and 2½ years, half had eaten more than an estimated 121 grams of chips. For each of raw carrots, other raw and salad vegetables (not tomatoes), green beans, and leafy green vegetables, the median amount eaten by consumers was less than 30 grams. The median amounts of diet and non-diet soft drinks consumed by the youngest group of children were 1205 grams and 1506 grams respectively. Although drinks formulated specially for young children and infants were consumed relatively infrequently, by only 8% of the youngest children, they were taken in quite large amounts by those having them, a median quantity of 936 grams.

The mean amounts of the different types of fats consumed generally increased with age, for example for butter from 23 grams for children aged 1½ to 2½ years to 32 grams for those aged 3½ to 4½ years (p<0.05), and for 'polyunsaturated' margarine from 29 grams to 41 grams (p<0.01). As foods, rather than nutrients, these represent fats used mainly for spreading and hence this increase will be associated mainly with the greater quantities of bread consumed by the older children.

4.3.1 Differences between boys and girls in the oldest age group

It was thought that by the age of 3½ years there might be some significant differences between boys and girls in the mean amounts of various types of foods being eaten. Table 4.15 shows, for boys and girls separately, the proportions aged 3½ to 4½ years consuming the various types of foods and the mean and median quantities consumed by consumers. *(Table 4.15)*

The data show not only no differences between boys and girls aged 3½ to 4½ years in the types of foods they ate, but also very few significant differences in the mean amounts of the various types of foods consumed. Significant differences were only found in respect of three food subgroups where boys, on average, consumed greater amounts than girls; these were wholegrain and high fibre breakfast cereals (p<0.05), biscuits (p<0.01) and bananas (p<0.05).

However there were a few more general patterns of differences between boys and girls in the data, which, with a larger or less clustered sample design, might have

reached the level of statistical significance. For example, girls were consuming greater median amounts of pasta and rice, and salad and raw vegetables, whereas boys had higher median intakes of other, more traditional carbohydrates, such as non-high fibre and wholegrain breakfast cereals, buns, cakes and pastries, and white and wholemeal bread. Apart from fruit juice, where boys and girls drank similar amounts, this oldest group of boys consumed greater median amounts than girls of most drinks, including tea and coffee.

4.4 Variation by social class of head of household

In Table 4.16 as elsewhere in this Report the social class of the head of household has been categorised as either manual or non-manual; the table shows for these two groups the proportion of children consuming the foods of various types, and the estimated mean and median amounts eaten by consumers. *(Table 4.16)*

The survey data show very clear patterns and differences in the types of foods consumed by children from manual and non-manual backgrounds; indeed for almost every food type there is at least one food subgroup where there is a significant difference in the proportion of consumers from manual and non-manual home backgrounds. Overall the pattern suggests a diet among children from a manual background with less emphasis on fruit and whole grain cereals; however the same subgroup of children were also less likely to be eating buns, cakes and pastries.

Among cereals and cereal products, children whose head of household was in a non-manual social class group were more likely to have eaten rice, wholemeal bread, wholegrain and high fibre breakfast cereals, and buns, cakes and pastries (p<0.01), although their mean consumption was not significantly different from children from a manual background who were eating these foods. However for white bread and non-wholegrain/high fibre breakfast cereals, children from a manual home background were not only more likely to be eating these foods (p<0.05) but they were also eating significantly greater quantities; for non-wholegrain and high fibre breakfast cereals, p<0.05 and for white bread, p<0.01.

Among milks and milk products there were no differences for any food subgroup in the average quantities consumed between the two groups of children, although children from the non-manual group were more likely to have eaten ice cream (p<0.05), fromage frais and cheese other than cottage cheese (p<0.01).

Overall there were also no significant differences in the average amounts of fats and oils consumed by children from different home backgrounds, although the data show a tendency for children from the manual group to be eating greater average quantities. There were nevertheless some differences in the types of fats consumed; children from a non-manual home were more likely to have eaten butter and 'polyunsaturated' margarine, whereas children from a manual background were more likely to eat non-polyunsaturated soft margarine (p<0.01) and reduced fat spreads (p<0.05).

Children from a manual home background were more likely to eat and ate greater average amounts of meat pies and pastries, whereas children from a non-manual background were more likely to eat and ate greater average amounts of chicken and turkey (all differences: p<0.05). For other meats there were no differences in the average consumption although children whose head of household was classified in the non-manual group were more likely to have eaten bacon and ham (p<0.05) and coated chicken (p<0.01), and less likely to have eaten burgers and kebabs (p<0.01).

Oily fish and white fish (not fried) were more likely to have been eaten by children from the non-manual group (p<0.01).

There were no differences between the two groups of children in the average amounts of vegetables consumed (excluding potatoes), but children from a non-manual home were more likely to have eaten salad and raw vegetables (for raw carrots: p<0.01; for raw tomatoes and other raw and salad vegetables: p<0.05). Children from a manual home background were not only more likely to have eaten potato chips (p<0.01), they also consumed significantly greater average quantities of both chips and savoury snacks such as crisps (p<0.01).

Almost all types of fruit, including fruit canned in juice, were more likely to have been eaten by children from a non-manual social class background (for apples and pears, and canned fruit in juice: p<0.05; for other fruits: p<0.01). There were however no significant differences in the average amounts of the different fruits consumed between the two groups of children.

Children from the manual group were more likely to have consumed table sugar (p<0.01) and sugar confectionery (p<0.05) and they also ate significantly greater average amounts of these foods. For example, an estimated average of 40 grams of table sugar (about 10 level teaspoons) and 125 grams of sugar confectionery was eaten by children from the manual group, compared with 24 grams of table sugar—about 6 level teaspoons (p<0.01)—and 103 grams of sugar confectionery (p<0.05) consumed by children from the non-manual group. As well as eating greater average quantities of sugar confectionery, children from a manual home background also on average ate greater quantities of chocolate confectionery — 109 grams compared with 91 grams (p<0.01).

Of the beverages, fruit juice was drunk by nearly half the children in the non-manual group (48%) compared with only a quarter (26%) of the manual group, and 6% of the non-manual group of children were drinking mineral or tonic water compared with only 2% of other children (p<0.01). In both cases there was no significant difference in the average amounts being consumed. However this was not the case for either tea or coffee, where not only were children from a manual home background significantly more likely to drink these beverages (tea: p<0.01; coffee: p<0.05) but they were also consuming them in larger average amounts (p<0.05). For example, the 44% of children in the manual group who were drinking tea were consuming an average of 767 grams (about four cups in seven days) compared with an average of 559 grams (about three cups) consumed by the 29% of children from the non-manual group. Information from the interview on the proportions of children who drank sweetened tea and coffee is given in Chapter 6 with data on carbohydrate intake (Table 6.12).

4.5 Variation by fieldwork wave in the foods eaten

Although generally most foods are widely available throughout the year, there may nevertheless be some seasonality in diet. The proportion of consumers in each fieldwork wave who ate foods of various types, and the mean and median amounts eaten by consumers are shown in Table 4.17. (Table 4.17)

Although there are differences they are not as many as might have been expected[11]. Some are obviously related to the seasonal nature of the food or seasonal weather conditions; for example, raw tomatoes, salad and raw vegetables, ice cream and diet soft drinks were most likely to be consumed during the spring and early summer months, April to June (Wave 4 of fieldwork). Green beans, and other fruit, which is mainly soft fruit, were eaten by the greatest proportions of children in high and late summer, July to September (Wave 1 of fieldwork). October to December (Wave 3) saw the highest proportions consuming beef and dishes made with beef and in the following three months the traditional winter vegetables of carrots and leafy green vegetables were most likely to be eaten. During January to March, the proportion of children eating citrus fruits, oranges, satsumas, clementines and similar was highest.

For some other foods the reasons for apparent seasonal differences are less obvious; for example, between July and September the proportion of children eating rice and eating sugar confectionery was higher than at any other time of the year; white bread was consumed most frequently during the period October to December; non-diet soft drinks were most popular during January to March, and fromage frais was eaten by a higher proportion of children during April to June than at any other time of the year.

4.6 Variation by region in the foods eaten

Table 4.18 gives similar information on the types of foods eaten by children in each of the four main regions used throughout this Report. (Table 4.18)

Although there are a large number of differences between regions in the proportions of children eating the various foods, patterns of eating behaviour associated with region are not always clear or as might be expected.[12]

For example, children in Scotland were the most likely to be eating chips, beef and veal, canned fruit in syrup and drinking non-diet soft drinks, and were the least likely to be eating cheese, most types of vegetable, other fruit (mainly soft fruit), drinking fruit juice and consuming reduced fat spread (not polyunsaturated). However they were also the most likely to be drinking semi-skimmed milk, and the least likely to be eating biscuits, lamb, fried white fish, and table sugar.

The data show some evidence that children in the Northern region of England were eating more traditional foods, particularly when compared with children living in London and the South East. For example, children in the Northern region were the most likely, and children in London and South East the least likely, to be eating meat pies and products (36% compared with 21%), baked beans (54% and 45%), and 'other' potatoes — boiled, mashed and jacket (82% and 71%)—and to be drinking coffee (12% and 3%). Children in the Northern region were also significantly more likely than children in Scotland to be consuming fried white fish and biscuits. In contrast they were the least likely group to be eating rice, fromage frais, coated chicken, raw and salad vegetables (not tomatoes or carrots), and nuts and fruit and nut mixes.

Some of these differences between children in Scotland and the Northern region of England and other children in the survey are likely, in part at least, to be a reflection of social class differences in the composition of the regions. As Table 3.19 showed, the proportion of children with heads of household in the manual social class group in both Scotland and the Northern region was significantly greater than in London and the South East.

Children in the Central and South West regions of England and in Wales were more likely than children elsewhere in Great Britain to be eating most types of vegetable; for example, 58% were eating peas, 10% green beans, 42% leafy green vegetables and 61% carrots compared with children in Scotland where the proportions consuming these vegetables were 36%, 1%, 19% and 28% respectively (p<0.01).

Nearly half of these children from the Central and South West regions and Wales (48%) had drunk tea and 8% had drunk coffee during the recording period, significantly higher proportions compared with children in London and the South East, where less than a third (29%) were tea drinkers and only 3% drank coffee (p<0.01 and p<0.05). The children from the Central region, the South West and Wales were also more likely than other children to be consuming table sugar, although the mean amounts they consumed were not significantly different from the mean amounts consumed by other children.

The data clearly suggest a much less traditional pattern of eating by children in London and the South East than elsewhere, particularly as compared with children in the North of England and Scotland. For example, children in London and the South East were the most likely to be consuming rice, wholemeal bread, cheese, fromage frais, raw tomatoes and salad and other raw vegetables, fruit juice, 'other' fruit — mainly soft fruits, nuts and fruit and nut mixes. Correspondingly they were the least likely to be eating white bread and non-wholegrain/high fibre breakfast cereals. They were less likely than other children to be having soft, non-polyunsaturated margarine,

but more likely to be consuming butter. Of the meats and meat products they were the least likely consumers of meat pies and pastries, and of beef, veal and dishes, but they were the group most likely to be eating coated chicken. About two thirds (65%) of children in London and the South East had eaten chips compared with more than three quarters (78%) of children in Scotland (p<0.05), but for other fried and roast potatoes the position was reversed with London and South Eastern children being more likely consumers than Scottish children (42% compared with 24% — p<0.01). Children in London and the South East were also the most likely to have eaten non-fried white fish and oily fish and were the lowest proportion of consumers of sugar confectionery, non-diet soft drinks and, as noted above, of tea and coffee.

4.7 Consumption of dietary supplements and artificial sweeteners

4.7.1 Dietary supplements
In the interview which preceded keeping the dietary record, 21% of children were reported as taking dietary supplements, that is vitamin or mineral preparations, including fluoride preparations[13] (see *Tables 3.50 to 3.54*).

Tables 4.19 and 4.20 give information on supplement taking from the four-day dietary records. Over the recording period 11% of children had taken dietary supplements as tablets, 3% as syrups or oils and 5% had taken supplements as drops[14].

Information from the dietary records showed that the oldest group of children were more likely than the youngest to be taking dietary supplements in tablet form (p<0.01), although there were no differences associated with age in the proportions taking supplements as drops or syrup.

An earlier survey of the diets and nutritional status of British adults found that supplement taking was strongly and positively associated with the social class of the head of the household[15]. There is a similar relationship for children; thus although children from a non-manual home background were more likely to be consuming foods which are rich sources of vitamins and minerals, such as fruit juice, salad and raw vegetables and nearly all types of fruit, they were also significantly more likely to be taking dietary supplements; for example among the children in the non-manual group 15% were taking supplements in tablet form, 5% as syrup and 7% as drops; among children from a manual home background the corresponding proportions were 7%, 2% and 4% (comparing difference between the non-manual and manual groups, for tablets: p<0.01; for syrup and drops: p<0.05).   *(Tables 4.19 and 4.20)*

4.7.2 Artificial sweeteners
From the interview 1% of children were reported as drinking tea sweetened with an artificial sweetener and 1% drank coffee sweetened in this way (see *Chapter 6, Table 6.13*). The data also showed that a very small proportion of children were having artificial sweeteners either added to their food at the table, for example, on

breakfast cereals, or in home cooked food, such as stewed fruit or in baking. Overall 2% of children were reported to be consuming artificial sweeteners either added at the table or in cooking *(table not shown)*.

Information taken from the dietary records confirmed this low usage by children; over the four recording days only 1% of children consumed artificial sweeteners which were either being used at the table or added in cooking. However the total consumption of artificial sweeteners by children is likely to be much higher than these data suggest since many low calorie and diet products, such as soft drinks and yogurts, are sweetened artificially and as has been shown in this Chapter these products were being consumed by significant proportions of children, and for low calorie soft drinks in quite large quantities.

Preliminary estimates of the likely intakes of each of the sweeteners from these sources indicate that even high-level consumers, as represented by the 97.5 percentile level of consumption, are within the respective Acceptable Daily Intakes (ADIs)[16]. Nonetheless this is clearly an area which will require continued careful surveillance by MAFF.

References and notes

1 Thomas M, Goddard E, Hickman M, Hunter P, *1992 General Household Survey.* HMSO (London, 1994), Table 2.38.
2 For further information on the possible effects of this re-weighting on estimates of the proportions of consumers and on estimates of the total mean and median amounts of foods eaten over a seven-day period see Appendix J.
3 None of the children in the sample were reported as consuming any spirits or liqueurs during the recording period. Information about these and about the consumption of food supplements and artificial sweeteners is not shown in the tables leaving data for 94 of the 99 food subgroups.
4 'Other white fish and dishes' includes, apart from fish dishes, any fish that is *not* coated or fried, for example fish that has been steamed, poached or grilled.
5 'Coated white fish' includes white fish coated with batter or egg and crumb, fried *or* grilled, for example, grilled, crumbed fish fingers.
6 Information based on answers from all 1859 respondents who co-operated with the interview, including 184 who did not complete a full four-day dietary record for their child.

7 Department of Health. Report on Health and Social Subjects: 45. *Weaning and the Weaning Diet.* HMSO (London, 1994).
8 Follow-on milks are manufactured products intended for giving only after the age of 6 months as the milk component in a mixed diet. See Department of Health. Report on Health and Social Subjects: 45. *Weaning and the Weaning Diet.* HMSO (London, 1994).
9 White A, Freeth S and O'Brien M. *Infant feeding 1990.* HMSO (London, 1992), Table 2.27.
10 If more than one allergic reaction was reported, all were coded. No order of priority was assigned in coding reactions.
11 All differences commented on are significantly different at least at the p<0.05 level, and are based on comparisons between the two waves with the highest and lowest proportions of consumers.
12 All differences commented on are significant at least at the p<0.05 level, and are based on comparisons between the two regions with the highest and lowest proportions of consumers.
13 Fluoride preparations are not nutritional supplements; the term 'fluoride supplements' reflects common usage in the dental profession.
14 Interviewers were told to check carefully for consistency between the information on the use of dietary supplements given in the dietary record and during the interview. Differences may be due to dietary supplements only being taken on some days—not dietary recording days; mothers forgetting to give the child their supplement; and dietary records not being kept for some children who took supplements.
15 Gregory J, Foster K, Tyler H, Wiseman M. *The Dietary and Nutritional Survey of British Adults.* HMSO (London, 1990).
16 *Acceptable Daily Intakes (ADIs) for Intense Sweeteners:* The intense sweeteners permitted in the UK are acesulfame-K, aspartame, saccharin and thaumatin. Thaumatin is not much used and has no ADI. The ADIs and references to the other three are as follows:
Acesulfame-K ADI = 0–9mg/kg body weight/day.
  Ref: *Reports of the Scientific Committee for Food, 16th Series.* Commission of the European Communities, 1985.
Aspartame ADI = 0–40mg/kg body weight/day.
  Ref: *Committees on the Toxicity, Mutagenicity and Carcinogenicity of Chemicals in Food, Consumer Products and the Environment, 1992 Annual Report.* HMSO (London, 1993).
Saccharin ADI = 0–5mg/kg body weight/day.
  Ref: MAFF Press Release, 16 August 1990.

Table 4.1 Household access to amenities and domestic appliances

Amenities and domestic appliances	NDNS: Children aged 1½–4½ years	GHS 1992*	
		Small family**	Large family**
With access to a garden	91%	n/a	n/a
With a separate kitchen†	100%	100%	100%
Owns or has use of:			
refrigerator	96%	n/a	n/a
freezer	95%	93%	93%
microwave	72%	70%	72%
car or van	78%	78%	80%
Base = 100%	1859††	1942	608

General Household Survey 1992. HMSO (London, 1994) Table 2.38
**Small family: 1 or 2 persons aged 16 or over and 1 or 2 persons aged under 16. Large family: 1 or more persons aged 16 or over and 3 or more persons aged under 16, or 3 or more persons aged 16 or over and 2 persons aged under 16.
†Includes a small number of cases where the kitchen was shared with other households.
††Base = all informants. Percentages based on informants keeping a dietary record were the same as shown in this table.
n/a Not available

Table 4.2 Proportion of households with selected food items in the home at the time of the interview

(a) Prompted food item	% with item in the house at the time of interview
A breakfast cereal	98
Bread or bread rolls	98
Milk including infant formula	99
A tin of baked beans or spaghetti	94
Eggs	91
Biscuits of any kind	87
Potatoes	95

(b) Number of items in the house at time of interview	% of households
All 7 items	72
6 items	20
5 items	6
4 items	2
3 items	0
2 items	0
1 item	–
None available	–
Base = 100%	1859

Table 4.3 Total quantities (grams) of food consumed as estimated for seven days by sex of child
Four days' intake re-weighted

Type of food	Consumers Boys			Consumers Girls			Consumers All			Total sample All	
	Mean	Median	% consumers	Mean	Median	% consumers	Mean	Median	% who ate	Mean	Median
	g	g	%	g	g	%	g	g	%	g	g
Pasta	234	176	49	261	192	52	248	180	51	127	14
Rice	193	138	18	188	134	18	190	135	18	35	0
Pizza	156	115	15	154	105	13	155	108	14	22	0
Other cereals	83	40	23	71	34	24	77	38	24	18	0
White bread	233	206	85	218	180	85	226	191	86	194	155
Wholemeal bread	170	139	27	153	109	27	162	119	27	44	0
Soft grain bread	147	97	7	161	132	6	154	111	7	10	0
Other bread	120	87	32	104	74	26	113	80	30	33	0
Wholegrain & high fibre b'fast cereals	135	101	63	113	88	58	125	95	61	77	36
Other breakfast cereals	95	79	66	89	70	64	92	74	66	61	35
Biscuits	127	106	89	109	92	86	118	98	88	105	87
Fruit pies	104	78	5	93	71	6	99	77	6	6	0
Buns, cakes & pastries	124	93	56	117	92	53	121	92	55	66	27
Milk puddings	273	200	27	222	150	23	249	169	25	62	0
Ice cream	138	107	40	137	95	45	137	100	43	59	0
Sponge type puddings	171	117	3	162	102	3	166	110	3	5	0
Other puddings	206	150	29	190	126	28	198	140	30	57	0
Whole milk	1935	1624	84	1805	1509	80	1872	1575	83	1551	1241
Semi-skimmed milk	1192	831	31	1237	831	32	1215	831	32	390	0
Skimmed milk	669	370	5	741	464	4	701	425	4	30	0
Infant formula	2818	3200	2	2103	1743	2	2438	1814	2	47	0
Other milk & cream	211	53	15	318	60	11	256	55	13	34	0
Cottage cheese	89	53	1	60	58	1	71	56	1	1	0
Other cheese	71	54	56	67	50	60	69	52	59	40	17
Fromage frais	234	160	24	203	168	27	218	162	26	56	0
Yogurt	337	300	40	374	301	38	355	300	40	141	0
Eggs & egg dishes	122	88	42	132	98	48	127	94	46	58	0
Butter	28	20	31	27	19	28	28	20	30	8	0
'Polyunsaturated' margarine	34	27	36	35	27	35	35	27	36	12	0
'Polyunsaturated' oil	6	3	1	8	4	1	7	3	1	0	0
'Polyunsaturated' low fat spread	28	22	9	27	20	8	27	21	9	2	0
Other low fat spread	36	25	14	37	32	13	37	28	14	5	0
Block margarine	44	46	1	24	21	1	34	30	1	0	0
Soft margarine, not polyunsaturated	33	24	17	30	20	17	32	22	17	5	0
'Polyunsaturated' reduced fat spread	30	21	7	27	17	9	28	20	8	2	0
Other reduced fat spread	33	28	17	31	21	17	32	25	17	5	0
Other fats & oils not polyunsaturated	7	4	4	9	5	5	8	5	5	0	0
Bacon & ham	57	38	36	56	37	43	57	37	40	23	0
Beef, veal & dishes	202	137	44	170	110	48	185	119	47	86	0
Lamb & dishes	94	39	15	92	48	15	93	43	15	14	0
Pork & dishes	65	39	18	72	42	18	68	42	18	13	0
Coated chicken	127	102	17	104	80	19	115	90	18	21	0
Chicken & turkey dishes	85	53	53	93	59	49	89	57	52	46	5
Liver, liver products & dishes	79	44	5	65	38	3	73	43	4	3	0
Burgers & kebabs	104	92	25	96	75	22	100	85	24	24	0
Sausages	123	100	53	114	83	52	119	90	53	63	15
Meat pies & pastries	154	113	29	142	117	26	149	115	28	42	0
Other meat products	106	58	26	96	62	27	100	60	27	27	0

35

Table 4.3 Total quantities (grams) of food consumed as estimated for seven days by sex of child *(continued)*
Four days' intake re-weighted

Type of food	Consumers Boys			Consumers Girls			Consumers All			Total sample All	
	Mean	Median	% consumers	Mean	Median	% consumers	Mean	Median	% who ate	Mean	Median
	g	g	%	g	g	%	g	g	%	g	g
Coated & fried white fish	113	98	*40*	117	95	*36*	115	97	*38*	44	0
Shellfish	99	55	*2*	57	28	*3*	76	40	*3*	2	0
Other white fish & dishes	111	62	*11*	122	85	*9*	116	76	*10*	12	0
Oily fish	76	47	*14*	66	48	*17*	70	48	*16*	11	0
Raw carrots	62	37	*10*	57	29	*10*	60	32	*10*	6	0
Other raw and salad vegetables	69	38	*20*	73	44	*28*	72	41	*24*	17	0
Raw tomatoes	75	47	*14*	83	54	*20*	79	50	*17*	14	0
Peas	65	42	*52*	59	40	*52*	62	40	*53*	33	6
Green beans	27	16	*7*	50	32	*7*	39	24	*7*	3	0
Baked beans	176	134	*50*	166	119	*47*	171	125	*49*	84	0
Leafy green vegetables	48	33	*34*	58	36	*37*	53	35	*39*	19	0
Carrots (not raw)	63	42	*55*	57	40	*52*	60	40	*54*	32	6
Fresh tomatoes (not raw)	56	31	*2*	62	58	*2*	59	41	*2*	1	0
Other vegetables (not raw)	102	60	*61*	102	68	*61*	102	63	*62*	63	21
Potato chips	209	150	*71*	192	140	*69*	200	147	*71*	142	86
Fried/roast potatoes	76	50	*39*	72	47	*35*	74	49	*37*	28	0
Other potato products	98	76	*13*	95	82	*10*	97	78	*12*	11	0
Other potatoes	200	146	*76*	206	154	*77*	203	150	*77*	157	99
Savoury snacks	87	70	*77*	82	67	*77*	85	70	*78*	66	50
Apples & pears	231	158	*50*	206	155	*48*	219	157	*50*	108	0
Citrus fruits	187	141	*24*	209	145	*28*	199	144	*26*	52	0
Bananas	245	200	*45*	222	180	*45*	234	194	*46*	107	0
Canned fruit in juice	131	86	*6*	125	88	*6*	128	86	*6*	8	0
Canned fruit in syrup	142	93	*8*	130	86	*8*	136	89	*8*	11	0
Nuts, fruit & nut mixes	34	28	*14*	39	25	*12*	37	26	*13*	5	0
Other fruit	182	120	*31*	190	128	*34*	186	125	*33*	62	0
Sugar	35	20	*54*	32	17	*52*	33	18	*54*	18	2
Preserves	29	21	*43*	30	21	*33*	29	21	*38*	11	0
Sweet spreads, fillings & icings	24	15	*8*	22	15	*10*	23	15	*9*	2	0
Sugar confectionery	116	88	*59*	114	75	*55*	115	81	*58*	67	20
Chocolate confectionery	105	77	*73*	98	78	*73*	101	78	*74*	75	52
Fruit juice	690	475	*35*	756	492	*36*	724	482	*36*	258	0
Diet soft drinks	1824	1325	*50*	1494	1028	*46*	1666	1160	*49*	810	0
Other soft drinks	2175	1749	*86*	2004	1568	*83*	2092	1635	*86*	1793	1295
Mineral & tonic water	520	225	*3*	765	392	*4*	664	312	*4*	25	0
Wine	20	15	*1*	46	51	*1*	31	25	*1*	0	0
Fortified wine	18	18	*0*	–	–	–	18	18	*0*	0	0
Beers	67	64	*0*	6	6	*0*	55	52	*0*	0	0
Cider & perry	60	60	*0*	110	110	*0*	93	60	*0*	0	0
Coffee, as consumed	740	589	*6*	479	321	*8*	599	327	*7*	43	0
Tea, as consumed	683	457	*33*	695	465	*41*	690	463	*37*	259	0
Tap water	2426	2052	*92*	2171	1771	*90*	2300	1910	*92*	2120	1742
Miscellaneous	282	117	*89*	257	118	*88*	270	118	*90*	242	94
Commercial infant foods	295	207	*4*	299	203	*4*	297	203	*4*	13	0
Commercial infant drinks	845	566	*2*	1304	916	*3*	1110	900	*2*	25	0

Table 4.4   Whether child ever had cows' milk as a drink by sex and age of child

Whether ever had cows' milk as a drink	Sex of child		Age of child (in years)			
	Boys	Girls	1½–2½	2½–3½	3½–4½	All
	%	%	%	%	%	%
Never had cows' milk to drink	4	5	6	5	3	5
Had cows' milk to drink:						
but no longer having	7	8	8	8	7	8
still having	89	86	86	88	90	88
Base = 100%*	943	916	648	668	543	1859

*Base = all informants.

Table 4.5   Type of milk child usually had as a drink by sex and age of child

Type of milk child usually had as a drink	Sex of child		Age of child (in years)			
	Boys	Girls	1½–2½	2½–3½	3½–4½	All
	%	%	%	%	%	%
Did not have milk as a drink	7	8	9	8	7	8
Whole milk	70	66	74	66	63	68
Semi-skimmed milk	18	21	12	21	25	19
Skimmed milk	1	1	0	1	2	1
Powdered baby milk	1	0	1	0	0	0
Other*	1	1	2	1	1	1
Unknown	2	3	2	3	3	3
Base = 100%	943	916	648	668	543	1859

*Includes soya milk and cows' milk where fat content was not known.

Table 4.6   Types of milk used on breakfast cereal and in cooking by sex and age of child

Types of milk used on cereal and in cooking	Sex of child		Age of child (in years)			
	Boys	Girls	1½–2½	2½–3½	3½–4½	All
	%	%	%	%	%	%
Whole milk	77	73	82	74	67	75
Semi-skimmed milk	27	30	19	27	35	27
Skimmed milk	3	2	2	2	5	3
Powdered baby milk	1	0	1	0	–	0
Other*	2	1	2	2	1	2
Base = 100%**	943	916	648	668	543	1859

*Includes soya milk and cows' milk where fat content was not known.
**Percentages add to more than 100 as some children were having more than one type of milk.

Table 4.7   Age of child when first had cows' milk as a drink by sex of child

Age first had cows' milk as a drink	Sex of child		
	Boys	Girls	All
	%	%	%
Under 6 months	4	2	3
6 months but less than 9 months	25	28	27
9 months but less than 12 months	27	28	27
12 months but less than 18 months	35	31	33
18 months but less than 24 months	5	5	5
24 months or more	2	3	2
Don't know/can't remember	2	3	3
Base = 100%*	901	868	1769

*Base = number of children who ever had cows' milk as a drink.

Table 4.8   Age of child when first had semi-skimmed milk as a drink by sex of child

Age child started having semi-skimmed milk as a drink	Sex of child		
	Boys	Girls	All
	%	%	%
Never had semi-skimmed milk	82	80	80
Under 6 months	–	–	–
6 months but less than 9 months	1	2	2
9 months but less than 12 months	2	2	2
12 months but less than 18 months	3	3	3
18 months but less than 24 months	3	3	3
24 months or more	6	10	8
Don't know/can't remember	2	1	2
Base = 100%*	901	868	1769

*Base = number of children who ever had cows' milk as a drink.

Table 4.9   Duration of breast-feeding up to age nine months by sex of child

Duration of breast-feeding	Sex of child		
	Boys	Girls	All
	%	%	%
Percentage of mothers breast-feeding at:			
Birth	59	60	59
1 week	51	51	51
2 weeks	47	47	47
6 weeks	37	39	38
4 months	23	26	24
6 months	16	19	18
9 months	9	10	10
Base = 100%	943	916	1859

Table 4.10   Whether child ever had infant formula or follow-on milk and duration of formula-feeding by sex of child

Whether ever had formula milk and duration of formula-feeding	Sex of child		
	Boys	Girls	All
	%	%	%
Had infant formula or follow-on milk	88	87	88
Percentage of children having formula milk at:			
2 months	88	86	87
6 months	84	83	83
9 months	63	61	62
12 months	38	34	36
18 months	7	7	7
Base = 100%	943	916	1859

Table 4.11 Age of child when first had cows' milk as a drink by age when stopped formula or follow-on milk

Age of child (in months) when when stopped formula-feeding	Age of child (in months) when first had cows' milk as a drink							All*
	under 3	3– under 6	6– under 9	9– under 12	12– under 18	18– under 24	24 and over	
under 2	0%	–	0%	–	0%	0%	0%	1%
2–under 6	0%	2%	1%	0%	0%	0%	0%	4%
6–under 9	–	0%	20%	3%	1%	0%	0%	24%
9–under 12	–	0%	2%	23%	4%	1%	0%	31%
12–under 18	–	–	2%	2%	27%	2%	0%	33%
18 months or older	–	0%	0%	1%	2%	2%	1%	7%
All*	0%	3%	26%	29%	35%	5%	2%	Base 100% = 1514

*All children who were formula fed and had ever had cows' milk as a drink, excluding informants not answering or unable to remember age of child at time started cows' milk and/or stopped formula.
  Boxed areas show estimated percentage of children who were no longer having formula feeds at the time they started having cows' milk as a drink.

Table 4.12 Age of child when first had cows' milk as a drink by age when stopped breast-feeding

Age of child (in months) when stopped breast-feeding	Age of child (in months) when first had cows' milk as a drink							All*
	under 3	3– under 6	6– under 9	9– under 12	12– under 18	18– under 24	24 and over	
under 1 week	–	0%	3%	4%	5%	1%	0%	14%
1 week–under 2 weeks	–	0%	2%	2%	2%	–	0%	7%
2 weeks–under 6 weeks	–	0%	3%	5%	6%	1%	0%	16%
6 weeks–under 4 months	–	0%	6%	6%	9%	1%	0%	22%
4 months–under 6 months	–	0%	4%	2%	4%	0%	0%	12%
6 months–9 months	0%	0%	4%	4%	5%	1%	0%	14%
over 9 months	–	0%	3%	2%	8%	1%	0%	15%
All*	0%	2%	26%	26%	39%	5%	2%	Base 100% = 1514

*All children who were breast-fed and had ever had cows' milk as a drink, excluding informants not answering or unable to remember age of child at time started cows' milk and/or stopped breast-feeding.
  Boxed areas show estimated percentage of children who were no longer having breast feeds at the time they started having cows' milk as a drink.

Table 4.13 Proportion of children reported to be allergic to certain foods and nature of allergic reaction by sex and age of child

Whether any food allergy and nature of reaction	Sex of child		Age of child (in years)			All
	Boys	Girls	1½–2½	2½–3½	3½–4½	
	%	%	%	%	%	%
Allergic to certain foods of whom:	16	11	13	12	16	14
allergy diagnosed by a doctor	6	4	5	4	6	5
Type of reaction:						
hyperactivity/behavioural problems	8	4	4	5	10	6
rash/blotches	2	3	4	2	3	3
eczema	2	2	2	2	1	2
wheezing/asthma	2	0	1	1	1	1
upset stomach/diarrhoea/vomiting	3	2	3	2	1	2
swelling	0	0	0	0	1	0
weight loss/failure to thrive	0	–	0	–	–	0
allergic rhinitis**	0	–	–	0	–	0
other	1	1	0	1	1	1
Base = 100%	943	916	648	668	543	1859

*If more than one allergic reaction was reported, all were coded. No order of priority was assigned in coding reactions.
**Itchy eyes and runny nose or other nasal symptoms.

Table 4.14 Total quantities (grams) of food consumed as estimated for seven days by age of child
Four days' intake re-weighted

Type of food	Age of child (years)								
	1½–2½			2½–3½			3½–4½		
	Mean	Median	% consumers	Mean	Median	% consumers	Mean	Median	% consumers
	g	g	%	g	g	%	g	g	%
Pasta	232	165	54	237	174	50	284	210	49
Rice	175	115	17	217	150	19	175	134	19
Pizza	152	102	12	147	112	15	167	118	16
Other cereals	77	31	22	70	36	24	83	45	26
White bread	181	143	83	227	200	87	273	244	88
Wholemeal bread	152	113	29	148	110	27	192	142	26
Soft grain bread	114	72	7	165	104	6	189	173	7
Other bread	97	70	30	126	89	32	115	77	26
Wholegrain & high fibre b'fast cereals	119	93	64	134	101	62	121	94	58
Other breakfast cereals	78	63	62	96	73	65	103	88	72
Biscuits	101	80	86	123	108	91	133	114	88
Fruit pies	81	75	5	94	70	6	121	89	6
Buns, cakes & pastries	94	69	50	131	109	55	135	101	61
Milk puddings	229	152	25	248	165	26	275	200	23
Ice cream	126	90	35	135	100	47	149	110	48
Sponge type puddings	85	41	2	185	110	4	191	155	4
Other puddings	178	130	29	200	141	28	220	149	30
Whole milk	2233	2115	86	1772	1456	82	1543	1286	80
Semi-skimmed milk	1297	688	23	1261	945	35	1103	805	38
Skimmed milk	550	321	3	853	376	4	670	462	7
Infant formula	2327	1743	4	2639	3250	1	3329	3329	0
Other milk & cream	397	38	12	221	63	12	175	50	17
Cottage cheese	57	48	2	73	84	1	99	64	1
Other cheese	65	49	60	67	50	58	76	58	57
Fromage frais	248	191	26	197	145	27	209	158	23
Yogurt	369	307	43	341	286	42	353	307	33
Eggs & egg dishes	115	86	45	132	96	45	135	100	47
Butter	23	16	29	28	20	31	32	21	29
'Polyunsaturated' margarine	29	20	36	35	29	37	41	35	34
'Polyunsaturated' oil	7	3	1	6	30	1	7	5	1
'Polyunsaturated' low fat spread	25	21	9	27	19	8	31	25	8
Other low fat spread	34	23	13	32	20	14	45	35	15
Block margarine	12	12	0	27	29	0	47	46	1
Soft margarine, not polyunsaturated	29	17	16	32	22	19	34	29	17
'Polyunsaturated' reduced fat spread	21	19	8	29	18	7	35	25	9
Other reduced fat spread	28	18	15	32	25	18	36	30	19
Other oils and fats not polyunsaturated	8	5	5	9	40	4	7	5	5
Bacon & ham	46	31	34	55	38	41	67	47	46
Beef, veal & dishes	184	114	48	185	119	46	186	128	46
Lamb & dishes	72	31	14	111	55	16	91	50	15
Pork & dishes	60	35	17	74	40	19	71	48	19
Coated chicken	91	67	16	124	117	16	125	92	24
Chicken & turkey dishes	81	48	52	91	52	51	95	62	52
Liver, liver products & dishes	97	47	4	74	49	4	43	20	4
Burgers & kebabs	90	70	22	96	77	24	116	103	26
Sausages	111	77	51	111	82	54	136	115	54
Meat pies & pastries	133	102	28	148	103	29	166	127	27
Other meat products	83	52	23	98	62	28	119	66	30
Coated & fried white fish	101	85	39	119	105	38	128	105	38
Shellfish	93	44	2	36	24	3	102	68	3
Other white fish & dishes	118	69	13	117	77	8	112	80	9
Oily fish	60	45	15	77	45	17	73	59	15
Raw carrots	34	20	8	48	28	10	89	57	13
Other raw and salad vegetables	53	25	21	70	46	24	91	50	27
Raw tomatoes	67	36	18	85	50	17	88	67	17
Peas	56	40	57	63	38	52	69	50	48
Green beans	28	16	7	47	33	7	40	21	6
Baked beans	167	112	52	173	135	50	175	123	45
Leafy green vegetables	47	29	38	54	29	36	60	47	33
Carrots (not raw)	53	40	57	64	40	51	65	40	53
Fresh tomatoes (not raw)	33	34	2	34	20	2	117	87	2
Other vegetables (not raw)	94	60	64	102	63	60	112	70	61

Type of food	Age of child (years)								
	1½–2½			2½–3½			3½–4½		
	Mean	Median	% consumers	Mean	Median	% consumers	Mean	Median	% consumers
	g	g	%	g	g	%	g	g	%
Potato chips	174	121	66	203	150	71	225	175	76
Fried/roast potatoes	67	48	34	71	49	37	84	51	41
Other potato products	90	66	12	99	76	11	103	91	12
Other potatoes	193	137	80	200	150	75	220	165	77
Savoury snacks	73	60	73	90	78	80	90	74	81
Apples & pears	205	129	48	217	164	51	236	163	49
Citrus fruits	220	144	25	196	149	28	177	135	24
Bananas	220	179	53	242	200	43	245	200	40
Canned fruit in juice	126	47	5	129	102	7	129	100	6
Canned fruit in syrup	103	78	7	149	97	8	151	100	9
Nuts, fruit & nut mixes	26	24	12	38	27	13	46	33	15
Other fruit	161	116	33	184	120	34	221	150	32
Sugar	35	17	50	30	17	55	35	22	57
Preserves	24	18	35	28	22	40	37	27	40
Sweet spreads, fillings & icings	24	15	6	25	16	11	20	12	12
Sugar confectionery	94	60	46	117	86	62	130	92	67
Chocolate confectionery	86	65	70	105	84	76	113	82	76
Fruit juice	761	482	34	761	499	37	635	464	36
Diet soft drinks	1717	1205	41	1591	1086	52	1710	1239	52
Other soft drinks	1998	1506	80	2085	1586	88	2197	1842	90
Mineral & tonic water	486	225	4	711	400	4	860	390	3
Wine	19	19	0	41	29	1	29	28	1
Fortified wine	18	18	0	–	–	–	–	–	–
Beers	–	–	–	48	7	1	64	64	0
Cider & perry	–	–	–	32	32	0	124	124	0
Coffee, as consumed	499	314	6	672	386	8	598	467	8
Tea, as consumed	755	522	38	665	456	36	641	428	38
Tap water	2525	2133	92	2256	1892	90	2092	1685	94
Miscellaneous	281	118	88	268	108	91	258	129	90
Commercial infant foods	345	238	4	251	134	3	113	96	2
Commercial infant drinks	1067	936	8	1350	877	2	471	471	0

Table 4.15 Total quantities (grams) of food consumed as estimated for seven days by sex of child: children aged 3½ to 4½ years
Four days' intake re-weighted

Type of food	Sex of child								
	Boys			Girls			All aged 3½ to 4½ years		
	Mean	Median	% consumers	Mean	Median	% consumers	Mean	Median	% consumers
	g	g	%	g	g	%	g	g	%
Pasta	241	165	49	320	241	53	284	210	49
Rice	143	115	18	204	170	20	175	134	19
Pizza	146	105	14	186	182	17	167	118	16
Other cereals	89	58	27	77	40	25	83	45	26
White bread	285	254	88	261	224	89	273	244	88
Wholemeal bread	210	175	25	173	111	27	192	142	26
Soft grain bread	173	131	7	208	216	6	189	173	7
Other bread	113	74	30	118	77	22	115	77	26
Wholegrain & high fibre b'fast cereals	141	100	59	99	83	57	121	94	58
Other breakfast cereals	106	95	70	99	79	74	103	88	72
Biscuits	150	133	88	114	97	87	133	114	88
Fruit pies	127	72	6	116	108	7	121	89	6
Buns, cakes & pastries	146	110	64	122	96	58	135	101	61
Milk puddings	311	242	24	237	151	23	275	200	23
Ice cream	143	111	43	154	100	52	149	110	48
Sponge type puddings	139	125	4	239	187	4	191	155	4
Other puddings	218	150	32	221	147	28	220	149	30
Whole milk	1576	1316	82	1509	1266	79	1543	1286	80
Semi-skimmed milk	1075	778	38	1138	806	37	1103	805	38
Skimmed milk	594	345	8	767	746	6	670	462	7
Infant formula	3329	3329	1	–	–	–	3329	3329	0
Other milk & cream	147	46	20	219	65	14	175	50	17
Cottage cheese	174	174	1	49	64	1	99	64	1
Other cheese	78	54	55	74	61	59	76	58	57
Fromage frais	217	156	21	203	161	26	209	158	23
Yogurt	366	312	33	340	300	33	353	307	33
Eggs & egg dishes	134	104	46	136	99	49	135	100	47
Butter	33	21	28	32	21	30	32	21	29
'Polyunsaturated' margarine	46	42	34	37	24	34	41	35	34
'Polyunsaturated' oil	7	5	1	7	7	2	7	5	1
'Polyunsaturated' low fat spread	35	29	9	26	19	7	31	25	8
Other low fat spread	48	35	14	42	35	16	45	35	15
Block margarine	48	59	2	45	45	0	47	46	1
Soft margarine, not polyunsaturated	39	30	16	29	26	17	34	29	17
'Polyunsaturated' reduced fat spread	39	31	8	31	16	11	35	25	9
Other reduced fat spread	35	30	20	37	30	19	36	30	19
Other oils and fats not polyunsaturated	8	5	4	6	5	6	7	5	5
Bacon & ham	61	45	44	73	50	47	67	47	46
Beef, veal & dishes	193	135	44	180	126	48	186	128	46
Lamb & dishes	101	63	14	83	49	17	91	50	15
Pork & dishes	71	46	22	70	49	17	71	48	19
Coated chicken	134	91	25	115	93	22	125	92	24
Chicken & turkey dishes	91	60	56	99	66	49	95	62	52
Liver, liver products & dishes	42	20	5	44	21	2	43	20	4
Burgers & kebabs	119	103	30	112	100	23	116	103	26
Sausages	139	115	51	133	116	56	136	115	54
Meat pies & pastries	182	150	28	149	123	27	166	127	27
Other meat products	118	67	31	119	65	29	119	66	30
Coated & fried white fish	119	92	40	138	111	36	128	105	38
Shellfish	115	84	3	87	60	3	102	68	3
Other white fish & dishes	96	50	10	133	127	8	112	80	9
Oily fish	80	65	12	69	47	17	73	59	15
Raw carrots	80	55	14	99	66	11	89	57	13
Other raw and salad vegetables	83	50	24	97	59	31	91	50	27
Raw tomatoes	81	60	11	92	74	22	88	67	17
Peas	70	58	46	67	42	51	69	50	48
Green beans	23	15	6	62	40	5	40	21	6
Baked beans	176	132	45	174	120	45	175	123	45
Leafy green vegetables	61	50	35	58	44	31	60	47	33
Carrots (not raw)	70	44	57	58	40	49	65	40	53
Fresh tomatoes (not raw)	187	155	1	82	81	2	117	87	2
Other vegetables (not raw)	109	63	59	114	84	62	112	70	61

Table 4.15 Total quantities (grams) of food consumed as estimated for seven days by sex of child: children aged 3½ to 4½ years *(continued)*
Four days' intake re-weighted

Type of food	Sex of child								
	Boys			Girls			All aged 3½ to 4½ years		
	Mean	Median	% consumers	Mean	Median	% consumers	Mean	Median	% consumers
	g	g	%	g	g	%	g	g	%
Potato chips	213	155	76	238	203	76	225	175	76
Fried/roast potatoes	90	54	45	77	49	37	84	51	41
Other potato products	108	101	14	96	91	9	103	91	12
Other potatoes	211	152	78	229	173	76	220	165	77
Savoury snacks	94	75	80	87	71	81	90	74	81
Apples & pears	255	176	48	217	150	50	236	163	49
Citrus fruits	157	117	22	195	145	26	177	135	24
Bananas	284	215	39	207	170	42	245	200	40
Canned fruit in juice	159	95	6	101	100	7	129	100	6
Canned fruit in syrup	162	106	8	142	86	11	151	100	9
Nuts, fruit & nut mixes	39	27	16	53	43	13	46	33	15
Other fruit	195	125	32	248	163	31	221	150	32
Sugar	39	26	56	32	20	59	35	22	57
Preserves	40	28	43	34	26	36	37	27	40
Sweet spreads, fillings & icings	21	13	10	19	12	13	20	12	12
Sugar confectionery	137	105	67	124	75	67	130	92	67
Chocolate confectionery	115	82	74	111	82	77	113	82	76
Fruit juice	695	464	34	579	462	38	635	464	36
Diet soft drinks	1830	1402	56	1568	1032	49	1710	1239	52
Other soft drinks	2376	1986	89	2015	1635	90	2197	1842	90
Mineral & tonic water	100	100	0	914	391	6	860	390	3
Wine	16	6	1	41	51	1	29	28	1
Fortified wine	–	–	–	–	–	–	–	–	–
Beers	64	64	1	–	–	–	64	64	0
Cider & perry	60	60	1	187	187	0	124	124	0
Coffee, as consumed	617	553	8	579	327	8	598	467	8
Tea, as consumed	734	468	35	559	380	41	641	428	38
Tap water	2260	1858	96	1915	1557	93	2092	1685	94
Miscellaneous	269	140	88	248	127	92	258	129	90
Commercial infant foods	102	94	2	133	180	2	113	96	2
Commercial infant drinks	42	42	0	900	900	0	471	471	0

Table 4.16 Total quantities (grams) of food consumed as estimated for seven days by social class of head of household
Four days' intake re-weighted

Type of food	Non-manual			Manual			All*		
	Mean	Median	% consumers	Mean	Median	% consumers	Mean	Median	% consumers
	g	g	%	g	g	%	g	g	%
Pasta	246	185	56	250	182	47	248	180	51
Rice	173	132	23	207	141	15	190	135	20
Pizza	164	124	14	148	97	14	155	108	14
Other cereals	84	44	20	68	30	27	77	38	24
White bread	199	159	83	245	217	88	226	191	86
Wholemeal bread	165	130	38	155	111	19	162	119	27
Soft grain bread	170	133	8	130	86	5	154	111	7
Other bread	108	75	33	119	84	28	113	80	30
Wholegrain & high fibre b'fast cereals	127	94	67	121	95	57	125	95	61
Other breakfast cereals	85	68	62	97	80	69	92	74	66
Biscuits	119	104	91	118	95	87	118	98	88
Fruit pies	117	90	5	86	67	6	99	77	6
Buns, cakes & pastries	123	93	61	118	90	51	121	92	55
Milk puddings	232	151	28	266	194	23	249	169	25
Ice cream	127	90	47	147	110	40	137	100	43
Sponge type puddings	167	135	3	169	99	3	166	110	3
Other puddings	205	143	31	196	142	28	198	140	3
Whole milk	1841	1598	83	1909	1570	83	1872	1575	83
Semi-skimmed milk	1347	861	33	1086	787	31	1215	831	32
Skimmed milk	620	380	5	735	450	4	701	425	4
Infant formula	3093	3250	1	2095	1680	2	2438	1814	2
Other milk & cream	265	57	13	248	53	14	256	55	13
Cottage cheese	89	78	1	50	42	1	71	56	1
Other cheese	69	54	64	67	50	54	69	52	59
Fromage frais	227	162	32	207	158	21	218	162	26
Yogurt	361	293	43	350	307	37	355	300	40
Eggs & egg dishes	129	99	47	124	89	45	127	94	46
Butter	25	20	34	30	19	25	28	20	30
'Polyunsaturated' margarine	35	27	41	34	25	32	35	27	36
'Polyunsaturated' oil	7	3	2	7	3	1	7	3	1
'Polyunsaturated' low fat spread	26	20	9	29	24	8	27	21	9
Other low fat spread	37	28	15	37	28	13	37	28	14
Block margarine	21	19	0	43	37	1	34	30	1
Soft margarine, not polyunsaturated	27	17	13	35	27	21	32	22	17
'Polyunsaturated' reduced fat spread	24	17	8	31	23	8	28	20	8
Other reduced fat spread	30	19	14	34	27	20	32	25	17
Other oils and fats not polyunsaturated	8	4	6	8	5	4	8	5	5
Bacon & ham	58	40	44	54	37	37	57	37	40
Beef, veal & dishes	183	122	47	183	117	46	185	119	47
Lamb & dishes	99	55	15	88	35	16	93	43	15
Pork & dishes	60	45	17	73	39	19	68	42	18
Coated chicken	110	79	22	120	98	15	115	90	18
Chicken & turkey dishes	99	62	56	79	47	48	89	57	52
Liver, liver products & dishes	80	50	4	69	24	3	73	43	4
Burgers & kebabs	98	79	19	104	90	27	100	85	24
Sausages	115	90	50	121	93	56	119	90	53
Meat pies & pastries	127	87	25	162	123	31	149	115	28
Other meat products	86	51	26	112	67	27	100	60	27
Coated & fried white fish	115	97	40	116	98	37	115	97	38
Shellfish	56	38	3	105	53	2	76	40	3
Other white fish & dishes	112	71	13	108	66	7	116	76	10
Oily fish	64	46	20	78	50	12	70	48	16
Raw carrots	59	40	13	64	30	7	60	32	10
Other raw and salad vegetables	72	45	28	69	37	21	72	41	24
Raw tomatoes	83	57	21	76	45	15	79	50	17
Peas	61	43	50	62	40	54	62	40	53
Green beans	41	25	6	35	22	7	39	24	7
Baked beans	173	120	48	167	127	51	171	125	49
Leafy green vegetables	53	34	37	54	36	34	53	35	39
Carrots (not raw)	66	42	54	56	40	53	60	40	54
Fresh tomatoes (not raw)	71	47	2	43	22	1	59	41	2
Other vegetables (not raw)	111	70	66	91	60	58	102	63	62

43

Table 4.16 Total quantities (grams) of food consumed as estimated for seven days by social class of head of household *(continued)*
Four days' intake re-weighted

Type of food	Social class of head of household								
	Non-manual			Manual			All*		
	Mean	Median	% consumers	Mean	Median	% consumers	Mean	Median	% consumers
	g	g	%	g	g	%	g	g	%
Potato chips	176	128	63	217	168	77	200	147	71
Fried/roast potatoes	72	51	34	72	44	39	74	49	37
Other potato products	89	64	13	102	91	11	97	78	12
Other potatoes	203	144	75	203	151	79	203	150	77
Savoury snacks	77	62	77	91	75	79	85	70	78
Apples & pears	229	162	54	207	147	46	219	157	50
Citrus fruits	188	145	31	206	140	22	199	144	26
Bananas	239	200	53	228	170	40	234	194	46
Canned fruit in juice	132	90	8	124	85	4	128	86	6
Canned fruit in syrup	130	85	9	143	90	7	136	89	8
Nuts, fruit & nut mixes	35	25	17	40	28	10	37	26	13
Other fruit	185	128	45	181	119	23	186	125	33
Sugar	24	13	48	40	24	59	33	18	54
Preserves	27	20	43	32	23	35	29	21	38
Sweet spreads, fillings & icings	19	13	11	28	17	8	23	15	9
Sugar confectionery	103	70	54	125	93	62	115	81	58
Chocolate confectionery	91	70	74	109	85	74	101	78	74
Fruit juice	768	501	48	657	462	26	724	482	36
Diet soft drinks	1633	1146	52	1713	1201	46	1666	1160	49
Other soft drinks	1999	1525	83	2153	1770	87	2092	1635	86
Mineral & tonic water	742	328	6	454	295	2	664	312	4
Wine	18	15	1	50	51	1	31	25	1
Fortified wine	–	–	–	18	18	0	18	18	0
Beers	–	–	–	67	64	0	55	52	0
Cider & perry	32	32	0	124	124	0	93	60	0
Coffee, as consumed	377	164	5	715	524	9	599	327	7
Tea, as consumed	559	350	29	767	521	44	690	463	37
Tap water	2361	1968	94	2246	1831	90	2300	1910	92
Miscellaneous	241	109	89	296	128	90	270	118	90
Commercial infant foods	295	189	6	294	235	3	297	203	4
Commercial infant drinks	1242	906	4	741	877	1	1110	900	2

*Includes those in the Armed Forces, those where the HOH had never worked, and others where social class could not be derived.

Table 4.17 Total quantities (grams) of food consumed as estimated for seven days by fieldwork wave
Four days' intake re-weighted

Type of food	Fieldwork wave											
	Wave 1: July–September			Wave 2: October–December			Wave 3: January–March			Wave 4: April–June		
	Mean	Median	% con-sumers	Mean	Median	% con-sumers	Mean	Median	% con-sumers	Mean	Median	% con-sumers
	g	g	%	g	g	%	g	g	%	g	g	%
Pasta	233	165	50	245	189	51	259	182	52	254	197	50
Rice	196	142	24	188	125	20	193	139	15	183	118	16
Pizza	144	107	15	166	108	11	166	108	15	144	115	16
Other cereals	89	41	21	71	39	26	63	37	24	88	32	25
White bread	243	207	83	218	186	90	229	196	83	215	173	88
Wholemeal bread	149	112	28	144	108	24	174	158	30	174	113	27
Soft grain bread	112	78	7	172	131	6	169	138	6	157	105	7
Other bread	133	75	25	110	80	32	106	82	28	108	80	33
Wholegrain & high fibre b'fast cereals	128	98	56	128	102	64	122	90	63	122	91	62
Other breakfast cereals	93	73	66	88	71	65	93	75	65	95	76	67
Biscuits	114	90	84	124	107	90	119	97	88	115	99	90
Fruit pies	82	70	5	95	77	5	109	78	6	103	73	6
Buns, cakes & pastries	128	93	52	121	90	55	111	88	56	125	98	57
Milk puddings	252	171	23	292	210	23	199	128	27	266	189	26
Ice cream	153	120	49	133	84	37	119	90	34	141	100	53
Sponge type puddings	158	158	1	134	71	3	179	125	5	180	175	3
Other puddings	182	132	28	185	130	27	205	149	30	216	143	31
Whole milk	1870	1617	84	1923	1573	83	1920	1687	82	1765	1351	83
Semi-skimmed milk	1077	843	29	1277	880	30	1312	937	34	1157	764	35
Skimmed milk	1030	550	5	606	482	4	570	344	5	564	359	3
Infant formula	2977	3227	2	2987	3200	2	1904	1362	1	1694	1512	3
Other milk & cream	221	67	15	235	60	13	224	60	13	353	39	13
Cottage cheese	88	62	2	67	84	1	66	50	2	31	31	0
Other cheese	72	53	56	66	53	57	65	51	58	73	51	63
Fromage frais	230	170	22	213	151	21	245	189	26	190	148	33
Yogurt	366	295	42	349	307	40	336	277	37	369	312	39
Eggs & egg dishes	127	99	52	116	89	44	143	107	45	120	88	43
Butter	29	17	28	28	20	27	26	20	28	27	20	36
'Polyunsaturated' margarine	35	27	39	36	27	37	34	28	36	33	26	32
'Polyunsaturated' oil	3	2	1	11	11	1	8	4	2	4	2	1
'Polyunsaturated' low fat spread	32	26	7	28	23	10	26	18	8	25	18	9
Other low fat spread	37	28	13	39	31	15	34	25	16	36	21	11
Block margarine	58	58	1	34	32	1	21	21	0	18	18	0
Soft margarine, not polyunsaturated	33	23	17	26	17	16	34	24	18	32	25	17
'Polyunsaturated' reduced fat spread	26	23	4	29	20	8	29	18	10	28	20	10
Other reduced fat spread	29	21	18	31	21	16	33	26	18	34	30	18
Other fats & oils, not polyunsaturated	12	6	5	7	2	5	9	5	4	5	4	0
Bacon & ham	53	37	40	54	38	39	60	40	40	59	38	42
Beef, veal & dishes	149	109	45	207	130	52	199	131	49	173	108	40
Lamb & dishes	82	36	18	120	82	13	80	37	17	98	42	13
Pork & dishes	63	45	14	82	44	20	54	35	19	73	42	20
Coated chicken	120	96	16	124	90	16	111	88	20	108	74	22
Chicken & turkey dishes	90	61	49	95	60	57	77	45	50	93	52	50
Liver, liver products & dishes	107	56	4	53	40	3	75	28	4	57	49	0
Burgers & kebabs	116	97	26	99	94	25	92	76	23	95	80	24
Sausages	118	95	53	116	87	53	116	83	52	125	103	54
Meat pies & pastries	161	130	29	147	104	29	147	122	27	140	93	28
Other meat products	93	59	25	94	59	25	110	60	30	102	69	28
Coated & fried white fish	112	96	37	115	94	39	114	93	39	120	104	38
Shellfish	91	80	3	80	33	3	32	30	2	84	56	3
Other white fish & dishes	133	79	9	120	125	8	111	85	11	106	53	12
Oily fish	61	42	16	70	41	14	67	51	17	84	60	15
Raw carrots	66	45	9	79	37	8	55	38	13	46	25	10
Other raw and salad vegetables	71	42	26	71	40	18	69	39	22	75	40	31
Raw tomatoes	86	55	20	86	65	13	59	43	16	86	53	21

Table 4.17 Total quantities (grams) of food consumed as estimated for seven days by fieldwork wave *(continued)*
Four days' intake re-weighted

Type of food	Wave 1: July–September			Wave 2: October–December			Wave 3: January–March			Wave 4: April–June		
	Mean	Median	% con-sumers	Mean	Median	% con-sumers	Mean	Median	% con-sumers	Mean	Median	% con-sumers
	g	g	%	g	g	%	g	g	%	g	g	%
Peas	62	40	52	63	42	53	61	40	55	63	40	51
Green beans	38	26	11	41	23	7	41	22	5	33	20	5
Baked beans	173	132	52	173	124	49	167	125	49	173	120	47
Leafy green vegetables	65	42	30	54	38	38	50	34	42	45	27	31
Carrots (not raw)	53	40	51	64	42	52	61	42	62	61	40	50
Fresh tomatoes (not raw)	63	42	2	65	34	2	57	31	2	47	45	0
Other vegetables (not raw)	101	60	63	88	55	62	104	72	60	114	71	63
Potato chips	209	150	70	194	145	71	192	136	73	210	151	69
Fried/roast potatoes	65	53	32	82	50	40	74	43	41	73	50	35
Other potato products	108	93	11	88	62	10	92	82	13	100	90	12
Other potatoes	187	137	77	207	151	76	202	150	78	214	150	78
Savoury snacks	78	62	80	85	69	77	87	70	77	87	78	78
Apples & pears	213	141	45	222	148	53	215	171	52	225	162	48
Citrus fruits	196	139	13	194	157	29	219	146	39	162	120	20
Bananas	249	202	49	219	181	41	221	167	44	246	202	50
Canned fruit in juice	111	70	6	209	105	4	98	94	7	130	76	7
Canned fruit in syrup	129	100	7	149	90	8	118	82	7	143	83	10
Nuts, fruit & nut mixes	39	27	16	41	26	11	29	23	13	39	30	14
Other fruit	249	175	43	140	94	28	168	120	30	171	113	33
Sugar	36	22	52	36	21	53	34	16	56	28	16	53
Preserves	30	22	36	33	25	38	26	19	37	28	20	42
Sweet spreads, fillings & icings	22	15	10	21	12	9	28	18	8	21	15	11
Sugar confectionery	137	91	65	98	70	57	94	71	53	134	100	59
Chocolate confectionery	92	71	67	103	78	71	106	84	80	102	74	75
Fruit juice	817	535	38	685	446	35	648	466	34	756	499	37
Diet soft drinks	1648	979	45	1543	1084	45	1688	1242	50	1761	1356	55
Other soft drinks	2432	2111	87	2013	1628	86	1862	1400	89	2131	1587	82
Mineral & tonic water	813	309	4	413	212	4	790	352	3	670	458	5
Wine	27	34	1	51	51	0	28	28	0	27	15	1
Fortified wine	18	18	0	–	–	–	–	–	–	–	–	–
Beers	69	69	1	77	77	0	–	–	–	29	29	0
Cider & perry	93	60	1	–	–	–	–	–	–	–	–	–
Coffee, as consumed	617	524	7	726	360	6	660	419	8	377	262	7
Tea, as consumed	680	453	35	644	392	38	778	572	42	628	462	34
Tap water	2423	2058	93	2166	1849	93	2188	1749	89	2447	2163	94
Miscellaneous	260	94	90	283	112	91	279	147	91	252	122	87
Commercial infant foods	354	208	4	354	159	5	208	132	3	248	232	4
Commercial infant drinks	1405	1065	3	1140	525	2	901	755	2	971	990	3

Table 4.18 Total quantities (grams) of food consumed as estimated for seven days by region
Four days' intake re-weighted

Type of food	Region											
	Scotland			Northern			Central, South West and Wales			London and South East		
	Mean	Median	% con-sumers	Mean	Median	% con-sumers	Mean	Median	% con-sumers	Mean	Median	% con-sumers
	g	g	%	g	g	%	g	g	%	g	g	%
Pasta	235	176	48	258	194	51	265	178	50	228	167	53
Rice	170	95	19	191	148	15	177	135	18	207	132	23
Pizza	203	163	18	182	130	14	133	94	14	138	107	13
Other cereals	185	98	15	61	37	30	71	32	25	78	40	20
White bread	236	210	88	230	199	87	241	214	88	200	162	82
Wholemeall bread	146	146	16	146	100	27	158	111	26	178	136	33
Soft grain bread	157	96	8	153	101	4	140	100	7	166	124	8
Other bread	101	75	28	103	79	33	133	97	24	108	71	33
Wholegrain and high fibre b'fast cereals	140	87	57	135	103	61	110	92	62	128	92	62
Other breakfast cereals	110	95	77	90	71	66	94	75	67	85	69	61
Biscuits	121	112	79	121	104	92	118	95	89	117	97	88
Fruit pies	68	41	5	71	62	6	118	98	7	108	85	4
Buns, cakes & pastries	109	68	48	116	90	51	118	93	57	129	93	58
Milk puddings	352	300	27	228	141	25	243	169	27	236	187	22
Ice cream	109	79	44	168	119	45	129	92	41	129	100	43
Sponge type puddings	68	87	2	139	120	4	224	172	4	103	63	2
Other puddings	134	103	25	243	192	28	189	133	30	191	132	30
Whole milk	1689	1444	82	1899	1600	82	1848	1572	85	1935	1607	82
Semi-skimmed milk	1178	888	39	1105	806	30	1261	805	31	1264	861	33
Skimmed milk	421	253	3	1000	501	5	504	370	4	700	425	4
Infant formula	–	–	–	2185	1574	2	2590	3200	2	2516	1976	2
Other milk & cream	196	33	9	158	46	15	282	95	13	331	57	14
Cottage cheese	–	–	–	99	63	1	55	42	2	67	60	1
Other cheese	68	47	50	64	51	55	67	44	60	74	60	63
Fromage frais	232	200	23	233	156	16	222	157	24	207	162	35
Yogurt	391	351	43	349	300	41	342	294	39	361	300	38
Eggs & egg dishes	179	146	52	109	79	44	129	99	45	121	91	46
Butter	29	20	34	27	17	28	29	20	25	27	20	34
'Polyunsaturated' margarine	33	25	31	35	27	41	36	30	35	34	25	35
'Polyunsaturated' oil	12	12	1	5	3	1	6	3	1	7	4	2
'Polyunsaturated' low fat spread	17	13	8	23	18	7	36	25	9	25	24	10
Other low fat spread	28	16	17	32	29	11	39	31	16	40	27	13
Block margarine	32	32	1	27	18	1	28	21	1	58	58	0
Soft margarine, not polyunsaturated	31	27	22	32	22	21	32	25	18	30	20	12
'Polyunsaturated' reduced fat spread	22	17	7	31	22	8	26	20	9	31	22	7
Other reduced fat spread	26	18	10	28	20	15	34	25	22	33	29	16
Other fats & oils, not polyunsaturated	7	4	5	10	7	3	9	5	5	7	4	6
Bacon & ham	82	48	39	52	36	42	53	37	39	56	37	40
Beef, veal & dishes	170	131	56	177	105	49	189	126	46	195	121	42
Lamb & dishes	76	50	4	87	44	16	95	42	17	97	48	17
Pork & dishes	67	42	15	70	43	21	68	40	20	68	41	16
Coated chicken	97	74	19	124	114	15	98	74	16	127	90	23
Chicken & turkey dishes	80	62	44	73	47	47	86	56	55	105	66	55
Liver, liver products & dishes	82	23	3	72	48	4	98	65	4	45	25	4
Burgers & kebabs	129	97	25	92	78	24	105	100	23	94	80	25
Sausages	125	102	58	120	92	53	114	82	53	120	103	51
Meat pies & pastries	133	87	26	183	150	36	144	120	29	112	69	21
Other meat products	101	85	33	115	63	28	99	60	27	87	50	24
Coated & fried white fish	112	83	31	121	102	45	112	92	36	114	101	38
Shellfish	116	50	5	64	37	2	62	51	2	70	36	4
Other white fish & dishes	153	79	7	122	98	10	97	61	8	118	82	14
Oily fish	84	56	13	51	45	14	75	52	17	75	54	17
Raw carrots	66	49	8	64	28	11	60	33	10	55	34	11
Other raw and salad vegetables	90	42	21	60	35	19	66	36	23	78	52	30
Raw tomatoes	72	54	17	68	48	13	65	42	17	99	70	21
Peas	59	41	36	70	48	55	62	39	58	56	40	51
Green beans	94	94	1	34	21	6	41	25	10	35	24	7
Baked beans	131	95	44	185	129	54	177	145	51	162	122	45
Leafy green vegetables	57	47	19	51	35	34	53	36	42	55	33	36
Carrots (not raw)	42	32	28	61	42	56	65	42	61	57	40	52
Fresh tomatoes (not raw)	38	38	1	54	20	1	92	60	1	51	40	3
Other vegetables (not raw)	129	71	53	76	46	59	100	73	61	115	70	68

47

Table 4.18   Total quantities (grams) of food consumed as estimated for seven days by region *(continued)*
Four days' intake re-weighted

Type of food	Region											
	Scotland			Northern			Central, South West and Wales			London and South East		
	Mean	Median	% con-sumers	Mean	Median	% con-sumers	Mean	Median	% con-sumers	Mean	Median	% con-sumers
	g	g	%	g	g	%	g	g	%	g	g	%
Potato chips	228	152	78	222	165	73	198	145	72	173	128	65
Fried/roast potatoes	71	47	24	68	49	32	79	47	41	74	51	42
Other potato products	89	85	11	101	91	11	94	76	13	100	64	11
Other potatoes	185	140	77	191	134	82	218	163	80	203	151	71
Savoury snacks	93	75	81	76	60	77	92	76	79	80	65	76
Apples & pears	259	227	50	203	148	49	216	160	48	221	150	51
Citrus fruits	192	150	27	196	138	26	187	124	27	218	157	25
Bananas	261	205	45	232	199	44	218	176	43	242	200	50
Canned fruit in juice	110	100	9	119	85	6	118	69	6	156	100	6
Canned fruit in syrup	130	86	15	134	90	7	130	60	6	145	107	8
Nuts, fruit & nut mixes	27	14	12	45	25	9	38	30	13	34	26	17
Other fruit	219	169	25	173	127	30	177	112	32	196	124	39
Sugar	32	21	44	34	19	54	36	19	60	30	17	50
Preserves	39	26	32	31	24	39	29	21	38	26	19	41
Sweet spreads, fillings & icings	17	14	5	26	17	8	23	14	10	21	13	11
Sugar confectionery	134	102	70	128	101	62	106	77	56	106	62	53
Chocolate confectionery	101	84	76	112	82	73	100	78	78	93	69	69
Fruit juice	642	462	28	649	462	33	673	479	33	831	504	43
Diet soft drinks	1602	959	50	1618	1146	45	1812	1304	48	1572	1095	52
Other soft drinks	1637	1387	92	2285	1801	87	2131	1727	85	2041	1592	83
Mineral and tonic water	193	123	2	495	260	2	721	480	3	715	324	7
Wine	5	5	1	58	58	1	46	46	0	17	11	1
Fortified wine	–	–	–	–	–	–	18	18	0	–	–	–
Beers	–	–	–	29	29	0	–	–	–	71	77	1
Cider & perry	–	–	–	187	187	0	60	60	0	32	32	0
Coffee, as consumed	432	262	5	682	508	12	595	327	8	454	327	3
Tea, as consumed	580	434	43	720	475	36	767	523	48	581	360	29
Tap water	1603	1128	85	2297	1830	92	2353	1904	91	2443	2241	96
Miscellaneous	415	286	81	255	114	88	244	123	91	267	93	92
Commercial infant foods	186	154	4	306	92	4	304	212	5	311	211	4
Commercial infant drinks	1853	525	2	1026	1104	1	1035	855	2	1064	792	3

Table 4.19   Proportion of children taking dietary supplements during four-day recording period by age and sex of child

Proportion of children taking dietary supplements as:	Sex of child		Age of child (years)			
	Boys	Girls	1½–2½	2½–3½	3½–4½	All
	%	%	%	%	%	%
tablets	10	11	7	11	15	11
syrup/oil	3	3	3	4	3	3
drops	4	6	7	4	4	5
Base = 100%	*848*	*606*	*493*	*848*	*827*	*1675*

Table 4.20   Proportion of children taking dietary supplements during four-day recording period by social class of head of household

Proportion of children taking dietary supplements as:	Social class of head of household	
	Non-manual	Manual
	%	%
tablets	15	7
syrup/oil	5	2
drops	7	4
Base = 100%	*748*	*867*

5 Food energy intake

5.1 Introduction

In this and the following four chapters, data are presented on the intakes of energy and nutrients by the children. As described in Chapter 2, these intake data are derived from the dietary records for those children for whom a four-day weighed intake record was kept, which covered both weekend days, a total of 1675 children. Intakes of energy and nutrients are presented for children in each of the three age cohorts; for the oldest group of children, those aged 3½ to 4½ years, data for boys and girls are shown separately. Variation in intake of energy and the various nutrients according to the main socio-demographic characteristics of the sample is also discussed, and for energy and selected nutrients the percentage of the total intake derived from different food types is also shown.

Where appropriate, intake levels for groups of children are compared with the Dietary Reference Values (DRVs) as defined by the Department of Health in the Report *Dietary Reference Values for Food Energy and Nutrients for the United Kingdom*[1].

Intake data are presented as average daily amounts; that is, the four-day intake derived from the dietary record, weighted to represent intake for seven days (five weekdays plus two weekend days) and then averaged to produce a daily amount[2]. For energy and each nutrient the data are presented in the form of cumulative distributions, making it possible readily to identify the proportions of children with intakes above or below different values. Values for mean and median daily intakes and intakes at the upper and lower 2.5 percentiles are also shown.

For energy, the majority of the tables show intakes expressed as kilojoules (kJ)[3]; key tables and textual figures also give kilocalorie values (kcal).

5.2 Intake of energy

Boys between the ages of 1½ and 4½ years had an average daily energy intake of 4930kJ (1172kcal), significantly higher than that of girls in the sample, 4663kJ (1108kcal) (p<0.01). For both boys and girls values for median intakes were close to the mean values. However for both sexes, and in each of the three age cohorts, the range of intakes was large, energy intakes for the top 2.5 percentile of children being more than twice those of the lowest 2.5 percentile. For example, among children aged between 2½ and 3½ years, 2.5% of children had intakes below 3039kJ (720kcal), while 2.5% had intakes above 6991mJ (1663kcal).

As expected, mean intakes of energy increased with age; from 4393kJ (1045kcal) for the youngest children, to 4882kJ (1160kcal) for those aged between 2½ and 3½ years (p<0.01). In the oldest group, boys had mean recorded intakes 380kJ (90kcal) above that of the oldest group of girls, 5356kJ (1273kcal) compared with 4976kJ (1183kcal) (p<0.01). At the lower extreme of the energy intake distribution, 2.5% of children aged between 1½ and 2½ years had energy intakes at or below 2634kJ (625kcal); for children in the middle age cohort the equivalent value was 3039kJ (720kcal), for the oldest group of boys, 3349kJ (795kcal) and for the oldest group of girls, 3207kJ (761kcal). At the upper end of the distribution 2.5% of the youngest children had reported daily energy intakes at or above 6596kJ (1569kcal); for children aged 2½ to 3½ years the equivalent value was 6991kJ (1663kcal); for boys aged 3½ to 4½ years, 8085kJ (1928kcal) and for girls aged 3½ to 4½ years, 7372kJ (1753kcal).   *(Tables 5.1 and 5.2; Figs 5.1 and 5.2)*

5.2.1 Children who were unwell

Over a quarter (27%) of the children were reported by their mothers as being unwell at some time during the dietary recording period, and for 16% of children their eating was reported as being affected by being unwell. It would be expected therefore that these children would have significantly lower intakes of energy and many nutrients than either children who were not unwell or who were unwell but whose eating was not affected. Table 5.3 shows that this was indeed the case; mean energy intake for children who were unwell and whose eating was affected was about 6% lower than that for children who were unwell whose eating was not affected, and about 13% lower than the mean intake for children who were not unwell (p<0.05 and p<0.01). Despite it being reported that being unwell had not affected the eating habits of some children, energy intakes for this group were also significantly lower than for children not reported as being unwell (p<0.05).   *(Table 5.3)*

5.3 Energy intake and estimated average requirements

Estimates of energy requirements of different population groups are termed 'Estimated Average Requirements' (EARs)[1]. Interpolated values of the EARs for boys and girls in the age range covered by this survey were calculated and plotted together with the mean energy intakes at three-monthly age intervals for children in the survey; these are shown in Figures 5.3 and 5.4. The mean energy intakes, as measured by the survey, were below the EARs; for example, the average energy intake for girls aged between 3½ and 4½ years was 4976kJ (1183kcal) and the EAR for the same group is 5930kJ (1415kcal), lower by almost 1000kJ (230kcal).

Similarly the difference between mean energy intake and the EAR for boys in the age group 3½ to 4½ years was 1124kJ (272kcal). Figures 5.3 and 5.4 show that the divergence between EARs and the mean energy intakes increased with age. This divergence could arise from inadequate energy intake, a biased low measure of intake, or an exaggerated estimate of energy requirement.

In the pilot study of this survey, measurements of energy intake using the same dietary recording method were compared with measurements of energy expenditure using the doubly-labelled water technique[4]. On average the measures of energy intake and energy expenditure were extremely close and were below the EARs. The mean relative bias between the techniques was 154kJ/d. In the older children, aged between 3½ and 4½ years, the mean relative bias was only 37kJ/d. One would expect that since the same method of collecting energy intake data was adopted in this main study, values with a similarly small order of bias would result. This suggests that the divergence between the EARs and energy intakes cannot be ascribed to methodological errors in assessing children's energy intakes.   *(Figs 5.3 and 5.4)*

The EARs use 'standard' values for weight as one of the bases for calculation which results in the same EARs expressed as body weight for boys and girls up to the age of three years (440kJ/kg or 95kcal/kg). The needs may differ a little after the age of three years resulting in an EAR of 385kJ/kg (92kcal/kg) for girls between 3 and 4 years, and 405kJ/kg (97kcal/kg) for boys. When interpolated to the age group 3½ to 4½ years they become 375kJ/kg (90kcal/kg) for girls and 400kJ/kg (95kcal/kg) for boys (Table 5.4). Table 5.5 gives information on the energy intake per kilogram body weight by age and sex. The mean values for energy intakes expressed as body weight were 90% of the EARs for boys and girls aged between 1½ and 2½ years, 84% for boys and girls aged 2½ to 3½ years, and 82% for boys and girls aged between 3½ and 4½ years. These results suggest that the EARs for these age groups may be an overestimate of energy requirements. Alternatively the children may not have been consuming sufficient energy. However anthropometric measures (see *Chapter 11*) suggest that energy intakes were adequate as reflected in the increasing heights and weights of British children.

(Tables 5.4 and 5.5)

5.4 Contribution of main food types to food energy[5] intake

Table 5.6 shows the contribution of the major food types to food energy intake for children in the three age cohorts and for boys and girls separately.

For boys and girls and in each age cohort the largest contribution to recorded food energy intake was from cereals and cereal products, providing 30% of the overall mean intake. In this respect children resemble adults; the 1986/7 survey of the diets and nutritional status of British adults[6] found that cereals and cereal products contributed 30% of total average recorded energy intake. Moreover, the children in this survey, like the

adults in the earlier survey, were getting about one third of this energy from cereal products from biscuits, buns, cakes and pastries (9%). Breads contributed a further 9% and breakfast cereals 6%.

Overall, about one fifth of food energy was obtained from milk and milk products, a larger proportion than for adults (11%). For children, the proportion of energy from milk and milk products reduced as the children got older, from 26% for the youngest group aged 1½ to 2½ years, to about 16% for the oldest children (p<0.01). Most of the energy from milk products was obtained from cows' milk, providing 19% of the food energy of the youngest group and 12% for the oldest children (NS).

Vegetables, including potatoes and savoury snacks, were the next largest contributors to overall energy intake, providing 12% of food energy followed by meat, meat products and dishes, providing 10%. Again these proportions were similar to those for adults (16% and 12%). There was no significant difference by age in the proportions of energy provided by either vegetables or the meat food types. The majority of the energy derived from vegetables came from the consumption of potato chips and savoury snacks, for example crisps, each providing about 4% of the overall energy intake.

Chocolate confectionery contributed 5% of food energy intake, and table sugars, preserves and confectionery contributed a further 3%, giving a total of 8% overall for the food type. Again there was no significant difference in this proportion associated with the age or sex of the child.

At all ages 8% of food energy was obtained from beverages, 6% coming from soft drinks (not low calorie).

Consumption of fruit and nuts by children only provided 3% of their food energy intake, and this proportion was constant across all age groups; bananas contributed 1%.

Commercial infant foods and drinks did not make a major contribution to food energy intake; even for the youngest group only 1% of the total was derived from this source.   *(Table 5.6; Figs 5.5 and 5.6)*

Figures 5.5 to 5.9 show the contribution of the main food types to average energy intake for different subgroups in the sample. Figures 5.5 and 5.6 present the data in Table 5.6 as histograms. Figures 5.7, 5.8 and 5.9 present similar data for children by region, social class of head of household and by mother's highest educational qualification level.

It has already been shown that there was some variation in the types and quantities of different foods eaten by children living in different parts of Great Britain (see *Chapter 4*). For example children living in Scotland and the Northern region of England were more likely than other children, particularly those living in London and the South East, to be consuming potato chips, meat pies and soft drinks. They were also less likely to be eating most types of vegetable except potatoes. Although the composition of their diet differed this does not necessarily mean that either their intake of food energy or individual nutrients would differ, or that the contribution made by the different main food types to overall intake would differ significantly by region.

Figure 5.7 (regional data) reflects to a limited extent, the regional differences in the proportions of children consuming different types and quantities of foods. The differences were small, and none were statistically significant, although this may be a function of the relatively small size of some of the regional subgroups. The data suggest however that children living in Scotland and the Northern region were deriving slightly more of their energy from meat and meat products, and from sugars, preserves and confectionery and less of their energy from milk and milk products than children living elsewhere.

The data also suggest (*Figure 5.8*) that children whose head of household was in the manual social class group derived a slightly higher proportion of their energy from vegetables, potatoes and savoury snacks, and from sugars, preserves and confectionery than children from a non-manual home background, but again the differences between the two groups were not significant.

For some food types there appeared to be a systematic association between the contribution to energy intake and the highest educational qualification obtained by the child's mother (*Figure 5.9*). For example, the proportion of energy derived from cereals and cereal products was highest for children whose mothers had qualifications above GCE 'A' level equivalent, 32%, compared with 29% for children whose mothers had no formal qualifications (NS). A similar pattern can be seen for milk and milk products (22% and 20%), for fruit and nuts (5% and 2%), and for beverages (8% and 6%). Conversely the proportion of energy derived from meat and meat products, from vegetables, potatoes and savoury snacks, and from sugars, preserves and confectionery, fell as the educational level of the child's mother increased. Comparing children whose mothers had no qualifications with those whose mothers had the highest educational qualifications, the proportions of energy derived from these three food types for the two groups of children were 11% and 8% (meat), 14% and 10% (vegetables), and 9% and 6% (sugars). *(Figs 5.7 to 5.9)*

5.5 Variation in energy intake

Tables 5.7 to 5.12 show the distribution of energy intake for different subgroups in the sample of children.

Region
As noted above differences in the foods eaten by children living in different parts of Great Britain will not necessarily be reflected in differences in average daily energy intake. Table 5.7 shows that although mean energy intake was lowest among children living in London and the South East (4708kJ, 1119kcal) and highest for children in the Northern region (4860kJ, 1155kcal), these regional differences in mean intake were small (NS). However differences were greater among children at the upper 2.5 percentile of the distribution; for children in London and the South East average daily intake was 7084kJ (1682kcal) compared with 7459kJ (1773kcal) for children living in Scotland. *(Table 5.7)*

Socio-economic characteristics
Although the data show that the mean energy intake for children from a manual home background was above that of children from a non-manual background (4830kJ, 1148kcal compared with 4767kJ, 1132kcal) the difference was not statistically significant. Neither did the small differences associated with the employment status of the head of household reach the level of significance, where the highest mean intake was for children whose head of household was economically inactive (4923kJ, 1171kcal) and lowest for children from households where the head was working (4768kJ, 1133kcal). Given the relatively small size of both the unemployed and economically inactive groups quite large differences would have been required to reach statistical significance levels. Table 5.9 suggests however that the range of intakes was much greater among the unemployed group than among either the working or economically inactive groups. Among the unemployed group, children at or above the upper 2.5 percentile of the distribution had an average energy intake about 6000kJ above that of children at or below the lower 2.5 percentile. Among the working group the difference was only about 4000kJ and for children from homes where the head of household was economically inactive the difference in intakes was about 4700kJ. *(Tables 5.8 and 5.9)*

Families receiving state benefits
Differences in the types of foods consumed by children whose parents were receiving Family Credit and/or Income Support were not reflected in significant differences in mean energy intake. Nor were intakes at either the lowest or highest ends of the distribution markedly different although in cases where these benefits were being received, the 2.5% of children at the lowest end of the distribution had intakes somewhat lower than the corresponding children whose parents were not receiving benefits, 2665kJ (634kcal) compared with 2889kJ (687kcal). Although these differences in mean energy intake between the two groups are not statistically significant, this pattern is consistent with energy values for other subgroups classified by other measures indicative of economic status. For example, both among children in households whose head was unemployed or economically inactive, and among children from a manual home background, mean energy intakes were higher and intakes at the lower 2.5 percentile lower than for other children. The higher mean energy intakes may derive from differences in the types and/or amounts of foods eaten by these children. Variations between subgroups in the sample in intakes of nutrients and their principal food sources are considered in subsequent chapters. *(Table 5.10)*

Family type
There were no significant differences in mean energy intake according to family type, although the data suggest that intakes of children in lone parent families

tended to be higher than for children of married (or cohabiting) couples. This again conforms to the pattern described above of higher energy intakes by groups variously categorised as of lower economic status and is also, at least in part, a reflection of the interrelationships among the various socio-economic characteristics; for example, lone parents being more likely to receive benefits than married couples (see *Table 3.40*)[7]. The range of energy intakes for children in lone parent families, particularly where there was only one child, was large; between the lower and upper 2.5 percentiles more than 5500kJ for single children in lone parent families. Among married couples, children with siblings had a mean energy intake somewhat higher than that of singleton children (4802kJ, 1141kcal compared with 4680kJ, 1112kcal, p: NS).   *(Table 5.11)*

Mother's highest educational qualification

The data show no systematic differences in mean energy intake associated with mothers' educational level, as measured by their highest qualification. Although the lowest intake, 4760kJ (1131kcal), was for children whose mothers had higher level educational qualifications, above GCE 'A' level and equivalent, and the highest mean intake was for children whose mothers had no formal educational qualifications, 4893kJ (1164kcal), the difference in mean intakes was not significant.

(Table 5.12)

5.6 Intake of energy from foods eaten outside the home

The data presented above represent the energy intake by the child from foods consumed both in and out of the home. The data in Table 5.13 show mean intakes for all children from foods eaten away from home. Children who did not eat away from home during the four-day dietary recording period (11% of children) thus had nil energy intake from foods eaten outside the home.

In this survey, eating away from home is defined as any eating occasion outside the subject's own home, including occasions when the food eaten outside the home was prepared at home. It thus includes eating in other private households, for example, and particularly for this age group, having tea with friends, eating at playgroup or toddlers' club, including eating a packed lunch or snack taken from home, as well as eating in commercial establishments. 'Takeaway' items eaten at home are not classified as eating away from home.

The distribution of energy intakes from foods eaten away from home was skewed, with median values being between about 240kJ to 280kJ (55kcal to 65kcal) lower than mean values; intakes ranged from nil to 3610kJ at the upper 2.5 percentile (nil to 859kcal).

Overall, children in the sample derived about one fifth of their mean energy intake from foods eaten away from home; 1043kJ (248kcal) out of 4798kJ (1141kcal) (see *Tables 5.1 and 5.2*). There were only small differences in the proportion of mean energy intake derived from foods eaten away from home between boys and girls and between children in different age groups. For example,

among the youngest age group 19% of energy came from foods eaten away from home compared with 22% for boys aged 3½ to 4½ years and 25% for girls aged 3½ to 4½ years.

The differences found between the age groups in total mean energy intake are reflected in intakes of energy from foods eaten away from home.   *(Table 5.13)*

5.7 Comparisons with other studies

In this section the data on energy intakes for children aged 1½ to 4½ years from this survey are compared with data from a national survey carried out 25 years ago and with data from a more contemporary study.

5.7.1 Comparisons with the nutrition survey of preschool children, 1967/8[8]

A brief account of the methodology of this earlier national dietary survey of preschool children and a table showing mean intakes of energy and some nutrients is given in Appendix P.

Twenty five years ago, mean energy intakes for children were significantly higher than for children in the current survey (p<0.01); in each of the three age cohorts, children in the earlier survey had mean intakes about 17% higher than children today (see *Table 5.14*). A similar reduction in energy intake has been noted in other recent studies[9].

Energy is required for basic metabolic functions, for keeping warm, for activity and also for growth in the young. Energy intake is generally closely matched to these requirements. Life today, compared with that 25 years ago, is probably less physically active; small children spend more time than previously in sedentary activities, such as watching television, they are more likely to travel by car, and the trend towards smaller families may also have led to there being less active play by small children than when there were a larger number of siblings in the family. Energy needs for keeping warm are less because most homes generally are better heated. Furthermore the additional and high requirements for energy at the time of infectious disease are probably less today with the lower frequency of such diseases compared with 25 years ago. It appears that mean energy intakes have fallen in line with current requirements for energy expenditure.

In other respects the data from the 1967/8 survey show remarkable similarities to that from this survey. For example, the earlier survey, like the present one, found that energy intakes were higher in children whose head of household was in a manual social class group, and in children whose mothers had the lowest educational background. Children in the lowest income families also had energy intakes greater than those from higher income groups. Neither have the main sources of energy changed markedly over the period, with the cereals and milk food types being the main sources then as today. However the proportion of energy derived from biscuits, buns, cakes and pastries and from sugars, preserves and confectionery, is today only about half that of the 1967/8 proportions.

5.7.2 Comparisons with other studies

There are few contemporary studies of the diets and nutrition of preschool age children with survey designs and dietary methodologies sufficiently similar to allow comparisons with this current survey. Most have focused on special populations, for example, ethnic minority groups and particular economic status groups, and while these provide useful data for comparing with subgroups in this national sample, they are not representative of the population of preschool children.

One source of comparative data is from the study of 153 healthy children aged between 2 and 5 years living in Edinburgh, Scotland and carried out between May 1988 and April 1990, which used a seven-day weighed inventory methodology for assessing food and nutrient intake (Payne and Belton)[9].

Payne and Belton reported mean energy intakes for boys and girls which are very close to estimates from this study *(Table 5.14)*. Moreover similar patterns for energy intake by different subgroups to those found by this survey were reported, in particular an increase in average daily intake with age and boys had slightly higher intakes than girls. The Edinburgh study, like this national survey, found a wide range of daily energy intakes, with a difference of over 100% between the highest and lowest intakes. They also reported, although data were not shown, that differences in the proportions of children eating different types and amounts of foods generally had little effect on food energy intake. In the commentary on their findings, Payne and Belton discussed the significance of the apparently low energy intakes of the children studied, 60% to 85% of current UK EARs, and come to conclusions similar to those in this Report (see *Section 5.3*).   *(Table 5.14)*

References and notes

1 Department of Health. Report on Health and Social Subjects: 41. *Dietary Reference Values for Food Energy and Nutrients for the United Kingdom.* HMSO (London, 1991).
2 Mean daily intake =
[(Σ intake on two weekend days)+(Σ intake on two weekdays * 2.5)] ÷ 7 See *Chapter 4* and *Appendix J*.
3 Energy intakes for adults are conventionally expressed as megajoules (MJ). For young children ranges of energy intakes expressed as megajoules would not provide sufficient level of detail, and kilojoules have therefore been the preferred unit for presentation in this Report. 1MJ = 1000kJ.
4 Davies PSW, Coward WA, Gregory J, White A, Mills A. Total energy expenditure and energy intake in the preschool child: a comparison. *Brit J Nutr* 194; **72(1):** 13–20.
5 For this age group 'food energy' is equivalent to total energy (there is negligible energy obtained from alcohol). Throughout this Report references to 'total energy' are for total **food** energy, unless explicitly stated otherwise.
6 Gregory J, Foster K, Tyler H, Wiseman M. *The Dietary and Nutritional Survey of British Adults.* HMSO (London, 1990).
7 Chapter 3 includes information on the inter-relationships between the main classificatory variables, including the various indicators of socio-economic status.
8 Department of Health and Social Security. Report on Health and Social Subjects: 10. *A Nutrition Survey of Pre-School Children 1967–68.* HMSO (London, 1975).
9 Payne JA, Belton NR. Nutrient intake and growth in preschool children. Comparison of energy intake and sources of energy with growth. *J Hum Nutr & Dietetics.* 1992; **5:** 287–298.

Figure 5.1 Average daily energy intake (kJ) by sex of child

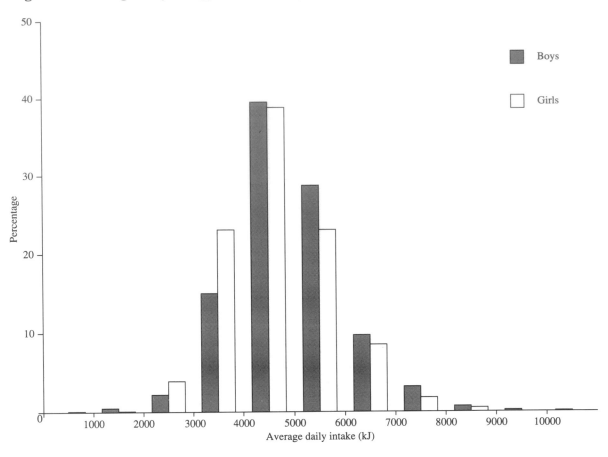

Figure 5.2 Average daily energy intake (kJ) by age of child

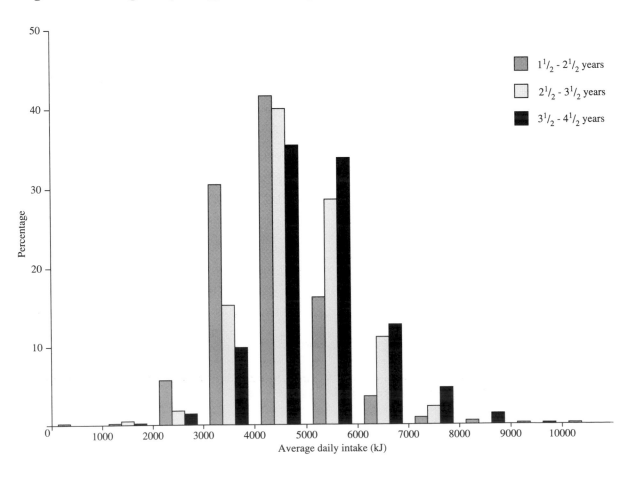

Figure 5.3 Average daily energy intake (kJ) ± standard error* plotted against Estimated Average Requirements: boys

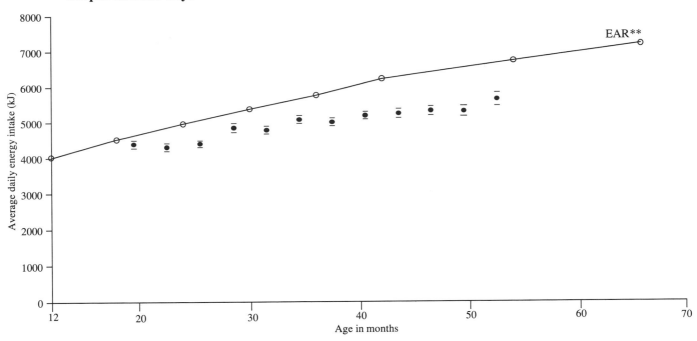

* Plotted at 3-monthly age intervals
** EAR values interpolated from values given in Department of Health. Report on Health and Social Subjects: 41. *Reference values for Food Energy and Nutrients for the United Kingdom.* HMSO (London, 1991).

Figure 5.4 Average daily energy intake (kJ) ± standard error* plotted against Estimated Average Requirements: girls

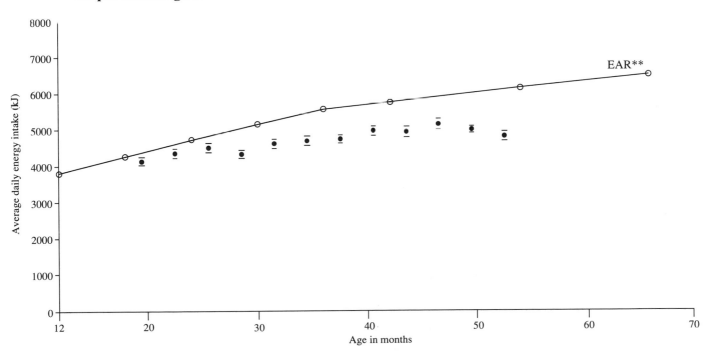

* Plotted at 3-monthly age intervals
** EAR values interpolated from values given in Department of Health. Report on Health and Social Subjects: 41. *Reference values for Food Energy and Nutrients for the United Kingdom.* HMSO (London, 1991).

Figure 5.5 Percentage contribution of food types to average daily energy intake by sex of child

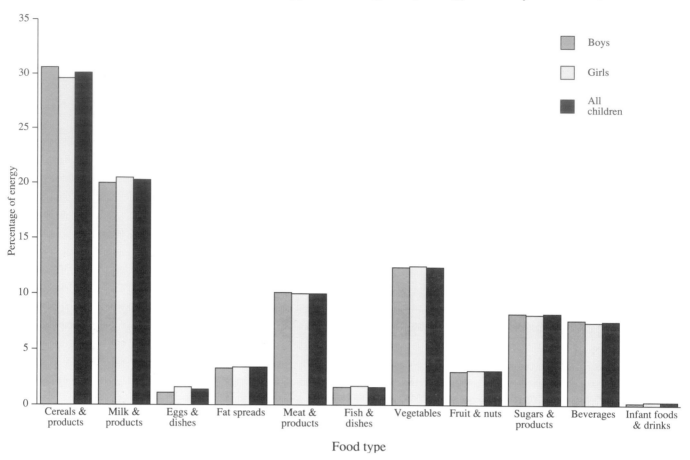

Figure 5.6 Percentage contribution of food types to average daily energy intake by age of child

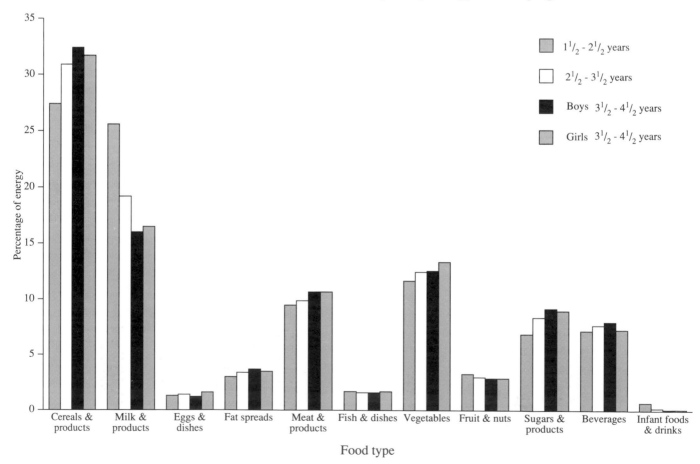

Figure 5.7 Percentage contribution of food types to average daily energy intake by region

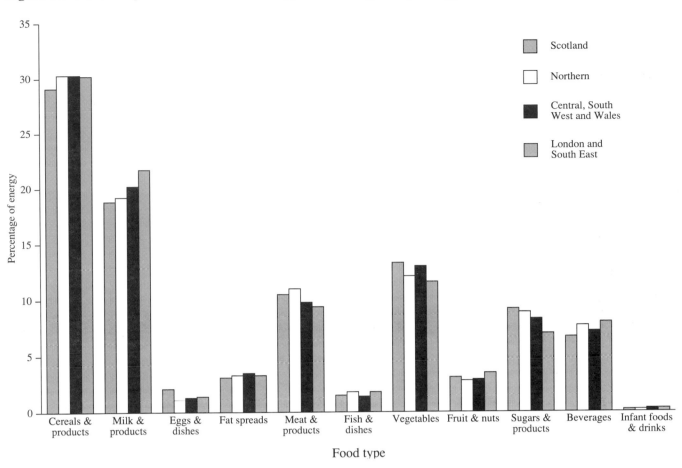

Figure 5.8 Percentage contribution of food types to average daily energy intake by social class of head of household (as defined by occupation)

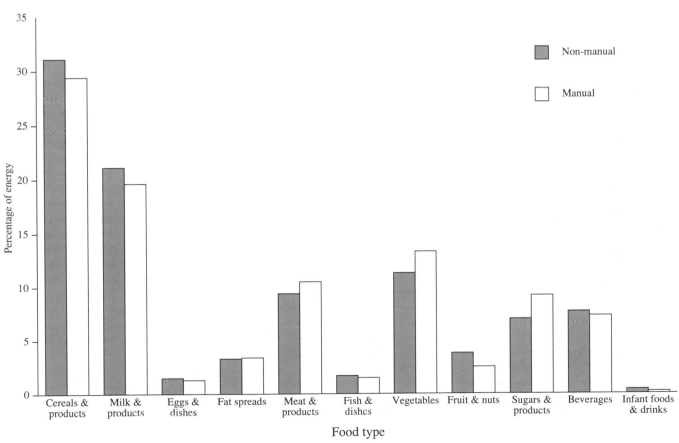

Figure 5.9 Percentage contribution of food types to average daily energy intake by mother's highest educational qualification

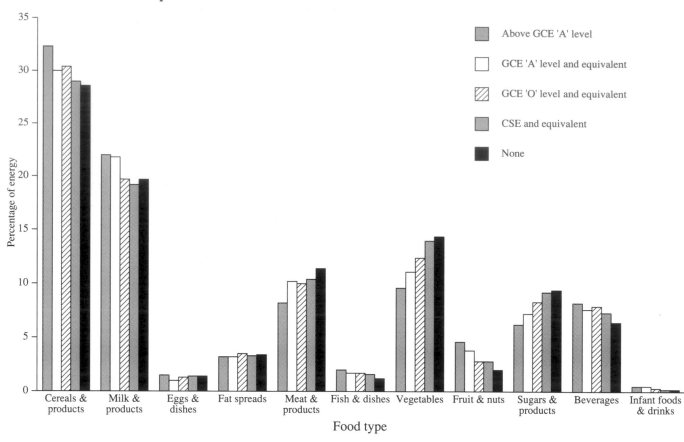

Table 5.1 Average daily energy intake (kJ) by age and sex of child

Energy intake (kJ)	Age and sex of child						
	All aged 1½ – 2½ years	All aged 2½ – 3½ years	All aged 3½ – 4½ years		All boys	All girls	All
			Boys	Girls			
	cum %	cum %	cum %	cum %	cum %	cum %	cum %
Less than 3000	6	2	1	2	3	4	3
Less than 4000	37	18	8	15	18	27	22
Less than 5000	78	58	39	56	51	66	62
Less than 6000	95	86	78	84	86	89	88
Less than 7000	98	98	92	96	96	98	97
Less than 8000	99	100	97	99	99	99	99
All	100		100	100	100	100	100
Base	*576*	*606*	*250*	*243*	*848*	*827*	*1675*
Mean (average value)	4393	4882	5356	4976	4930	4663	4798
Median value	4310	4837	5236	4879	4866	4587	4744
Lower 2.5 percentile	2634	3039	3349	3207	2899	2739	2823
Upper 2.5 percentile	6596	6991	8085	7372	7270	6985	7150
Standard error of the mean	42.8	41.2	70.8	65.6	37.6	36.9	26.5

Table 5.2 Average daily energy intake (kcal) by age and sex of child

Energy intake (kcal)	Age and sex of child						
	All aged 1½ – 2½ years	All aged 2½ – 3½ years	All aged 3½ – 4½ years		All boys	All girls	All
			Boys	Girls			
	cum %	cum %	cum %	cum %	cum %	cum %	cum %
Less than 750	8	4	2	2	4	6	5
Less than 1000	46	25	14	21	25	35	30
Less than 1250	85	67	51	66	67	74	71
Less than 1500	96	90	83	91	89	93	91
Less than 1750	99	99	95	97	98	99	98
Less than 2000	99	100	99	99	99	99	99
All	100		100	100	100	100	100
Base	*576*	*606*	*250*	*243*	*848*	*827*	*1675*
Mean (average value)	1045	1160	1273	1183	1172	1108	1141
Median value	1025	1149	1245	1159	1156	1090	1128
Lower 2.5 percentile	625	720	795	761	689	651	671
Upper 2.5 percentile	1569	1663	1928	1753	1735	1662	1698
Standard error of the mean	10.2	9.8	16.8	15.6	8.9	8.8	6.3

Table 5.3 Average daily energy intake (kJ) by whether child was reported as being unwell during dietary recording period

Energy intake (kJ)	Whether unwell during period		
	Unwell and eating affected	Unwell and eating not affected	Not unwell
	cum %	cum %	cum %
Less than 3000	11	2	2
Less than 4000	39	29	18
Less than 5000	77	68	57
Less than 6000	92	90	86
Less than 7000	97	97	97
Less than 8000	99	100	99
All	100		100
Base	*266*	*190*	*1219*
Mean (average value)	4298	4637	4932
Median value	4226	4400	4855
Lower 2.5 percentile	2060	3073	3101
Upper 2.5 percentile	7115	7115	7162
Standard error of the mean	71.9	72.2	30.0

Table 5.3(a) Average daily energy intake (kcal) by whether child was reported as being unwell during dietary recording period

Energy intake (kcal)	Whether unwell during period		
	Unwell and eating affected	Unwell and eating not affected	Not unwell
	cum %	cum %	cum %
Less than 750	15	4	3
Less than 1000	50	40	24
Less than 1250	83	77	67
Less than 1500	94	93	90
Less than 1750	99	99	98
Less than 2000	100	100	99
All			100
Base	*266*	*190*	*1219*
Mean (average value)	1022	1102	1172
Median value	1005	1046	1154
Lower 2.5 percentile	489	729	736
Upper 2.5 percentile	1690	1686	1702
Standard error of the mean	17.1	17.2	7.1

Table 5.4 Estimated average requirements for energy intakes per kilogram body weight for boys and girls by age*

Age (in years)	Estimated average requirement per kg of body weight – kJ (kcal)/kg/d for:			
	Boys		Girls	
under 3½ years	400	(95)	400	(95)
3½ – 4½ years	400	(95)	375	(90)

*Values have been interpolated for children 3½ to 4½ years from values given in Department of Health and Social Subjects: 41. *Dietary Reference Values for Food Energy and Nutrients for the United Kingdom.* HMSO (London, 1991).

Table 5.5 Average daily energy intake per kilogram body weight (kJ/kg) by age and sex of child

Energy intake per kilogram body weight (kJ/kg)	Age and sex of child						
	All aged 1½–2½ years	All aged 2½–3½ years	All aged 3½–4½ years		All boys	All girls	All
			Boys	Girls			
Mean (average value)	361	337	326	306	341	337	339
Median value	354	336	325	302	338	329	334
Lower 2.5 percentile	212	202	195	191	209	191	198
Upper 2.5 percentile	569	497	462	461	510	527	516
Standard error of the mean	3.7	3.1	4.5	4.4	2.6	2.9	2.0
*No of cases**	*538*	*578*	*237*	*239*	*793*	*799*	*1592*

*Excludes children not weighed or where weight measurement was invalid (see Chapter 11).

Table 5.6(a) Contribution of food types to average daily energy intake (kJ) by age and sex of child

Food types	Age and sex of child						
	All aged 1½–2½ years	All aged 2½–3½ years	All aged 3½–4½ years		All boys	All girls	All
			Boys	Girls			
	kJ	kJ	kJ	kJ	kJ	kJ	kJ
Cereals & cereal products	1202	1507	1735	1576	1510	1381	1446
of which:							
breads	*335*	*417*	*505*	*457*	*422*	*394*	*408*
breakfast cereals	*247*	*286*	*319*	*272*	*298*	*253*	*275*
biscuits, buns, cakes & pastries	*351*	*486*	*591*	*454*	*481*	*419*	*450*
Milk & products	1125	936	858	821	989	955	973
of which:							
cows' milk	*845*	*704*	*630*	*601*	*748*	*704*	*726*
Eggs & egg dishes	57	69	65	78	57	75	66
Fat spreads	133	167	198	176	164	159	161
Meat & meat products	417	485	573	531	497	466	482
of which:							
sausages	*96*	*104*	*120*	*127*	*110*	*104*	*107*
Fish & fish dishes	74	78	84	84	80	77	78
Vegetables, potatoes & savoury snacks	513	613	374	669	610	581	595
of which:							
potato chips	*144*	*182*	*203*	*225*	*186*	*170*	*178*
savoury snacks	*166*	*223*	*233*	*220*	*207*	*201*	*204*
Fruit & nuts	144	148	157	145	148	147	148
of which:							
bananas	*64*	*56*	*60*	*47*	*60*	*56*	*58*
Sugar, preserves & confectionery	305	410	492	446	407	376	391
of which:							
chocolate confectionery	*174*	*229*	*244*	*249*	*219*	*212*	*215*
Beverages	314	375	431	364	374	347	361
of which:							
soft drinks (not low calorie)	*248*	*299*	*365*	*303*	*309*	*275*	*292*
Commercial infant foods & drinks	29	8	3	3	12	15	14
Miscellaneous	80	86	85	83	83	83	83
Average daily intake (kJ)	**4393**	**4882**	**5356**	**4976**	**4930**	**4663**	**4798**
Total no of children	**576**	**606**	**250**	**243**	**848**	**827**	**1675**

Table 5.6(b)   Percentage contribution of food types to average daily energy intake (kJ) by age and sex of child

Food types	Age and sex of child						
	All aged 1½–2½ years	All aged 2½–3½ years	All aged 3½–4½ years		All boys	All girls	All
			Boys	Girls			
	%	%	%	%	%	%	%
Cereals & cereal products	27	31	32	32	31	30	30
of which:							
breads	*8*	*9*	*9*	*9*	*9*	*9*	*9*
breakfast cereals	*6*	*6*	*6*	*6*	*6*	*5*	*6*
biscuits, buns, cakes & pastries	*8*	*10*	*11*	*9*	*10*	*9*	*9*
Milk & milk products	26	19	16	16	20	21	20
of which:							
cows' milk	*19*	*14*	*12*	*12*	*15*	*15*	*15*
Eggs & egg dishes	1	1	1	2	1	2	1
Fat spreads	3	3	4	4	3	3	3
Meat & meat products	10	10	11	11	10	10	10
of which:							
sausages	*2*	*2*	*2*	*3*	*2*	*2*	*2*
Fish & fish dishes	2	2	2	2	2	2	2
Vegetables, potatoes and savoury snacks	12	12	13	13	12	12	12
of which:							
potato chips	*3*	*4*	*4*	*5*	*3*	*4*	*4*
savoury snacks	*4*	*5*	*4*	*4*	*4*	*4*	*4*
Fruit & nuts	3	3	3	3	3	3	3
of which:							
bananas	*2*	*1*	*1*	*1*	*1*	*1*	*1*
Sugar, preserves & confectionery	7	8	9	9	8	8	8
of which:							
chocolate confectionery	*4*	*5*	*5*	*5*	*4*	*5*	*5*
Beverages	7	8	8	7	8	7	8
of which:							
soft drinks (not low calorie)	*6*	*6*	*7*	*6*	*6*	*7*	*6*
Commercial infant foods & drinks	1	0	0	0	0	0	0
Miscellaneous	2	2	2	2	2	2	2
Average daily intake (kJ)	**4393**	**4882**	**5356**	**4976**	**4930**	**4663**	**4798**
Total no of children	**576**	**606**	**250**	**243**	**848**	**827**	**1675**

Table 5.7(a)   Average daily energy intake (kJ) by region

Energy intake (kJ)	Region			
	Scotland	Northern	Central, South West and Wales	London and South East
	cum %	cum %	cum %	cum %
Less than 3000	4	3	3	4
Less than 4000	21	22	21	24
Less than 5000	60	59	59	67
Less than 6000	87	86	87	90
Less than 7000	96	97	97	97
Less than 8000	99	99	99	99
All	100	100	100	100
Base	*165*	*427*	*563*	*520*
Mean (average value)	4800	4860	4834	4708
Median value	4708	4794	4818	4621
Lower 2.5 percentile	2780	2769	2917	2774
Upper 2.5 percentile	7459	7217	7153	7084
Standard error of the mean	86.7	53.9	44.4	47.7

Table 5.7(b) Average daily energy intake (kcal) by region

Energy intake (kJ)	Region			
	Scotland	Northern	Central, South West and Wales	London and South East
	cum %	cum %	cum %	cum %
Less than 750	6	4	5	5
Less than 1000	30	28	29	32
Less than 1250	70	67	70	76
Less than 1500	92	90	91	93
Less than 1750	97	98	99	98
Less than 2000	99	99	99	99
All	100	100	100	100
Base	*165*	*427*	*563*	*520*
Mean (average value)	1141	1155	1149	1119
Median value	1120	1142	1146	1099
Lower 2.5 percentile	660	658	693	658
Upper 2.5 percentile	1773	1710	1701	1682
Standard error of the mean	20.6	12.8	10.6	11.4

Table 5.8 Average daily energy intake by social class of head of household

Energy intake (kJ)	Social class of head of household		
	Non-manual	Manual	All*
	cum %	cum %	cum %
Less than 3000	3	4	3
Less than 4000	22	21	22
Less than 5000	64	60	62
Less than 6000	89	87	88
Less than 7000	97	97	97
Less than 8000	99	99	99
All	100	100	100
Base	*748*	*867*	*1675*
Mean (average value)	4767	4830	4798
Median value	4701	4794	4744
Lower 2.5 percentile	2909	2785	2823
Upper 2.5 percentile	7104	7211	7150
Standard error of the mean	38.1	37.9	26.5

*Includes those in the Armed Forces, those where the HOH had never worked, and others where social class could not be derived.

Table 5.9 Average daily energy intake (kJ) by employment status of head of household

Energy intake (kJ)	Employment status of head of household		
	Working	Unemployed	Economically inactive
	cum %	cum %	cum %
Less than 3000	3	7	1
Less than 4000	22	23	23
Less than 5000	63	60	58
Less than 6000	88	85	85
Less than 7000	97	97	93
Less than 8000	99	97	98
All	100	100	100
Base	*1249*	*167*	*259*
Mean (average value)	4768	4830	4923
Median value	4718	4730	4881
Lower 2.5 percentile	2865	2335	3101
Upper 2.5 percentile	7044	8401	7815
Standard error of the mean	29.2	101.4	73.5

Table 5.10 Average daily energy intake (kJ) by whether child's parents were receiving Income Support or Family Credit

Energy intake (kJ)	Whether receiving benefit(s)	
	Receiving benefit(s)	Not receiving benefits
	cum %	cum %
Less than 3000	4	3
Less than 4000	22	23
Less than 5000	58	63
Less than 6000	85	89
Less than 7000	95	97
Less than 8000	98	99
All	100	100
Base	*534*	*1140*
Mean (average value)	4871	4763
Median value	4841	4717
Lower 2.5 percentile	2665	2889
Upper 2.5 percentile	7560	7070
Standard error of the mean	52.2	30.4

Table 5.11 Average daily energy intake (kJ) by family type

Energy intake (kJ)	Family type			
	Married or cohabiting couple		Lone parent	
	One child	More than one child	One child	More than one child
	cum %	cum %	cum %	cum %
Less than 3000	4	3	4	2
Less than 4000	24	22	23	23
Less than 5000	67	62	50	60
Less than 6000	90	88	84	85
Less than 7000	97	97	93	94
Less than 8000	99	99	96	99
All	100	100	100	100
Base	*366*	*1011*	*121*	*177*
Mean (average value)	4680	4802	4959	4911
Median value	4608	4752	5014	4867
Lower 2.5 percentile	2783	2802	2560	3064
Upper 2.5 percentile	6995	7077	8341	7816
Standard error of the mean	53.5	33.5	118.4	86.4

Table 5.12 Average daily energy intake (kJ) by mother's highest educational qualification level

Energy intake (kJ)	Mother's highest educational qualification level					
	Above GCE 'A' level	GCE 'A' level and equivalent	GCE 'O' level and equivalent	CSE and equivalent	None	All*
	cum %	cum %	cum %	cum %	cum %	cum %
Less than 3000	2	3	3	5	4	3
Less than 4000	22	21	24	22	21	22
Less than 5000	63	60	63	63	58	62
Less than 6000	89	85	88	89	87	88
Less than 7000	99	97	96	98	94	97
Less than 8000	100	100	99	100	98	99
All			100		100	100
Base	*305*	*183*	*390*	*236*	*358*	*1675*
Mean (average value)	4760	4793	4777	4759	4893	4798
Median value	4676	4778	4715	4788	4837	4744
Lower 2.5 percentile	3049	2641	2824	2823	2614	2823
Upper 2.5 percentile	6916	7010	7150	6955	7830	7150
Standard error of the mean	54.3	79.3	45.0	68.3	64.1	26.5

*Includes those where there was no mother in the household and those not answering qualification level.

Table 5.13(a) Foods eaten away from home: average daily energy intake (kJ) by age and sex of child

Energy intake (kJ)	Age and sex of child						
	All aged 1½ – 2½ years	All aged 2½ – 3½ years	All aged 3½ – 4½ years		All boys	All girls	All
			Boys	Girls			
Mean (average value)	839	1100	1191	1228	1052	1033	1043
Median value	598	865	928	972	776	756	761
Lower 2.5 percentile*	–	–	–	–	–	–	–
Upper 2.5 percentile	3175	3619	4428	3812	3663	3603	3610
Standard error of the mean	36.6	41.2	70.2	65.4	35.1	33.8	24.4
No of cases	576	606	250	243	848	827	1675

*Nil intakes (–) at the lower 2.5 percentile represent children who did not eat away from home during the dietary recording period.

Table 5.13(b) Foods eaten away from home: average daily energy intake (kcal) by age and sex of child

Energy intake (kcal)	Age and sex of child						
	All aged 1½ – 2½ years	All aged 2½ – 3½ years	All aged 3½ – 4½ years		All boys	All girls	All
			Boys	Girls			
Mean (average value)	200	262	283	292	250	246	248
Median value	143	206	222	231	185	180	181
Lower 2.5 percentile*	–	–	–	–	–	–	–
Upper 2.5 percentile	753	863	1052	907	871	857	859
Standard error of the mean	8.7	9.8	16.7	15.6	8.3	8.0	5.8
No of cases	576	606	250	243	848	827	1675

*Nil intakes (–) at the lower 2.5 percentile represent children who did not eat away from home during the dietary recording period.

Table 5.14 Average daily energy intake: comparisons between other studies and the NDNS of children aged 1½ to 4½ years

Study	Subjects		No of children	Average daily intake	NDNS children aged 1½ to 4½ years		
					Subjects		Average daily energy intake
DHSS: 1967/8 (GB)[1] (7–day weighed intake)	All	1½ – 2½ yrs	394	1262kcal 5.3MJ	All	1½ – 2½ yrs	1045kcal 4.4MJ
	All	2½ – 3½ yrs	407	1401kcal 5.9MJ	All	2½ – 3½ yrs	1160kcal 4.9MJ
	All	3½ – 4½ yrs	319	1468kcal 6.1MJ	All	3½ – 4½ yrs	1228kcal 5.2MJ
Payne & Belton: 1988/90 (Edinburgh)[2] (7–day weighed intake)	Boys	2 yrs	31	4504kJ	All	1½ – 2½ yrs	4393kJ
	Girls	2 yrs	42	4390kJ			
	Boys	3 yrs	31	5009kJ	All	2½ – 3½ yrs	4881kJ
	Girls	3 yrs	38	4757kJ			
	Boys	4 yrs	35	5300kJ	Boys	3½ – 4½ yrs	5356kJ
	Girls	4 yrs	30	5062kJ	Girls	3½ – 4½ yrs	4976kJ

[1] Department of Health and Social Security (1975).
[2] Payne JA, Belton NR (1992).

6 Protein and carbohydrate intake

6.1 Introduction

In this and the following chapter data are presented on intakes of protein, carbohydrates, total fat and fatty acids, and on the percentage of food energy provided by each. Intakes are expressed as daily averages, calculated from re-weighting to a seven-day daily average, intakes for the 1675 children for whom a dietary record covering two weekdays and two weekend days was obtained[1]. Protein and carbohydrates are considered in this chapter; for carbohydrates information is shown separately for total available carbohydrate, starch, total sugars, non-milk extrinsic sugars, intrinsic and milk sugars and starch, and non-starch polysaccharides ('fibre')[2].

6.2 Protein

Average daily protein intake for children aged between 1½ and 4½ years was 36.8g (median 35.9g). Average intake increased slightly with age, being lowest among those aged 1½ to 2½ years, 35.4g, and highest among boys aged 3½ to 4½ years, 39.4g (NS).

(Table 6.1 and Figs 6.1 and 6.2)

The current UK Reference Nutrient Intake (RNI) for protein for children aged 1 to 3 years is 14.5g/d and for children aged 4 to 6 years 19.7g/d[3]. Only 1% of children aged under 4 years and 2% of those aged 4 and over had intakes below the appropriate RNI for their age group. As Table 6.2 shows most children had intakes of protein well in excess of the RNI; mean protein intake for children under 4 years was 251% of the RNI and for those aged 4 and over 200% of the RNI. *(Table 6.2)*

As shown in Table 6.3, overall, protein provided about 13% of the food energy intake of the children in the survey. The youngest children, those aged 1½ to 2½ years, obtained a slightly higher proportion of their energy from protein than older children, and had somewhat higher protein intakes per megajoule energy, but for the oldest cohort there were no significant differences in either measure between boys and girls *(Table 6.4)*. Table 6.3 also shows that the proportion of food energy obtained from protein by those at the upper extreme of the distribution was more than twice that of children at the lower extreme; for example, the upper 2.5 percentile of children aged between 2½ and 3½ years obtained 18.2% of their food energy from protein compared with only 8.3% for those at the lower 2.5 percentile. *(Tables 6.3 and 6.4)*

The energy contribution of the macronutrients, protein, carbohydrates and total fat to total food energy intake for children in the sample is shown in Table 6.5 and Figure 6.3. *(Table 6.5 and Fig 6.3)*

As Table 6.6 shows, more than three quarters of the protein consumed was derived from three main food types. Milk and milk products were the major sources, providing 33% overall, with cows' milk contributing between 20% and 29% depending on the age of the child; cereals and cereal products provided a further 23% and meat and meat products 22%. Compared with older children the youngest children obtained significantly more protein from milk and milk products, (p<0.05) and somewhat less from cereals and cereal products and meat and meat products (NS).

(Table 6.6)

In 1967/8, the survey of preschool children reported mean protein intakes for each of the age cohorts which were slightly higher than those for children in this NDNS survey[4]. The contribution from milk and cream to protein intake was also somewhat higher in 1967/8 than for children in the current survey, both in terms of absolute intake and percentage contribution. For example, in 1967/8 children aged between 1½ and 2½ years had an average daily protein intake of 38.0g, of which 12.3g, 32%, was contributed by milk and milk products. Children aged 1½ to 2½ years in this NDNS had an average daily intake of 35.4g protein, of which 10.7g, 30%, came from milk and milk products. Table 6.7 shows that there were similar differences for the other age cohorts.

(Table 6.7)

6.3 Carbohydrates

The average daily intake of total available carbohydrate was 155g (median 151g). Mean intake varied with age, the lowest intakes being recorded for the youngest children in the sample, 139g, rising to 162g for girls aged 3½ to 4½ years and 177g for boys in the same age group (p<0.01). For each age group the range in carbohydrate intake was large; for example, among children aged between 1½ and 2½ years the lowest 2.5 percentile of children were consuming 80g carbohydrate or less a day compared with 218g a day consumed by those at the upper 2.5 percentile. *(Table 6.8 and Figs 6.4 and 6.5)*

About 51% of total food energy was derived from carbohydrates. There were no significant differences between the age groups in the percentage of food energy obtained from total carbohydrate (see also *Fig 6.3*). At the lower 2.5 percentile in each age group children were obtaining about 40% of their food energy from carbohydrates and at the upper 2.5 percentile at least 60% of energy was derived from this source. *(Table 6.9)*

The main sources of carbohydrates did not vary by age

group nor differ between boys and girls. Cereals and cereal products were the major source, contributing 39% overall to total intake, with white bread and breakfast cereals each providing 9%, and biscuits 6%. Fourteen per cent of total carbohydrate intake was obtained from beverages, with soft drinks, not low calorie, contributing the major part (12%). Milk and milk products contributed a further 12% to total carbohydrate intake. For the youngest children this food type provided a slightly greater proportion of carbohydrate (16%) than the overall average (NS). *(Table 6.10)*

6.3.1 Sugars

As well as showing intakes of total sugars for the children in the survey, information is also given on their intakes of *non-milk extrinsic sugars* and *intrinsic and milk sugars*.

Extrinsic sugars are any sugars which are not contained within the cellular structure of the food, whether natural and unprocessed, or refined. Examples are the sugars in honey, table sugar and lactose in milk and milk products. Non-milk extrinsic sugars are therefore all extrinsic sugars *excluding* lactose in milk and milk products, which are seen to be a special case.

Intrinsic sugars are those contained within the cellular structure of the food; milk sugars include extrinsic milk sugars, that is lactose in milk and milk products. As in the COMA Report on Dietary Reference Values[3] information on intakes of intrinsic and milk sugars is combined with information on intakes of starch for presentation purposes.

Total sugars
The average daily intake of total sugars was 87g (median 83.0g). Overall total sugars intake for boys was higher than for girls (p<0.01) and intakes increased significantly with age between the two younger age cohorts (p<0.01), and again for the oldest group of boys as compared with all children aged 2½ to 3½ years (p<0.05). For all groups the range of intakes was large; for example, among boys aged 3½ to 4½ years intakes ranged between 42g at the lower 2.5 percentile and 175g at the upper 2.5 percentile.

(Table 6.11 and Figs 6.6 and 6.7)

Most of the differences in intakes were accounted for by differences in energy intakes. As Table 6.4a shows, overall the mean daily total sugars intake per megajoule was 18.1g, with no differences between the age cohorts or between boys and girls. Thus sugars contributed a relatively constant proportion of food energy intake of boys and girls and in each of the three age cohorts.

Beverages contributed one quarter of the total sugars intake in the children's diets, with soft drinks providing 21% overall and 23% in the diets of boys aged 3½ to 4½ years. Cereals and cereal products, milk and milk products, table and added sugars, and preserves and confectionery each contributed about 20% to the intake of total sugars in the children's diets. The consumption of cows' milk provided 16% of the total sugars intake (mainly as lactose) and again this proportion fell as the

children got older, from 19% for those aged 1½ to 2½ years to about 12% for those aged 3½ to 4½ years (p<0.05). Sugar confectionery and chocolate confectionery each contributed 7% to overall intake and although the differences are not statistically significant, the proportion of total intake coming from the consumption of sugar confectionery showed some increase with age. *(Table 6.12)*

The initial interview which preceded keeping the dietary record, also collected information on the use of sugar in tea and coffee. It can be seen from Table 6.13 that just over half the children who drank tea and about 60% of those who drank coffee, usually drank it sweetened with sugar; thus overall 33% of children were drinking tea sweetened with sugar and 14% were drinking coffee sweetened with sugar. There were no differences in the use of sugar in tea or coffee between boys and girls or between children of different ages. *(Table 6.13)*

Non-milk extrinsic sugars
The average daily consumption of non-milk extrinsic sugars by children in this survey was 57g (median 53g), representing about 65% of the total sugars consumption. Intake increased significantly with age, from a mean of 48g for children aged 1½ to 2½ years to 60g for those aged 2½ to 3½ years (p<0.01). Consumption by girls aged between 3½ and 4½ years was not significantly above that of children in the middle age cohort, but among the oldest boys intakes again rose to a mean of 69g (p<0.05). In each age cohort intakes at the upper 2.5 percentile were on average at least twice that at the median, and at the lower 2.5 percentile intakes ranged from 10g for children aged 1½ to 2½ years, to 22g for children aged 3½ to 4½ years. *(Table 6.14 and Figs 6.8 and 6.9)*

The current UK recommendation is that for groups of people the intake of non-milk extrinsic sugars should contribute no more than an average of about 10% of total dietary energy. This level is intended for the general population and is based on a goal of reduced dental caries. The Working Group of the Committee on the Medical Aspects of Food Policy on the Weaning Diet considered that this value is applicable to preschool children, who are a group at high risk of dental caries[5]. As Table 6.15 shows, the mean value for all children in this survey and in each age cohort was above the current recommendation. For example, children aged 2½ to 3½ years were deriving, on average 19.3% of their total food energy from non-milk extrinsic sugars. Children at the upper 2.5 percentile of the distribution were obtaining at least a third of their energy from this source.

(Table 6.15)

As Table 6.4b shows, differences between the age cohorts in mean intake of non-milk extrinsic sugars were not entirely the consequence of differences in energy intake. Thus while the youngest cohort had an average intake of non-milk extrinsic sugars of 11.0g per megajoule food energy, this rose to 12.8g per megajoule for boys aged between 3½ and 4½ years (p<0.05).

For each age cohort the main sources of non-milk extrinsic sugars were beverages (39%), sugars, preserves and confectionery (27%) and cereals and cereal products (23%). Of the 39% contribution to total intake made by beverages, 32% came from the consumption of soft drinks (not low calorie). Chocolate and sugar confectionery each contributed about 10% to total intake of non-milk extrinsic sugars.

There was a trend for the contribution of cereals and cereal products and sugars, preserves and confectionery to total intake of non-milk extrinsic sugars to increase with age; for example, among children aged 1½ to 2½ years 25% of total intake came from the sugars, preserves and confectionery group, compared with 29% for boys and girls aged 3½ to 4½ years (NS).   (Table 6.16)

6.3.2 Starch

The average daily starch intake by children in the survey was 68g (median 67g), representing about 44% of total carbohydrate intake and contributing 22% of total food energy. For the total sample the range in intakes between the lower and upper 2.5 percentiles was between 30g and 116g. There was a consistent trend for starch intake to increase with age, and the oldest boys had mean intakes greater than the oldest girls (p<0.05). The same pattern can be seen in Table 6.4b, which adjusts for variation in energy intake; intakes of total starch per megajoule food energy intake increased with age from a mean value of 13.4g/mJ among children aged 1½ to 2½ years, to 14.9g/mJ for boys aged 3½ to 4½ years and 15.1g/mJ for girls in the same age cohort.
                        (Table 6.17 and Figs 6.10 and 6.11)

Nearly two thirds of the total starch intake was obtained from the consumption of cereals and cereal products with white bread contributing 19% and wholemeal bread 4%. Breakfast cereals contributed 16% of the total intake, with high fibre and wholemeal types accounting for half of this. The only other group contributing more than 10% to total starch intake was vegetables, including potatoes and savoury snacks, 26%. Each age cohort derived about 10% of their total starch intake from fried potatoes, mainly as chips.
                                            (Table 6.18)

6.3.3 Intrinsic sugars, milk sugars and starch

This group includes starch and all sugars with the exception of non-milk extrinsic sugars as previously defined (see 6.3.1 above); that is, total available carbohydrate minus non-milk extrinsic sugars.

The COMA Panel on Dietary Reference Values proposed that starches and intrinsic and milk sugars should provide on average 39% of total food energy for the population and that this should apply to children over 2 years old[3].

Table 6.19 shows on average children in this survey were obtaining about 32% of their total food energy intake from this group of carbohydrates. Neither the mean value nor values at the upper and lower percentiles of

the distribution showed any association with either age or sex. Children at the lower 2.5 percentile of the distribution obtained about 22% of their energy from intrinsic and milk sugars and starch, while values for those at the upper 2.5 percentile were about 44% of food energy.
                                            (Table 6.19)

6.3.4 Non-starch polysaccharides (NSP)

Adult dietary intakes of NSP in the UK are estimated to be between 11g/d and 13g/d, and the COMA Panel on Dietary Reference Values proposed that the diet of the adult population should contain on average 18g/d non-starch polysaccharide, with a range of 12 to 24g/d, from a variety of foods. The Panel made no recommendation about NSP intakes for children, except that children should have proportionately lower intakes which were probably best related to their lower body size. They recommended that children of less than 2 years should not take foods rich in NSP at the expense of more energy-rich foods which they require for adequate growth[3].

The average daily intake of NSP by the total sample of children was 6.1g (median 5.8g). Mean intakes increased with age from 5.5g among the youngest cohort to 6.8g for the oldest boys and 6.4g for the oldest girls (p<0.01). Children with the lowest daily intakes (at the lower 2.5 percentile of the distribution) had an average NSP consumption ranging between 2.0g (those aged 1½ to 2½ years) and 2.9g (boys aged 3½ to 4½ years). Those with the highest intakes (at the upper 2.5 percentile) were, on average, consuming about twice the median amount. Nevertheless mean daily intakes of NSP per megajoule food energy were low, 1.3g/mJ, and showed no variation with either age or sex (see Tables 6.4a and 6.4b).
                        (Table 6.20 and Figs 6.12 and 6.13)

The main source of NSP is cereals, particularly wholegrain foods, and, as Table 6.21b shows, children in this survey obtained more than 40% of their NSP intake from the consumption of cereals and cereal products. High fibre and wholegrain breakfast cereals provided between 10% and 14% of total intake depending on age and sex and overall wholemeal and white bread provided 6% and 7% of the total respectively. A further 35% of total intake was derived from the consumption of vegetables, including potatoes and savoury snacks, and another 11% from fruit.   (Table 6.21)

6.4 Bowel movements

During the four days when the dietary record was being completed mothers were asked also to keep a record of the number of bowel movements their child had each day. A copy of the recording document with the instructions to mothers is given in Appendix A.

The purpose of collecting this information was primarily to establish normative values for the population of children aged between 1½ to 4½ years, which are not available from other sources, and to be able to relate the information on the number (and type) of bowel movement to other information collected, principally dietary data. Information is presented here on the average number of bowel movements per day for children in the survey (Table 6.22) and Table 6.23 shows the mean NSP intake for children according to their number of bowel movements.

Overall about 80% of the children had at least one bowel movement a day; 13% had two or more bowel movements per day on average over the recording period. The data suggest that after the age of 2½ years, the frequency of bowel movements declines somewhat; only 13% of children in the youngest cohort did not have a bowel movement each day, compared with 23% of those aged 2½ to 3½ years and 26% of boys and 30% of girls in the oldest age group. It should be noted, however, that it is more likely that the older children were able to go to the toilet unassisted and hence it is more likely that some bowel movements may have gone unrecorded by their mother or other carer.

Nevertheless Table 6.23 shows a positive association between the recorded number of bowel movements and the mean daily intake of NSP. Thus children who did not have a bowel movement every day had a mean NSP intake of 5.6g; those with one movement a day had a mean NSP intake of 6.1g (p<0.05), and those with more than two bowel movements per day an intake of 6.6g (p<0.01). *(Tables 6.22 and 6.23)*

6.5 Variation in intake of protein and carbohydrates

Tables 6.24 to 6.30 show mean and median intakes of protein and carbohydrates for different groups of children in the sample.

Children reported as being unwell
It was shown in the previous chapter that children who were reported as being unwell during the dietary recording period had lower average daily energy intakes than other children. Those whose eating was reported as being affected had the lowest energy intakes, but even among those whose eating was said not to have been affected by being unwell, energy intakes were lower compared with those of children not reported as being unwell.

Table 6.24 shows that children whose eating was reported as being affected by their being unwell had significantly lower intakes of protein and all carbohydrates than children who were not unwell (p<0.01). For each nutrient, intakes were on average about 13% lower among the unwell group than for those who were not unwell. Even among those who were reported as being unwell but whose eating was said not to have been affected, intakes of total carbohydrates, total sugars, non-milk extrinsic sugars and starch were lower than those of children who were not unwell, by between 6% and 9% (carbohydrate: p<0.01; total sugars, non-milk extrinsic sugars and starch: p<0.05). However, although the absolute intakes of nutrients were lower for unwell children, the proportion of food energy provided by carbohydrates was similar for all three groups of children, suggesting that in respect of carbohydrates the reduced consumption was due to the reduced energy

intake and not to any selective preference for carbohydrates by the children who were not reported as being unwell. *(Table 6.24)*

Region
In general there were quite small differences between children in different regions in their average intakes of protein and carbohydrates. Only intakes of NSP and starch varied significantly by region, intakes of starch being lowest for children living in London and the South East and highest among those from the Central and South West regions of England and Wales (p<0.01). Intakes of NSP were also highest for children in the Central and South West regions and Wales, but were lowest among Scottish children (p<0.05).

There was almost no variation between children living in different parts of Great Britain in either their average daily protein intake, or in the proportion of energy they derived from carbohydrates. *(Table 6.25)*

Socio-economic characteristics
As described in Chapter 3, a number of measures of the socio-economic status of the child's household were derived from the interview data which were obtained prior to keeping the dietary record. It has also been noted that many of these measures were interrelated; for example, households receiving Family Credit and Income Support were more likely to have a head of household who was from the manual, rather than non-manual, social class group. Bearing such associations in mind the data show that although there was no difference in the total carbohydrate intake between children from different social backgrounds, there was a difference between the groups in average intakes of different types of carbohydrates. The tables show a clear trend for children from households of lower economic status to have lower average intakes of total sugars but higher starch intakes than other children.

For example, average intakes of total sugars were lowest for children whose mothers had qualifications below GCE 'O' level standard *(Table 6.26)*; intakes were also lower for children from households where the head was not working *(Table 6.27)* and where the family was in receipt of either Family Credit or Income Support *(Table 6.29)*. However children from these same groups had higher starch intakes than other children.

In the Report of the dental survey, which was carried out as a follow up to this diet and nutrition survey, relationships between the dental health of these children and their intakes of sugars are discussed[6].

There was also a tendency for children from a manual social class background to have lower intakes of protein (p<0.05) *(Table 6.28)*. *(Tables 6.26 to 6.29)*

Family type
Overall there was no significant variation in the average daily intake of total carbohydrates, NSP or protein associated with family type nor did the proportion of energy derived from carbohydrates vary significantly. However, as with the measures of socio-economic status

described above, there were similar differences associated with family type in intakes of the different types of carbohydrate. In particular, children from lone parent families where there was more than one child in the family had significantly higher intakes of starch than other children, but somewhat lower intakes of total sugars and non-milk extrinsic sugars (as compared with children from two-parent families with more than one child: for starch, p<0.01; for total sugars and non-milk extrinsic sugars, p<0.05).   *(Table 6.30)*

References and notes

1 Mean daily intake =
[(Σ intake on two weekend days) + (Σ intake on two week-days * 2.5)] ÷ 7 See *Chapter 4* and *Appendix J*.
2 Non-starch polysaccharides refer to non alpha-glucans as measured by the technique of Englyst and Cummings. Englyst HN, Cummings JH. Improved method for measurement of dietary fiber as non-starch polysaccharides in plant foods. *J Ass Off Anal Chem* 1988; **71**: 808–814.
3 Department of Health. Report on Health and Social Subjects: 41. *Dietary Reference Values for Food Energy and Nutrients for the United Kingdom*. HMSO (London, 1991).
4 Department of Health and Social Security. Report on Health and Social Subjects: 10. *A Nutrition Survey of Pre-school Children, 1967–8*. HMSO (London, 1975). See also *Appendix P*.
5 Department of Health. Report on Health and Social Subjects: 45. *Weaning and the Weaning Diet*. HMSO (London, 1994).
6 Hinds K and Gregory J. *National Diet and Nutrition Survey: Children aged 1½ to 4½ years. Volume 2: Report of the Dental Survey*. HMSO (London, 1995).

Figure 6.1 Average daily protein intake by sex of child

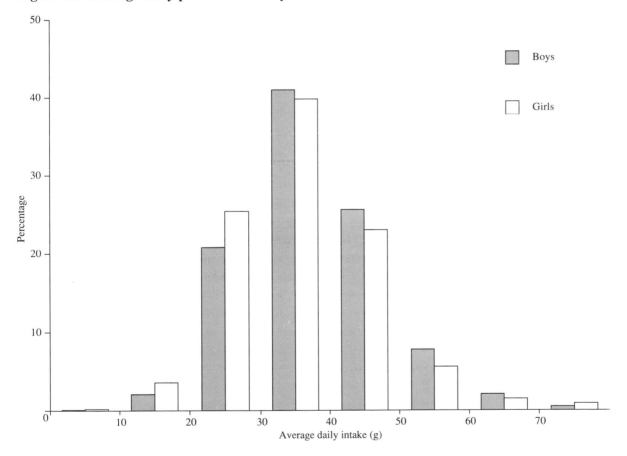

Figure 6.2 Average daily protein intake by age of child

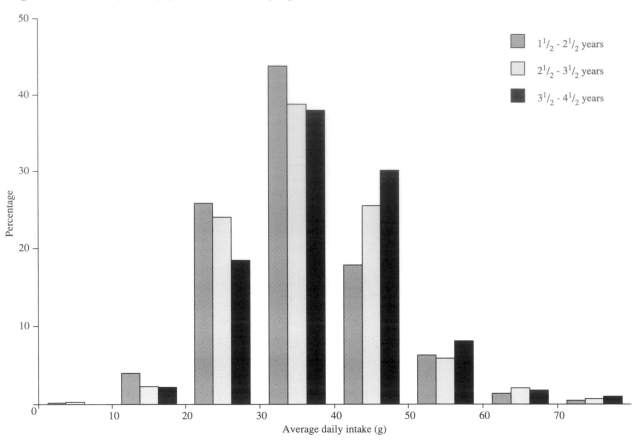

Figure 6.3 Contribution to food energy intake from total fat, carbohydrate and protein by age and sex

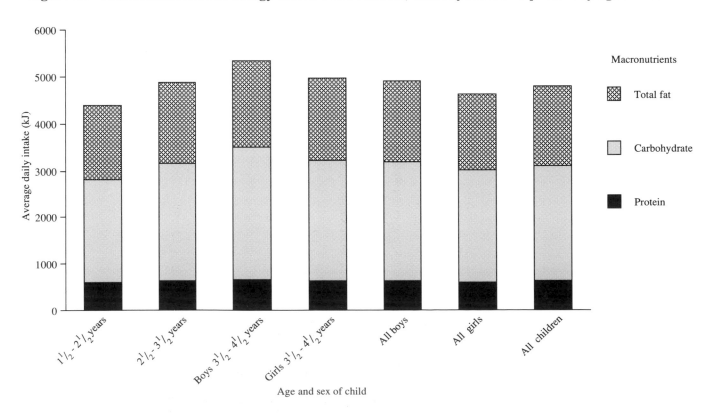

Figure 6.4 Average daily carbohydrate intake by sex of child

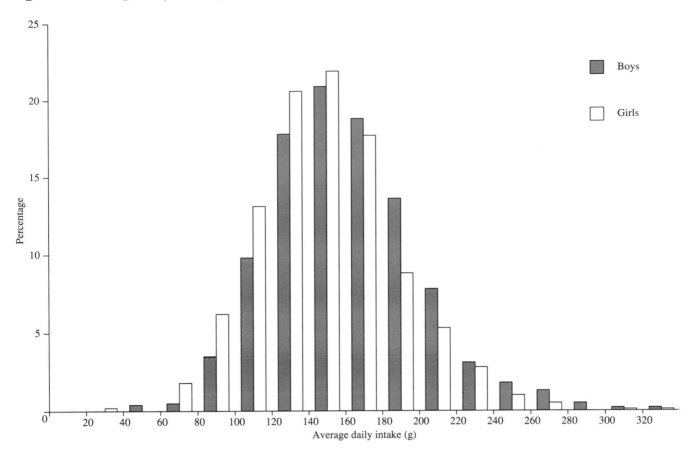

Figure 6.5 Average daily carbohydrate intake by age of child

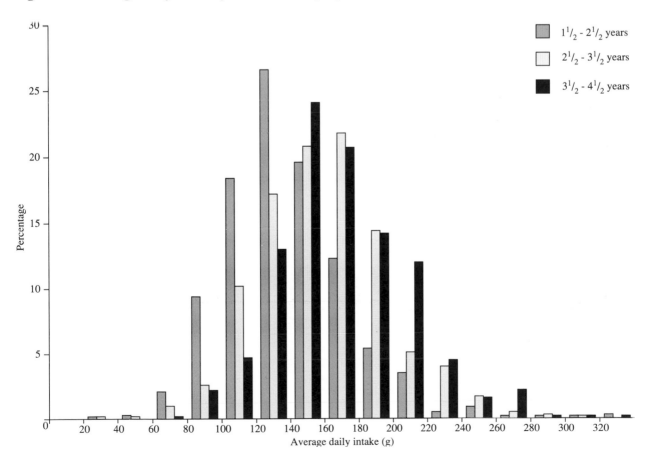

71

Figure 6.6 Average daily total sugars intake by sex of child

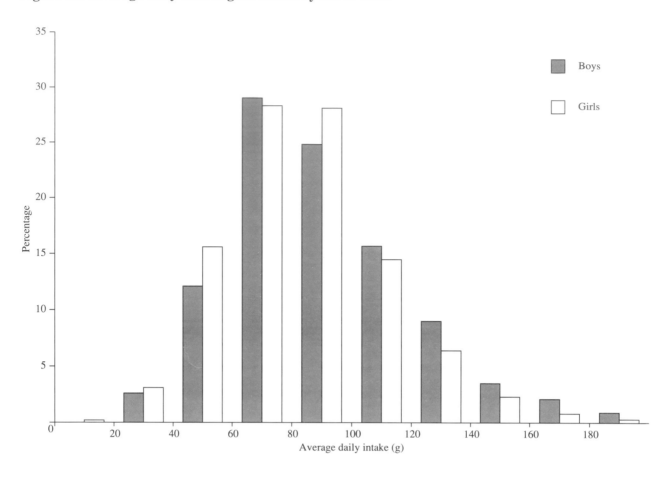

Figure 6.7 Average daily total sugars intake by age of child

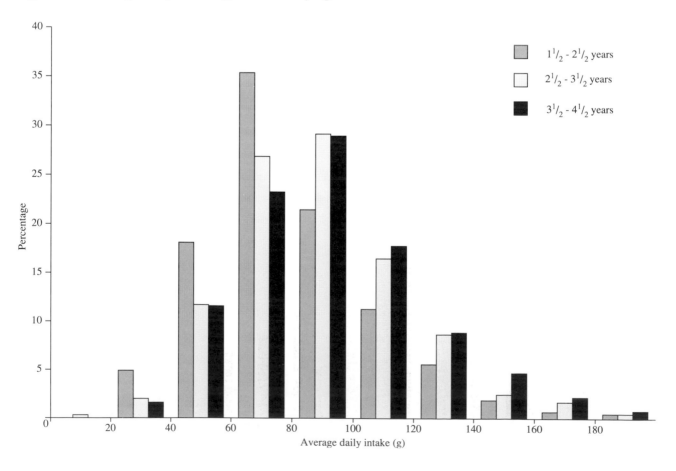

Figure 6.8 Average daily non-milk extrinsic sugars intake by sex of child

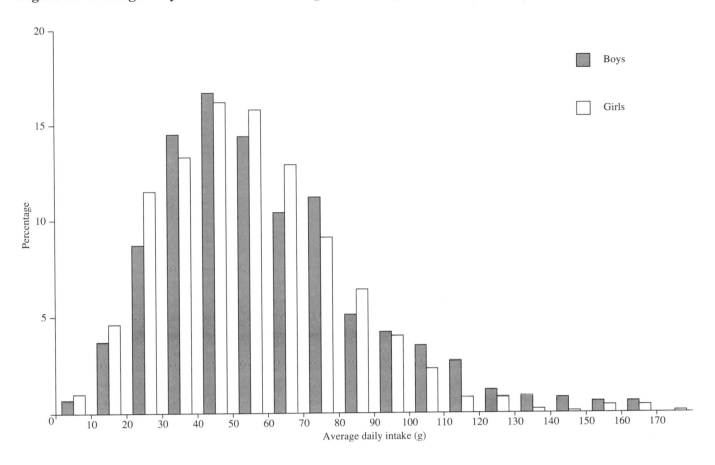

Figure 6.9 Average daily non-milk extrinsic sugars intake by age of child

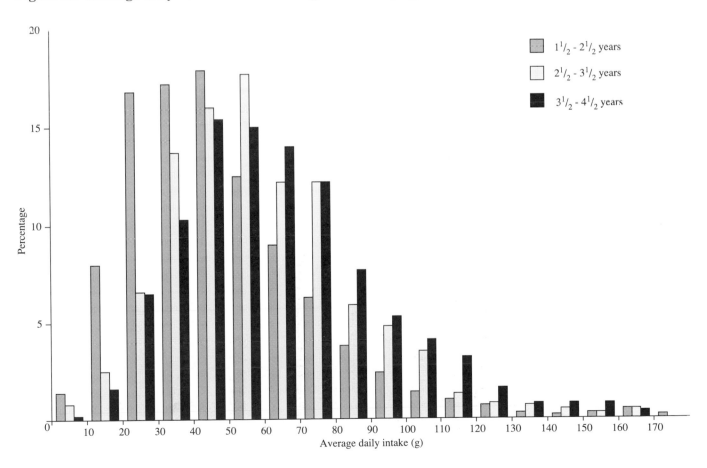

73

Figure 6.10 Average daily starch intake by sex of child

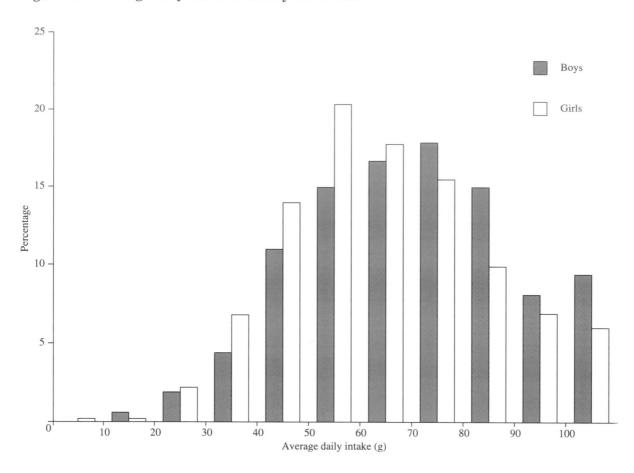

Figure 6.11 Average daily starch intake by age of child

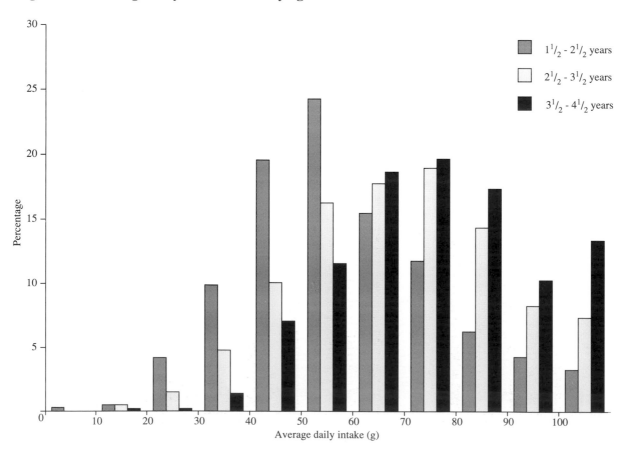

Figure 6.12 Average daily intake of non-starch polysaccharides by sex of child

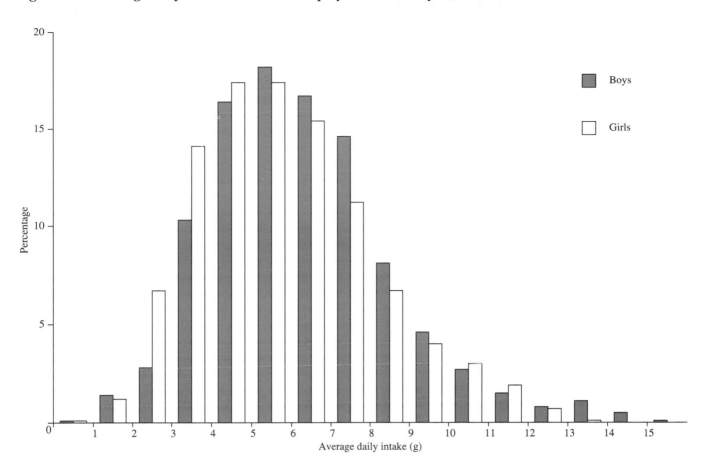

Figure 6.13 Average daily intake of non-starch polysaccharides by age of child

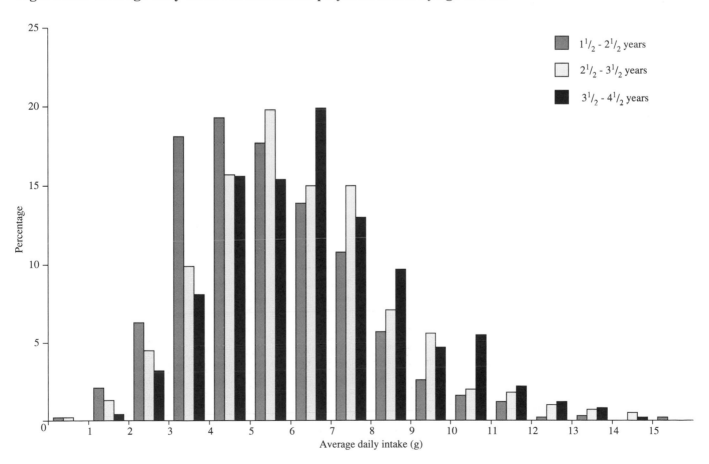

Table 6.1   Average daily protein intake (g) by age and sex of child

Average daily protein intake (g)	Age and sex of child								
	All aged 1½ – 2½ years	All aged 2½ – 3½ years	All aged 3½ – 4½ years		All under 4 years	All 4 years and over	All boys	All girls	All
			Boys	Girls					
	cum %	cum %	cum %	cum %	cum %	cum %	cum %	cum %	cum %
Less than 14.5*	1	1	1	0	1	1	1	1	1
Less than 19.7**	4	2	2	2	3	1	2	3	3
Less than 25	12	11	7	9	11	7	9	12	10
Less than 30	30	27	18	23	27	19	23	29	26
Less than 35	52	47	34	42	48	34	44	47	46
Less than 40	74	66	53	65	68	58	64	69	66
Less than 45	84	82	73	79	82	74	79	83	87
All	100	100	100	100	100	100	100	100	100
Base	576	606	250	243	1457	218	848	827	1675
Mean (average value)	35.4	36.8	39.4	37.7	36.4	39.4	37.4	36.2	36.8
Median value	34.6	35.9	39.1	37.5	35.6	38.6	36.4	35.6	35.9
Lower 2.5 percentile	18.4	20.0	20.3	19.7	19.2	20.9	20.1	18.2	19.3
Upper 2.5 percentile	59.2	61.1	60.2	63.5	59.4	62.8	60.4	60.2	60.4
Standard error of the mean	0.42	0.42	0.66	0.67	0.27	0.72	0.35	0.36	0.25

*RNI for children aged between 1 and 3 years
**RNI for children aged between 4 and 6 years

Table 6.2   Average daily protein intake as percentage of Reference Nutrient Intake (RNI) by age and sex of child

Age and sex of child	Average daily intake as % of RNI			
	Mean	Median	se	Base
All aged 1½ – 2½ years	244	239	2.9	576
All aged 2½ – 3½ years	254	248	2.9	606
Aged 3½ – 4½ years*:				
Boys	241	235	4.4	250
Girls	227	212	4.7	243
All aged under 4 years	251	245	1.9	1457
All aged 4 years and over	200	196	3.6	218
All boys	249	240	2.4	848
All girls	240	234	2.5	825
All	244	238	1.7	1675

* Protein intake as a percentage of the RNI was calculated at individual child level: thus in this age group values for children under 4 years of age used 14.5g/d as the RNI and for children aged 4 and over 19.7g/d was taken as the RNI. The values for all children aged 3½ to 4½ years were then pooled to give a mean, median and se for the age group.

Table 6.3   Percentage of food energy from protein by age and sex of child

Percentage of food energy from protein	Age and sex of child						
	All aged 1½ – 2½ years	All aged 2½ – 3½ years	All aged 3½ – 4½ years		All boys	All girls	All
			Boys	Girls			
	cum %	cum %	cum %	cum %	cum %	cum %	cum %
Less than 10	8	12	13	13	11	10	11
Less than 12	25	40	45	41	37	34	35
Less than 14	59	72	78	70	70	66	68
Less than 16	83	91	92	92	89	87	88
Less than 18	95	97	98	97	97	96	97
All	100	100	100	100	100	100	100
Base	576	606	250	243	848	827	1675
Mean (average value)	13.6	12.7	12.4	12.7	12.8	13.1	13.0
Median value	13.4	12.5	12.3	12.6	12.7	12.9	12.8
Lower 2.5 percentile	8.9	8.3	8.2	8.6	8.2	8.4	8.5
Upper 2.5 percentile	19.0	18.2	17.9	18.7	18.3	18.8	18.6
Standard error of the mean	0.11	0.10	0.15	0.16	0.09	0.09	0.06

Table 6.4(a) Average daily intake of protein and carbohydrates (g) per MJ food energy by sex of child

Nutrient	Sex of child								
	Boys			Girls			All		
Intake (g) per MJ energy:	*Mean*	*Median*	*se*	*Mean*	*Median*	*se*	*Mean*	*Median*	*se*
Protein	7.6	7.5	0.05	7.8	7.7	0.05	7.7	7.6	0.04
Total carbohydrate	51.4	51.5	0.21	50.8	51.2	0.21	51.1	51.4	0.15
Total sugars	18.2	17.7	0.16	18.1	17.9	0.15	18.1	17.8	0.11
Starch	14.4	14.4	0.12	14.1	14.1	0.12	14.2	14.3	0.08
Non-milk extrinsic sugars	12.0	11.1	0.17	11.8	11.5	0.16	11.9	11.3	0.12
Non-starch polysaccharides	1.3	1.2	0.01	1.3	1.2	0.01	1.3	1.2	0.01
Base		848			827			1675	

Table 6.4(b) Average daily intake of protein and carbohydrates (g) per MJ food energy by age of child

Nutrient	Age and sex of child											
	All aged 1½–2½ years			All aged 2½–3½ years			All aged 3½–4½ years					
							Boys			Girls		
Intake (g) per MJ energy:	*Mean*	*Median*	*se*	*Mean*	*Median*	*se*	*Mean*	*Median*	*se*	*Mean*	*Median*	*se*
Protein	8.1	8.0	0.06	7.5	7.5	0.06	7.4	7.3	0.09	7.6	7.5	0.09
Total carbohydrate	49.9	50.3	0.27	51.5	51.8	0.24	52.3	52.1	0.37	51.7	51.7	0.37
Total sugars	18.2	17.5	0.19	18.3	18.2	0.17	18.2	17.6	0.30	17.7	17.7	0.27
Starch	13.4	13.2	0.15	14.4	14.5	0.14	14.9	15.0	0.21	15.1	14.8	0.21
Non-milk extrinsic sugars	11.0	10.4	0.21	12.2	11.9	0.19	12.8	11.9	0.31	12.1	12.0	0.29
Non-starch polysaccharides	1.3	1.2	0.02	1.3	1.2	0.02	1.3	1.2	0.03	1.3	1.2	0.03
Base		576			606			250			242	

Table 6.5 Macronutrient contribution to food energy intake by age and sex of child

	Age and sex of child						
	All aged 1½ – 2½ years	All aged 2½ – 3½ years	All aged 3½ – 4½ years		All boys	All girls	All
			Boys	Girls			
Average daily intake:							
Total food energy (kcal)	1045	1160	1273	1183	1172	1108	1141
Total food energy (kJ)	4393	4882	5356	4976	4930	4663	4798
Protein (g)	35.4	36.8	39.4	37.7	37.4	36.2	36.8
Carbohydrate (g)	139	159	177	162	160	150	155
Total fat (g)	42.5	46.3	50.1	47.2	46.7	44.6	45.7
Percentage food energy from:							
Protein (%)	13.6	12.7	12.4	12.7	12.8	13.1	13.0
Carbohydrate (%)	49.9	51.5	52.3	51.7	51.4	50.8	51.1
Fat (%)	36.4	35.8	35.3	35.5	35.7	36.1	35.9

Table 6.6(a) Contribution of food types to average daily protein intake (g) by age and sex of child

Food types	All aged 1½ – 2½ years	All aged 2½ – 3½ years	All aged 3½ – 4½ years		All boys	All girls	All
			Boys	Girls			
	g	g	g	g	g	g	g
Cereals & cereal products	7.3	8.8	10.1	9.4	8.9	8.2	8.6
of which:							
white bread	*1.8*	*2.4*	*3.0*	*2.7*	*2.4*	*2.3*	*2.3*
wholemeal bread	*0.6*	*0.6*	*0.7*	*0.6*	*0.6*	*0.6*	*0.6*
breakfast cereals	*1.4*	*1.6*	*1.7*	*1.4*	*1.7*	*1.4*	*1.5*
biscuits	*0.8*	*1.0*	*1.2*	*1.0*	*1.0*	*0.9*	*1.0*
Milk & milk products	13.6	11.8	10.9	10.5	12.3	11.9	12.1
of which:							
cows' milk	*10.3*	*8.9*	*8.0*	*7.7*	*9.3*	*8.8*	*9.1*
other milk & cream	*0.4*	*0.2*	*0.2*	*0.2*	*0.3*	*0.2*	*0.3*
cheese	*1.3*	*1.3*	*1.4*	*1.5*	*1.3*	*1.4*	*1.4*
fromage frais & yogurt	*1.6*	*1.4*	*1.2*	*1.2*	*1.4*	*1.4*	*1.4*
Eggs & egg dishes	0.9	1.1	1.1	1.2	0.9	1.2	1.0
Fat spreads	0.1	0.1	0.1	0.1	0.1	0.1	0.1
Meat & meat products	7.1	8.2	9.9	9.1	8.3	8.1	8.2
of which:							
bacon & ham	*0.5*	*0.7*	*0.8*	*1.0*	*0.6*	*0.7*	*0.7*
beef, veal & dishes	*1.6*	*1.7*	*1.7*	*1.7*	*1.7*	*1.7*	*1.7*
chicken & turkey	*1.8*	*2.0*	*2.9*	*2.3*	*2.2*	*2.0*	*2.1*
Fish & fish dishes	1.4	1.5	1.6	1.6	1.5	1.5	1.5
Vegetables, potatoes & savoury snacks	2.7	3.1	3.3	3.4	3.1	3.0	3.1
of which:							
vegetables, excluding potatoes	*1.2*	*1.3*	*1.3*	*1.3*	*1.3*	*1.3*	*1.3*
potatoes	*1.1*	*1.2*	*1.4*	*1.5*	*1.2*	*1.2*	*1.2*
savoury snacks	*0.4*	*0.6*	*0.6*	*0.6*	*0.5*	*0.5*	*0.5*
Fruit and nuts	0.5	0.6	0.6	0.6	0.5	0.6	0.5
Sugars, preserves & confectionery	0.7	0.9	1.0	1.0	0.9	0.8	0.9
Beverages	0.3	0.3	0.3	0.2	0.2	0.3	0.3
Commercial infant foods & drinks	0.2	0.0	0.0	0.0	0.1	0.1	0.1
Miscellaneous	0.5	0.5	0.4	0.5	0.5	0.5	0.5
Average daily intake (g)	**35**	**37**	**39**	**38**	**37**	**36**	**37**
Total number of children	**576**	**606**	**250**	**243**	**848**	**827**	**1675**

Table 6.6(b) Percentage contribution of food types to average daily protein intake by age and sex of child

Food types	Age and sex of child						
	All aged 1½ – 2½ years	All aged 2½ – 3½ years	All aged 3½ – 4½ years		All boys	All girls	All
			Boys	Girls			
	%	%	%	%	%	%	%
Cereals & cereal products	21	24	26	25	24	23	23
of which:							
white bread	5	6	8	7	6	6	6
wholemeal bread	2	1	2	2	2	2	2
breakfast cereals	4	4	4	4	4	4	4
biscuits	2	3	3	2	3	2	3
Milk & milk products	38	32	28	28	32	33	33
of which:							
cows' milk	29	24	20	20	25	24	25
other milk & cream	1	0	0	0	1	1	1
cheese	4	4	4	4	3	4	4
fromage frais & yogurt	4	4	3	3	4	4	4
Eggs & egg dishes	3	3	3	3	2	3	3
Fat spreads	0	0	0	0	0	0	0
Meat & meat products	20	22	25	24	22	22	22
of which:							
bacon & ham	1	2	2	3	2	2	2
beef, veal & dishes	5	5	4	4	5	5	5
chicken & turkey	5	5	7	6	6	6	6
Fish & fish dishes	4	4	4	4	4	4	4
Vegetables, potatoes & savoury snacks	8	8	8	9	8	8	8
of which:							
vegetables, excluding potatoes	3	4	3	3	4	3	3
potatoes	3	3	3	4	3	3	3
savoury snacks	1	2	1	1	1	1	1
Fruit and nuts	1	1	1	1	1	1	1
Sugars, preserves & confectionery	2	2	3	3	2	2	2
Beverages	1	1	1	1	1	1	1
Commercial infant foods & drinks	0	0	0	0	0	0	0
Miscellaneous	1	1	1	1	1	1	1
Average daily intake (g)	**35**	**37**	**39**	**38**	**37**	**36**	**37**
Total number of children	**576**	**606**	**250**	**243**	**848**	**827**	**1675**

Table 6.7 Protein intakes (g) and milk as a source of protein; 1967/8* and NDNS children aged 1½ to 4½ years

	Age of child					
	1½ – 2½ years		2½ – 3½ years		3½ – 4½ years	
	1967/8 survey	NDNS 1992/3	1967/8 survey	NDNS 1992/3	1967/8 survey	NDNS 1992/3
Mean intake (g)	38.0	35.4	40.7	36.8	41.6	38.5
Contribution from milk and cream (g)	12.3	10.7	10.9	9.1	10.8	8.0
% contribution from milk and cream	32	30	27	24	26	20
Base	*349*	*576*	*407*	*606*	*319*	*493*

* Department of Health and Social Security. Report on Health and Social Subjects: 10. *A Nutrition Survey of Pre-school Children, 1967–68.* HMSO (London, 1975), Table A28.

Table 6.8 Average daily carbohydrate intake (g) by age and sex of child

Carbohydrate intake (g)	Age and sex of child						
	All aged 1½ – 2½ years	All aged 2½ – 3½ years	All aged 3½ – 4½ years		All boys	All girls	All
			Boys	Girls			
	cum %	cum %	cum %	cum %	cum %	cum %	cum %
Less than 100	12	4	2	3	4	8	6
Less than 130	44	20	12	14	22	30	26
Less than 160	77	52	36	53	53	64	58
Less than 190	92	83	64	80	79	87	83
Less than 210	96	92	80	93	89	94	91
All	100	100	100	100	100	100	100
Base	576	606	250	243	848	827	1675
Mean (average value)	139	159	177	162	160	150	155
Median value	135	157	173	159	157	146	151
Lower 2.5 percentile	80	96	106	96	94	85	88
Upper 2.5 percentile	218	242	275	238	253	230	243
Standard error of the mean	1.5	1.5	2.6	2.1	1.4	1.3	1.0

Table 6.9 Percentage of food energy from carbohydrate by age and sex of child

Percentage of food energy from carbohydrate	Age and sex of child						
	All aged 1½ – 2½ years	All aged 2½ – 3½ years	All aged 3½ – 4½ years		All boys	All girls	All
			Boys	Girls			
	cum %	cum %	cum %	cum %	cum %	cum %	cum %
Less than 40	7	3	0	2	3	5	4
Less than 45	23	11	10	11	15	16	15
Less than 50	48	37	36	39	40	43	41
Less than 55	78	73	71	74	74	76	75
Less than 60	93	92	89	92	91	94	92
All	100	100	100	100	100	100	100
Base	576	606	250	243	848	827	1675
Mean (average value)	49.9	51.5	52.3	51.7	51.4	50.8	51.1
Median value	50.3	51.8	52.1	51.7	51.5	51.2	51.4
Lower 2.5 percentile	36.6	38.8	41.1	39.9	39.3	37.1	38.5
Upper 2.5 percentile	62.3	63.5	64.1	65.3	64.1	63.0	63.7
Standard error of the mean	0.27	0.24	0.37	0.37	0.21	0.21	0.15

Table 6.10(a) Contribution of food types to average daily carbohydrate intake (g) by age and sex of child

Food types	Age and sex of child						
	All aged 1½ – 2½ years	All aged 2½ – 3½ years	All aged 3½ – 4½ years		All boys	All girls	All
			Boys	Girls			
	g	g	g	g	g	g	g
Cereals & cereal products	50.5	62.8	72.6	66.0	63.2	57.7	60.5
of which:							
white bread	*10.9*	*14.3*	*18.1*	*16.6*	*14.3*	*13.8*	*14.0*
wholemeal bread	*2.7*	*2.5*	*3.3*	*3.0*	*2.8*	*2.7*	*2.8*
high fibre & wholegrain							
breakfast cereals	*6.8*	*7.1*	*7.4*	*5.4*	*7.6*	*6.0*	*6.8*
other breakfast cereals	*6.1*	*7.8*	*9.5*	*9.3*	*8.0*	*7.4*	*7.7*
biscuits	*7.9*	*10.3*	*12.2*	*9.1*	*10.4*	*8.8*	*9.6*
Milk & milk products	21.8	18.4	16.5	15.9	19.1	18.8	18.9
of which:							
cows' milk	*15.5*	*13.5*	*12.1*	*11.8*	*14.0*	*13.4*	*13.7*
fromage frais & yogurt	*4.7*	*4.3*	*3.6*	*3.5*	*4.0*	*4.4*	*4.2*
Eggs & egg dishes	0.1	0.2	0.2	0.2	0.2	0.2	0.2
Fat spreads	0.0	0.0	0.0	0.0	0.0	0.0	0.0
Meat & meat products	3.8	4.6	5.4	4.7	4.7	4.2	4.4
Fish & fish dishes	1.1	1.2	1.2	1.3	1.2	1.1	1.2
Vegetables, potatoes & savoury snacks	17.2	20.1	22.0	22.1	20.1	19.3	19.7
of which:							
vegetables, excluding potatoes	*3.4*	*3.6*	*3.6*	*3.6*	*3.7*	*3.4*	*3.5*
potatoes, fried	*5.8*	*7.1*	*8.3*	*8.5*	*7.4*	*6.7*	*7.0*
other potatoes	*3.7*	*3.7*	*4.1*	*4.3*	*3.7*	*4.0*	*3.9*
savoury snacks	*4.3*	*5.7*	*6.0*	*5.7*	*5.3*	*5.2*	*5.2*
Fruit and nuts	7.7	7.6	7.8	7.1	7.7	7.5	7.6
of which:							
fruit	*7.6*	*7.5*	*7.7*	*6.9*	*7.6*	*7.4*	*7.5*
nuts, fruit & nut mixes	*0.1*	*0.1*	*0.1*	*0.2*	*0.1*	*0.1*	*0.1*
Sugars, preserves & confectionery	13.1	17.7	21.9	19.2	17.8	16.1	17.0
of which:							
sugar	*2.6*	*2.5*	*3.3*	*2.8*	*2.8*	*2.5*	*2.7*
preserves	*0.9*	*1.3*	*1.9*	*1.4*	*1.4*	*1.2*	*1.3*
sugar confectionery	*4.2*	*6.8*	*9.1*	*7.3*	*6.7*	*5.9*	*6.3*
chocolate confectionery	*5.4*	*7.2*	*7.6*	*7.7*	*6.9*	*6.5*	*6.7*
Beverages	19.3	23.0	26.5	22.4	23.0	21.3	22.2
of which:							
fruit juice	*3.4*	*3.6*	*3.1*	*2.8*	*3.1*	*3.6*	*3.4*
soft drinks, not low calorie	*15.4*	*18.6*	*22.7*	*18.8*	*19.2*	*17.1*	*18.2*
Commercial infant foods & drinks	1.4	0.4	0.2	0.2	0.6	0.7	0.6
Miscellaneous	2.8	2.9	2.7	2.8	2.8	2.8	2.8
Average daily intake (g)	**139**	**159**	**177**	**162**	**160**	**150**	**155**
Total number of children	**576**	**606**	**250**	**243**	**848**	**827**	**1675**

Table 6.10(b)   Percentage contribution of food types to average daily carbohydrate intake by age and sex of child

Food types	Age and sex of child						
	All aged 1½ – 2½ years	All aged 2½ – 3½ years	All aged 3½ – 4½ years		All boys	All girls	All
			Boys	Girls			
	%	%	%	%	%	%	%
Cereals & cereal products	36	39	41	41	39	38	39
of which:							
white bread	*8*	*9*	*10*	*10*	*9*	*9*	*9*
wholemeal bread	*2*	*2*	*2*	*2*	*2*	*2*	*2*
high fibre & wholegrain							
breakfast cereals	*5*	*4*	*4*	*3*	*5*	*4*	*4*
other breakfast cereals	*4*	*5*	*5*	*6*	*5*	*5*	*5*
biscuits	*6*	*6*	*7*	*6*	*6*	*6*	*6*
Milk & milk products	16	12	9	10	12	12	12
of which:							
cows' milk	*11*	*8*	*7*	*7*	*9*	*9*	*9*
fromage frais & yogurt	*3*	*3*	*2*	*2*	*2*	*3*	*3*
Eggs & egg dishes	0	0	0	0	0	0	0
Fat spreads	0	0	0	0	0	0	0
Meat & meat products	3	3	3	3	3	3	3
Fish & fish dishes	1	1	1	1	1	1	1
Vegetables, potatoes & savoury snacks	12	13	12	14	12	13	13
of which:							
vegetables, excluding potatoes	*2*	*2*	*2*	*2*	*2*	*2*	*2*
potatoes, fried	*4*	*4*	*5*	*5*	*5*	*4*	*4*
other potatoes	*3*	*2*	*2*	*3*	*2*	*3*	*2*
savoury snacks	*3*	*4*	*3*	*3*	*3*	*3*	*3*
Fruit and nuts	5	5	4	4	5	5	5
of which:							
fruit	*5*	*5*	*4*	*4*	*5*	*5*	*5*
nuts, fruit & nut mixes	*0*	*0*	*0*	*0*	*0*	*0*	*0*
Sugars, preserves & confectionery	9	11	12	12	11	11	11
of which:							
Sugar	*2*	*1*	*2*	*2*	*2*	*2*	*2*
preserves	*1*	*1*	*1*	*1*	*1*	*1*	*1*
sugar confectionery	*3*	*4*	*5*	*4*	*4*	*4*	*4*
chocolate confectionery	*4*	*4*	*4*	*5*	*4*	*4*	*4*
Beverages	14	14	15	14	14	14	14
of which:							
fruit juice	*2*	*2*	*2*	*2*	*2*	*2*	*2*
soft drinks, not low calorie	*11*	*12*	*13*	*12*	*12*	*11*	*12*
Commercial infant foods & drinks	1	0	0	0	0	0	0
Miscellaneous	2	2	1	2	2	2	2
Average daily intake (g)	**139**	**159**	**177**	**162**	**160**	**150**	**155**
Total number of children	**576**	**606**	**250**	**243**	**848**	**827**	**1675**

Table 6.11   Average daily total sugars intake (g) by age and sex of child

Total sugars intake (g)	Age and sex of child						
	All aged 1½ – 2½ years	All aged 2½ – 3½ years	All aged 3½ – 4½ years		All boys	All girls	All
			Boys	Girls			
	cum %	cum %	cum %	cum %	cum %	cum %	cum %
Less than 50	12	6	4	5	7	8	8
Less than 70	39	26	20	25	28	31	29
Less than 90	72	53	45	56	56	62	59
Less than 110	87	78	67	84	76	85	80
Less than 130	94	92	84	94	90	94	91
All	100	100	100	100	100	100	100
Base	*576*	*606*	*250*	*243*	*848*	*827*	*1675*
Mean (average value)	80	89	98	88	90	84	87
Median value	76	88	94	86	84	82	83
Lower 2.5 percentile	36	40	42	42	40	38	38
Upper 2.5 percentile	148	152	175	153	164	146	156
Standard error of the mean	1.2	1.1	2.1	1.7	1.1	0.1	0.7

Table 6.12(a) Contribution of food types to average daily sugars intake by age and sex of child

Food types	Age and sex of child						
	All aged 1½ – 2½ years	All aged 2½ – 3½ years	All aged 3½ – 4½ years		All boys	All girls	All
			Boys	Girls			
	g	g	g	g	g	g	g
Cereals & cereal products	13.6	18.1	21.1	18.9	17.9	16.3	17.1
of which:							
white bread	*0.7*	*0.9*	*1.1*	*1.0*	*0.9*	*0.8*	*0.8*
wholemeal bread	*0.1*	*0.1*	*0.1*	*0.1*	*0.1*	*0.1*	*0.1*
high fibre & wholegrain							
* breakfast cereals*	*1.0*	*1.1*	*1.3*	*1.0*	*1.1*	*1.0*	*1.1*
other breakfast cereals	*1.7*	*2.1*	*3.0*	*2.7*	*2.3*	*2.1*	*2.2*
biscuits	*3.5*	*4.9*	*5.6*	*4.2*	*4.8*	*4.1*	*4.4*
Milk & milk products	21.7	18.4	16.5	15.9	19.1	18.7	18.9
of which:							
cows' milk	*15.5*	*13.5*	*12.1*	*11.8*	*14.0*	*13.4*	*13.7*
fromage frais & yogurt	*4.7*	*4.3*	*3.6*	*3.5*	*4.0*	*4.4*	*4.2*
Eggs & egg dishes	0.0	0.0	0.0	0.0	0.0	0.0	0.0
Fat spreads	0.0	0.0	0.0	0.0	0.0	0.0	0.0
Meat & meat products	0.4	0.6	0.6	0.6	0.6	0.6	0.6
Fish & fish dishes	0.0	0.0	0.0	0.0	0.0	0.0	0.0
Vegetables, potatoes & savoury snacks	2.1	2.2	2.4	2.4	2.2	2.2	2.2
of which:							
vegetables, excluding potatoes	*1.5*	*1.6*	*1.7*	*1.7*	*1.6*	*1.6*	*1.6*
potatoes, fried	*0.2*	*0.3*	*0.3*	*0.3*	*0.3*	*0.2*	*0.3*
other potatoes	*0.2*	*0.2*	*0.2*	*0.2*	*0.2*	*0.2*	*0.2*
savoury snacks	*0.1*	*0.2*	*0.2*	*0.2*	*0.2*	*0.2*	*0.2*
Fruit and nuts	7.3	7.3	7.4	6.8	7.3	7.1	7.2
of which:							
fruit	*7.2*	*7.2*	*7.3*	*6.7*	*7.2*	*7.1*	*7.2*
nuts, fruit & nut mixes	*0.0*	*0.0*	*0.1*	*0.1*	*0.0*	*0.0*	*0.0*
Sugars, preserves & confectionery	12.8	17.2	21.2	18.6	17.3	15.6	16.5
of which:							
sugar	*2.6*	*2.5*	*3.3*	*2.8*	*2.8*	*2.5*	*2.7*
preserves	*0.9*	*1.3*	*1.9*	*1.4*	*1.4*	*1.1*	*1.3*
sugar confectionery	*4.0*	*6.6*	*8.9*	*7.2*	*6.6*	*5.6*	*6.2*
chocolate confectionery	*5.2*	*6.8*	*7.2*	*7.3*	*6.5*	*6.2*	*6.4*
Beverages	19.3	23.0	26.5	22.4	23.0	21.3	22.2
of which:							
fruit juice	*3.4*	*3.6*	*3.1*	*2.8*	*3.1*	*3.6*	*3.4*
soft drinks, not low calorie	*15.4*	*18.6*	*22.7*	*18.8*	*19.2*	*17.1*	*18.2*
Commercial infant foods & drinks	0.8	0.3	0.1	0.1	0.3	0.5	0.4
Miscellaneous	1.7	1.8	1.7	1.7	1.7	1.7	1.7
Average daily intake (g)	**80**	**89**	**98**	**88**	**90**	**84**	**87**
Total number of children	**576**	**606**	**250**	**243**	**848**	**827**	**1675**

Table 6.12(b)   Percentage contribution of food types to average daily sugars intake by age and sex of child

Food types	Age and sex of child						
	All aged 1½ – 2½ years	All aged 2½ – 3½ years	All aged 3½ – 4½ years		All boys	All girls	All
			Boys	Girls			
	%	%	%	%	%	%	%
Cereals & cereal products	17	20	22	22	20	19	20
of which:							
white bread	*1*	*1*	*1*	*1*	*1*	*1*	*1*
wholemeal bread	*0*	*0*	*0*	*0*	*0*	*0*	*0*
high fibre & wholegrain							
* breakfast cereals*	*1*	*1*	*1*	*1*	*1*	*1*	*1*
other breakfast cereals	*2*	*2*	*3*	*3*	*3*	*2*	*2*
biscuits	*4*	*5*	*6*	*5*	*5*	*5*	*5*
Milk & milk products	27	21	17	18	21	22	22
of which:							
cows' milk	*19*	*15*	*12*	*13*	*16*	*16*	*16*
fromage frais & yogurt	*6*	*5*	*4*	*4*	*4*	*5*	*5*
Eggs & egg dishes	0	0	0	0	0	0	0
Fat spreads	0	0	0	0	0	0	0
Meat & meat products	1	1	1	1	1	1	1
Fish & fish dishes	0	0	0	0	0	0	0
Vegetables, potatoes & savoury snacks	3	2	2	3	2	3	2
of which:							
vegetables, excluding potatoes	*2*	*2*	*2*	*2*	*2*	*2*	*2*
potatoes, fried	*0*	*0*	*0*	*0*	*0*	*0*	*0*
other potatoes	*0*	*0*	*0*	*0*	*0*	*0*	*0*
savoury snacks	*0*	*0*	*0*	*0*	*0*	*0*	*0*
Fruit and nuts	9	8	8	8	8	8	8
of which:							
fruit	*9*	*8*	*7*	*8*	*8*	*8*	*8*
nuts, fruit & nut mixes	*0*	*0*	*0*	*0*	*0*	*0*	*0*
Sugars, preserves & confectionery	16	19	22	21	19	18	19
of which:							
sugar	*3*	*3*	*3*	*3*	*3*	*3*	*3*
preserves	*1*	*1*	*2*	*1*	*1*	*1*	*1*
sugar confectionery	*5*	*7*	*9*	*8*	*7*	*7*	*7*
chocolate confectionery	*6*	*8*	*7*	*8*	*7*	*7*	*7*
Beverages	24	26	27	26	26	25	25
of which:							
fruit juice	*4*	*4*	*3*	*3*	*3*	*4*	*4*
soft drinks, not low calorie	*19*	*21*	*23*	*21*	*21*	*20*	*21*
Commercial infant foods & drinks	1	0	0	0	0	1	0
Miscellaneous	2	2	2	2	2	2	2
Average daily intake (g)	**80**	**89**	**98**	**88**	**90**	**84**	**87**
Total number of children	**576**	**606**	**250**	**243**	**848**	**827**	**1675**

Table 6.13   Use of sugar and artificial sweeteners in tea and coffee by age and sex of child

Use of sugar and artificial sweeteners	Age of child			Sex of child		All children
	1½–2½ years	2½–3½ years	3½–4½ years	Boys	Girls	
	%	%	%	%	%	%
Tea drinking						
Drinks tea:	58	59	63	58	63	61
with sugar	29	33	36	33	32	33
with artificial sweetener	1	1	1	1	1	1
unsweetened	29	25	26	24	30	27
Does not drink tea	42	40	37	42	37	39
Coffee drinking						
Drinks coffee:	19	23	27	23	23	23
with sugar	11	14	16	15	13	14
with artificial sweetener	0	1	1	1	0	1
unsweetened	7	8	10	7	10	8
Does not drink coffee	81	77	73	78	77	77
*Base: number of children**	*648*	*668*	*543*	*943*	*916*	*1859*

*All children including those for whom no dietary record was available.

Table 6.14 Average daily non-milk extrinsic sugars intake (g) by age and sex of child

Non-milk extrinsic sugars intake (g)	Age and sex of child						
	All aged 1½ – 2½ years	All aged 2½ – 3½ years	All aged 3½ – 4½ years		All boys	All girls	All
			Boys	Girls			
	cum %	cum %	cum %	cum %	cum %	cum %	cum %
Less than 30	26	10	7	10	13	17	15
Less than 45	53	31	22	30	36	38	37
Less than 60	74	57	44	54	59	62	60
Less than 75	86	75	66	76	75	80	78
Less than 90	93	88	77	89	85	91	88
All	100	100	100	100	100	100	100
Base	576	606	250	243	848	827	1675
Mean (average value)	48	60	69	60	59	55	57
Median value	43	56	65	58	54	53	53
Lower 2.5 percentile	10	17	22	22	16	14	15
Upper 2.5 percentile	117	123	145	121	136	114	124
Standard error of the mean	1.1	1.1	1.9	1.6	1.0	0.9	0.7

Table 6.15 Percentage of food energy from non-milk extrinsic sugars by age and sex of child

Percentage of food energy from non-milk extrinsic sugars	Age and sex of child						
	All aged 1½ – 2½ years	All aged 2½ – 3½ years	All aged 3½ – 4½ years		All boys	All girls	All
			Boys	Girls			
	cum %	cum %	cum %	cum %	cum %	cum %	cum %
Less than 10	20	9	7	8	12	13	12
Less than 15	43	30	25	29	34	32	33
Less than 20	67	57	56	55	61	59	60
Less than 25	84	80	74	83	80	82	81
Less than 30	93	91	86	93	90	92	91
All	100	100	100	100	100	100	100
Base	576	606	250	243	848	827	1675
Mean (average value)	17.3	19.3	20.3	19.2	18.8	18.6	18.7
Median value	16.4	18.8	18.8	18.9	17.5	18.2	17.8
Lower 2.5 percentile	5.1	6.4	7.8	8.0	6.1	5.4	5.8
Upper 2.5 percentile	36.5	34.7	37.4	35.6	37.0	34.5	35.6
Standard error of the mean	0.34	0.30	0.49	0.45	0.27	0.26	0.19

Table 6.16(a)   Contribution of food types to average daily intake of non-milk extrinsic sugars (g) by age and sex of child

Food types	Age and sex of child						
	All aged 1½ – 2½ years	All aged 2½ – 3½ years	All aged 3½ – 4½ years		All boys	All girls	All
			Boys	Girls			
	g	g	g	g	g	g	g
Cereals & cereal products	10.3	14.1	16.4	14.6	13.9	12.6	13.2
of which:							
white bread	0.0	0.0	0.0	0.0	0.0	0.0	0.0
wholemeal bread	0.0	0.0	0.0	0.0	0.0	0.0	0.0
high fibre & wholegrain							
* breakfast cereals*	0.6	0.8	1.0	0.8	0.8	0.8	0.8
other breakfast cereals	1.4	1.8	2.6	2.4	2.0	1.8	1.9
biscuits	3.3	4.7	5.3	4.0	4.6	3.9	4.2
Milk & milk products	3.2	2.8	2.6	2.5	2.8	2.9	2.9
of which:							
cows' milk	0.0	0.1	0.1	0.3	0.1	0.2	0.1
fromage frais & yogurt	2.6	2.4	2.0	1.9	2.2	2.4	2.3
Eggs & egg dishes	0.0	0.0	0.0	0.0	0.0	0.0	0.0
Fat spreads	—	—	—	—	—	—	—
Meat & meat products	0.1	0.1	0.1	0.2	0.1	0.1	0.1
Fish & fish dishes	0.0	0.0	0.0	0.0	0.0	0.0	0.0
Vegetables, potatoes & savoury snacks	0.6	0.6	0.6	0.6	0.6	0.6	0.6
of which:							
vegetables, excluding potatoes	0.6	0.6	0.6	0.6	0.6	0.6	0.6
potatoes, fried	0.0	0.0	0.0	0.0	0.0	0.0	0.0
other potatoes	0.0	0.0	0.0	0.0	0.0	0.0	0.0
savoury snacks	0.0	0.0	0.0	0.0	0.0	0.0	0.0
Fruit and nuts	0.6	0.6	0.6	0.6	0.6	0.6	0.6
of which							
fruit	0.5	0.6	0.6	0.5	0.6	0.6	0.6
nuts, fruit & nut mixes	0.0	0.0	0.0	0.1	0.0	0.0	0.0
Sugars, preserves & confectionery	12.1	16.4	20.3	17.7	16.5	14.8	15.7
of which:							
sugar	2.6	2.5	3.3	2.8	2.8	2.5	2.7
preserves	0.9	1.3	1.8	1.3	1.4	1.1	1.2
sugar confectionery	4.0	6.6	8.9	7.1	6.6	5.7	6.2
chocolate confectionery	4.5	6.0	6.2	6.4	5.7	5.4	5.6
Beverages	19.3	23.0	26.5	22.4	23.0	21.3	22.2
of which:							
fruit juice	3.4	3.6	3.1	2.8	3.1	3.6	3.4
soft drinks, not low calorie	15.4	18.6	22.7	18.8	19.2	17.1	18.2
Commercial infant foods & drinks	0.8	0.3	0.0	0.1	0.3	0.5	0.4
Miscellaneous	1.5	1.6	1.6	1.6	1.6	1.5	1.5
Average daily intake (g)	**48**	**60**	**69**	**60**	**59**	**55**	**57**
Total number of children	**576**	**606**	**250**	**243**	**848**	**827**	**1675**

Table 6.16(b)   Percentage contribution of food types to average daily intake of non-milk extrinsic sugars by age and sex of child

Food types	Age and sex of child						
	All aged 1½ – 2½ years	All aged 2½ – 3½ years	All aged 3½ – 4½ years		All boys	All girls	All
			Boys	Girls			
	%	%	%	%	%	%	%
Cereals & cereal products	21	24	24	24	23	23	23
of which:							
white bread	—	—	—	—	—	—	—
wholemeal bread	*0*	*0*	*0*	—	*0*	*0*	*0*
high fibre & wholegrain							
breakfast cereals	*1*	*1*	*1*	*1*	*1*	*1*	*1*
other breakfast cereals	*3*	*3*	*4*	*4*	*3*	*3*	*3*
biscuits	*7*	*8*	*8*	*7*	*8*	*7*	*7*
Milk & milk products	7	5	4	4	5	5	5
of which:							
cows' milk	*0*	*0*	*0*	*0*	*0*	*0*	*0*
fromage frais & yogurt	*5*	*4*	*3*	*3*	*4*	*4*	*4*
Eggs & egg dishes	0	0	0	0	0	0	0
Fat spreads	—	—	—	—	—	—	—
Meat & meat products	0	0	0	0	0	0	0
Fish & fish dishes	0	0	0	0	0	0	0
Vegetables, potatoes & savoury snacks	1	1	1	1	1	1	1
of which:							
vegetables, excluding potatoes	*1*	*1*	*1*	*1*	*1*	*1*	*1*
potatoes, fried	*0*	*0*	—	—	*0*	*0*	*0*
other potatoes	*0*	*0*	*0*	*0*	*0*	*0*	*0*
savoury snacks	*0*	*0*	*0*	*0*	*0*	*0*	*0*
Fruit and nuts	1	1	1	1	1	1	1
of which:							
fruit	*1*	*1*	*1*	*1*	*1*	*1*	*1*
nuts, fruit & nut mixes	*0*	*0*	*0*	*0*	*0*	*0*	*0*
Sugars, preserves & confectionery	25	27	29	28	27	27	27
of which:							
sugar	*5*	*4*	*5*	*5*	*5*	*5*	*5*
preserves	*2*	*2*	*3*	*2*	*2*	*2*	*2*
sugar confectionery	*8*	*11*	*13*	*12*	*11*	*10*	*11*
chocolate confectionery	*9*	*10*	*9*	*11*	*10*	*10*	*10*
Beverages	40	39	38	37	39	39	39
of which:							
fruit juice	*7*	*6*	*4*	*5*	*5*	*7*	*6*
soft drinks, not low calorie	*32*	*31*	*33*	*32*	*32*	*31*	*32*
Commercial infant foods & drinks	2	0	0	0	0	1	1
Miscellaneous	3	3	2	3	3	3	3
Average daily intake (g)	**48**	**60**	**69**	**60**	**59**	**55**	**57**
Total number of children	**576**	**606**	**250**	**243**	**848**	**827**	**1675**

Table 6.17   Average daily starch intake (g) by age and sex of child

Starch intake (g)	Age and sex of child						
	All aged 1½ – 2½ years	All aged 2½ – 3½ years	All aged 3½ – 4½ years		All boys	All girls	All
			Boys	Girls			
	cum %	cum %	cum %	cum %	cum %	cum %	cum %
Less than 40	15	7	2	1	7	9	8
Less than 50	34	17	8	10	18	23	21
Less than 70	74	51	34	45	49	62	55
Less than 85	90	80	64	73	77	82	80
Less than 100	97	93	84	89	90	94	92
All	100	100	100	100	100	100	100
Base	*576*	*606*	*250*	*243*	*848*	*827*	*1675*
Mean (average value)	59	70	79	74	71	66	68
Median value	56	70	79	72	70	64	67
Lower 2.5 percentile	24	31	40	42	30	29	30
Upper 2.5 percentile	103	115	125	120	116	115	116
Standard error of the mean	0.8	0.9	1.4	1.3	0.8	0.7	0.5

Table 6.18(a) Contribution of food types to average daily intake of starch (g) by age and sex of child

Food types	Age and sex of child						
	All aged 1½ – 2½ years	All aged 2½ – 3½ years	All aged 3½ – 4½ years		All boys	All girls	All
			Boys	Girls			
	g	g	g	g	g	g	g
Cereals & cereal products	36.7	44.7	51.5	47.0	45.2	41.4	43.3
of which:							
white bread	*10.2*	*13.4*	*17.0*	*15.6*	*13.4*	*12.9*	*13.2*
wholemeal bread	*2.6*	*2.4*	*3.2*	*2.8*	*2.7*	*2.6*	*2.6*
high fibre & wholegrain							
breakfast cereals	*5.7*	*6.0*	*6.1*	*4.4*	*6.4*	*5.0*	*5.7*
other breakfast cereals	*4.4*	*5.7*	*6.5*	*6.6*	*5.7*	*5.3*	*5.5*
biscuits	*4.3*	*5.4*	*6.6*	*4.9*	*5.6*	*4.7*	*5.1*
Milk & milk products	0.0	0.0	0.0	0.0	0.0	0.0	0.0
of which:							
cows' milk	*0.0*	*0.0*	*0.0*	*0.0*	*0.0*	*0.0*	*0.0*
fromage frais & yogurt	*0.0*	*0.0*	*0.0*	*0.0*	*0.0*	*0.0*	*0.0*
Eggs & egg dishes	0.1	0.2	0.2	0.1	0.1	0.1	0.1
Fat spreads	0.0	0.0	0.0	0.0	0.0	0.0	0.0
Meat & meat products	3.3	4.0	4.8	4.1	4.1	3.6	3.9
Fish & fish dishes	1.0	1.1	1.2	1.3	1.2	1.1	1.1
Vegetables, potatoes & savoury snacks	15.2	17.9	19.6	19.7	17.8	17.1	17.5
of which:							
vegetables, excluding potatoes	*1.9*	*2.0*	*1.9*	*1.9*	*2.0*	*1.8*	*1.9*
potatoes, fried	*5.6*	*6.8*	*8.1*	*8.2*	*7.1*	*6.4*	*6.8*
other potatoes	*3.5*	*3.5*	*3.9*	*4.1*	*3.5*	*3.8*	*3.7*
savoury snacks	*4.1*	*5.5*	*5.8*	*5.5*	*5.2*	*5.0*	*5.1*
Fruit and nuts	0.4	0.4	0.4	0.4	0.4	0.4	0.4
of which							
fruit	*0.4*	*0.3*	*0.4*	*0.3*	*0.4*	*0.3*	*0.3*
nuts, fruit & nut mixes	*0.0*	*0.0*	*0.0*	*0.1*	*0.0*	*0.0*	*0.0*
Sugars, preserves & confectionery	0.4	0.5	0.6	0.6	0.5	0.5	0.5
of which:							
sugar	*0.0*	*0.0*	*0.0*	*0.0*	*0.0*	*0.0*	*0.0*
preserves	*0.0*	*0.0*	*0.0*	*0.0*	*0.0*	*0.0*	*0.0*
sugar confectionery	*0.1*	*0.1*	*0.2*	*0.1*	*0.1*	*0.1*	*0.1*
chocolate confectionery	*0.2*	*0.4*	*0.4*	*0.4*	*0.4*	*0.3*	*0.4*
Beverages	0.0	0.0	0.0	0.0	0.0	0.0	0.0
of which:							
fruit juice	*0.0*	*0.0*	*0.0*	*0.0*	*0.0*	*0.0*	*0.0*
soft drinks, not low calorie	*0.0*	*0.0*	*0.0*	*0.0*	*0.0*	*0.0*	*0.0*
Commercial infant foods & drinks	0.5	0.1	0.1	0.1	0.2	0.2	0.2
Miscellaneous	1.1	1.1	1.0	1.1	1.1	1.1	1.1
Average daily intake (g)	**59**	**70**	**79**	**74**	**71**	**66**	**68**
Total number of children	**576**	**606**	**250**	**243**	**848**	**827**	**1675**

Table 6.18(b)   Percentage contribution of food types to average daily intake of starch by age and sex of child

Food types	All aged 1½–2½ years	All aged 2½–3½ years	All aged 3½–4½ years		All boys	All girls	All
			Boys	Girls			
	%	%	%	%	%	%	%
Cereals & cereal products	62	64	65	63	64	63	64
of which:							
white bread	17	19	21	21	19	20	19
wholemeal bread	4	3	4	4	4	4	4
high fibre & wholegrain							
breakfast cereals	10	9	8	6	9	8	8
other breakfast cereals	7	8	8	9	8	8	8
biscuits	7	8	8	7	8	7	7
Milk & milk products	0	0	0	0	0	0	0
of which:							
cows' milk	—	—	—	—	—	—	—
fromage frais & yogurt	0	0	0	0	0	0	0
Eggs & egg dishes	0	0	0	0	0	0	0
Fat spreads	—	—	—	—	—	—	—
Meat & meat products	6	6	6	5	6	5	6
Fish & fish dishes	2	2	1	2	2	2	2
Vegetables, potatoes & savoury snacks	26	25	25	26	25	26	26
of which:							
vegetables, excluding potatoes	3	3	2	3	3	3	3
potatoes, fried	9	10	10	11	10	10	10
other potatoes	6	5	5	5	5	6	5
savoury snacks	7	8	7	7	7	8	7
Fruit and nuts	1	1	1	1	1	1	1
of which:							
fruit	1	0	0	0	0	0	0
nuts, fruit & nut mixes	0	0	0	0	0	0	0
Sugars, preserves & confectionery	1	1	1	1	1	1	1
of which:							
sugar	—	0	—	—	0	0	0
preserves	0	0	0	0	0	0	0
sugar confectionery	0	0	0	0	0	0	0
chocolate confectionery	0	0	1	1	0	0	0
Beverages	0	0	0	0	0	0	0
of which:							
fruit juice	—	0	—	0	0	0	0
soft drinks, not low calorie	—	—	—	—	—	—	—
Commercial infant foods & drinks	1	0	0	0	0	0	0
Miscellaneous	2	2	1	1	1	2	2
Average daily intake (g)	**59**	**70**	**79**	**74**	**71**	**65**	**68**
Total number of children	**576**	**606**	**250**	**243**	**848**	**827**	**1675**

Table 6.19   Percentage of food energy from intrinsic and milk sugars and starch by age and sex of child

Percentage of food energy from intrinsic sugars, milk sugars and starch	All aged 1½–2½ years	All aged 2½–3½ years	All aged 3½–4½ years		All boys	All girls	All
			Boys	Girls			
	cum %	cum %	cum %	cum %	cum %	cum %	cum %
Less than 25	7	8	7	7	7	8	7
Less than 30	30	35	35	34	31	36	33
Less than 35	68	70	73	68	69	70	70
Less than 40	93	92	93	91	93	92	93
Less than 44	98	99	99	99	99	99	99
All	100	100	100	100	100	100	100
Base	576	606	250	243	848	827	1675
Mean (average value)	32.6	32.2	32.0	32.5	32.5	32.2	32.4
Median value	32.6	32.1	31.8	32.0	32.5	31.9	32.2
Lower 2.5 percentile	21.0	22.1	21.1	23.0	21.4	21.9	21.7
Upper 2.5 percentile	43.7	43.4	44.1	44.2	43.7	43.5	43.5
Standard error of the mean	0.23	0.22	0.34	0.35	0.19	0.19	0.13

Table 6.20 Average daily non-starch polysaccharides intake (g) by age and sex of child

Non-starch polysaccharides intake (g)	Age and sex of child						
	All aged 1½ – 2½ years	All aged 2½ – 3½ years	All aged 3½ – 4½ years		All boys	All girls	All
			Boys	Girls			
	cum %	cum %	cum %	cum %	cum %	cum %	cum %
Less than 3	8	6	3	4	4	8	6
Less than 5	46	31	23	32	31	40	35
Less than 7	77	66	60	65	66	72	69
Less than 9	94	88	84	87	89	90	89
Less than 11	98	96	94	97	96	97	97
All	100	100	100	100	100	100	100
Base	*576*	*606*	*250*	*243*	*848*	*827*	*1675*
Mean (average value)	5.5	6.2	6.8	6.4	6.3	5.9	6.1
Median value	5.2	6.0	6.5	6.2	6.0	5.9	5.8
Lower 2.5 percentile	2.0	2.6	2.9	2.7	2.6	2.4	2.5
Upper 2.5 percentile	10.5	12.0	12.5	11.3	12.0	11.3	11.4
Standard error of the mean	0.09	0.09	0.15	0.14	0.08	0.08	0.06

Table 6.21(a) Contributions of food types to average daily intake of non-starch polysaccharides (g) by age and sex of child

Food types	Age and sex of child						
	All aged 1½ – 2½ years	All aged 2½ – 3½ years	All aged 3½ – 4½ years		All boys	All girls	All
			Boys	Girls			
	%	%	%	%	%	%	%
Cereals & cereal products	2.4	2.7	3.1	2.7	2.8	2.5	2.6
of which:							
white bread	*0.3*	*0.4*	*0.6*	*0.5*	*0.4*	*0.4*	*0.4*
wholemeal bread	*0.4*	*0.3*	*0.4*	*0.4*	*0.4*	*0.4*	*0.4*
high fibre & wholegrain							
breakfast cereals	*0.8*	*0.8*	*0.9*	*0.6*	*0.9*	*0.7*	*0.8*
other breakfast cereals	*0.1*	*0.1*	*0.1*	*0.1*	*0.1*	*0.1*	*0.1*
biscuits	*0.2*	*0.3*	*0.4*	*0.3*	*0.3*	*0.2*	*0.3*
Milk & milk products	0.0	0.0	0.0	0.0	0.0	0.0	0.0
Eggs & egg dishes	0.0	0.0	0.0	0.0	0.0	0.0	0.0
Fat spreads	—	—	—	—	—	—	—
Meat & meat products	0.2	0.3	0.3	0.3	0.3	0.2	0.2
Fish & fish dishes	0.0	0.0	0.0	0.0	0.0	0.0	0.0
Vegetables, potatoes & savoury snacks	1.9	2.2	2.4	2.4	2.2	2.1	2.2
of which:							
vegetables, excluding potatoes	*1.0*	*1.0*	*1.1*	*1.1*	*1.0*	*1.0*	*1.0*
potatoes, fried	*0.4*	*0.5*	*0.6*	*0.6*	*0.5*	*0.5*	*0.5*
other potatoes	*0.3*	*0.3*	*0.3*	*0.3*	*0.3*	*0.3*	*0.3*
savoury snacks	*0.3*	*0.4*	*0.4*	*0.4*	*0.4*	*0.3*	*0.4*
Fruit and nuts	0.7	0.7	0.7	0.7	0.7	0.7	0.7
of which:							
fruit	*0.6*	*0.0*	*0.7*	*0.6*	*0.7*	*0.7*	*0.7*
nuts, fruit & nut mixes	*0.0*	*0.0*	*0.0*	*0.0*	*0.0*	*0.0*	*0.0*
Sugars, preserves & confectionery	0.1	0.1	0.2	0.1	0.1	0.1	0.1
Beverages	0.0	0.0	0.0	0.0	0.0	0.0	0.0
Commercial infant foods & drinks	0.0	0.0	0.0	0.0	0.0	0.0	0.0
Miscellaneous	0.1	0.1	0.1	0.1	0.1	0.1	0.1
Average daily intake (g)	**5**	**6**	**7**	**6**	**6**	**6**	**6**
Total number of children	**576**	**606**	**250**	**243**	**848**	**827**	**1675**

Table 6.21(b) Percentage contribution of food types to average daily intake of non-starch polysaccharides by age and sex of child

Food types	All aged 1½ – 2½ years	All aged 2½ – 3½ years	All aged 3½ – 4½ years		All boys	All girls	All
			Boys	Girls			
	%	%	%	%	%	%	%
Cereals & cereal products	43	43	45	42	44	42	43
of which:							
white bread	*6*	*7*	*8*	*8*	*7*	*7*	*7*
wholemeal bread	*7*	*5*	*6*	*6*	*6*	*6*	*6*
high fibre & wholegrain							
breakfast cereals	*14*	*13*	*13*	*10*	*14*	*11*	*12*
other breakfast cereals	*1*	*1*	*2*	*2*	*2*	*1*	*2*
biscuits	*4*	*5*	*5*	*4*	*5*	*4*	*5*
Milk & milk products	1	1	1	1	1	1	1
Eggs & egg dishes	0	0	0	0	0	0	0
Fat spreads	—	—	—	—	—	—	—
Meat & meat products	4	4	4	4	4	3	4
Fish & fish dishes	0	1	1	1	1	1	1
Vegetables, potatoes & savoury snacks	35	35	35	37	35	36	35
of which:							
vegetables, excluding potatoes	*18*	*17*	*16*	*17*	*16*	*17*	*17*
potatoes, fried	*7*	*8*	*9*	*9*	*8*	*8*	*8*
other potatoes	*5*	*4*	*4*	*5*	*4*	*5*	*5*
savoury snacks	*5*	*6*	*6*	*6*	*6*	*6*	*6*
Fruit and nuts	12	12	10	11	11	12	11
of which:							
fruit	*12*	*11*	*10*	*10*	*10*	*11*	*11*
nuts, fruit & nut mixes	*0*	*1*	*1*	*1*	*1*	*1*	*1*
Sugars, preserves & confectionery	1	2	2	2	2	2	2
Beverages	0	1	0	0	0	1	0
Commercial infant foods & drinks	1	0	0	0	0	0	0
Miscellaneous	2	2	1	2	1	2	2
Average daily intake (g)	**5**	**6**	**7**	**6**	**6**	**6**	**6**
Total number of children	**576**	**606**	**250**	**243**	**848**	**827**	**1675**

Table 6.22 Average number of bowel movements per day during dietary recording period by age and sex of child

Average number of bowel movements per day	All aged 1½ – 2½ years	All aged 2½ – 3½ years	All aged 3½ – 4½ years		All boys	All girls	All
			Boys	Girls			
	%	%	%	%	%	%	%
Fewer than 1 a day	13	23	26	30	19	23	21
1 a day	22	27	28	26	24	26	25
More than 1, fewer than 2 a day	45	36	35	36	40	38	39
2 a day	6	6	5	2	6	4	5
More than 2, fewer than 3 a day	10	5	3	4	7	6	6
3 or more a day	2	1	2	2	1	2	2
Not known	2	2	2	1	2	1	2
Base = 100%	*576*	*606*	*250*	*243*	*848*	*827*	*1675*

Table 6.23 Average number of bowel movements per day during dietary recording period by average daily intake of non-starch polysaccharides (g)

Average number of bowel movements per day	Average daily intake of non-starch polysaccharides (g)			
	Mean	*Median*	*se*	*Base*
Fewer than 1 a day	5.6	5.3	0.11	*353*
1 a day	6.1	5.8	0.12	*420*
More than 1, fewer than 2 a day	6.2	6.0	0.09	*653*
2 a day	6.4	6.1	0.29	*89*
More than 2, fewer than 3 a day	6.6	6.5	0.22	*108*
3 or more a day	6.7	6.1	0.54	*27*
All children*	6.1	5.8	0.06	*1675*

*Includes those for whom number of bowel movements was not known.

Table 6.24 Average daily intake of protein and carbohydrates (g) by whether child was reported as being unwell during dietary recording period

Nutrient	Whether child reported as unwell during dietary recording period								
	Unwell and eating affected			Unwell and eating not affected			Not unwell		
	Mean	*Median*	*se*	*Mean*	*Median*	*se*	*Mean*	*Median*	*se*
Protein (g)	34	33	0.7	36	35	0.7	38	36	0.3
Carbohydrate (g)	138	137	2.5	150	144	2.5	160	156	1.1
Carbohydrate as % food energy	51	51	0.4	51	51	0.4	51	51	0.2
Total sugars (g)	77	74	1.8	85	79	1.9	90	86	0.8
Non-milk extrinsic sugars (g)	50	46	1.6	54	50	1.7	59	56	0.8
Starch (g)	61	59	1.3	65	62	1.5	70	69	0.6
Non-starch polysaccharides (g)	5.4	5.1	0.13	6.1	5.8	0.17	6.2	6.0	0.07
Base	*266*			*190*			*1219*		

Table 6.25 Average daily intake of protein and carbohydrates (g) by region

Nutrient	Region											
	Scotland			Northern			Central, South West and Wales			London and South East		
	Mean	*Median*	*se*	*Mean*	*Median*	*se*	*Mean*	*Median*	*se*	*Mean*	*Median*	*se*
Protein (g)	37	36	0.8	36	36	0.5	37	36	0.4	37	36	0.4
Carbohydrate (g)	155	152	3.0	158	156	2.0	157	152	1.6	152	147	1.7
Carbohydrate as % food energy	51	51	0.5	51	51	0.3	51	52	0.3	51	51	0.3
Total sugars (g)	87	83	2.3	89	83	1.5	86	84	1.2	86	82	1.3
Non-milk extrinsic sugars (g)	57	54	2.0	60	55	1,4	57	53	1.1	56	52	1.3
Starch (g)	69	67	1.7	69	67	1.1	70	68	1.0	65	64	0.9
Non-starch polysaccharides (g)	5.7	5.4	0.17	6.1	5.9	0.11	6.2	6.0	0.09	6.0	5.7	0.10
Base	*165*			*427*			*563*			*520*		

Table 6.26 Average daily intake of protein and carbohydrates (g) by mother's highest educational qualification level

Nutrient	Mother's highest educational qualification level														
	Above GCE 'A' level			GCE 'A' level and equivalent			GCE 'O' level and equivalent			CSE and equivalent			None		
	Mean	*Median*	*se*	*Mean*	*Median*	*se*	*Mean*	*Median*	*se*	*Mean*	*Median*	*se*	*Mean*	*Median*	*se*
Protein (g)	38	38	0.5	38	37	0.8	36	35	0.4	36	35	0.7	37	36	0.6
Carbohydrate (g)	155	153	2.1	154	149	2.8	156	151	1.7	154	150	2.6	155	151	2.1
Carbohydrate as % food energy	51	51	0.4	51	51	0.5	52	52	0.2	51	52	0.4	50	50	0.3
Total sugars (g)	91	87	1.6	88	87	2.1	88	82	1.3	84	80	1.9	84	80	1.5
Non-milk extrinsic sugars (g)	57	54	1.5	56	53	2.0	59	54	1.2	56	54	1.8	56	51	1.4
Starch (g)	64	63	1.1	66	63	1.5	68	67	0.9	70	68	1.5	72	70	1.2
Non-starch polysaccharides (g)	6.7	6.3	0.14	6.5	6.7	0.18	5.9	5.7	0.089	5.9	5.6	0.15	5.7	5.5	0.11
Base	*305*			*183*			*590*			*236*			*358*		

Table 6.27 Average daily intake of protein and carbohydrates (g) by employment status of head of household

Nutrient	Employment status of head of household								
	Working			Unemployed			Economically inactive		
	Mean	*Median*	*se*	*Mean*	*Median*	*se*	*Mean*	*Median*	*se*
Protein (g)	37	36	0.3	37	36	1.0	37	36	0.7
Carbohydrate (g)	155	150	1.1	154	153	3.3	157	155	2.6
Carbohydrate as % food energy	51	52	0.2	50	51	0.5	50	51	0.4
Total sugars (g)	89	84	0.8	83	80	2.3	82	79	1.8
Non-milk extrinsic sugars (g)	58	54	0.8	55	53	2.1	54	50	1.6
Starch (g)	66	65	0.6	72	68	2.0	76	76	1.5
Non-starch polysaccharides (g)	6.1	5.8	0.06	5.9	5.6	0.19	6.1	5.8	0.14
Base		*1249*			*167*			*259*	

Table 6.28 Average daily intake of protein and carbohydrates (g) by social class of head of household

Nutrient	Social class of head of household					
	Non-manual			Manual		
	Mean	*Median*	*se*	*Mean*	*Median*	*se*
Protein (g)	38	36	0.4	36	36	0.4
Carbohydrate (g)	154	150	1.4	156	153	1.3
Carbohydrate as % food energy	51	51	0.2	51	52	0.2
Total sugars (g)	88	84	1.1	87	83	1.0
Non-milk extrinsic sugars (g)	56	52	1.0	59	55	1.0
Starch (g)	66	65	0.8	70	68	0.8
Non-starch polysaccharides (g)	6.4	6.0	0.09	5.8	5.6	0.07
Base		*748*			*867*	

Table 6.29 Average daily intake of protein and carbohydrates (g) by whether child's parents were receiving Income Support or Family Credit

Nutrient	Whether receiving benefit(s)					
	Receiving benefit(s)			Not receiving benefits		
	Mean	*Median*	*se*	*Mean*	*Median*	*se*
Protein (g)	37	36	0.5	37	36	0.3
Carbohydrate (g)	157	155	1.8	154	150	1.1
Carbohydrate as % food energy	51	51	0.3	51	51	0.2
Total sugars (g)	83	81	1.3	89	84	0.9
Non-milk extrinsic sugars (g)	55	52	1.2	58	54	0.8
Starch (g)	74	71	1.0	66	64	0.6
Non-starch polysaccharides (g)	6.0	5.7	0.10	6.1	5.9	0.07
Base		*534*			*1140*	

Table 6.30 Average daily intake of protein and carbohydrates (g) by family type

Nutrient	Family type											
	Married or cohabiting couple						Lone parent					
	1 child			More than one child			1 child			More than one child		
	Mean	*Median*	*se*	*Mean*	*Median*	*se*	*Mean*	*Median*	*se*	*Mean*	*Median*	*se*
Protein (g)	37	37	0.5	36	36	0.3	38	38	1.1	37	36	0.8
Carbohydrate (g)	150	148	2.0	156	153	1.2	159	156	4.1	158	155	3.1
Carbohydrate as % food energy	51	51	0.3	51	52	0.2	51	50	0.5	51	52	0.5
Total sugars (g)	88	84	1.5	88	84	0.9	86	82	3.0	81	76	2.2
Non-milk extrinsic sugars (g)	55	50	1.5	59	55	0.9	57	54	2.7	53	48	2.0
Starch (g)	62	61	1.0	68	67	0.7	74	72	2.1	77	76	1.9
Non-starch polysaccharides (g)	5.9	5.7	0.12	6.1	5.9	0.07	6.3	6.0	0.22	6.1	5.7	0.17
Base		*366*			*1011*			*121*			*177*	

7 Nutrient intake: fat and fatty acids

7.1 Introduction: current recommendations on fat intake for adults and children

Dietary fat is a high density source of energy and carrier of fat soluble vitamins. In the diets of infant and young children, it helps to ensure that even small eaters obtain adequate energy intakes without having to consume a bulky diet.

Breast-fed infants derive about 50% food energy from fat[1]. Adults in this country derive about 40% energy from fat but there is considerable individual variation[2]. The kinds and amounts of fats in the diet directly influence levels of cholesterol in the blood. As a result, several expert groups, including COMA in 1991[3] and 1994[4] have recommended moderation in total fat and in saturated fatty acid intakes to the extent that total fat contributes an average of about 35% of food energy and saturated fatty acids an average of about 10%. Consumption of *trans* fatty acids is recommended not to rise further than the current average of about 2% of food energy.

These recommendations were formulated for adults. Dietary fat intake in children, its relationship with plasma cholesterol and the significance of any long-term effects are less well researched, but some data are available. It is recommended that these dietary patterns of fat intake are appropriate for the whole population of children by the age of 5 years. Thus, between the age of infancy to the age of 5 years there is an expectation that the proportion of energy from dietary fat will fall from 50%, as supplied by breast feeding or infant formula, to 35% and that the rate of change will depend on individual factors. Dietary manipulation for the purpose of moderating dietary fat intake should not begin below the age of 2 years[5]. A flexible approach is encouraged to the timing and extent of dietary change for individual children between the age of 2 and 5 years. The maintenance of adequate energy intakes must be paramount in determining the composition of the diet at these ages. While some children from 2 years may consume a diverse diet and can accept a planned reduction in fat intake, for example by the consumption of semi-skimmed rather than whole cows' milk, others may best delay dietary changes until closer to the age of 5 years if their energy requirements for growth and health are to be maintained.

This chapter presents data on the children's intakes of total fat, saturated, *trans* and *cis* monounsaturated, and polyunsaturated fatty acids and cholesterol. Figure 7.1 shows the intakes of fat and fatty acids by children in the survey[6]. In Figure 7.2 the proportional contribution of each of the fatty acids to the food energy derived from fat is shown. *(Figs 7.1 and 7.2)*

The intakes of the individual fatty acids and the proportion of food energy derived from them are discussed in the sections below. Results are also given which show the food sources of total fat and fatty acids and variations in intake by demographic and socio-economic characteristics of the children and their households.

7.2 Total fat

The average daily total fat intake for all children in the sample was 45.7g (median 44.4g). Mean intakes increased with age, with the difference in intake between the two youngest cohorts being particularly marked (p<0.01); overall, boys had somewhat higher average daily total fat intakes than girls (p<0.05). Children at the lower 2.5 percentile of the distribution had intakes about half the median amount while those at the upper 2.5 percentile had intakes ranging between 68.6g for children aged 1½ to 2½ years to 82.4g for boys aged 3½ to 4½ years. *(Table 7.1; Figs 7.3 and 7.4)*

Overall an average of 36% of energy was derived from fat. Although older children had higher dietary intakes of total fat, they tended to derive a smaller proportion of their energy from fat than those in the younger groups; for example 56% of children aged between 2½ and 4½ years derived 35% or more food energy from total fat compared with 61% of younger children (NS). Table 7.2 shows that overall about 5% of children were deriving 45% or more of their energy from fat. *(Table 7.2)*

The contribution of total fat, and the other macro-nutrients (protein and carbohydrate) to total food energy is shown in Figure 6.3 and Table 6.5.

Table 7.3 shows mean total fat intake for children in four surveys carried out since the early 1950s; in 1951[7], 1963[8], 1967/8[9] and this current NDNS in 1992/3. Although the age groupings used on the different surveys are not fully comparable, the data suggest that between 1951 and 1992/3[10] the mean intake of total fat by preschool age children declined and there was an accompanying reduction in the proportion of energy derived from fat of the order of 3% to 4%. *(Table 7.3)*

7.3 Saturated fatty acids

About 45% of the total fat intake of children in this survey came from saturated fatty acids. Thus the mean saturated fatty acid intake was 20.6g (median 20.0g), and like total fat intake, intakes of saturated fatty acids tended to increase with age. Differences by age cohort

were more marked at the higher intakes; for example at the upper 2.5 percentile children aged 1½ to 2½ years had an average intake of 33.4g compared with 36.9g by boys aged 3½ to 4½ years. There was no significant difference in mean intake between boys and girls in the sample.
(Table 7.4)

Table 7.5 shows overall children in this survey were deriving 16% of their food energy from saturated fatty acids. As was found in relation to total fat, for saturated fatty acids the proportion of energy derived from this source tended to be higher among the younger children; for example, among children aged 1½ to 2½ years 16.9% of energy was derived from saturated fatty acids compared with 15.5% for children aged 3½ to 4½ years (p<0.01). *(Table 7.5)*

7.4 Trans unsaturated fatty acids *(trans* fatty acids)

Mean intake of *trans* fatty acids by children in the survey was 2.2g (median 2.0g), representing about 5% of total fat intake ranging between the lower and upper 2.5 percentiles from 0.8g to 4.6g. Boys had greater mean intakes than girls (p<0.01). Intakes increased significantly with age, especially at higher intakes; thus 25% of boys aged 3½ to 4½ years had an average daily intake of 3g or more compared with 12% of children aged 1½ to 2½ years (p<0.01). *(Table 7.6)*

Table 7.7 shows that children were, on average, deriving 1.7% of their food energy from the consumption of *trans* fatty acids and that despite the marked variation in absolute intakes by age and sex there was no similar variation with respect to the percentage of energy derived from this source. *(Table 7.7)*

7.5 *Cis* monounsaturated fatty acids

The average daily intake of *cis* monounsaturated fatty acids by children in the sample was 14.2g (median 13.7g) representing about 30% of total fat intake. In common with total fat and other fatty acids average intakes of *cis* monounsaturated fatty acids increased with age and boys had higher average intakes than girls (p<0.05). Average intakes at the lower 2.5 percentile were about half the median value. *(Table 7.8)*

Table 7.9 shows that overall children were deriving about 11% of their food energy from *cis* monounsaturated fatty acids.

Again although there were significant variations in absolute intake associated with age and sex, these were largely associated with differences in energy intake and not the result of differences in the nutrient density of *cis* monounsaturated fatty acids in the foods eaten by different groups of children. *(Table 7.9)*

7.6 Polyunsaturated fatty acids

Cis polyunsaturated fatty acids can be divided into two groups, *cis* n-3 and *cis* n-6 polyunsaturates. Fish oils are the richest source of cis n-3 polyunsaturates; *cis* n-6 polyunsaturated fatty acids are mainly found in plant oils, including soya, corn and sunflower oils.

7.6.1 Cis n-3 polyunsaturated fatty acids

Average daily intakes of *cis* n-3 polyunsaturated fatty acids ranged from 0.8g for children aged 1½ to 2½ years to 1.0g for boys aged 3½ to 4½ years (p<0.05), with a mean for all children in the survey of 0.9g (median 0.8g). *(Table 7.10)*

Overall only about 0.7% of food energy was derived from *cis* n-3 polyunsaturated fatty acids; there was no difference in this proportion between boys and girls nor any significant variation by age.

The COMA Panel on Dietary Reference Values in its Report[3] recommended that '...for infants, children and adults linoleic acid (*cis* n-6) should provide at least 1% of total energy and alpha linolenic acid (*cis* n-3) at least 0.2% of total energy'. Less than 0.5% of children in this survey recorded intakes of total *cis* n-3 polyunsaturated fatty acids below this. *(Table 7.11)*

7.6.2 Cis n-6 polyunsaturated fatty acids

Average intakes of *cis* n-6 polyunsaturated fatty acids were much higher than intakes of *cis* n-3 polyunsaturated fatty acids. The overall mean intake was 5.0g (median 4.7g) representing about 11% of total fat intake. As with *cis* n-3 polyunsaturates, mean intakes of *cis* n-6 polyunsaturated fatty acids increased with age from 4.3g among the youngest children to 5.8g by boys aged 3½ to 4½ years (p<0.01). *(Table 7.12)*

The differences between the age groups were not attributable solely to variation in energy intake, since, as can be seen from Table 7.13, they remained after adjusting for this variation. Thus the oldest group of children were deriving 4.1% of their food energy from *cis* n-6 polyunsaturated fatty acids, compared with 3.7% for children aged between 1½ and 2½ years (p<0.01). Overall, children in this survey were deriving just under 4% of their energy from this source. At the lower 2.5 percentile 1.8% of food energy was from *cis* n-6 polyunsaturated fatty acids, which is above the DRV individual minimum for children recommended by the Panel on Dietary Reference Values (1%)[3]. *(Table 7.13)*

Total intake of *cis* polyunsaturated fatty acids (*cis* n-3 plus *cis* n-6) and the percentage of energy they provided for children in the survey is shown in Table 7.14.
(Table 7.14)

7.7 Cholesterol

Dietary cholesterol has a small effect on plasma cholesterol levels. There are no DRVs for cholesterol.

The average daily intake of cholesterol was 138mg (median 125mg). Mean intakes again increased with age (p<0.05), but overall boys and girls had very similar mean intakes. *(Table 7.15)*

7.8 Sources of fat in the diet

Tables 7.16 to 7.21 show the sources of total fat and fatty acids in the diets of the children by age and sex and their contribution to total fat intake.

7.8.1 Total fat, saturated, trans unsaturated and cis monounsaturated fatty acids

The three main sources of total fat, saturated, *trans* unsaturated ('*trans* fatty acids'), and *cis* monounsaturated fatty acids, were milk and milk products, cereals and cereal products, and meat and meat products. The contribution made by both milk and milk products, and by cereals and cereal products to intakes of total fat and these fatty acids showed a consistent trend associated with age. For milk and milk products the contribution fell as the children got older while for cereals and cereal products the reverse was seen with the proportion of the intake derived from this source increasing with age.

Overall milk and milk products accounted for 27% of total fat intake (*Table 7.16 b*), a similar proportion of the total intake of *trans* fatty acids (*Table 7.18 b*), and a slightly smaller proportion of *cis* monounsaturated fatty acids intake (23%) (*Table 7.19 b*); for saturated fatty acids the proportion of intake derived from milk and milk products was higher, 38% (*Table 7.17 b*). In each case the major part of the contribution came from the consumption of cows' milk.

Compared with children in the 1967/8 survey[9], children in 1992/3 were getting about the same proportion of their total fat intake from meat and meat products, but biscuits and cakes, fats and oils and eggs and eggs dishes all accounted for much smaller proportions of dietary fat intake than in 1967/8. In both surveys cows' milk was the main contributor to total fat intake, and although the proportion contributed to total fat intake by milk for the youngest children was about the same in both surveys, for other children the proportional contribution made by cows' milk has become less since 1967/8.

(Figs 7.5 to 7.7)

Overall children in the survey were deriving about 20% of their intake of total fat, saturated and *cis* monounsaturated fatty acids from cereals and cereal products. Milk and milk products and cereals and cereal products each contributed 28% of total *trans* fatty acids intake.

Meat and meat products contributed a slightly greater proportion to total *cis* monounsaturated fatty acids intake than did cereal products, 20% and 18% respectively. For total fat, saturated, and *trans* fatty acids about 15% of total intake came from the consumption of meat and meat products. Except for *trans* fatty acids there was an indication that in each case the contribution made by meat and meat products to total intake increased slightly with age (NS).

Vegetables, especially fried potatoes and savoury snacks, also contributed significant amounts to the intake of total fat, saturated and *cis* monounsaturated fatty acids (13%, 10% and 16% respectively). In each case the consumption of fried potatoes (mainly as chips[11]) and savoury snacks accounted for nearly all of this.

The consumption of fat spreads by the children contributed 14% to the overall total intake of *trans* fatty acids and the data suggest that the proportion increased with age. For total fat, saturated and *cis* monounsaturated fatty acids the contribution made to total intake by fat spreads was much smaller, no more than 9%.

(Tables 7.16 to 7.19)

7.8.2 Cis n-3 and n-6 polyunsaturated fatty acids

The principal contribution to total intake of *cis* n-3 polyunsaturated fatty acids, accounting for 28%, came from the consumption of vegetables, including potatoes and savoury snacks. The vegetables food type was also the main contributor to total intake of *cis* n-6 polyunsaturated fatty acids (24%). The contribution from all vegetables to total *cis* n-3 fatty acids intake was 0.24g/d compared with 1.2g/d for *cis* n-6 fatty acids.

The other principal sources of *cis* n-3 fatty acids were cereals and cereal products (14%), fish and fish dishes (13%) and milk and milk products (11%). Of these, only the milks food type showed any marked association with age, the proportion of total intake decreasing as the children got older.

The consumption of cereals and cereal products also made a significant contribution to the total average daily intake of *cis* n-6 fatty acids (22%). Fat spreads accounted for a similar proportion (20%) and meat and meat products, a further 14% overall. The contribution to total intake made by these three main food types showed no clear association with age. *(Tables 7.20 and 7.21)*

7.9 Variation in intake of fat

Children reported as being unwell

Children who were reported as being unwell had lower mean daily intakes of total fat and all fatty acids than other children; this generally applied whether or not their eating was reported to have been affected by their illness[12]. For example, the average daily intake of total fat by children whose eating was affected was 41g, compared with 44g for those whose eating was not affected (p<0.05) and 47g for those who were not reported as being unwell (p<0.01).

However when variation in energy intake was controlled, these differences were no longer evident.

(Table 7.22)

Region

There were very few differences in average intake of fat or fatty acids between children living in different parts of Great Britain. Compared with average values for all children, absolute intakes of *trans* fatty acids were higher for children living in the Northern region of England (p<0.01) and children in London and the South East had significantly lower intakes of *cis* monounsaturated fatty acids than other children (p<0.05). However most of these differences were associated with differences in energy intake between children living in different parts of Great Britain and not differences in the nutrient density of their diet in relation to fatty acids.

(Table 7.23)

Socio-economic characteristics

The data showed a generally consistent pattern for intakes of total fat and certain fatty acids to be higher for children from less economically advantaged backgrounds. In particular both the absolute intake and the percentage of energy derived from *cis* monounsaturated fatty acids was significantly higher among children from a manual home background, from households where Family Credit or Income Support were being received, where the head was economically inactive and from households where the mother had no formal educational qualifications (compared to all children: p<0.01). Absolute intakes of total fat were generally higher for these children, but apart from the group whose mothers had no formal educational qualifications, who derived significantly more energy from total fat than other children, the percentage energy from total fat was similar to that of other groups of children in the survey. Children from households on benefit and where the head was economically inactive also had higher average daily intakes of both *cis* n-3 and *cis* n-6 polyunsaturated fatty acids, but the percentage of energy derived from these was not markedly higher than for other children.

(Tables 7.24 to 7.27)

Family type

Table 7.28 shows a pattern of higher intakes of total fat and each fatty acid by children in lone parent families compared with children in two-parent families, and a general tendency for children with sisters or brothers to have somewhat higher intakes than children with no siblings. Some differences in the percentage of energy derived from total fat and fatty acids between the groups were evident but were small except in respect of *cis* monounsaturated fatty acids, where children from lone parent families with brothers or sisters were obtaining 11.7% energy compared with 11.0% for all children in two-parent households (p<0.01). *(Table 7.28)*

7.10 Variation in sources of fat in the diet

Tables 7.29 to 7.46 compare the sources of fat in the diet of children within the sample, by region, social class of head of household, and mother's highest educational qualification level.

Tables 7.29 to 7.34 show that there were differences in the contribution made by different food types to the total intake of fat and individual fatty acids for children living in different parts of Great Britain.

For example, children in London and the South East obtained more of their total intake of total fat, saturated, *trans* and *cis* monounsaturated fatty acids from milk and milk products than other children. These same children also derived more of their *trans* and *cis* n-6 fatty acid intake from cereals and cereal products, the differences largely being attributable to their consumption of buns, cakes and pastries. Compared with other children, those living in Scotland and the Northern region of England derived a larger proportion of their intake of total fat, saturated and *trans* fatty acids from meat and meat products. For children in Scotland, compared with those living in London and the South East, the consumption of

fried potatoes also contributed a greater proportion of their total intake of total fat, and all the individual fatty acids. *(Tables 7.29 to 7.34)*

Generally there were few statistically significant differences in the sources of total fat and fatty acids associated with the social class of the child's head of household, although the data suggest some consistent trends and there were some associations with the mother's highest educational qualification level. For example, there was a tendency for milk and milk products and cereals and cereal products to contribute more to the overall intake of total fat and individual fatty acids of children from a non-manual background than a manual home background. Conversely the contribution made by meat and meat products to total intake was greater for children from manual rather than non-manual backgrounds (NS). For all three major food types associations were also found with the mother's educational level; thus children whose mothers had no formal qualifications generally derived more of their intake of fatty acids from meat and meat products and less from cereals and cereal products, and from milk and milk products than children whose mothers had higher level qualifications. For *trans* fatty acids these differences in the contribution made by both cereals and cereal products and by meat and meat products were particularly marked (p<0.05).

Vegetables tended to be a more important source of total fat and all fatty acids except *trans* fatty acids, for both the manual group and children whose mothers had no qualifications with almost all the difference between these children and others being accounted for by the contribution to intake from the consumption of chips and other fried potatoes and savoury snacks.

(Tables 7.35 to 7.46)

References and notes

1 Department of Health and Social Security. Report on Health and Social Subjects: 12. *The Composition of Mature Human Milk.* HMSO (London, 1977).

2 Gregory J, Foster K, Tyler H, Wiseman M. *The Dietary and Nutritional Survey of British Adults.* HMSO (London, 1990).

3 Department of Health and Social Security. Report on Health and Social Subjects: 41. *Dietary Reference Values for Food Energy and Nutrients for the United Kingdom.* HMSO (London, 1991).

4 Department of Health. Report on Health and Social Subjects: 46. *Nutritional Aspects of Cardiovascular Disease.* HMSO (London, 1994).

5 Department of Health. Report on Health and Social Subjects: 45. *Weaning and the Weaning Diet.* HMSO (London, 1994).

6 The fat in most foods is a mixture of triglycerides (1 unit glycerol with 3 fatty acids), phospholipids, sterols and related compounds. Total fat relates to all of these and not just the fatty acids measured separately in the survey.

7 Bransby ER and Fothergill JE. The diets of young children. *Br J Nutr.* 1954; **8:** 195–204.

8 Ministry of Health. Reports on Public Health and Medical Subjects: 118. *A Pilot Survey of the Nutrition of Young Children in 1963.* HMSO (London, 1968).

9 Department of Health. Report on Health and Social Subjects: 10. *A Nutrition Survey of Pre-school Children, 1967–68.* HMSO (London, 1975).

10 The 1951 survey was a small study of only 461 children living in a small number of areas and fieldwork covered only one month of the year. Rationing was still in force at the time of the survey and the food composition tables used were different from those subsequently used. The 1963 survey was a pilot study for the later 1967/8 national survey. Estimates from the 1967/8 survey are likely to be more reliable than those from either the 1951 or 1963 surveys.

11 The average amount of 'fried potatoes' eaten by children, who consumed them during the dietary recording period was 27g; 20g of this amount was chips. The remainder was consumed as other fried potatoes, such as croquettes, waffles, Hash Browns, and roast potatoes, which because of their fat content are classified to this subgroup.

12 Average daily intakes for children reported as being unwell whose eating was affected were significantly lower than those of children not reported as being unwell: p<0.01 for total fat and all fatty acids except *cis* n– 3 polyunsaturated fatty acids where p<0.05.

Comparisons between those whose eating was apparently unaffected by illness and those not unwell generally showed less marked differences: p<0.05 for total fat, saturated and *trans* fatty acids; p<0.05 for *cis* monounsaturated fatty acids; for *cis* polyunsaturated fatty acids p>0.05 (NS).

Figure 7.1 Intake of fat and fatty acids (g) by age and sex of child

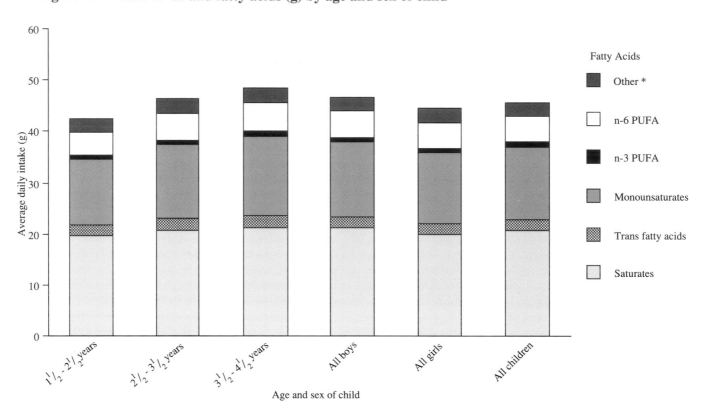

* See note (6) to text

Figure 7.2 Contribution of fatty acids to energy derived from total fat intake (per cent): all children

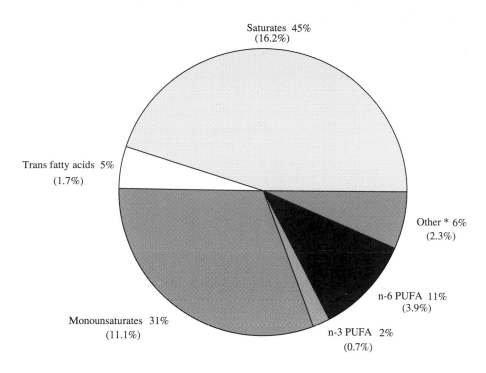

Saturates 45%
(16.2%)

Trans fatty acids 5%
(1.7%)

Other * 6%
(2.3%)

n-6 PUFA 11%
(3.9%)

n-3 PUFA 2%
(0.7%)

Monounsaturates 31%
(11.1%)

% in brackets = contribution to total food energy intake; total fat provided 36% of food energy

* See note (6) to text

Figure 7.3 Average daily fat intake by sex of child

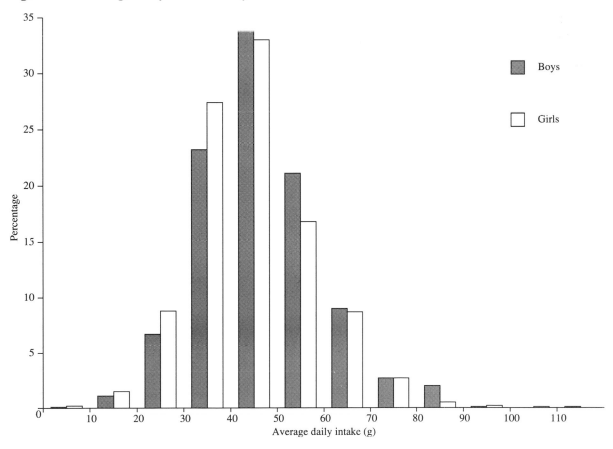

Boys

Girls

Percentage

Average daily intake (g)

Figure 7.4 Average daily fat intake by age of child

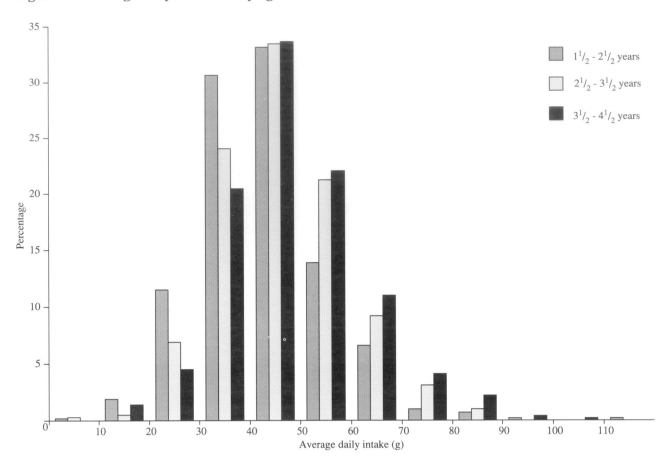

Legend:
- 1½ - 2½ years
- 2½ - 3½ years
- 3½ - 4½ years

Y-axis: Percentage
X-axis: Average daily intake (g)

Figure 7.5 Percentage contribution of some food types to total fat intake, 1992/3* and 1967/8: children aged 1½ - 2½ years**

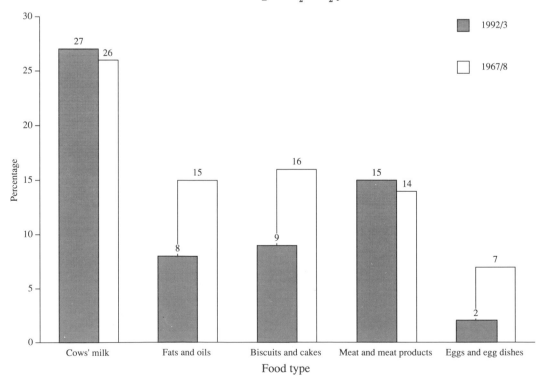

Legend:
- 1992/3
- 1967/8

Y-axis: Percentage
X-axis: Food type

Categories and values:
- Cows' milk: 27, 26
- Fats and oils: 8, 15
- Biscuits and cakes: 9, 16
- Meat and meat products: 15, 14
- Eggs and egg dishes: 2, 7

* NDNS 1992/3
** Department of Health and Social Security (1975)

Figure 7.6 Percentage contribution of some food types to total fat intake, 1992/3* and 1967/8**: children aged $2^1/_2$ - $3^1/_2$ years

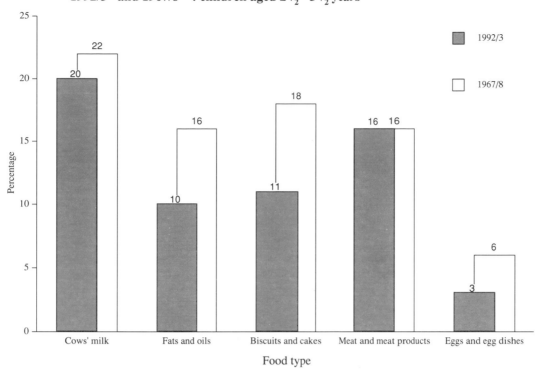

* NDNS 1992/3
** Department of Health and Social Security (1975)

Figure 7.7 Percentage contribution of some food types to total fat intake, 1992/3* and 1967/8**: children aged $3^1/_2$ - $4^1/_2$ years

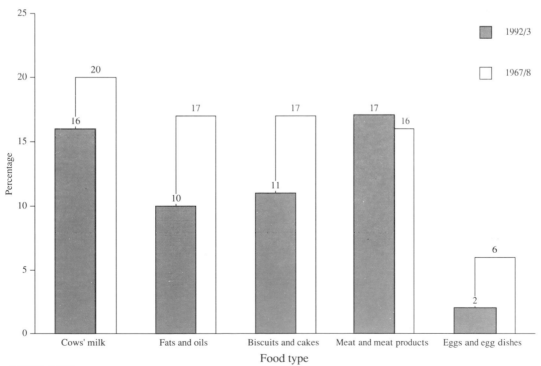

* NDNS 1992/3
** Department of Health and Social Security (1975)

Table 7.1 Average daily total fat intake (g) by age and sex of child

Total fat intake (g)	Age and sex of child						
	All aged 1½ – 2½ years	All aged 2½ – 3½ years	All aged 3½ – 4½ years		All boys	All girls	All
			Boys	Girls			
	cum %	cum %	cum %	cum %	cum %	cum %	cum %
Less than 25	6	3	2	2	3	4	3
Less than 35	28	17	8	16	16	23	19
Less than 45	62	49	40	49	49	56	52
Less than 55	86	79	69	74	77	81	79
Less than 65	95	92	86	88	92	92	92
All	100	100	100	100	100	100	100
Base	576	606	250	243	848	827	1675
Mean (average value)	42.5	46.3	50.1	47.2	46.7	44.6	45.7
Median value	41.5	45.2	48.4	45.2	45.1	43.5	44.4
Lower 2.5 percentile	20.2	23.9	28.9	22.9	24.1	22.4	23.2
Upper 2.5 percentile	68.6	73.7	82.4	74.2	78.0	72.3	74.8
Standard error of the mean	0.52	0.50	0.85	0.87	0.45	0.45	0.32

Table 7.2 Percentage food energy intake from total fat by age and sex of child

Percentage food energy intake from total fat	Age and sex of child						
	All aged 1½ – 2½ years	All aged 2½ – 3½ years	All aged 3½ – 4½ years		All boys	All girls	All
			Boys	Girls			
	cum %	cum %	cum %	cum %	cum %	cum %	cum %
Less than 25	3	1	3	2	3	2	2
Less than 30	13	11	15	14	14	11	13
Less than 35	39	44	44	44	42	42	42
Less than 40	73	81	84	81	79	78	79
Less than 45	94	95	97	97	96	95	95
All	100	100	100	100	100	100	100
Base	576	606	250	243	848	827	1675
Mean (average value)	36.4	35.8	35.3	35.5	35.7	36.1	35.9
Median value	36.6	35.9	35.7	35.8	36.0	36.1	36.0
Lower 2.5 percentile	24.7	25.3	23.9	24.6	24.6	25.2	25.0
Upper 2.5 percentile	47.2	46.2	45.2	45.2	45.6	46.7	46.0
Standard error of the mean	0.23	0.21	0.32	0.32	0.18	0.18	0.13

Table 7.3 Mean daily total fat intake and percentage of food energy from fat for children in four surveys: 1951 (Bransby and Fothergill, 1954); 1963 (Ministry of Health, 1968); 1967/8 (Department of Health, 1975) and 1992/3 (this NDNS survey)

	1951 B & F	1963 MoH	1967/8 DH	1992/3 NDNS	1951 B & F	1963 MoH	1967/8 DH	1992/3 NDNS	1951 B & F	1963 MoH	1967/8 DH	1992/3 NDNS
	1 to 2 years*		1½ to 2½ years*		2 to 3 years*		2½ to 3½ years*		3 to 4 years*		3½ to 4½ years*	
Fat (g)	59	51	54.4	42.5	69	61	59.7	46.3	70	58	61.9	48.6
Energy (kcal)	1330	1117	1262	1045	1540	1349	1401	1160	1590	1341	1468	1228
% energy from fat	39.9	41.1	38.3	36.4	40.3	40.7	38.4	35.8	39.6	38.9	37.9	35.4

*The different age groupings in the different surveys should be taken into account when making comparisions between the four surveys.

Bransby ER, Fothergill JE. The diets of young children, *Br J Nutr. 8: 195–204.*
Ministry of Health. *A Pilot Survey of the Nutrition of Young Children in 1963.*
  Reports on Public Health and Medical Subjects: 118. HMSO (London, 1968).
Department of Health and Social Security. Report on Health and Social Subjects: 10.
  A Nutrition Survey of Pre-school Children, 1967–68. HMSO (London, 1975).

Table 7.4 Average daily intake of saturated fatty acids (g) by age and sex of child

Intake of saturated fatty acids (g)	Age and sex of child						
	All aged 1½ – 2½ years	All aged 2½ – 3½ years	All aged 3½ – 4½ years		All boys	All girls	All
			Boys	Girls			
	cum %	cum %	cum %	cum %	cum %	cum %	cum %
Less than 10	4	2	1	2	2	3	3
Less than 15	21	17	11	19	16	23	19
Less than 20	54	49	44	50	47	53	50
Less than 25	82	78	72	78	77	81	79
Less than 30	93	92	90	92	91	93	92
All	100	100	100	100	100	100	100
Base	*576*	*606*	*250*	*243*	*848*	*827*	*1675*
Mean (average value)	19.7	20.8	21.9	20.6	21.1	20.0	20.6
Median value	19.2	20.2	21.0	20.1	20.4	19.4	20.0
Lower 2.5 percentile	8.7	10.0	11.4	9.9	10.0	9.0	9.4
Upper 2.5 percentile	33.4	34.5	36.9	34.0	35.2	33.9	34.7
Standard error of the mean	0.27	0.26	0.41	0.42	0.22	0.22	0.16

Table 7.5 Percentage food energy intake from saturated fatty acids by age and sex of child

Percentage food energy intake from saturated fatty acids	Age and sex of child						
	All aged 1½ – 2½ years	All aged 2½ – 3½ years	All aged 3½ – 4½ years		All boys	All girls	All
			Boys	Girls			
	cum %	cum %	cum %	cum %	cum %	cum %	cum %
Less than 12	9	8	10	12	9	10	9
Less than 15	29	40	46	43	38	38	38
Less than 17	63	76	82	81	72	74	73
Less than 20	81	90	92	93	88	87	87
Less than 22	92	96	99	98	96	95	95
All	100	100	100	100	100	100	100
Base	*576*	*606*	*250*	*243*	*848*	*827*	*1675*
Mean (average value)	16.9	16.0	15.4	15.5	16.2	16.2	16.2
Median value	16.9	15.7	15.2	15.6	16.1	15.9	16.1
Lower 2.5 percentile	10.4	10.6	9.8	9.5	10.1	10.0	10.0
Upper 2.5 percentile	24.3	23.5	21.6	21.7	23.1	23.7	23.5
Standard error of the mean	0.15	0.13	0.19	0.19	0.11	0.12	0.08

Table 7.6 Average daily intake of *trans* fatty acids (g) by age and sex of child

Intake of *trans* fatty acids (g)	Age and sex of child						
	All aged 1½ – 2½ years	All aged 2½ – 3½ years	All aged 3½ – 4½ years		All boys	All girls	All
			Boys	Girls			
	cum %	cum %	cum %	cum %	cum %	cum %	cum %
Less than 1.5	29	19	14	19	19	24	22
Less than 2.0	57	47	38	44	46	52	49
Less than 2.5	79	69	61	71	69	75	72
Less than 3.0	88	84	75	83	83	86	84
Less than 3.5	93	90	84	92	89	92	90
All	100	100	100	100	100	100	100
Base	*576*	*606*	*250*	*243*	*848*	*827*	*1675*
Mean (average value)	2.0	2.2	2.4	2.3	2.3	2.1	2.2
Median value	1.9	2.0	2.3	2.1	2.1	2.0	2.0
Lower 2.5 percentile	0.8	0.9	0.9	0.8	0.8	0.8	0.8
Upper 2.5 percentile	4.3	4.5	4.8	5.1	4.5	4.7	4.6
Standard error of the mean	0.04	0.04	0.06	0.06	0.03	0.03	0.02

Table 7.7 Percentage food energy intake from *trans* fatty acids by age and sex of child

Percentage food energy intake from *trans* fatty acids	Age and sex of child						
	All aged 1½ – 2½ years	All aged 2½ – 3½ years	All aged 3½ – 4½		All boys	All girls	All
			Boys	Girls			
	cum %	cum %	cum %	cum %	cum %	cum %	cum %
Less than 1.0	4	5	6	6	5	5	5
Less than 1.5	35	37	37	37	36	37	36
Less than 2.0	78	77	75	78	77	78	77
Less than 2.5	92	92	92	93	93	92	92
Less than 3.0	96	97	98	97	97	96	96
All	100	100	100	100	100	100	100
Base	*576*	*606*	*250*	*243*	*848*	*827*	*1675*
Mean (average value)	1.7	1.7	1.7	1.7	1.7	1.7	1.7
Median value	1.6	1.6	1.7	1.6	1.6	1.6	1.6
Lower 2.5 percentile	0.9	0.9	0.8	0.9	0.9	0.9	0.9
Upper 2.5 percentile	3.2	3.2	3.1	3.1	3.1	3.2	3.2
Standard error of the mean	0.02	0.02	0.04	0.04	0.02	0.02	0.01

Table 7.8 Average daily intake of *cis* monounsaturated fatty acids (g) by age and sex of child

Intake of *cis* monounsaturated fatty acids (g)	Age and sex of child						
	All aged 1½ – 2½ years	All aged 2½ – 3½ years	All aged 3½ – 4½ years		All boys	All girls	All
			Boys	Girls			
	cum %	cum %	cum %	cum %	cum %	cum %	cum %
Less than 10	20	12	6	11	12	15	14
Less than 12	43	27	20	30	28	36	32
Less than 14	66	49	36	49	49	57	53
Less than 16	80	70	60	65	69	73	71
Less than 18	90	84	76	79	83	85	84
All	100	100	100	100	100	100	100
Base	*576*	*606*	*250*	*243*	*848*	*827*	*1675*
Mean (average value)	13.0	14.4	15.7	14.8	14.5	13.9	14.2
Median value	12.8	14.0	15.1	14.3	14.0	13.4	13.7
Lower 2.5 percentile	6.0	7.4	8.0	6.9	7.2	6.6	6.9
Upper 2.5 percentile	21.9	23.8	26.4	24.0	24.8	23.7	24.0
Standard error of the mean	0.17	0.16	0.28	0.29	0.15	0.15	0.10

Table 7.9 Percentage food energy intake from *cis* monounsaturated fatty acids by age and sex of child

Percentage food energy intake from *cis* monounsaturated fatty acids	Age and sex of child						
	All aged 1½ – 2½ years	All aged 2½ – 3½ years	All aged 3½ – 4½ years		All boys	All girls	All
			Boys	Girls			
	cum %	cum %	cum %	cum %	cum %	cum %	cum %
Less than 9	12	12	13	12	13	11	12
Less than 10	27	27	30	25	29	25	27
Less than 11	47	49	48	46	48	47	48
Less than 12	68	70	66	67	69	67	68
Less than 13	83	85	85	85	85	83	84
All	100	100	100	100	100	100	100
Base	*576*	*606*	*250*	*243*	*848*	*827*	*1675*
Mean (average value)	11.2	11.1	11.1	11.1	11.1	11.2	11.1
Median value	11.1	11.0	11.1	11.1	11.1	11.1	11.1
Lower 2.5 percentile	7.3	7.5	7.2	7.4	7.3	7.5	7.4
Upper 2.5 percentile	15.5	15.2	14.8	14.8	15.0	15.1	15.0
Standard error of the mean	0.08	0.08	0.12	0.12	0.07	0.07	0.05

Table 7.10 Average daily intake of *cis* n–3 polyunsaturated fatty acids (g) by age and sex of child

Intake of *cis* n–3 polyunsaturated fatty acids (g)	Age and sex of child						
	All aged 1½ – 2½ years	All aged 2½ – 3½ years	All aged 3½ – 4½ years		All boys	All girls	All
			Boys	Girls			
	cum %	cum %	cum %	cum %	cum %	cum %	cum %
Less than 0.3	4	2	0	1	2	2	2
Less than 0.6	40	30	21	25	28	34	31
Less than 0.9	71	64	56	54	61	66	64
Less than 1.2	87	82	78	77	81	84	83
Less than 1.5	94	91	89	90	91	92	93
All	100	100	100	100	100	100	100
Base	*576*	*606*	*250*	*243*	*848*	*827*	*1675*
Mean (average value)	0.8	0.9	1.0	1.0	0.9	0.8	0.9
Median value	0.7	0.8	0.8	0.8	0.8	0.7	0.8
Lower 2.5 percentile	0.3	0.3	0.4	0.3	0.3	0.3	0.3
Upper 2.5 percentile	1.8	2.2	2.8	2.6	2.2	2.1	2.2
Standard error of the mean	0.02	0.02	0.04	0.04	0.17	0.17	0.01

Table 7.11 Percentage total energy intake from *cis* n–3 polyunsaturated fatty acids by age and sex of child

Percentage total energy intake from *cis* n–3 polyunsaturated fatty acids	Age and sex of child						
	All aged 1½ – 2½ years	All aged 2½ – 3½ years	All aged 3½ – 4½ years		All boys	All girls	All
			Boys	Girls			
	cum %	cum %	cum %	cum %	cum %	cum %	cum %
Less than 0.3	11	12	9	11	11	11	11
Less than 0.5	51	49	52	40	49	48	49
Less than 0.7	76	76	74	70	74	76	75
Less than 0.9	89	88	87	86	87	89	88
All	100	100	100	100	100	100	100
Base	*576*	*606*	*250*	*243*	*848*	*827*	*1675*
Mean (average value)	0.7	0.7	0.7	0.7	0.7	0.7	0.7
Median value	0.6	0.6	0.6	0.6	0.6	0.6	0.6
Lower 2.5 percentile	0.3	0.3	0.3	0.3	0.3	0.3	0.3
Upper 2.5 percentile	1.6	1.7	1.8	1.9	1.6	1.7	1.7
Standard error of the mean	0.01	0.01	0.02	0.02	0.01	0.01	0.01

Table 7.12 Average daily intake of *cis* n–6 polyunsaturated fatty acids (g) by age and sex of child

Intake of *cis* n–6 polyunsaturated fatty acids (g)	Age and sex of child						
	All aged 1½ – 2½ years	All aged 2½ – 3½ years	All aged 3½ – 4½ years		All boys	All girls	All
			Boys	Girls			
	cum %	cum %	cum %	cum %	cum %	cum %	cum %
Less than 3	26	12	6	8	15	16	15
Less than 5	72	54	39	50	55	60	57
Less than 7	92	81	76	79	84	83	83
Less than 9	98	95	90	92	95	95	95
All	100	100	100	100	100	100	100
Base	*576*	*606*	*250*	*243*	*848*	*827*	*1675*
Mean (average value)	4.3	5.1	5.8	5.5	5.1	4.9	5.0
Median value	3.9	4.9	5.4	5.0	4.8	4.5	4.7
Lower 2.5 percentile	1.6	1.9	2.6	2.3	1.8	1.8	1.8
Upper 2.5 percentile	9.0	9.9	11.4	11.5	10.2	10.5	10.3
Standard error of the mean	0.08	0.08	0.15	0.14	0.07	0.07	0.05

Table 7.13 Percentage food energy intake from *cis* n–6 polyunsaturated fatty acids by age and sex of child

Percentage food energy intake from *cis* n–6 polyunsaturated fatty acids	Age and sex of child						
	All aged 1½ – 2½ years	All aged 2½ – 3½ years	All aged 3½ – 4½ years		All boys	All girls	All
			Boys	Girls			
	cum %	cum %	cum %	cum %	cum %	cum %	cum %
Less than 2	7	4	0	2	5	3	4
Less than 3	36	26	17	18	28	25	27
Less than 4	64	56	49	53	57	57	57
Less than 5	84	80	79	77	82	79	81
Less than 6	93	91	92	90	92	90	91
All	100	100	100	100	100	100	100
Base	576	606	250	243	848	827	1675
Mean (average value)	3.7	4.0	4.1	4.1	3.9	4.0	3.9
Median value	3.5	3.8	4.0	3.9	3.7	3.7	3.7
Lower 2.5 percentile	1.7	1.8	2.1	2.0	1.8	1.9	1.8
Upper 2.5 percentile	6.8	7.4	7.4	7.8	7.0	7.6	7.3
Standard error of the mean	0.06	0.06	0.08	0.09	0.05	0.05	0.03

Table 7.14 Average daily intake (g) and percentage of energy from polyunsaturated fatty acids (*cis* n–3 + *cis* n–6) by age and sex of child

cis n–3 + n–6 polyunsaturated fatty acids	Age and sex of child						
	All aged 1½ – 2½ years	All aged 2½ – 3½ years	All aged 3½ – 4½ years		All boys	All girls	All
			Boys	Girls			
	cum %	cum %	cum %	cum %	cum %	cum %	cum %
Average daily intake (g):							
Mean	5.1	6.0	6.8	6.4	6.0	5.8	5.9
Median	4.7	5.6	6.4	5.9	5.6	5.4	5.5
Lower 2.5 percentile	2.1	2.4	3.1	2.9	2.4	2.3	2.3
Upper 2.5 percentile	10.8	11.4	13.1	12.6	11.6	11.9	11.7
Standard error of the mean	0.09	0.09	0.16	0.16	0.08	0.08	0.06
Percentage energy from cis n–3 + n–6 polyunsaturated fatty acids							
Mean (average value)	4.4	4.7	4.8	4.9	4.6	4.7	4.6
Median value	4.1	4.4	4.7	4.6	4.4	4.4	4.4
Lower 2.5 percentile	2.2	2.2	2.7	2.6	2.2	2.4	2.3
Upper 2.5 percentile	8.0	8.1	8.5	8.9	8.0	8.4	8.2
Standard error of the mean	0.06	0.06	0.09	0.10	0.05	0.05	0.04
Base	576	606	250	243	848	827	1675

Table 7.15 Average daily intake of cholesterol (mg) by age and sex of child

Intake of cholesterol (mg)	Age and sex of child						
	All aged 1½ – 2½ years	All aged 2½ – 3½ years	All aged 3½ – 4½ years		All boys	All girls	All
			Boys	Girls			
	cum %	cum %	cum %	cum %	cum %	cum %	cum %
Less than 60	7	7	3	7	19	24	6
Less than 100	33	32	22	26	46	52	30
Less than 140	65	61	56	58	69	75	61
Less than 180	83	80	76	76	83	86	80
Less than 220	91	89	89	88	89	92	90
All	100	100	100	100	100	100	100
Base	576	606	250	243	848	827	1675
Mean (average value)	133	137	147	144	137	139	138
Median value	119	121	134	129	124	125	125
Lower 2.5 percentile	41	47	48	44	45	42	45
Upper 2.5 percentile	318	324	332	345	316	333	322
Standard error of the mean	2.9	2.8	4.2	4.6	2.2	2.5	1.7

Table 7.16(a) Contribution of food types to average daily intake of total fat (g) by age and sex of child

Food types	Age and sex of child						
	All aged 1½ – 2½ years	All aged 2½ – 3½ years	All aged 3½ – 4½ years		All boys	All girls	All
			Boys	Girls			
	g	g	g	g	g	g	g
Cereals & cereal products	7.3	9.5	10.9	9.7	9.4	8.6	9.0
of which:							
biscuits	*2.6*	*3.5*	*4.1*	*3.1*	*3.4*	*2.9*	*3.2*
buns, cakes & pastries	*1.1*	*1.8*	*2.2*	*1.8*	*1.7*	*1.6*	*1.6*
Milk & milk products	14.8	11.9	11.1	10.5	12.9	12.3	12.6
of which:							
cows' milk	*11.4*	*9.1*	*8.1*	*7.6*	*9.9*	*9.2*	*9.5*
other milk & cream	*0.8*	*0.3*	*0.4*	*0.3*	*0.5*	*0.5*	*0.5*
cheese	*1.7*	*1.7*	*1.9*	*1.9*	*1.7*	*1.8*	*1.8*
fromage frais & yogurt	*0.8*	*0.7*	*0.6*	*0.7*	*0.7*	*0.8*	*0.8*
Eggs & egg dishes	1.1	1.3	1.2	1.5	1.0	1.4	1.2
Fat spreads	3.5	4.5	5.3	4.7	4.4	4.2	4.3
of which:							
butter	*0.8*	*1.0*	*1.1*	*1.1*	*1.0*	*0.9*	*1.0*
polyunsaturated margarine	*1.2*	*1.5*	*1.8*	*1.5*	*1.4*	*1.5*	*1.5*
Meat & meat products	6.4	7.4	8.6	8.1	7.6	7.1	7.3
of which:							
sausages	*1.8*	*2.0*	*2.2*	*2.4*	*2.1*	*2.0*	*2.0*
beef, veal & dishes	*1.0*	*0.9*	*1.0*	*1.0*	*1.0*	*0.9*	*1.0*
all chicken & turkey	*0.6*	*0.8*	*1.0*	*0.8*	*0.8*	*0.7*	*0.7*
Fish & fish dishes	0.9	0.9	1.0	1.0	1.0	0.9	0.9
Vegetables, potatoes & savoury snacks	5.1	6.4	7.2	7.0	6.4	6.0	6.2
of which:							
vegetables, excluding potatoes	*0.5*	*0.6*	*0.6*	*0.6*	*0.6*	*0.5*	*0.6*
potatoes, fried	*1.9*	*2.4*	*2.8*	*2.8*	*2.5*	*2.3*	*2.4*
other potatoes	*0.2*	*0.2*	*0.3*	*0.3*	*0.2*	*0.3*	*0.2*
savoury snacks	*2.4*	*3.3*	*3.4*	*3.2*	*3.0*	*2.9*	*3.0*
Fruit & nuts	0.3	0.5	0.6	0.6	0.4	0.5	0.5
of which:							
fruit	*0.1*	*0.1*	*0.1*	*0.1*	*1.0*	*0.1*	*0.1*
nuts, fruit & nut mixes	*0.2*	*0.4*	*0.5*	*0.5*	*0.4*	*0.4*	*0.4*
Sugar, preserves & confectionery	2.3	3.0	3.3	3.3	2.9	2.8	2.8
of which:							
chocolate confectionery	*2.1*	*2.7*	*2.9*	*3.0*	*2.6*	*2.6*	*2.6*
Beverages	0.0	0.0	0.0	0.0	0.0	0.0	0.0
Commercial infant foods & drinks	0.1	0.0	0.0	0.0	0.0	0.0	0.1
Miscellaneous	0.6	0.8	0.9	0.7	0.7	0.8	0.7
Average daily intake (g)	**42.5**	**46.3**	**50.1**	**47.2**	**46.7**	**44.6**	**45.7**
Total number of children	**576**	**606**	**250**	**243**	**848**	**827**	**1675**

Table 7.16(b) Percentage contribution of food types to average daily intake of total fat by age and sex of child

Food types	All aged 1½ – 2½ years	All aged 2½ – 3½ years	All aged 3½ – 4½ years		All boys	All girls	All
			Boys	Girls			
	%	%	%	%	%	%	%
Cereals & cereal products	17	20	22	21	20	19	20
of which:							
biscuits	*6*	*7*	*8*	*6*	*7*	*7*	*7*
buns, cakes & pastries	*3*	*4*	*4*	*4*	*4*	*3*	*4*
Milk & milk products	35	26	22	22	27	27	27
of which:							
cows' milk	*27*	*20*	*16*	*16*	*21*	*21*	*21*
other milk & cream	*2*	*1*	*1*	*1*	*1*	*1*	*1*
cheese	*4*	*4*	*4*	*4*	*4*	*4*	*4*
fromage frais & yogurt	*2*	*2*	*1*	*1*	*2*	*2*	*2*
Eggs & egg dishes	2	3	2	3	2	3	3
Fat spreads	8	10	11	10	9	9	9
of which:							
butter	*2*	*2*	*2*	*2*	*2*	*2*	*2*
polyunsaturated margarine	*3*	*3*	*4*	*3*	*3*	*3*	*3*
Meat & meat products	15	16	17	17	16	16	16
of which:							
sausages	*4*	*4*	*4*	*5*	*4*	*4*	*4*
beef, veal & dishes	*2*	*2*	*2*	*2*	*2*	*2*	*2*
all chicken & turkey	*1*	*2*	*2*	*2*	*2*	*2*	*2*
Fish & fish dishes	2	2	2	2	2	2	2
Vegetables, potatoes & savoury snacks	12	14	14	15	14	13	13
of which:							
vegetables, excluding potatoes	*1*	*1*	*1*	*1*	*1*	*1*	*1*
potatoes, fried	*5*	*5*	*6*	*6*	*5*	*5*	*5*
other potatoes	*1*	*0*	*0*	*1*	*0*	*1*	*0*
savoury snacks	*6*	*7*	*7*	*7*	*6*	*7*	*7*
Fruit & nuts	1	1	1	1	1	1	1
of which:							
fruit	*0*	*0*	*0*	*0*	*0*	*0*	*0*
nuts, fruit & nut mixes	*1*	*1*	*1*	*1*	*1*	*1*	*1*
Sugar, preserves & confectionery	5	6	7	7	6	6	6
of which:							
chocolate confectionery	*5*	*6*	*6*	*6*	*6*	*6*	*6*
Beverages	1	1	1	1	1	1	1
Commercial infant foods & drinks	0	0	0	0	0	0	0
Miscellaneous	1	2	2	2	2	2	2
Average daily intake (g)	**42.5**	**46.3**	**50.1**	**47.2**	**46.7**	**44.6**	**45.7**
Total number of children	**576**	**606**	**250**	**243**	**848**	**827**	**1675**

Table 7.17(a) Contribution of food types to average daily intake of saturated fatty acids (g) by age and sex of child

Food types	Age and sex of child						
	All aged 1½ – 2½ years	All aged 2½ – 3½ years	All aged 3½ – 4½ years		All boys	All girls	All
			Boys	Girls			
	g	g	g	g	g	g	g
Cereals & cereal products	3.1	4.2	4.7	4.2	4.1	3.7	3.9
of which:							
biscuits	1.2	1.7	2.0	1.5	1.7	1.4	1.6
buns, cakes & pastries	0.4	0.7	0.8	0.6	0.6	0.6	0.6
Milk & milk products	9.1	7.4	6.9	6.6	8.0	7.6	7.8
of which:							
cows' milk	7.2	5.7	5.1	4.8	6.2	5.8	6.0
other milk & cream	0.3	0.2	0.2	0.2	0.2	0.2	0.2
cheese	1.1	1.1	1.2	1.2	1.1	1.1	1.1
fromage frais & yogurt	0.5	0.4	0.4	0.4	0.4	0.4	0.4
Eggs & egg dishes	0.3	0.4	0.4	0.6	0.3	0.4	0.4
Fat spreads	1.2	1.5	1.8	1.6	1.5	1.4	1.5
of which:							
butter	0.5	0.7	0.7	0.7	0.7	0.6	0.6
polyunsaturated margarine	0.2	0.3	0.3	0.3	0.3	0.3	0.3
Meat & meat products	2.4	2.8	3.2	3.1	2.9	2.7	2.8
of which:							
sausages	0.7	0.7	0.8	0.9	0.8	0.7	0.8
beef, veal & dishes	0.4	0.4	0.4	0.4	0.4	0.4	0.4
all chicken & turkey	0.2	0.2	0.3	0.2	0.2	0.2	0.2
Fish & fish dishes	0.2	0.2	0.2	0.2	0.2	0.2	0.2
Vegetables, potatoes & savoury snacks	1.7	2.1	2.4	2.2	2.1	1.9	2.0
of which:							
vegetables, excluding potatoes	0.1	0.1	0.1	0.1	0.1	0.1	0.1
potatoes, fried	0.5	0.6	0.7	0.7	0.6	0.6	0.6
other potatoes	0.1	0.9	0.1	0.1	0.1	0.1	0.1
savoury snacks	1.0	1.3	1.4	1.3	1.2	1.2	1.2
Fruit & nuts	0.1	0.1	0.1	0.1	0.1	0.1	0.1
of which:							
fruit	0.0	0.0	0.0	0.0	0.0	0.0	0.0
nuts, fruit & nut mixes	0.0	0.1	0.1	0.1	0.1	0.1	0.1
Sugar, preserves & confectionery	1.3	1.7	1.9	1.8	1.6	1.6	1.6
of which:							
chocolate confectionery	1.2	1.6	1.7	1.7	1.5	1.5	1.5
Beverages	0.0	0.0	0.0	0.0	0.0	0.0	0.0
Commercial infant foods & drinks	0.0	0.0	0.0	0.0	0.0	0.0	0.0
Miscellaneous	0.3	0.3	0.3	0.3	0.3	0.3	0.3
Average daily intake (g)	**19.7**	**20.8**	**21.9**	**20.6**	**21.1**	**20.0**	**20.6**
Total number of children	**576**	**606**	**250**	**243**	**848**	**827**	**1675**

Table 7.17(b)   Percentage contribution of food types to average daily intake of saturated fatty acids by age and sex of child

Food types	Age and sex of child						
	All aged 1½ – 2½ years	All aged 2½ – 3½ years	All aged 3½ – 4½ years		All boys	All girls	All
			Boys	Girls			
	%	%	%	%	%	%	%
Cereals & cereal products	16	20	21	20	19	18	19
of which:							
biscuits	*6*	*8*	*9*	*7*	*8*	*7*	*8*
buns, cakes & pastries	*2*	*3*	*4*	*3*	*3*	*3*	*3*
Milk & milk products	46	36	31	32	38	38	38
of which:							
cows' milk	*36*	*27*	*23*	*23*	*29*	*29*	*29*
other milk & cream	*2*	*1*	*1*	*1*	*1*	*1*	*1*
cheese	*6*	*5*	*5*	*6*	*5*	*5*	*5*
fromage frais & yogurt	*2*	*2*	*2*	*2*	*2*	*2*	*2*
Eggs & egg dishes	2	2	2	2	1	2	2
Fat spreads	6	7	8	8	7	7	7
of which:							
butter	*3*	*3*	*3*	*3*	*3*	*3*	*3*
polyunsaturated margarine	*1*	*1*	*1*	*1*	*1*	*1*	*1*
Meat & meat products	12	13	15	15	14	13	14
of which:							
sausages	*3*	*3*	*4*	*4*	*4*	*4*	*4*
beef, veal & dishes	*2*	*2*	*2*	*2*	*2*	*2*	*2*
all chicken & turkey	*1*	*1*	*1*	*1*	*1*	*1*	*1*
Fish & fish dishes	1	1	1	1	1	1	1
Vegetables, potatoes & savoury snacks	8	10	11	11	10	10	10
of which:							
vegetables, excluding potatoes	*1*	*1*	*1*	*1*	*1*	*1*	*1*
potatoes, fried	*2*	*3*	*3*	*3*	*3*	*3*	*3*
other potatoes	*0*	*0*	*0*	*0*	*0*	*0*	*0*
savoury snacks	*5*	*6*	*6*	*6*	*6*	*6*	*6*
Fruit & nuts	0	0	1	1	1	1	1
of which:							
fruit	*0*	*0*	*0*	*0*	*0*	*0*	*0*
nuts, fruit & nut mixes	*0*	*0*	*0*	*0*	*0*	*0*	*0*
Sugar, preserves & confectionery	6	8	8	9	8	8	8
of which:							
chocolate confectionery	*6*	*8*	*8*	*8*	*7*	*7*	*7*
Beverages	0	0	0	0	0	0	0
Commercial infant foods & drinks	0	0	0	0	0	0	0
Miscellaneous	1	1	1	1	1	1	1
Average daily intake (g)	**19.7**	**20.8**	**21.9**	**20.6**	**21.1**	**20.0**	**20.6**
Total number of children	**576**	**606**	**250**	**243**	**848**	**827**	**1675**

Table 7.18(a)   Contribution of food types to average daily intake of *trans* fatty acids (g) by age and sex of child

Food types	Age and sex of child						
	All aged 1½ – 2½ years	All aged 2½ – 3½ years	All aged 3½ – 4½ years		All boys	All girls	All
			Boys	Girls			
	g	g	g	g	g	g	g
Cereals & cereal products	0.49	0.66	0.78	0.69	0.65	0.60	0.62
of which:							
biscuits	0.23	0.30	0.36	0.25	0.30	0.25	0.28
buns, cakes & pastries	0.13	0.19	0.25	0.20	0.19	0.18	0.18
Milk & milk products	0.72	0.58	0.54	0.51	0.62	0.59	0.61
of which:							
cows' milk	0.56	0.45	0.40	0.37	0.48	0.45	0.47
other milk & cream	0.04	0.02	0.02	0.01	0.02	0.02	0.02
cheese	0.08	0.08	0.09	0.09	0.08	0.08	0.08
fromage frais & yogurt	0.04	0.03	0.03	0.03	0.03	0.04	0.04
Eggs & egg dishes	0.02	0.03	0.02	0.03	0.02	0.03	0.03
Fat spreads	0.25	0.32	0.38	0.33	0.31	0.30	0.31
of which:							
butter	0.03	0.04	0.05	0.05	0.04	0.04	0.04
polyunsaturated margarine	0.08	0.10	0.11	0.09	0.09	0.09	0.09
Meat & meat products	0.33	0.36	0.39	0.37	0.37	0.34	0.36
of which:							
sausages	0.02	0.02	0.02	0.02	0.02	0.02	0.02
beef, veal & dishes	0.04	0.03	0.04	0.04	0.04	0.03	0.04
all chicken & turkey	0.01	0.02	0.03	0.03	0.02	0.02	0.02
Fish & fish dishes	0.04	0.04	0.04	0.04	0.04	0.04	0.04
Vegetables, potatoes & savoury snacks	0.09	0.11	0.12	0.12	0.11	0.10	0.10
of which:							
vegetables, excluding potatoes	0.01	0.01	0.01	0.01	0.01	0.01	0.01
potatoes, fried	0.05	0.07	0.07	0.08	0.07	0.06	0.06
other potatoes	0.02	0.01	0.02	0.01	0.02	0.02	0.02
savoury snacks	0.02	0.02	0.02	0.02	0.02	0.02	0.02
Fruit & nuts	0.00	0.00	0.00	0.00	0.00	0.00	0.00
of which:							
fruit	0.00	—	—	—	—	0.00	0.00
nuts, fruit & nut mixes	0.00	0.00	0.00	0.00	0.00	0.00	0.00
Sugar, preserves & confectionery	0.07	0.12	0.16	0.14	0.12	0.11	0.11
of which:							
chocolate confectionery	0.06	0.10	0.11	0.11	0.10	0.08	0.09
Beverages	0.00	—	0.00	0.00	0.00	0.00	0.00
Commercial infant foods & drinks	0.01	0.00	0.00	0.00	0.00	0.00	0.00
Miscellaneous	0.02	0.01	0.01	0.01	0.01	0.01	0.01
Average daily intake (g)	**2.0**	**2.2**	**2.4**	**2.3**	**2.3**	**2.1**	**2.2**
Total number of children	**576**	**606**	**250**	**243**	**848**	**827**	**1675**

Table 7.18(b) Percentage contribution of food types to average daily intake of *trans* fatty acids by age and sex of child

Food types	All aged 1½ – 2½ years	All aged 2½ – 3½ years	All aged 3½ – 4½ years		All boys	All girls	All
			Boys	Girls			
	%	%	%	%	%	%	%
Cereals & cereal products	24	29	32	31	29	28	28
of which:							
biscuits	*11*	*13*	*15*	*11*	*13*	*12*	*13*
buns, cakes & pastries	*6*	*8*	*10*	*9*	*8*	*8*	*8*
Milk & milk products	35	26	22	23	27	28	28
of which:							
cows' milk	*28*	*20*	*16*	*16*	*21*	*21*	*21*
other milk & cream	*2*	*1*	*1*	*0*	*1*	*1*	*1*
cheese	*4*	*4*	*4*	*4*	*3*	*4*	*4*
fromage frais & yogurt	*2*	*1*	*1*	*1*	*1*	*2*	*2*
Eggs & egg dishes	1	1	1	1	1	1	1
Fat spreads	12	14	15	15	14	14	14
of which:							
butter	*1*	*2*	*2*	*2*	*2*	*2*	*2*
polyunsaturated margarine	*4*	*4*	*4*	*4*	*4*	*4*	*4*
Meat & meat products	16	16	16	16	16	16	16
of which:							
sausages	*1*	*1*	*1*	*1*	*1*	*1*	*1*
beef, veal & dishes	*2*	*1*	*1*	*2*	*2*	*1*	*2*
all chicken & turkey	*1*	*1*	*1*	*1*	*1*	*1*	*1*
Fish & fish dishes	2	2	2	2	2	2	2
Vegetables, potatoes & savoury snacks	4	5	5	5	5	5	4
of which:							
vegetables, excluding potatoes	*0*	*0*	*0*	*0*	*0*	*0*	*0*
potatoes, fried	*2*	*3*	*3*	*3*	*3*	*3*	*3*
other potatoes	*1*	*0*	*1*	*0*	*1*	*1*	*1*
savoury snacks	*1*	*1*	*1*	*0*	*1*	*1*	*1*
Fruit & nuts	0	0	0	0	0	0	0
of which:							
fruit	*0*	—	—	—	—	*0*	*0*
nuts, fruit & nut mixes	*0*	*0*	*0*	*0*	*0*	*0*	*0*
Sugar, preserves & confectionery	3	5	6	6	5	5	5
of which:							
chocolate confectionery	*3*	*4*	*4*	*5*	*4*	*4*	*4*
Beverages	0	—	—	—	0	0	0
Commercial infant foods & drinks	0	0	0	0	0	0	0
Miscellaneous	1	0	0	0	0	0	0
Average daily intake (g)	**2.0**	**2.2**	**2.4**	**2.3**	**2.3**	**2.1**	**2.2**
Total number of children	**576**	**606**	**250**	**243**	**848**	**827**	**1675**

Table 7.19(a) Contribution of food types to average daily intake of *cis* monounsaturated fatty acids by age and sex of child

Food types	All aged 1½ – 2½ years	All aged 2½ – 3½ years	All aged 3½ – 4½ years		All boys	All girls	All
			Boys	Girls			
	g	g	g	g	g	g	g
Cereals & cereal products	2.1	2.7	3.1	2.7	2.6	2.4	2.5
of which:							
biscuits	*0.7*	*1.0*	*1.2*	*0.9*	*1.0*	*0.8*	*0.9*
buns, cakes & pastries	*0.3*	*0.5*	*0.6*	*0.5*	*0.5*	*0.5*	*0.5*
Milk & milk products	3.8	3.0	2.8	2.6	3.2	3.1	3.2
of which:							
cows' milk	*2.9*	*2.3*	*2.0*	*1.9*	*2.5*	*2.3*	*2.4*
other milk & cream	*0.2*	*0.1*	*0.1*	*0.1*	*0.1*	*0.2*	*0.1*
cheese	*0.4*	*0.4*	*0.4*	*0.5*	*0.4*	*0.4*	*0.4*
fromage frais & yogurt	*0.2*	*0.2*	*0.2*	*0.2*	*0.2*	*0.2*	*0.2*
Eggs & egg dishes	0.4	0.5	0.5	0.6	0.4	0.6	0.5
Fat spreads	1.0	1.3	1.5	1.3	1.3	1.2	1.2
of which:							
butter	*0.2*	*0.2*	*0.2*	*0.2*	*0.2*	*0.2*	*0.2*
polyunsaturated margarine	*0.3*	*0.4*	*0.4*	*0.4*	*0.4*	*0.4*	*0.4*
Meat & meat products	2.5	2.9	3.4	3.2	2.9	2.8	2.9
of which:							
sausages	*0.8*	*0.9*	*1.0*	*1.0*	*0.9*	*0.9*	*0.9*
beef, veal & dishes	*0.4*	*0.4*	*0.4*	*0.4*	*0.4*	*0.4*	*0.4*
all chicken & turkey	*0.2*	*0.3*	*0.4*	*0.3*	*0.3*	*0.3*	*0.3*
Fish & fish dishes	0.3	0.3	0.3	0.3	0.3	0.3	0.3
Vegetables, potatoes & savoury snacks	1.9	2.4	2.7	2.6	2.4	2.2	2.3
of which:							
vegetables, excluding potatoes	*0.1*	*0.1*	*0.2*	*0.2*	*0.2*	*0.1*	*0.2*
potatoes, fried	*0.7*	*0.9*	*1.1*	*1.1*	*0.9*	*0.9*	*0.9*
other potatoes	*0.1*	*0.0*	*0.1*	*0.1*	*0.0*	*0.1*	*0.1*
savoury snacks	*1.0*	*1.3*	*1.4*	*1.3*	*1.2*	*1.2*	*1.2*
Fruit & nuts	0.1	0.2	0.2	0.2	0.2	0.2	0.2
of which:							
fruit	*0.0*	*0.0*	*0.0*	*0.0*	*0.0*	*0.0*	*0.0*
nuts, fruit & nut mixes	*0.1*	*0.2*	*0.2*	*0.2*	*0.2*	*0.2*	*0.2*
Sugar, preserves & confectionery	0.7	0.9	1.0	1.0	0.9	0.8	0.9
of which:							
chocolate confectionery	*0.6*	*0.8*	*0.9*	*0.9*	*0.8*	*0.8*	*0.8*
Beverages	0.0	0.0	0.0	0.0	0.0	0.0	0.0
Commercial infant foods & drinks	0.0	0.0	0.0	0.0	0.0	0.0	0.0
Miscellaneous	0.2	0.2	0.3	0.2	0.2	0.2	0.2
Average daily intake (g)	**13.0**	**14.4**	**15.7**	**14.8**	**14.5**	**13.9**	**14.2**
Total number of children	**576**	**606**	**250**	**243**	**848**	**827**	**1675**

113

Table 7.19(b) Percentage of average daily intake of *cis* monounsaturated fatty acids from food types by age and sex of child

Food types	Age and sex of child						
	All aged 1½ – 2½ years	All aged 2½ – 3½ years	All aged 3½ – 4½ years		All boys	All girls	All
			Boys	Girls			
	%	%	%	%	%	%	%
Cereals & cereal products	16	19	20	18	18	17	18
of which:							
biscuits	*6*	*7*	*8*	*6*	*7*	*6*	*6*
buns, cakes & pastries	*3*	*4*	*4*	*4*	*3*	*3*	*3*
Milk & milk products	29	21	18	17	22	22	23
of which:							
cows' milk	*22*	*16*	*13*	*13*	*17*	*17*	*17*
other milk & cream	*2*	*1*	*1*	*0*	*1*	*1*	*1*
cheese	*3*	*3*	*3*	*3*	*3*	*3*	*3*
fromage frais & yogurt	*2*	*1*	*1*	*1*	*1*	*1*	*1*
Eggs & egg dishes	3	3	3	4	3	4	3
Fat spreads	8	9	9	9	9	9	8
of which:							
butter	*1*	*1*	*1*	*1*	*1*	*1*	*1*
polyunsaturated margarine	*2*	*3*	*3*	*2*	*2*	*3*	*2*
Meat & meat products	19	20	22	22	20	20	20
of which:							
sausages	*6*	*6*	*6*	*7*	*6*	*6*	*6*
beef, veal & dishes	*3*	*2*	*2*	*3*	*3*	*3*	*3*
all chicken & turkey	*2*	*2*	*3*	*2*	*2*	*2*	*2*
Fish & fish dishes	2	2	2	2	2	2	2
Vegetables, potatoes & savoury snacks	15	17	17	17	16	16	16
of which:							
vegetables, excluding potatoes	*1*	*1*	*1*	*1*	*1*	*1*	*1*
potatoes, fried	*6*	*6*	*7*	*6*	*6*	*6*	*6*
other potatoes	*0*	*0*	*0*	*0*	*0*	*0*	*0*
savoury snacks	*7*	*9*	*9*	*9*	*8*	*9*	*8*
Fruit & nuts	1	1	1	2	1	1	1
of which:							
fruit	*0*	*0*	*0*	*0*	*0*	*0*	*0*
nuts, fruit & nut mixes	*1*	*1*	*1*	*1*	*1*	*1*	*1*
Sugar & confectionery	5	6	6	7	6	6	6
of which:							
chocolate confectionery	*5*	*6*	*5*	*6*	*5*	*5*	*5*
Beverages	0	0	0	0	0	0	0
Commercial infant foods & drinks	0	0	0	0	0	0	0
Miscellaneous	2	2	2	1	2	2	2
Average daily intake (g)	**13.0**	**14.4**	**15.7**	**14.8**	**14.5**	**13.9**	**14.2**
Total number of children	**576**	**606**	**250**	**243**	**848**	**827**	**1675**

Table 7.20(a) Contribution of food types to average daily intake of *cis* n-3 polyunsaturated fatty acids by age and sex of child

Food types	Age and sex of child						
	All aged 1½ – 2½ years	All aged 2½ – 3½ years	All aged 3½ – 4½ years		All boys	All girls	All
			Boys	Girls			
	g	g	g	g	g	g	g
Cereals & cereal products	0.10	0.13	0.13	0.13	0.13	0.12	0.12
of which:							
biscuits	*0.02*	*0.02*	*0.02*	*0.02*	*0.02*	*0.02*	*0.02*
buns, cakes & pastries	*0.01*	*0.02*	*0.03*	*0.02*	*0.02*	*0.02*	*0.02*
Milk & milk products	0.13	0.09	0.09	0.08	0.11	0.10	0.10
of which:							
cows' milk	*0.08*	*0.06*	*0.06*	*0.05*	*0.07*	*0.06*	*0.07*
other milk & cream	*0.02*	*0.01*	*0.01*	*0.00*	*0.01*	*0.01*	*0.01*
cheese	*0.02*	*0.02*	*0.02*	*0.02*	*0.02*	*0.02*	*0.02*
fromage frais & yogurt	*0.01*	*0.01*	*0.01*	*0.01*	*0.01*	*0.01*	*0.01*
Eggs & egg dishes	0.01	0.01	0.02	0.01	0.01	0.01	0.01
Fat spreads	0.05	0.07	0.08	0.07	0.07	0.06	0.07
of which:							
butter	*0.01*	*0.01*	*0.01*	*0.01*	*0.01*	*0.01*	*0.01*
polyunsaturated margarine	*0.01*	*0.01*	*0.01*	*0.01*	*0.01*	*0.01*	*0.01*
Meat & meat products	0.08	0.10	0.11	0.10	0.10	0.09	0.09
of which:							
sausages	*0.02*	*0.02*	*0.02*	*0.02*	*0.02*	*0.02*	*0.02*
beef, veal & dishes	*0.01*	*0.01*	*0.01*	*0.01*	*0.01*	*0.01*	*0.01*
all chicken & turkey	*0.02*	*0.02*	*0.03*	*0.03*	*0.02*	*0.02*	*0.02*
Fish & fish dishes	0.09	0.11	0.12	0.13	0.11	0.11	0.11
Vegetables, potatoes & savoury snacks	0.21	0.25	0.27	0.28	0.25	0.24	0.24
of which:							
vegetables, excluding potatoes	*0.05*	*0.06*	*0.06*	*0.05*	*0.06*	*0.05*	*0.05*
potatoes, fried	*0.12*	*0.15*	*0.17*	*0.18*	*0.15*	*0.14*	*0.15*
other potatoes	*0.01*	*0.01*	*0.01*	*0.01*	*0.01*	*0.01*	*0.01*
savoury snacks	*0.03*	*0.04*	*0.04*	*0.04*	*0.04*	*0.04*	*0.04*
Fruit & nuts	0.06	0.08	0.12	0.10	0.09	0.08	0.08
of which:							
fruit	*0.01*	*0.01*	*0.01*	*0.01*	*0.01*	*0.01*	*0.01*
nuts, fruit & nut mixes	*0.05*	*0.06*	*0.11*	*0.09*	*0.07*	*0.07*	*0.07*
Sugar, preserves & confectionery	0.00	0.01	0.02	0.02	0.01	0.01	0.01
of which:							
chocolate confectionery	*0.10*	*0.01*	*0.01*	*0.01*	*0.01*	*0.01*	*0.01*
Beverages	0.00	0.00	0.00	0.00	0.00	0.00	0.00
Commercial infant foods & drinks	0.00	0.00	0.00	0.00	0.00	0.00	0.00
Miscellaneous	0.01	0.02	0.02	0.02	0.02	0.02	0.02
Average daily intake (g)	**0.8**	**0.9**	**1.0**	**1.0**	**0.9**	**0.8**	**0.9**
Total number of children	**576**	**606**	**250**	**243**	**848**	**827**	**1675**

115

Table 7.20(b)   Percentage contribution of food types to average daily intake of *cis* n-3 polyunsaturated fatty acids by age and sex of child

Food types	Age and sex of child						
	All aged 1½ – 2½ years	All aged 2½ – 3½ years	All aged 3½ – 4½ years		All boys	All girls	All
			Boys	Girls			
	%	%	%	%	%	%	%
Cereals & cereal products	13	15	13	14	14	14	14
of which:							
biscuits	*3*	*2*	*2*	*2*	*2*	*2*	*2*
buns, cakes & pastries	*1*	*2*	*3*	*2*	*2*	*2*	*2*
Milk & milk products	17	10	9	8	12	12	11
of which:							
cows' milk	*10*	*7*	*6*	*5*	*8*	*7*	*8*
other milk & cream	*3*	*1*	*1*	*0*	*1*	*1*	*1*
cheese	*3*	*2*	*2*	*2*	*2*	*2*	*2*
fromage frais & yogurt	*1*	*1*	*1*	*1*	*1*	*1*	*1*
Eggs & egg dishes	1	1	2	1	1	1	1
Fat spreads	6	8	8	7	8	7	8
of which:							
butter	*1*	*1*	*1*	*1*	*1*	*1*	*1*
polyunsaturated margarine	*1*	*1*	*1*	*1*	*1*	*1*	*1*
Meat & meat products	10	11	11	10	11	11	10
of which:							
sausages	*3*	*2*	*2*	*2*	*2*	*2*	*2*
beef, veal & dishes	*1*	*1*	*1*	*1*	*1*	*1*	*1*
all chicken & turkey	*2*	*3*	*3*	*3*	*2*	*2*	*2*
Fish & fish dishes	11	12	12	14	12	13	13
Vegetables, potatoes & savoury snacks	27	28	27	29	28	28	28
of which:							
vegetables, excluding potatoes	*6*	*7*	*6*	*5*	*7*	*6*	*6*
potatoes, fried	*15*	*17*	*17*	*19*	*17*	*17*	*17*
other potatoes	*1*	*1*	*1*	*1*	*1*	*1*	*1*
savoury snacks	*4*	*5*	*4*	*4*	*4*	*5*	*5*
Fruit & nuts	8	9	12	10	10	10	9
of which:							
fruit	*1*	*1*	*1*	*1*	*1*	*1*	*1*
nuts, fruit & nut mixes	*6*	*7*	*11*	*9*	*8*	*8*	*8*
Sugar & confectionery	1	1	2	2	1	1	1
of which:							
chocolate confectionery	*1*	*1*	*1*	*1*	*1*	*1*	*1*
Beverages	0	0	0	0	0	0	0
Commercial infant foods & drinks	0	0	0	0	0	0	0
Miscellaneous	1	2	2	2	2	2	2
Average daily intake (g)	**0.8**	**0.9**	**1.0**	**1.0**	**0.9**	**0.8**	**0.9**
Total number of children	**576**	**606**	**250**	**243**	**848**	**827**	**1675**

Table 7.21(a)   Contribution of food types to average daily intake of *cis* n-6 polyunsaturated fatty acids by age and sex of child

Food types	Age and sex of child						
	All aged 1½ – 2½ years	All aged 2½ – 3½ years	All aged 3½ – 4½ years		All boys	All girls	All
			Boys	Girls			
	g	g	g	g	g	g	g
Cereals & cereal products	0.97	1.2	1.3	1.3	1.2	1.1	1.1
of which:							
biscuits	*0.19*	*0.24*	*0.29*	*0.22*	*0.24*	*0.21*	*0.23*
buns, cakes & pastries	*0.13*	*0.21*	*0.28*	*0.23*	*0.21*	*0.19*	*0.20*
Milk & milk products	0.32	0.20	0.20	0.17	0.24	0.23	0.24
of which:							
cows' milk	*0.16*	*0.12*	*0.11*	*0.10*	*0.14*	*0.13*	*0.13*
other milk & cream	*0.08*	*0.02*	*0.02*	*0.00*	*0.04*	*0.04*	*0.04*
cheese	*0.04*	*0.04*	*0.05*	*0.04*	*0.04*	*0.04*	*0.04*
fromage frais & yogurt	*0.02*	*0.02*	*0.02*	*0.02*	*0.02*	*0.02*	*0.02*
Eggs & egg dishes	0.14	0.15	0.17	0.20	0.13	0.18	0.16
Fat spreads	0.84	1.0	1.2	1.1	1.0	1.0	1.0
of which:							
butter	*0.01*	*0.01*	*0.01*	*0.01*	*0.01*	*0.01*	*0.01*
polyunsaturated margarine	*0.56*	*0.71*	*0.84*	*0.68*	*0.66*	*0.68*	*0.67*
Meat & meat products	0.60	0.73	0.86	0.79	0.74	0.69	0.71
of which:							
sausages	*0.21*	*0.23*	*0.27*	*0.28*	*0.24*	*0.23*	*0.24*
beef, veal & dishes	*0.07*	*0.07*	*0.06*	*0.07*	*0.07*	*0.07*	*0.07*
all chicken & turkey	*0.10*	*0.15*	*0.19*	*0.15*	*0.14*	*0.14*	*0.14*
Fish & fish dishes	0.18	0.20	0.22	0.21	0.20	0.19	0.20
Vegetables, potatoes & savoury snacks	0.98	1.2	1.4	1.4	1.2	1.1	1.2
of which:							
vegetables, excluding potatoes	*0.14*	*0.16*	*0.20*	*0.18*	*0.17*	*0.15*	*0.16*
potatoes, fried	*0.44*	*0.54*	*0.61*	*0.65*	*0.55*	*0.52*	*0.53*
other potatoes	*0.05*	*0.05*	*0.05*	*0.08*	*0.05*	*0.06*	*0.50*
savoury snacks	*0.35*	*0.47*	*0.49*	*0.46*	*0.44*	*0.42*	*0.43*
Fruit & nuts	0.05	0.07	0.07	0.08	0.06	0.07	0.07
of which:							
fruit	*0.02*	*0.02*	*0.02*	*0.02*	*0.02*	*0.02*	*0.02*
nuts, fruit & nut mixes	*0.03*	*0.06*	*0.05*	*0.07*	*0.04*	*0.05*	*0.05*
Sugar, preserves & confectionery	0.09	0.14	0.15	0.15	0.13	0.12	0.13
of which:							
chocolate confectionery	*0.08*	*0.11*	*0.12*	*0.12*	*0.10*	*0.10*	*0.10*
Beverages	0.01	0.01	0.01	0.01	0.01	0.01	0.01
Commercial infant foods & drinks	0.01	0.00	0.00	0.00	0.01	0.00	0.01
Miscellaneous	0.08	0.18	0.21	0.15	0.14	0.14	0.14
Average daily intake (g)	**4.3**	**5.1**	**5.8**	**5.5**	**5.1**	**4.9**	**5.0**
Total number of children	**576**	**606**	**250**	**243**	**848**	**827**	**1675**

Table 7.21(b)   Percentage contribution of food types to average daily intake of *cis* n-6 polyunsaturated fatty acids by age and sex of child

Food types	Age and sex of child						
	All aged 1½ – 2½ years	All aged 2½ – 3½ years	All aged 3½ – 4½ years		All boys	All girls	All
			Boys	Girls			
	%	%	%	%	%	%	%
Cereals & cereal products	23	23	22	24	24	22	22
of which:							
biscuits	4	5	5	4	5	4	5
buns, cakes & pastries	3	4	5	4	4	4	4
Milk & milk products	7	4	3	3	5	5	5
of which:							
cows' milk	4	2	2	2	3	3	3
other milk & cream	2	0	0	0	1	1	1
cheese	1	1	1	1	1	1	1
fromage frais & yogurt	0	0	0	0	0	0	0
Eggs & egg dishes	3	3	3	4	3	4	3
Fat spreads	20	19	20	20	20	20	20
of which:							
butter	0	0	0	0	0	0	0
polyunsaturated margarine	13	14	14	12	13	14	13
Meat & meat products	14	14	15	14	15	14	14
of which:							
sausages	5	4	5	5	5	5	5
beef, veal & dishes	2	1	1	1	1	1	1
all chicken & turkey	2	3	3	3	3	3	3
Fish & fish dishes	4	4	4	4	4	4	4
Vegetables, potatoes & savoury snacks	23	24	23	25	24	23	24
of which:							
vegetables, excluding potatoes	3	3	3	3	3	3	3
potatoes, fried	10	10	10	12	11	10	11
other potatoes	1	1	1	1	1	1	1
savoury snacks	8	9	8	8	9	8	9
Fruit & nuts	1	1	1	1	1	1	1
of which:							
fruit	0	0	0	0	0	0	0
nuts, fruit & nut mixes	1	1	1	1	1	1	1
Sugar & confectionery	2	3	3	3	3	2	3
of which:							
chocolate confectionery	2	2	2	2	2	2	2
Beverages	0	0	0	0	0	0	0
Commercial infant foods & drinks	0	0	0	0	0	0	0
Miscellaneous	2	3	4	3	3	3	3
Average daily intake (g)	**4.3**	**5.1**	**5.8**	**5.5**	**5.1**	**4.9**	**5.0**
Total number of children	**576**	**606**	**250**	**243**	**848**	**827**	**1675**

Table 7.22   Average daily intake of total fat and fatty acids by whether child was reported as being unwell during dietary recording period

Fatty acids (g)	Whether child was reported as being unwell during period								
	Unwell and eating affected			Unwell and eating not affected			Not unwell		
	Mean	Median	se	Mean	Median	se	Mean	Median	se
Total fat	41.0	40.8	0.83	44.0	41.4	0.87	47.0	45.5	0.37
Saturated fatty acids	18.5	18.6	0.41	19.8	19.0	0.43	21.1	20.5	0.18
Trans fatty acids	1.9	1.8	0.06	2.1	2.0	0.07	2.3	2.1	0.03
cis monounsaturated fatty acids	12.7	12.8	0.27	13.4	12.6	0.27	14.6	14.1	0.12
cis n–3 polyunsaturated fatty acids	0.7	0.6	0.03	0.8	0.7	0.04	0.9	0.8	0.01
cis n–6 polyunsaturated fatty acids	4.5	4.1	0.14	4.9	4.5	0.16	5.1	4.8	0.06
Percentage energy from:								
total fat	35.8	36.1	0.34	35.8	35.6	0.36	35.9	36.1	0.15
saturated fatty acids	16.2	16.1	0.21	16.2	16.2	0.24	16.2	16.0	0.09
trans fatty acids	1.6	1.6	0.03	1.7	1.6	0.04	1.7	1.6	0.02
cis monounsaturated fatty acids	11.1	10.9	0.12	10.9	10.8	0.13	11.2	11.1	0.06
cis n–3 polyunsaturated fatty acids	0.7	0.6	0.02	0.7	0.6	0.03	0.7	0.6	0.01
cis n–6 polyunsaturated fatty acids	3.9	3.6	0.10	4.0	3.7	0.11	3.9	3.8	0.04
Total number of children		266			190			1203	

Table 7.23 Average daily intake of total fat and fatty acids by region

Fatty acids (g)	Region										
	Scotland			Northern			Central, South West and Wales			London and South East		
	Mean	Median	se	Mean	Median	se	Mean	Median	se	Mean	Median	se
Total fat	45.7	44.5	1.1	46.3	44.9	0.65	46.1	45.1	0.53	44.7	43.8	0.56
Saturated fatty acids	20.3	19.1	0.53	20.8	20.4	0.32	20.7	20.2	0.26	20.3	19.6	0.28
Trans fatty acids	2.1	1.9	0.07	2.4	2.1	0.06	2.2	2.1	0.04	2.1	2.0	0.02
cis monounsaturated fatty acids	14.5	14.1	0.36	14.3	13.7	0.21	14.4	14.0	0.17	13.7	13.2	0.18
cis n–3 polyunsaturated fatty acids	0.8	0.8	0.03	0.9	0.7	0.03	0.9	0.8	0.02	0.9	0.7	0.02
cis n–6 polyunsaturated fatty acids	5.0	4.7	0.16	5.0	4.7	0.11	5.1	4.7	0.09	4.9	4.5	0.09
Percentage energy from:											
total fat	35.8	36.2	0.42	35.9	36.7	0.26	36.0	36.1	0.22	35.9	35.6	0.23
saturated fatty acids	15.9	15.6	0.24	16.2	16.2	0.16	17.2	16.1	0.13	16.3	16.1	0.15
trans fatty acids	1.6	1.5	0.04	1.8	1.7	0.03	1.7	1.6	0.02	1.7	1.6	0.02
cis monounsaturated fatty acids	11.4	11.3	0.16	11.1	11.0	0.10	11.2	11.2	0.08	11.1	10.8	0.08
cis n–3 polyunsaturated fatty acids	0.7	0.6	0.02	0.7	0.6	0.02	0.7	0.6	0.01	0.7	0.6	0.02
cis n–6 polyunsaturated fatty acids	3.9	3.8	0.10	3.9	3.7	0.07	4.0	3.8	0.06	4.0	3.7	0.06
Total number of children	165			427			563			520		

Table 7.24 Average daily intake of total fat and fatty acids by social class of head of household

Fatty acids (g)	Social class of head of household					
	Non-manual			Manual		
	Mean	Median	se	Mean	Median	se
Total fat	45.0	44.1	0.46	46.3	44.6	0.46
Saturated fatty acids	20.3	19.8	0.23	20.8	20.2	0.22
Trans fatty acids	2.1	2.0	0.03	2.2	2.1	0.03
cis monounsaturated fatty acids	13.8	13.4	0.15	14.5	14.0	0.15
cis n–3 polyunsaturated fatty acids	0.9	0.7	0.02	0.9	0.8	0.02
cis n–6 polyunsaturated fatty acids	5.0	4.7	0.08	5.0	4.6	0.07
Percentage energy from:						
total fat	35.6	35.8	0.19	36.1	36.2	0.18
saturated fatty acids	16.1	16.1	0.12	16.3	16.1	0.11
trans fatty acids	1.7	1.6	0.02	1.7	1.6	0.02
cis monounsaturated fatty acids	10.9	10.9	0.07	11.3	11.3	0.06
cis n–3 polyunsaturated fatty acids	0.7	0.6	0.01	0.7	0.6	0.01
cis n–6 polyunsaturated fatty acids	4.0	3.7	0.05	3.9	3.7	0.04
Total number of children	748			867		

Table 7.25 Average daily intake of total fat and fatty acids by whether child's parents were receiving Income Support or Family Credit

Fatty acids (g)	Whether receiving benefit(s)					
	Receiving benefit(s)			Not receiving benefits		
	Mean	Median	se	Mean	Median	se
Total fat	47.0	45.2	0.63	45.1	44.2	0.36
Saturated fatty acids	20.7	20.0	0.30	20.5	19.9	0.18
Trans fatty acids	2.3	2.1	0.05	2.2	2.0	0.03
cis monounsaturated fatty acids	14.9	14.2	0.21	13.8	13.4	0.12
cis n–3 polyunsaturated fatty acids	0.9	0.8	0.02	0.8	0.7	0.01
cis n–6 polyunsaturated fatty acids	5.2	4.9	0.10	4.9	4.5	0.06
Percentage energy from:						
total fat	36.3	36.4	0.24	35.7	35.9	0.15
saturated fatty acids	16.0	15.7	0.14	16.2	16.1	0.10
trans fatty acids	1.7	1.6	0.03	1.7	1.6	0.16
cis monounsaturated fatty acids	11.5	11.4	0.09	11.0	10.9	0.05
cis n–3 polyunsaturated fatty acids	0.7	0.6	0.02	0.7	0.6	0.01
cis n–6 polyunsaturated fatty acids	4.0	3.8	0.06	3.9	3.7	0.04
Total number of children	534			1140		

Table 7.26   Average daily intake of total fat and fatty acids by employment status of head of household

Fatty acids (g)	Employment status of head of household								
	Working			Unemployed			Economically inactive		
	Mean	Median	se	Mean	Median	se	Mean	Median	se
Total fat	45.0	44.2	0.35	47.0	45.1	1.2	47.9	45.9	0.89
Saturated fatty acids	20.4	19.9	0.17	20.9	19.9	0.61	20.9	20.4	0.42
Trans fatty acids	2.2	2.0	0.02	2.3	2.0	0.09	2.3	2.1	0.06
cis monounsaturated fatty acids	13.8	13.4	0.11	14.8	13.9	0.39	15.3	14.5	0.30
cis n–3 polyunsaturated fatty acids	0.8	0.7	0.01	0.9	0.8	0.05	1.0	0.8	0.03
cis n–6 polyunsaturated fatty acids	4.9	4.6	0.06	5.2	4.9	0.18	5.4	5.0	0.15
Percentage energy from:									
total fat	35.7	35.8	0.15	36.6	36.7	0.42	36.6	36.5	0.33
saturated fatty acids	16.2	16.1	0.93	16.3	16.1	0.26	16.0	15.8	0.20
trans fatty acids	1.7	1.6	0.02	1.7	1.6	0.05	1.7	1.7	0.04
cis monounsaturated fatty acids	11.0	10.9	0.05	11.5	11.4	0.16	11.7	11.7	0.13
cis n–3 polyunsaturated fatty acids	0.6	0.6	0.09	0.7	0.6	0.04	0.8	0.6	0.02
cis n–6 polyunsaturated fatty acids	3.9	3.7	0.39	4.1	3.7	0.12	4.1	3.9	0.09
Total number of children		1249			167			259	

Table 7.27   Average daily intake of total fat and fatty acids by mother's highest educational qualification level

Fatty acids (g)	Mother's highest educational qualification level														
	Above GCE 'A' level			GCE 'A' level and equivalent			GCE 'O' level and equivalent			CSE and equivalent			None		
	Mean	Median	se	Mean	Median	se	Mean	Median	se	Mean	Median	se	Mean	Median	se
Total fat	44.2	43.3	0.63	45.5	44.8	0.99	45.0	44.2	0.52	45.5	44.3	0.77	48.2	46.8	0.81
Saturated fatty acids	20.1	19.2	0.32	20.5	19.5	0.49	20.2	19.9	0.26	20.4	20.1	0.37	21.6	20.8	0.40
Trans fatty acids	2.1	2.0	0.05	2.2	2.0	0.07	2.2	2.0	0.04	2.2	2.0	0.07	2.3	2.1	0.06
cis monounsaturated fatty acids	13.3	12.9	0.20	14.1	13.8	0.32	14.0	13.5	0.17	14.3	13.8	0.26	15.3	14.8	0.27
cis n–3 polyunsaturated fatty acids	0.8	0.7	0.03	0.9	0.8	0.04	0.9	0.8	0.02	0.9	0.8	0.03	0.9	0.7	0.03
cis n–6 polyunsaturated fatty acids	4.9	4.6	0.12	5.0	4.4	0.17	4.9	4.6	0.09	5.0	4.8	0.14	5.1	4.8	0.12
Percentage energy from:															
total fat	35.1	35.0	0.29	35.7	35.8	0.40	35.6	35.7	0.22	36.2	36.3	0.34	37.0	37.0	0.28
saturated fatty acids	16.0	16.1	0.19	16.1	16.1	0.24	16.0	15.9	0.14	16.2	15.8	0.21	16.6	16.4	0.17
trans fatty acids	1.7	1.6	0.03	1.7	1.6	0.04	1.7	1.6	0.02	1.7	1.6	0.04	1.7	1.7	0.03
cis monounsaturated fatty acids	10.6	10.6	0.10	11.0	11.1	0.15	11.0	11.0	0.08	11.3	11.2	0.12	11.7	11.7	0.11
cis n–3 polyunsaturated fatty acids	0.7	0.6	0.02	0.7	0.6	0.03	0.7	0.6	0.01	0.7	0.6	0.02	0.7	0.6	0.02
cis n–6 polyunsaturated fatty acids	3.9	3.7	0.08	3.9	3.5	0.11	3.9	3.7	0.06	4.0	3.8	0.10	4.0	3.8	0.07
Total number of children		305			183			590			236			358	

Table 7.28   Average daily intake of total fat and fatty acids by family type

Fatty acids (g)	Family type											
	Married or cohabiting couple						Lone parent					
	One child			More than one child			One child			More than one child		
	Mean	Median	se	Mean	Median	se	Mean	Median	se	Mean	Median	se
Total fat	44.5	44.3	0.64	44.5	44.2	0.40	47.7	45.4	1.4	47.6	45.0	1.0
Saturated fatty acids	20.4	20.3	0.33	20.6	19.6	0.20	20.8	20.4	0.66	20.7	20.0	0.47
Trans fatty acids	2.1	2.0	0.05	2.2	2.0	0.03	2.3	2.1	0.10	2.3	2.1	0.07
cis monounsaturated fatty acids	13.7	13.3	0.21	14.0	13.7	0.13	15.0	14.6	0.45	15.3	14.2	0.36
cis n–3 polyunsaturated fatty acids	0.8	0.8	0.02	0.9	0.7	0.02	1.0	0.9	0.05	1.0	0.8	0.04
cis n–6 polyunsaturated fatty acids	4.7	4.3	0.10	5.0	4.7	0.07	5.5	5.0	0.23	5.4	5.0	0.19
Percentage energy from:												
total fat	35.9	35.7	0.29	35.8	35.9	0.16	36.1	36.9	0.50	36.5	36.3	0.41
saturated fatty acids	16.5	16.4	0.18	16.1	15.9	0.10	15.8	15.7	0.27	15.9	15.7	0.25
trans fatty acids	1.7	1.7	0.26	1.7	1.6	0.02	1.8	1.7	0.06	1.7	1.7	0.04
cis monounsaturated fatty acids	11.0	10.9	0.10	11.0	11.0	0.06	11.4	11.6	0.18	11.7	11.5	0.16
cis n–3 polyunsaturated fatty acids	0.7	0.6	0.02	0.7	0.6	0.01	0.8	0.6	0.04	0.7	0.7	0.03
cis n–6 polyunsaturated fatty acids	3.8	3.5	0.07	3.9	3.7	0.04	4.1	4.0	0.01	4.1	4.0	0.10
Total number of children		366			1011			121			177	

Table 7.29 Percentage of average daily intake of total fat (g) from food types by region

Food types	Region			
	Scotland	Northern	Central, South West and Wales	London and South East
	%	%	%	%
Cereals and cereal products	18	20	19	20
of which:				
biscuits	6	7	7	7
buns, cakes & pastries	3	3	4	4
Milk & milk products	25	26	27	30
of which:				
cows' milk	19	20	21	22
Eggs & egg dishes	4	2	3	3
Fat spreads	9	9	10	9
Meat & meat products	17	18	15	15
Fish & fish dishes	2	2	2	2
Vegetables, potatoes & savoury snacks	15	13	14	13
of which:				
potatoes, fried	7	6	5	4
savoury snacks	8	6	7	6
Fruit & nuts	1	1	1	1
Sugar, preserves & confectionery	7	7	6	5
of which:				
chocolate confectionery	6	6	6	5
Beverages	0	0	0	0
Commercial infant foods & drinks	0	0	0	0
Miscellaneous	2	1	2	1
Average daily intake (g)	**45.7**	**46.3**	**46.1**	**44.7**
Total number of children	**165**	**427**	**563**	**520**

Table 7.30 Percentage of average daily intake of saturated fatty acids from food types by region

Food types	Region			
	Scotland	Northern	Central, South West and Wales	London and South East
	%	%	%	%
Cereals and cereal products	18	20	18	19
of which:				
biscuits	7	8	7	8
buns, cakes & pastries	2	3	3	3
Milk & milk products	35	36	38	41
of which:				
cows' milk	27	28	29	30
cheese	4	5	5	6
Eggs & egg dishes	3	2	2	2
Fat spreads	7	7	7	7
of which:				
butter	4	3	3	3
polyunsaturated margarine	1	1	1	1
Meat & meat products	14	15	13	12
Fish & fish dishes	1	1	1	1
Vegetables, potatoes & savoury snacks	11	9	10	10
of which:				
potatoes, fried	4	3	3	3
savoury snacks	7	5	6	5
Fruit & nuts	0	0	0	1
Sugar, preserves & confectionery	8	8	8	7
of which:				
chocolate confectionery	7	8	7	6
Beverages	0	0	0	0
Commercial infant foods & drinks	0	0	0	0
Miscellaneous	2	1	2	1
Average daily intake (g)	**20.3**	**20.8**	**20.7**	**20.3**
Total number of children	**165**	**427**	**563**	**520**

Table 7.31 Percentage of average daily intake of *trans* fatty acids from food types by region

Food types	Region			
	Scotland	Northern	Central, South West and Wales	London and South East
	%	%	%	%
Cereals and cereal products	26	26	29	30
of which:				
biscuits	*12*	*12*	*13*	*13*
buns, cakes & pastries	*7*	*7*	*9*	*10*
Milk & milk products	27	24	28	31
of which:				
cows' milk	*21*	*19*	*21*	*23*
Eggs & egg dishes	1	1	1	1
Fat spreads	14	13	15	13
of which:				
butter	*2*	*2*	*2*	*2*
polyunsaturated margarine	*3*	*4*	*4*	*4*
Meat & meat products	15	23	15	12
Fish & fish dishes	1	2	1	2
Vegetables, potatoes & savoury snacks	6	4	5	5
of which:				
potatoes, fried	*4*	*3*	*3*	*3*
savoury snacks	*1*	*1*	*1*	*1*
Fruit & nuts	0	0	0	0
Sugar, preserves & confectionery	8	6	5	4
of which:				
chocolate confectionery	*5*	*4*	*4*	*3*
Beverages	–	–	0	0
Commercial infant foods & drinks	0	0	0	0
Miscellaneous	1	0	0	1
Average daily intake (g)	**2.1**	**2.4**	**2.1**	**2.1**
Total number of children	**165**	**427**	**563**	**520**

Table 7.32 Percentage of average daily intake of *cis* monounsaturated fatty acids from food types by region

Food types	Region			
	Scotland	Northern	Central, South West and Wales	London and South East
	%	%	%	%
Cereals and cereal products	17	18	18	18
of which:				
biscuits	*6*	*7*	*6*	*7*
buns, cakes & pastries	*2*	*3*	*3*	*4*
Milk & milk products	19	21	22	25
of which:				
cows' milk	*15*	*17*	*17*	*18*
Eggs & egg dishes	5	3	3	3
Fat spreads	8	9	9	8
Meat & meat products	21	22	20	19
Fish & fish dishes	2	2	2	2
Vegetables, potatoes & savoury snacks	19	16	17	17
of which:				
potatoes, fried	*8*	*7*	*6*	*5*
savoury snacks	*9*	*7*	*9*	*8*
Fruit & nuts	1	1	1	1
Sugar, preserves & confectionery	6	7	6	6
of which:				
chocolate confectionery	*5*	*6*	*5*	*5*
Beverages	0	0	0	0
Commercial infant foods & drinks	0	0	0	0
Miscellaneous	2	1	2	1
Average daily intake (g)	**14.5**	**14.3**	**14.4**	**13.7**
Total number of children	**165**	**427**	**563**	**520**

Table 7.33 Percentage of average daily intake of *cis* n−3 polyunsaturated fatty acids from food types by region

Food types	Region			
	Scotland	Northern	Central, South West and Wales	London and South East
	%	%	%	%
Cereals and cereal products	15	14	14	14
of which:				
biscuits	*2*	*2*	*2*	*2*
buns, cakes & pastries	*1*	*2*	*2*	*2*
Milk & milk products	10	12	13	12
of which:				
cows' milk	*7*	*8*	*8*	*8*
Eggs & egg dishes	2	1	1	1
Fat spreads	7	7	8	7
Meat & meat products	12	12	11	10
Fish & fish dishes	10	14	12	14
Vegetables, potatoes & savoury snacks	32	29	29	26
of which:				
vegetables, excluding potatoes	*5*	*6*	*7*	*7*
potatoes, fried	*21*	*18*	*17*	*15*
savoury snacks	*5*	*3*	*5*	*3*
Fruit & nuts	6	9	8	12
of which:				
fruit	*1*	*1*	*1*	*1*
nuts, fruits & nut mixes	*5*	*7*	*7*	*10*
Sugar, preserves & confectionery	1	1	1	1
of which:				
chocolate confectionery	*1*	*1*	*1*	*1*
Beverages	0	0	0	0
Commercial infant foods & drinks	0	0	0	0
Miscellaneous	4	1	1	2
Average daily intake (g)	**0.8**	**0.9**	**0.9**	**0.9**
Total number of children	**165**	**427**	**563**	**520**

Table 7.34 Percentage of average daily intake of *cis* n−6 polyunsaturated fatty acids from food types by region

Food types	Region			
	Scotland	Northern	Central, South West and Wales	London and South East
	%	%	%	%
Cereals and cereal products	21	23	23	24
of which:				
biscuits	*4*	*5*	*5*	*4*
buns, cakes & pastries	*2*	*3*	*4*	*5*
Milk & milk products	4	4	5	5
of which:				
cows' milk	*2*	*3*	*2*	*3*
Eggs & egg dishes	5	3	3	3
Fat spreads	17	21	21	20
of which:				
polyunsaturated margarine	*11*	*15*	*13*	*13*
Meat & meat products	15	15	14	14
Fish & fish dishes	4	4	3	4
Vegetables, potatoes & savoury snacks	27	23	24	22
of which:				
vegetables, excluding potatoes	*3*	*2*	*3*	*4*
potatoes, fried	*13*	*12*	*10*	*9*
savoury snacks	*10*	*8*	*9*	*8*
Fruit & nuts	1	1	1	2
Sugar, preserves & confectionery	3	3	3	2
of which:				
chocolate confectionery	*2*	*2*	*2*	*2*
Beverages	0	0	0	0
Commercial infant foods & drinks	0	0	0	0
Miscellaneous	4	2	2	3
Average daily intake (g)	**5.0**	**5.0**	**5.1**	**4.9**
Total number of children	**165**	**427**	**563**	**520**

Table 7.35 Percentage of average daily intake of total fat from food types by social class of head of household

Food types	Social class of head of household	
	Non-manual	Manual
	%	%
Cereals & cereal products	21	18
of which:		
biscuits	*7*	*7*
buns, cakes & pastries	*3*	*3*
Milk & milk products	29	27
of which:		
cows' milk	*21*	*21*
Eggs & egg dishes	3	2
Fat spreads	9	9
Meat & meat products	15	17
Fish & fish dishes	2	2
Vegetables, potatoes & savoury snacks	12	15
of which:		
potatoes, fried	*4*	*6*
savoury snacks	*6*	*7*
Fruit & nuts	1	1
Sugar, preserves & confectionery	6	7
of which:		
chocolate confectionery	*5*	*5*
Beverages	0	0
Commercial infant foods & drinks	0	0
Miscellaneous	2	1
Average daily intake (g)	**45.0**	**46.3**
Total number of children	**748**	**867**

Table 7.36 Percentage of average daily intake of saturated fatty acids from food types by social class of head of household

Food types	Social class of head of household	
	Non-manual	Manual
	%	%
Cereals & cereal products	20	18
of which:		
biscuits	*8*	*7*
buns, cakes & pastries	*3*	*3*
Milk & milk products	39	37
of which:		
cows' milk	*29*	*29*
cheese	*6*	*5*
Eggs & egg dishes	2	2
Fat spreads	7	7
of which:		
butter	*3*	*3*
polyunsaturated margarine	*1*	*1*
Meat & meat products	12	14
Fish & fish dishes	1	1
Vegetables, potatoes & savoury snacks	9	11
of which:		
potatoes, fried	*2*	*3*
savoury snacks	*5*	*6*
Fruit & nuts	1	0
Sugar, preserves & confectionery	7	8
of which:		
chocolate confectionery	*7*	*8*
Beverages	0	0
Commercial infant foods & drinks	0	0
Miscellaneous	1	1
Average daily intake (g)	**20.3**	**20.8**
Total number of children	**748**	**867**

Table 7.37 Percentage of average daily intake of *trans* fatty acids from food types by social class of head of household

Food types	Social class of head of household	
	Non-manual	Manual
	%	%
Cereals & cereal products	32	26
of which:		
biscuits	*14*	*12*
buns, cakes & pastries	*10*	*7*
Milk & milk products	29	27
of which:		
cows' milk	*22*	*21*
Eggs & egg dishes	1	1
Fat spreads	13	14
of which:		
butter	*2*	*2*
polyunsaturated margarine	*5*	*3*
Meat & meat products	13	19
Fish & fish dishes	2	2
Vegetables, potatoes & savoury snacks	4	5
of which:		
potatoes, fried	*3*	*3*
savoury snacks	*1*	*1*
Fruit & nuts	0	0
Sugar, preserves & confectionery	4	6
of which:		
chocolate confectionery	*3*	*4*
Beverages	0	0
Commercial infant foods & drinks	0	0
Miscellaneous	1	0
Average daily intake (g)	**2.1**	**2.2**
Total number of children	**748**	**867**

Table 7.38 Percentage of average daily intake of *cis* monounsaturated fatty acids from food types by social class of head of household

Food types	Social class of head of household	
	Non-manual	Manual
	%	%
Cereals & cereal products	19	17
of which:		
biscuits	*7*	*6*
buns, cakes & pastries	*4*	*3*
Milk & milk products	24	21
of which:		
cows' milk	*17*	*17*
Eggs & egg dishes	4	3
Fat spreads	8	9
Meat & meat products	19	21
Fish & fish dishes	2	2
Vegetables, potatoes & savoury snacks	14	18
of which:		
potatoes, fried	*5*	*7*
savoury snacks	*8*	*9*
Fruit & nuts	2	1
Sugar, preserves & confectionery	6	6
of which:		
chocolate confectionery	*5*	*6*
Beverages	0	0
Commercial infant foods & drinks	0	0
Miscellaneous	2	2
Average daily intake (g)	**13.8**	**14.5**
Total number of children	**748**	**867**

Table 7.39 Percentage of average daily intake of *cis* n–3 polyunsaturated fatty acids from food types by social class of head of household

Food types	Social class of head of household	
	Non-manual	Manual
	%	%
Cereals & cereal products	15	14
of which:		
biscuits	*2*	*2*
buns, cakes & pastries	*2*	*2*
Milk & milk products	13	12
of which:		
cows' milk	*8*	*8*
Eggs & egg dishes	1	1
Fat spreads	7	8
Meat & meat products	10	12
Fish & fish dishes	13	12
Vegetables, potatoes & savoury snacks	25	30
of which:		
vegetables, excluding potatoes	*7*	*6*
potatoes, fried	*15*	*18*
savoury snacks	*3*	*5*
Fruit & nuts	13	7
of which:		
fruit	*2*	*1*
nuts, fruits & nut mixes	*10*	*6*
Sugar, preserves & confectionery	1	1
of which:		
chocolate confectionery	*1*	*1*
Beverages	1	0
Commercial infant foods & drinks	0	0
Miscellaneous	2	2
Average daily intake (g)	**0.9**	**0.9**
Total number of children	**748**	**867**

Table 7.40 Percentage of average daily intake of *cis* n–6 polyunsaturated fatty acids from food types by social class of head of household

Food types	Social class of head of household	
	Non-manual	Manual
	%	%
Cereals & cereal products	24	22
of which:		
biscuits	*5*	*4*
buns, cakes & pastries	*5*	*4*
Milk & milk products	5	5
of which:		
cows' milk	*3*	*3*
Eggs & egg dishes	3	3
Fat spreads	21	19
of which:		
polyunsaturated margarine	*15*	*12*
Meat & meat products	14	15
Fish & fish dishes	4	4
Vegetables, potatoes & savoury snacks	21	25
of which:		
vegetables, excluding potatoes	*4*	*3*
potatoes, fried	*9*	*12*
savoury snacks	*8*	*10*
Fruit & nuts	2	1
Sugar, preserves & confectionery	2	3
of which:		
chocolate confectionery	*2*	*2*
Beverages	0	0
Commercial infant foods & drinks	0	0
Miscellaneous	3	2
Average daily intake (g)	**5.0**	**5.0**
Total number of children	**748**	**867**

Table 7.41 Percentage of average daily intake of total fat from food types by mother's highest educational qualification level

Food types	Mother's highest educational qualification level				
	Above GCE 'A' level	GCE 'A' level and equivalent	GCE 'O' level and equivalent	CSE and equivalent	None
	%	%	%	%	
Cereals & cereal products	23	20	20	18	17
of which:					
biscuits	*8*	*7*	*7*	*7*	*6*
buns, cakes & pastries	*4*	*4*	*4*	*3*	*3*
Milk & milk products	31	30	27	26	26
of which:					
cows' milk	*22*	*20*	*20*	*20*	*22*
Eggs & egg dishes	3	2	3	3	3
Fat spreads	9	9	10	9	9
Meat & meat products	13	16	16	17	18
Fish & fish dishes	2	2	2	2	1
Vegetables, potatoes & savoury snacks	10	12	14	15	16
of which:					
potatoes, fried	*3*	*4*	*5*	*6*	*6*
savoury snacks	*5*	*6*	*7*	*7*	*7*
Fruit & nuts	1	2	1	1	1
Sugar, preserves & confectionery	5	6	6	7	6
of which:					
chocolate confectionery	*5*	*5*	*6*	*6*	*6*
Beverages	0	0	0	0	0
Commercial infant foods & drinks	0	0	0	0	0
Miscellaneous	2	2	2	2	2
Average daily intake (g)	**44.2**	**45.5**	**45.0**	**45.5**	**48.2**
Total number of children	**305**	**183**	**590**	**236**	**358**

Table 7.42 Percentage of average daily intake of saturated fatty acids from food types by mother's highest educational qualification level

Food types	Above GCE 'A' level	GCE 'A' level and equivalent	GCE 'O' level and equivalent	CSE and equivalent	None
	%	%	%	%	
Cereals & cereal products	22	19	19	18	17
of which:					
biscuits	*8*	*7*	*8*	*8*	*7*
buns, cakes & pastries	*4*	*3*	*3*	*2*	*2*
Milk & milk products	42	40	37	36	36
of which:					
cows' milk	*30*	*28*	*28*	*29*	*30*
cheese	*7*	*6*	*5*	*5*	*4*
Eggs & egg dishes	2	1	2	2	2
Fat spreads	7	7	8	7	7
of which:					
butter	*3*	*3*	*4*	*2*	*2*
polyunsaturated margarine	*2*	*1*	*1*	*1*	*1*
Meat & meat products	10	13	13	14	16
Fish & fish dishes	1	1	1	1	1
Vegetables, potatoes & savoury snacks	7	9	10	11	11
of which:					
potatoes, fried	*2*	*2*	*3*	*3*	*4*
savoury snacks	*5*	*5*	*6*	*6*	*6*
Fruit & nuts	1	1	0	1	0
Sugar, preserves & confectionery	6	7	8	8	8
of which:					
chocolate confectionery	*6*	*7*	*8*	*8*	*7*
Beverages	0	0	0	0	0
Commercial infant foods & drinks	0	0	0	0	0
Miscellaneous	1	2	1	1	2
Average daily intake (g)	**20.1**	**20.5**	**20.2**	**20.4**	**21.6**
Total number of children	**305**	**183**	**590**	**236**	**358**

Table 7.43 Percentage of average daily intake of *trans* fatty acids from food types by mother's highest educational qualification level

Food types	Above GCE 'A' level	GCE 'A' level and equivalent	GCE 'O' level and equivalent	CSE and equivalent	None
	%	%	%	%	
Cereals and cereal products	34	30	28	26	24
of which:					
biscuits	*14*	*13*	*13*	*13*	*11*
buns, cakes & pastries	*12*	*10*	*8*	*7*	*7*
Milk & milk products	31	30	26	26	27
of which:					
cows' milk	*23*	*21*	*20*	*20*	*22*
Eggs & egg dishes	1	1	1	1	1
Fat spreads	12	13	15	14	15
of which:					
butter	*2*	*2*	*2*	*1*	*2*
polyunsaturated margarine	*5*	*5*	*4*	*4*	*3*
Meat & meat products	11	14	16	18	20
Fish & fish dishes	2	2	2	2	1
Vegetables, potatoes & savoury snacks	3	4	5	5	5
of which:					
potatoes, fried	*1*	*2*	*3*	*3*	*3*
savoury snacks	*1*	*1*	*1*	*1*	*1*
Fruit & nuts	0	0	0	0	–
Sugar, preserves & confectionery	4	5	5	6	6
of which:					
chocolate confectionery	*3*	*4*	*4*	*4*	*5*
Beverages	–	0	–	0	–
Commercial infant foods & drinks	0	0	0	0	0
Miscellaneous	1	1	1	1	0
Average daily intake (g)	**2.1**	**2.2**	**2.2**	**2.2**	**2.3**
Total number of children	**305**	**183**	**590**	**236**	**358**

Table 7.44   Percentage of average daily intake of *cis* monounsaturated fatty acids by mother's highest educational qualification level

Food types	Mother's highest educational qualification level				
	Above GCE 'A' level	GCE 'A' level and equivalent	GCE 'O' level and equivalent	CSE and equivalent	None
	%	%	%	%	
Cereals & cereal products	22	18	18	17	16
of which:					
biscuits	*7*	*6*	*7*	*6*	*6*
buns, cakes & pastries	*4*	*4*	*4*	*3*	*3*
Milk & milk products	26	25	22	21	21
of which:					
cows' milk	*18*	*17*	*16*	*16*	*17*
Eggs & egg dishes	4	3	3	3	4
Fat spreads	8	8	9	9	9
Meat & meat products	17	20	20	20	22
Fish & fish dishes	2	2	2	2	1
Vegetables, potatoes & savoury snacks	12	14	16	18	18
of which:					
potatoes, fried	*3*	*5*	*7*	*8*	*8*
savoury snacks	*7*	*7*	*8*	*9*	*9*
Fruit & nuts	2	2	1	1	1
Sugar, preserves & confectionery	5	6	6	7	6
of which:					
chocolate confectionery	*5*	*5*	*6*	*6*	*6*
Beverages	0	0	0	0	0
Commercial infant foods & drinks	0	0	0	0	0
Miscellaneous	2	2	2	1	2
Average daily intake (g)	**13.3**	**14.1**	**14.0**	**14.3**	**15.3**
Total number of children	**305**	**183**	**590**	**236**	**358**

Table 7.45   Percentage of average daily intake of *cis* n–3 polyunsaturated fatty acids from food types by mother's highest educational qualification level

Food types	Mother's highest educational qualification level				
	Above GCE 'A' level	GCE 'A' level and equivalent	GCE 'O' level and equivalent	CSE and equivalent	None
	%	%	%	%	
Cereals & cereal products	17	13	14	14	12
of which:					
biscuits	*2*	*2*	*2*	*2*	*2*
buns, cakes & pastries	*2*	*2*	*2*	*2*	*2*
Milk & milk products	13	14	12	11	11
of which:					
cows' milk	*8*	*6*	*7*	*7*	*8*
Eggs & egg dishes	1	1	1	1	1
Fat spreads	6	7	8	8	9
Meat & meat products	10	11	11	11	12
Fish & fish dishes	14	13	13	13	10
Vegetables, potatoes & savoury snacks	22	23	30	31	33
of which:					
vegetables, excluding potatoes	*7*	*5*	*6*	*6*	*7*
potatoes, fried	*11*	*13*	*19*	*19*	*20*
savoury snacks	*4*	*3*	*5*	*4*	*4*
Fruit & nuts	12	14	8	9	8
of which:					
fruit	*2*	*1*	*1*	*1*	*1*
nuts, fruits & nut mixes	*10*	*13*	*7*	*8*	*7*
Sugar, preserves & confectionery	1	1	1	1	1
of which:					
chocolate confectionery	*1*	*1*	*1*	*1*	*1*
Beverages	1	0	0	0	0
Commercial infant foods & drinks	0	0	0	0	0
Miscellaneous	2	2	1	1	2
Average daily intake (g)	**0.8**	**0.9**	**0.9**	**0.9**	**0.9**
Total number of children	**305**	**183**	**590**	**236**	**358**

Table 7.46 Percentage of average daily intake of *cis* n–6 polyunsaturated fatty acids from food types by mother's highest educational qualification level

Food types	Mother's highest educational qualification level				
	Above GCE 'A' level	GCE 'A' level and equivalent	GCE 'O' level and equivalent	CSE and equivalent	None
	%	%	%	%	
Cereals & cereal products	26	23	23	22	21
of which:					
biscuits	*5*	*5*	*4*	*5*	*4*
buns, cakes & pastries	*5*	*4*	*4*	*3*	*3*
Milk & milk products	5	6	4	4	4
of which:					
cows' milk	*3*	*3*	*3*	*3*	*3*
Eggs & egg dishes	3	2	3	3	3
Fat spreads	22	20	20	19	19
of which:					
polyunsaturated margarine	*16*	*15*	*13*	*12*	*11*
Meat & meat products	12	15	14	14	16
Fish & fish dishes	5	4	4	4	3
Vegetables, potatoes & savoury snacks	18	20	24	27	27
of which:					
vegetables, excluding potatoes	*4*	*3*	*3*	*3*	*3*
potatoes, fried	*6*	*9*	*11*	*12*	*13*
savoury snacks	*7*	*7*	*9*	*10*	*10*
Fruit & nuts	2	2	1	2	1
Sugar, preserves & confectionery	2	2	3	3	3
of which:					
chocolate confectionery	*2*	*2*	*2*	*2*	*2*
Beverages	1	0	0	0	0
Commercial infant foods & drinks	0	0	0	0	0
Miscellaneous	4	5	3	2	2
Average daily intake (g)	**4.9**	**5.0**	**4.9**	**5.0**	**5.1**
Total number of children	**305**	**183**	**590**	**236**	**358**

8 Vitamins

Vitamins are organic compounds which are required in small amounts for growth and metabolism. They are essential substances which, with the exception of vitamin D, cannot be synthesised in the body and are therefore required in the diet.

This chapter presents data on the average daily intakes of vitamins and some precursors, for example carotene, which were derived from quantities of foods and dietary supplements consumed. Average daily intakes of vitamins were derived from weighting to seven days the intakes for the 1675 children for whom complete four-day weighed intake records containing two weekend days and two weekdays were obtained.[1]

Dietary supplements may have a sizeable impact on the intakes of some vitamins; about one fifth of children for whom four-day dietary records were completed were taking dietary supplements (see *Table 4.19*). This included 5% of children who were taking supplements in the form of drops; some of these would have been Department of Health Children's Vitamin Drops, which contain vitamins A, C and D.[2,3] In this Chapter data are therefore presented for intakes including dietary supplements, referred to as intakes from all sources, and excluding dietary supplements, referred to as intakes from food sources.

For those vitamins where UK Reference Nutrient Intake (RNI—see Box) values have been published for children aged 1 to 3 years and 4 to 6 years[4], the proportion of children meeting the current RNIs and Lower Reference Nutrient Intakes (LRNIs) are shown, and average daily intakes are compared with current RNIs, which are shown in Table 8.1.

REFERENCE NUTRIENT INTAKE (RNI)

The RNI for a vitamin or mineral is an amount of the nutrient that is enough, or more than enough, for about 97% of people in that group. If the average intake of the group is at the RNI, then the risk of deficiency in the group is very small. However, if the average intake is considerably lower than the RNI then it is possible that some of the group will have an intake below their requirement. This is even more likely if a proportion of the group have an intake below the LRNI. The LRNI of a vitamin or mineral is the amount of that nutrient that is enough for only the few people in a group who have low needs. For further definitions of the RNI and LRNI see Department of Health (1991).[4]

Average daily vitamin intakes are also presented per 1000kcal food energy and per kilogram body weight.

8.1 Vitamin A (retinol and carotene)

Vitamin A as pre-formed retinol is only available from animal products, especially liver, kidneys, oily fish and dairy products. However a number of carotenoids can be converted to retinol in the body, and these are primarily found in the yellow and orange pigments of vegetables; carrots and dark green vegetables are rich sources.

8.1.1 Pre-formed retinol

Average daily intake of pre-formed retinol from all sources, for children aged between 1½ and 4½ years was 433µg (median 286µg). Average intake decreased with age, being highest among children aged 1½ to 2½ years, 456µg, and lowest among children aged 3½ to 4½ years; 396µg for boys, and 414µg for girls (NS).

Average daily intakes of pre-formed retinol from food sources were lower than from all sources; the overall mean intake was 363µg (median 268µg). Thus supplements provided 19% of the total average daily intake of retinol for all children aged 1½ to 4½ years. However comparing the intakes for children in the top 2.5 percentile of the distribution with and without the inclusion of dietary supplements suggests supplements providing pre-formed retinol were predominantly being taken by children whose average daily intake was already high. For example, among children in the top 2.5 percentile aged 1½ to 2½ years intakes were increased by at least 43% when intakes from supplements were included.

As was observed for average intakes from all sources, average intakes from food sources decreased with age (NS).

The range of pre-formed retinol intakes from food sources was wide, with children aged 1½ to 4½ years at the lower 2.5 percentile having intakes which were about one quarter of the median intake. Intakes for children aged 1½ to 4½ years at the upper 2.5 percentile were at least twice the median intake. The distribution of pre-formed retinol intakes was skewed, with median intakes being about three quarters the mean intake, irrespective of age.
(Table 8.2)

8.1.2 β-carotene, α-carotene and β-cryptoxanthin

ß-carotene, α-carotene and ß-cryptoxanthin are all carotenoids with vitamin A activity. Only a few of the more than 100 carotenoids have structures that enable them to serve as precursors of vitamin A; ß-carotene is the most important of these. α-carotene and ß-cryptoxanthin have approximately half the activity of ß-carotene.

Average daily intake of ß-carotene for children aged 1½ to 4½ years from food sources was 790µg (median 600µg). Mean intakes increased with age although these differences did not reach statistical significance.

(Table 8.3)

Mean intake for children aged 1½ to 4½ years for α-carotene from food sources was 147µg (median 70.8µg), and for ß-cryptoxanthin 16.5µg (median 8.9µg). There was a tendency for mean intakes of α-carotene and ß-cryptoxanthin to increase with age, although differences in intake by age did not reach statistical significance.

(Tables 8.4 and 8.5)

For all three carotenoids measured there was a wide range of intakes. For example, intakes of ß-carotene among children aged 1½ to 4½ years at the lower 2.5 percentile were only about a quarter of the median intake, whereas intakes for children at the upper 2.5 percentile were at least three times the median intake (from *Table 8.3*).

8.1.3 Total carotene (ß-carotene equivalents)

Total carotene is expressed as ß-carotene equivalents, that is the sum of ß-carotene and half the amount of α-carotene and ß-cryptoxanthin.

As the dietary supplements taken by children in this survey did not provide any carotene the data presented refer to that obtained from the diet. Average daily total carotene intake for children aged between 1½ and 4½ years was 872µg (median 648µg). Average intake increased with age, being lowest among children aged 1½ to 2½ years, 796µg, and highest among children aged 3½ to 4½ years; boys had a somewhat higher intake than girls in this age group, 1029µg compared with 884µg (NS).

There was a very large range of total carotene intakes, with children at the bottom 2.5 percentile having intakes which were between a fifth and a quarter of the median intake, depending on age. Children at the upper 2.5 percentile of the distribution had intakes which were between three and a half and six times the median intake, depending on age. The distribution was skewed, with median intakes being at least two thirds the mean intake, depending on age.

(Table 8.6 and Figs 8.1 and 8.2)

Differences between age groups and boys and girls in intakes of total carotene might be associated with differences in energy intakes. Tables 8.7a and 8.7b show there were no significant differences in total carotene intake per 1000kcal food energy between boys and girls or children of different ages suggesting that differences in total intakes were due to differences in energy intake. There were no significant differences in intakes per kilogram body weight. *(Tables 8.7 and 8.8)*

Over half, 56%, of all children's total carotene intake came from vegetables, potatoes and savoury snacks.

Cooked carrots were the single largest provider, accounting for 35% of mean intake. Raw carrots also contributed to total carotene intake; the proportion provided rising from 4% among children aged 1½ to 2½ years to 13% among boys and 14% among girls aged 3½ to 4½ years (p<0.01). The total carotene contribution from soft drinks, mainly as added ß-carotene in orange coloured drinks, was 14% of the mean intake for children aged 1½ to 4½ years. *(Table 8.9b)*

8.1.4 Vitamin A (retinol equivalents)

The total vitamin A content of the diet is usually expressed as retinol equivalents using the conversion factor, 6µg ß-carotene as equivalent to 1µg retinol.

The mean intake from all sources for children aged 1½ to 4½ years was 578µg (median 428µg). Average intakes tended to decrease very slightly with age, falling from 589µg for children aged 1½ to 2½ years to 568µg for boys and 561µg for girls aged 3½ to 4½ years (NS).

Supplements containing pre-formed retinol provided 14% of the mean intake of vitamin A for children aged 1½ to 4½ years. Supplements containing pre-formed retinol greatly increased intakes of vitamin A for children in the upper 2.5 percentile. However supplements did not increase intakes for children in the lower 2.5 percentile, and median intakes only increased slightly.

(Table 8.10 and Figs 8.3 and 8.4)

There was a wide range of intakes, with children at the bottom 2.5 percentile having intakes from food sources which were about a third of the median intake, across all ages. Intakes of vitamin A for children at the upper 2.5 percentile were at least three times the median intake. As was seen for pre-formed retinol and total carotene, intakes of vitamin A were skewed, with median intakes about three quarters of the mean intake, depending on age. One reason for the skewed intakes of vitamin A is that only a limited number of foods are sources of vitamin A as pre-formed retinol. Children in this survey were also low consumers of vegetables (see *Table 4.3*) which are the main source of carotenoids.

Table 8.1 shows the current UK RNI and LRNI values for vitamin A for children aged between 1 and 3 years and 4 and 6 years[4]. The average daily intake of vitamin A from food sources among children aged 1½ to 4½ years was 127% of the RNI (see *Table 8.11*). However half of all children aged between 1½ and 4½ years had average daily intakes from food sources below the RNI value of 400µg/d. Average intakes from food sources for all children in the upper 2.5 percentile were at least three times the RNI, whereas children in the lower 2.5 percentile had intakes below the LRNI of 200µg/d *(Table 8.10)*. Overall 8% of children had intakes below the LRNI.

After controlling for differences in energy intake and body weight, vitamin A intakes tended to decrease with age, although none of these age differences were found to be statistically significant (see *Tables 8.7a and 8.8a*).

The main sources of vitamin A for all children in this survey were cows' milk (27%), liver (16%) and vegetables, excluding potatoes (16%). Milk and liver were also the main sources of vitamin A for children in the 1967/8 preschool children's nutrition survey, however vegetables provided more vitamin A for children in the current survey than in 1967/8[5]. Overall milk and milk products contributed a third of the average daily intake of vitamin A in this survey; however, the proportion declined slightly with age, being highest among children aged 1½ to 2½ years, 39%, and lowest among girls aged 3½ to 4½ years, 30% (NS).

Meat and meat products provided a further 20% of the average daily intake of vitamin A for children aged 1½ to 4½ years. Intakes of vitamin A from meat and meat products also tended to decline with age. *(Table 8.12b)*

8.2 B vitamins

8.2.1 Thiamin (vitamin B₁)

The average intake of thiamin from all sources for children aged 1½ to 4½ years was 0.8mg (median 0.7mg). Average intakes varied only slightly with age, with both boys and girls aged 3½ to 4½ years having higher intakes 0.9mg, than children aged 1½ to 2½ years, 0.8mg (NS).

As dietary supplements provided very little additional thiamin, average daily intake from food sources for all children was very similar to that from all sources. However, intakes for children in the upper 2.5 percentile increased by at least 13% when intakes from supplements were included, whereas median intakes and intakes among children in the lower 2.5 percentile were unchanged, suggesting supplements providing thiamin were predominantly being taken by children with higher intakes. *(Table 8.13)*

Table 8.14 shows that the average intake of thiamin from food sources among children aged under 4 years was 154% of the RNI and for children aged 4 years and over mean thiamin intake was 123% of the RNI (see *Table 8.1*). Only 10% of children under 4 years of age had intakes from food sources below the RNI whereas 32% of children aged 4 years and over had intakes below the RNI (p<0.01)[6]. However less than 1% of children under 4 years of age and 1% of children aged 4 years and over had intakes from all sources below the LRNI, (see *Table 8.1*). *(Table 8.13)*

Thiamin requirements are related to energy and carbohydrate intakes. When differences in energy intake were adjusted for, mean intake for children aged 1½ to 4½ was 0.7mg/1000kcal, higher than the RNI of 0.4mg/1000kcal. There were no differences in average intake by age or sex when differences in energy intake and body weight were accounted for (see *Tables 8.7 and 8.8*).

8.2.2 Riboflavin (vitamin B₂)

Mean riboflavin intake from all sources for children aged 1½ to 4½ years was 1.2mg (median 1.2mg). There were no differences in mean intake between age cohorts or between boys and girls. Dietary supplements made a negligible difference to mean riboflavin intakes. *(Table 8.15)*

Table 8.16 shows that the average daily intake of riboflavin from food sources among children aged under 4 years was 197% of the RNI whereas for children aged 4 years and over mean intake was 147% of the RNI (see *Table 8.1*). A greater proportion of children aged 4 years and over were below the RNI, 21% compared with younger children, 6% (p<0.01).[6] However less than 1% of children in either age group were below the LRNI. *(Table 8.15)*

After adjusting for variation in energy intake the mean intake of riboflavin per 1000kcal for children aged 1½ to 4½ years was 1.0mg/1000kcal, with no differences in intakes between the sexes or age cohorts. However mean intakes per kilogram body weight decreased with age; overall the mean intake was 0.09mg/kg, but children aged 1½ to 2½ years had mean intakes of 0.1mg/kg compared with 0.07mg/kg for children aged 3½ to 4½ years (p<0.01). The decrease in riboflavin intakes per kilogram body weight with age can be accounted for by the decline in milk consumption with age (see *Tables 8.7 and 8.8*).

The main food source of riboflavin was milk and milk products, providing children aged 1½ to 4½ years with 51% of their intake. It has already been shown that milk consumption declined with age (see *Table 4.14*) and there was a corresponding decline in the mean riboflavin intake provided by milk and milk products; thus children aged 1½ to 2½ years obtained 56% of their mean intake from milk and milk products compared with 44% for boys and 45% for girls aged 3½ to 4½ years (p<0.05).

The other main source of riboflavin was cereals and cereal products, of which breakfast cereals provided 16% of the total mean intake. This proportion increased with age from 13% for the youngest cohort to 18% for boys in oldest cohort (NS). *(Table 8.17b)*

The main sources of riboflavin found by the 1967/68 preschool children's survey were also milk and cereal products.[5] These two sources contributed to overall riboflavin intake in roughly the same proportions as were found for children in this NDNS survey.

8.2.3 Niacin equivalents

The niacin content of foods is expressed in the form of niacin equivalents, defined as the total amount of niacin plus one sixtieth of the weight (in mg) of tryptophan, which together constitute a B vitamin collectively known as niacin. Mean intake from all sources for children aged 1½ to 4½ years was 16.3mg (median 15.7mg). Intakes increased with age; children aged 1½ to 2½ years had the lowest intakes, 14.9mg, boys aged 3½ to 4½ years the highest, 18.2mg (p<0.01).

Supplements made a difference of only 2% to niacin intakes; the mean intake of niacin from food sources for all children was 16.0mg (median 15.5mg). *(Table 8.18)*

Table 8.19 shows that average daily intakes of niacin for all children were generally much higher than the RNI (shown in *Table 8.1*); for children aged under 4 years the mean intake from food sources was 197% of the RNI

131

and for children aged 4 years and over mean intake was 163% of the RNI.[6] No children under 4 years of age had niacin intakes from food sources below the RNI; only 6% of children aged 4 years and over had intakes below the RNI. None of the children in this survey were found to have intakes below the LRNI. *(Table 8.18)*

Controlling for variations in energy intake, the overall mean niacin intake was 14.2mg/1000kcal. No significant differences in mean intakes were found between the age cohorts or boys and girls. When differences in body weight were adjusted for, overall the mean intake was 1.1mg/kg, with children in the youngest age cohort having slightly higher intakes, 1.2mg/kg, than those in the other age cohorts, 1.1mg/kg (NS). (See *Tables 8.7 and 8.8*)

8.2.4 Vitamin B_6

Average daily intake of vitamin B_6 from all sources for children aged 1½ to 4½ years was 1.2mg (median 1.2mg). Although there was no difference in mean intake by sex, mean intake increased with age, with children in the youngest age cohort having significantly lower intakes, 1.1mg, than those in the oldest age cohort, 1.4mg for boys and 1.3mg for girls (p<0.05).

Dietary supplements taken by children in this survey made no difference to the mean intake for children aged 1½ to 4½ years, or to the overall pattern of increasing intakes with age. *(Table 8.20)*

Table 8.20 shows that although the majority of children had intakes above the RNI, the proportion of children with intakes below the RNI increased with age; 9% of children aged under 4 years had intakes below the RNI compared with 17% of children aged 4 years and over (see *Table 8.1*) (p<0.05). Furthermore only 1% of children under 4 years had intakes below the LRNI compared with 5% of children aged 4 years and over. Average daily intake from food sources for children aged under 4 years was 170% of the RNI and for children aged 4 years and over the mean intake was 148% of the RNI.[6] *(Table 8.21)*

When differences in energy intake were accounted for, mean intake for all children was 1.1mg/1000kcal. There were no significant differences by age or sex. Controlling for body weight, mean intake for children aged 1½ to 4½ years was 0.09mg/kg. Again there were no significant differences by age and sex. (See *Tables 8.7 and 8.8*)

The main sources of vitamin B_6 for all children were milk and milk products, 25%, cereal and cereal products, 23%, and vegetables, potatoes and savoury snacks, 23%. As noted earlier, milk consumption decreased with age and there was an associated decline in the intake of vitamin B_6 from milk and milk products with age. However, cereal consumption increased with age, replacing milk and milk products as a major source of vitamin B_6. *(Table 8.22b)*

8.2.5 Vitamin B_{12}

Average daily intake of vitamin B_{12} from all sources for children aged 1½ to 4½ years was 2.8µg (median 2.5µg).

Dietary supplements taken by children on this survey provided very little additional vitamin B_{12}. *(Table 8.23)*

Table 8.23 shows intakes were well above the RNI, with children at the bottom 2.5 percentile having intakes higher than the RNI (see *Table 8.1*). Only 2% of children aged 4 years and over had intakes below the RNI, and none of the children in this survey had intakes below the LRNI. The mean intake from food sources of vitamin B_{12} as a percentage of the RNI was high, 360% for children aged 4 years and over and 560% for children under 4 years.[6] *(Table 8.24)*

Controlling for variation in energy intake, the mean intake of vitamin B_{12} for children aged 1½ to 4½ years was 2.5µg/1000kcal. Intakes declined slightly with age, from 2.7µg/1000kcal for children aged 1½ to 2½ years to 2.2µg/1000kcal for boys aged 3½ to 4½ years. When variation in body weight was taken into account no differences were found in intakes associated with differences in age or sex. (See *Tables 8.7 and 8.8*)

Almost all animal products provide food sources of vitamin B_{12} whilst fruit and vegetables provide very little. The main source of vitamin B_{12} on this survey was milk and milk products which provided 47% of the mean intake with cows' milk providing 39% of the mean intake for children aged 1½ to 4½ years. Meat and meat products provided an additional 20% of the average daily intake of vitamin B_{12} for all children. *(Table 8.25b)*

8.2.6 Folate

Average daily folate intake from all sources for children aged 1½ to 4½ years was 132µg (median 124µg). As was seen with niacin and vitamin B_6 intakes, mean folate intake increased with age. Children in the youngest age group had significantly lower mean intakes, 120µg, than those aged 2½ to 3½ years, 134µg (p<0.05). Dietary supplements provided very little additional folate. Mean intake from food sources for children aged 1½ to 4½ years was 131µg (median 123µg). *(Table 8.26)*

Folate intakes were well above the UK RNI, shown in Table 8.1, with children at the lower 2.5 percentile having intakes above the LRNI (from *Table 8.26*). However, as was seen for other vitamins, such as thiamin, a greater proportion of children aged 4 years and over had intakes below the RNI than younger children, 20% compared with 6% (p<0.01). Mean intake from food sources for children aged under 4 years was 184% of the RNI and for children aged 4 years and over mean intake was 143% of the RNI.[6] *(Table 8.27)*

Accounting for differences in energy intake, mean intake for children aged 1½ to 4½ years was 116µg/1000kcal. There were no significant differences in the folate density of children's diets by age or sex. When folate intakes were compared after controlling for body weight, children in the youngest age cohort were found to have the highest mean intake, 9.9µg/kg, compared with girls aged 3½ to 4½ years, who had the lowest, 8.6µg/kg (p<0.05) (see *Tables 8.7 and 8.8*).

Meat and green vegetables are the main sources of folate yet for children aged 1½ to 4½ years the most important sources were breakfast cereals, 21%, vegetables, excluding potatoes, 9%, and cows' milk, 12%.   *(Table 8.28)*

8.2.7 *Biotin and pantothenic acid*

Average daily intake of biotin for children aged 1½ to 4½ years was 17.1µg (median 16.1µg) and for pantothenic acid the average intake from all sources was 2.8mg (median 2.6mg). There were no significant differences in the intakes of these two vitamins by age and sex. The dietary supplements taken by children in this survey provided very little pantothenic acid and no biotin.

(Tables 8.29 and 8.30)

8.3 Vitamin C

Average daily intake of vitamin C for children aged 1½ to 4½ years from all sources was 51.8mg (median 39.8mg). Supplements contributed 7% of mean vitamin C intake for all children; the mean intake from food alone for children aged 1½ to 4½ years was 48.6mg (median 37.7mg). There were no significant differences in intakes between boys and girls or age cohorts.

(Table 8.31 and Figs 8.5 and 8.6)

Table 8.31 shows 38% of children aged 1½ to 4½ years had average daily vitamin C intakes from food sources below the RNI, which is the same for both children under 4 years of age and those aged 4 years and over (RNIs are shown in *Table 8.1*). Dietary supplements reduced the proportion of children aged 1½ to 4½ years with intakes below the RNI to 35%. However intakes for children in the upper 2.5 percentile were at least five to six times greater than the RNI, depending on age. Only 1% of all children had intakes below the LRNI. Average daily intake of vitamin C as a percentage of the RNI rose slightly with age; mean intake from food sources for children under 4 years of age was 160% of the RNI whereas for children aged 4 years and over mean intake was 174% of the RNI.   *(Table 8.32)*

After controlling for children's energy intake, no significant differences were found between age groups or between boys and girls, although the vitamin C density of the diet declined slightly with age, and girls had a slightly more vitamin C dense diet than boys. The same pattern was observed when differences in body weight were accounted for. (See *Tables 8.7 and 8.8*)

The main sources of vitamin C for children aged 1½ to 4½ years were fruit juice, providing 20% of mean intake of vitamin C, and soft drinks, which provided 30%. In a previous survey of adults living in Great Britain, the proportion of vitamin C derived from vegetables, potatoes and savoury snacks was 46%.[7] Among children this was significantly lower, with just under a fifth, 19%, of vitamin C coming from vegetables, potatoes and savoury snacks (p<0.01). Potatoes and savoury snacks alone provided 13% of vitamin C intake for children aged 1½ to 4½ years. Fruit and nuts contributed 15% to overall vitamin C intake for children in the survey.

(Table 8.33b)

Data presented in Table 4.3 showed that the majority of children in the survey did not eat fruit and vegetables, excluding potatoes and savoury snacks, during the seven-days, and that consumers only ate relatively small amounts. However potatoes, particularly chips, and savoury snacks were consumed by the majority of children in this survey, and hence provided a greater proportion of vitamin C than other vegetables.

8.4 Vitamin D

Most of the body's requirement of vitamin D can be synthesised by the skin in the presence of sunlight. A few foods naturally contain vitamin D, but these are all animal products, in particular fatty fish. However some foods such as margarines and fat spreads, some yogurts and breakfast cereals are fortified with vitamin D. The amount of vitamin D in meat is uncertain which may lead to an underestimate of intake from this source.

Mean intake of vitamin D from all sources for children aged 1½ to 4½ years was 1.9µg (median 1.1µg). Vitamin D intakes from dietary supplements increased average intakes by about half for all children. There were no significant differences between boys and girls or between age cohorts in intakes from food or from all sources.

The distribution of intakes was skewed with median intakes being between 15% and 25% lower than mean intakes from food sources, depending on age and sex. The range of intakes was very wide, with children at the lower 2.5 percentile having intakes from food sources which were between a quarter and a fifth of the median intake, and children in the upper 2.5 percentile having intakes between two and a half and five times the median intake, depending on age and sex.

(Table 8.34 and Figs 8.7 and 8.8)

Table 8.1 shows the current RNI for vitamin D for children aged between 1 and 3 years; there is no RNI for children aged between 4 and 6 years and hence Table 8.35 only compares mean intakes of vitamin D with the RNI for children aged under 4 years.

Although the mean intake from food sources for children aged under 4 years was only 18% of the RNI, as stated earlier, most of the body's requirement can be synthesised in the presence of sunlight and over 90% of children in this survey were reported to have access to a garden or communal play area (see *Table 4.1*).

(Table 8.35)

Table 8.7a shows that if variation in energy intake is taken into account, children in the youngest age group have significantly higher vitamin D intakes per 1000kcal energy intake than older children (p<0.05). This reflects the change in diet from one with higher intakes of infant formula and manufactured weaning foods which are fortified with vitamin D, to a more mixed diet, which will not be as rich in vitamin D (from *Table 8.36a*).

No significant differences were found between age groups or boys and girls in intake of vitamin D, when differences in body weight were accounted for (see *Table 8.8*).

Table 8.36b shows differences by age in the contribution of milk products, including infant formula, to vitamin D intake. Children in the youngest age cohort obtained 17% of their mean vitamin D intake from other milk and products, which includes infant formula, compared with boys in the oldest age cohort, who obtained only 5% (p<0.01). Vitamin D fortified fat spreads, 26%, and breakfast cereals, 17%, were the other main food sources of this vitamin for all children. *(Table 8.36)*

8.5 Vitamin E

Average daily intakes of vitamin E are shown in Table 8.37; the average intake from all sources for children aged 1½ to 4½ years was 4.4mg (median 4.0mg). Supplements made only a negligible difference to vitamin E intakes; the overall mean intake from food sources was 4.3mg (median 4.0mg). Children in the youngest age cohort had significantly lower intakes of vitamin E than older children (p<0.01). There were no significant differences in intake by sex. *(Table 8.37)*

After controlling for differences in energy intake and body weight differences in vitamin E intake were no longer apparent (see *Tables 8.7 and 8.8*).

Just under a quarter of the mean intake of vitamin E for children aged 1½ to 4½ years was provided by fat spreads. Vegetables, including potatoes and savoury snacks provided just over a quarter of the mean intake. Savoury snacks, including crisps, alone provided 12% of the average intake for all children. *(Table 8.38b)*

8.6 Vitamin intakes for children who were reported to be taking dietary supplements

So far in this chapter data have been presented on the average daily vitamin intake of children aged 1½ to 4½ years from all sources, including dietary supplements, and from food sources only. Vitamins derived from dietary supplements will, however, be an important source for the small group of children within the sample who were reported to have been taking supplements during the dietary recording period. (The characteristics of this group are discussed in *Chapter 3, section 3.4.*)

Table 8.39 shows average daily vitamin intakes from all sources for children who were reported to have been taking dietary supplements and for those who were not taking dietary supplements. For children who were reported to have been taking supplements intakes from food sources alone are also shown.

Intakes of most vitamins from food sources alone were higher in those children reported to have been taking supplements than in other children. In particular, intakes from food sources of vitamin C and niacin equivalents, vitamins B$_6$ and B$_{12}$ were significantly higher

(p<0.05, except vitamin C, p<0.01) for children reported as taking dietary supplements than for other children. *(Table 8.39)*

8.7 Variations in vitamin intakes

In this section variation in the average daily intake of vitamins from all sources and food sources in relation to the main characteristics of the sample is considered. Since mean vitamin intake may be related to energy intake the quality of the diet of different groups is compared by looking at vitamin intake from food sources per 1000kcal food energy.

Children reported as being unwell
Table 8.40 shows vitamin intakes from all sources and food sources by whether the child was reported to have been unwell during the four-day recording period. Children whose eating was affected by illness were a relatively small group, but they had significantly lower intakes from food sources than those who were not reported as being unwell of thiamin, niacin, vitamins B$_6$, B$_{12}$, folate and pantothenic acid (p<0.01) and vitamin E (p<0.05). Intakes of total carotene and vitamin C, were also lower among children whose eating had been affected by illness, although these differences did not reach statistical significance. *(Table 8.40)*

Vitamin intakes from all sources for children whose eating was affected by illness were also significantly lower than for those who had not been unwell. Children whose illness had not affected their eating had intakes generally very similar to those who were reported to have been well.

However as average vitamin intakes from food sources per 1000kcal food energy for those children whose eating had been affected by being unwell were similar to those for children who had not been unwell, the differences between these groups in intakes were therefore largely a reflection of differences in total energy intake. *(Table 8.41)*

Region
The data *(Tables 8.42 to 8.43)* show that there was some marked variation between children living in different parts of Great Britain in their absolute intakes of many vitamins and that in some cases these differences were still apparent after adjusting for any differences in energy intakes.[8]

For example, even after adjusting for variation in energy intakes, children in Scotland still had the lowest intakes of both total carotene and vitamin C. Low intakes of vitamin C and total carotene among children living in Scotland are consistent with data presented in Table 4.18 which showed that children in Scotland were the least likely to be consumers of all types of vegetables, other fruit (mainly soft fruit) and fruit juice. Children living in London and the South East together with children living in the Northern region of England were also having diets which gave them absolute and adjusted intakes of folate which were lower than those of other children.

The diets of children in some regions generally provided higher intakes of certain vitamins; for example, vitamin C and niacin in the diets of children living in London and the South East, total carotene in the diets of children in the Central and South West regions of England and Wales and vitamin A and folate in the diets of children living in Scotland.

Other variations in absolute intakes between children in the different regions were no longer evident, or were much smaller when any variation in energy intake was taken into account. *(Tables 8.42 and 8.43)*

Socio-economic factors
Tables 8.44 to 8.51 show absolute intakes of vitamins and intakes adjusted for variation in energy intake, for different groups of children according to various socio-economic characteristics.

Whether the child came from a non-manual or manual home background appeared to have an effect on the child's intake of most vitamins, with those from a manual background generally having lower absolute intakes of most vitamins. However only intakes of total carotene, niacin, and vitamins B_{12}, C and E were still lower among the manual group after adjusting for differences between the groups in energy intake.

There was generally much less variation in absolute intakes associated with the other socio-economic characteristics considered, the head of household's working status, whether the child's parents were receiving Income Support or Family Credit or the mother's education level. However there was clear evidence that the diets of the children in less advantaged homes were having lower absolute and adjusted intakes of total carotene, niacin, and vitamin C. Intakes of all three of these vitamins were markedly lower for children where the head of household was not working, where the parents were receiving benefits and where the child's mother had no formal educational qualifications.
(Tables 8.44–8.51)

Family type
Tables 8.52 and 8.53 compare the vitamin intakes of children in lone parent families with those of other children in the survey.

As has been noted before when other comparisons by family type have been discussed, many of the apparent differences between groups are not statistically significant and it has been suggested that this is at least partly a function of the small size of the subgroups; this is particularly likely when the number of children within each family type is also considered. However, bearing in mind the differences in absolute and adjusted intakes found for vitamin C and total carotene for other subgroups in the sample, it is likely that children in lone parent families were having lower intakes of these two vitamins.

Tables 8.52 and 8.53 show that children in lone parent families did have lower absolute and adjusted intakes of total carotene than other children, and that children in lone parent families with more than one child had the lowest absolute intakes of both total carotene and vitamin C. After adjusting for variation in energy intake vitamin C levels for children from lone parent families with more than one child were still lower than for other children. Children who had brothers or sisters, both in lone parent and other families, had lower intakes of most vitamins than other children. *(Tables 8.52 and 8.53)*

The analysis of the data by other socio-economic characteristics also found significant differences in intakes of niacin for different subgroups. In respect of the child's family type no significant differences in either absolute or adjusted niacin intakes were found.

References and notes

1 See *Chapter 5* and *Appendix J* for details of deriving average daily intakes.
2 The Welfare Food Scheme was introduced in 1940 to ensure that expectant mothers and young children were properly nourished. The Scheme has continued to this day with a number of modifications. Children under 5 years of age in families in receipt of Income Support receive free vitamin drops. For further details of current entitlement see: Department of Health. Report on Health and Social Subjects: 45. *Weaning and the Weaning Diet.* HMSO (London,1994).
A daily dose of Department of Health Children's Vitamin Drops provides:
  – 200µg of vitamin A (retinol equivalents)
  – 20mg of vitamin C
  – 7µg of vitamin D.
3 The Working Party on the Fortification of Yellow Fats endorsed the COMA Panel on Child Nutrition recommendation that 'vitamin supplements be given to infants and young children aged from six months to at least two years and preferably five years...'. Department of Health. Report on Health and Social Subjects: 40. *The Fortification of Yellow Fats with Vitamins A and D.* HMSO (London, 1991).
4 Department of Health. Report on Health and Social Subjects: 41. *Dietary Reference Values for Food Energy and Nutrients for the United Kingdom.* HMSO (London, 1991).
5 Department of Health and Social Security. Report on Health and Social Subjects: 10. *A Nutrition Survey of Pre-School Children 1967-68.* HMSO (London, 1975).
6 RNIs for the age group 4 to 6 years are often higher than those for the age group 1 to 3 years. The children in this survey in the age group 4 years and over (i.e. 4 to 4½ years) are at the bottom end of the age range of 4 to 6 years and might not have reached the maximum requirement for the nutrient under discussion. It is likely that a gradual increased requirement for a nutrient occurs rather than a distinct change in requirements at the age of 4 years which should be borne in mind when interpreting these results.
7 Gregory J, Foster K, Tyler H, Wiseman M. *The Dietary and Nutritional Survey of British Adults.* HMSO (London, 1990).
8 Comments on differences are based on comparisons between children in the regions with the highest and lowest intakes per 1000kcal energy and were significant at, at least, the p<0.05 level.

Figure 8.1 Average daily total carotene intake from food sources by sex of child

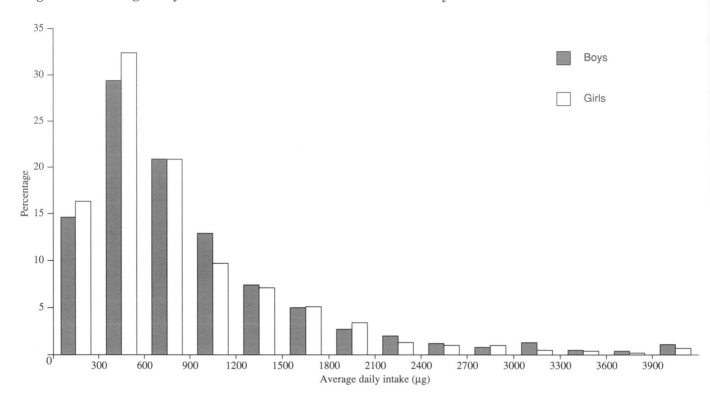

Figure 8.2 Average daily total carotene intake from food sources by age of child

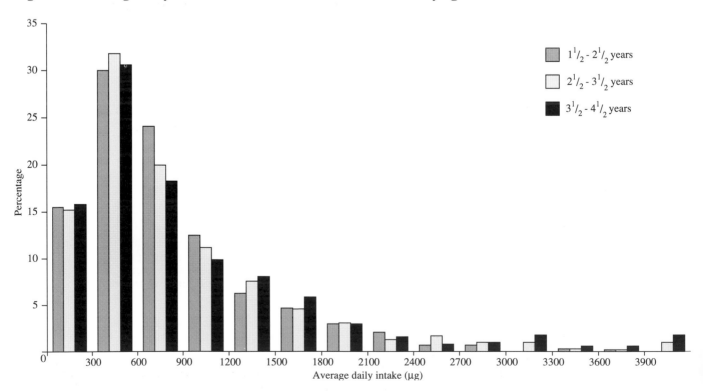

Figure 8.3a Average daily vitamin A (retinol equivalents) intake from all sources by sex of child

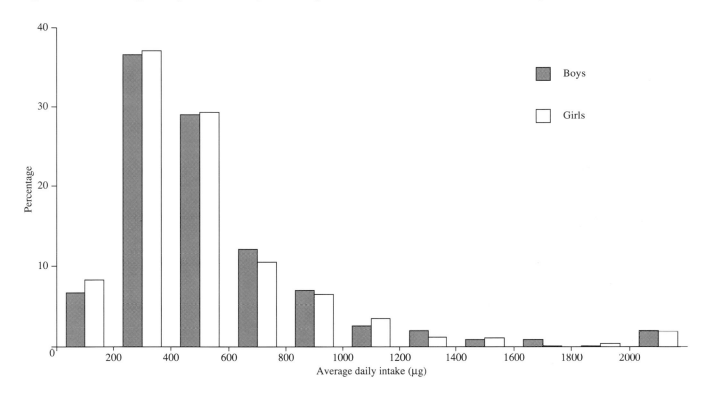

Figure 8.3b Average daily vitamin A (retinol equivalents) intake from food sources by sex of child

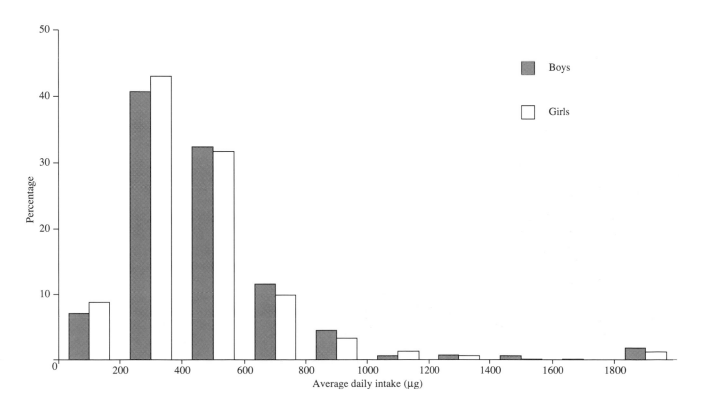

Figure 8.4a Average daily vitamin A (retinol equivalents) intake from all sources by age of child

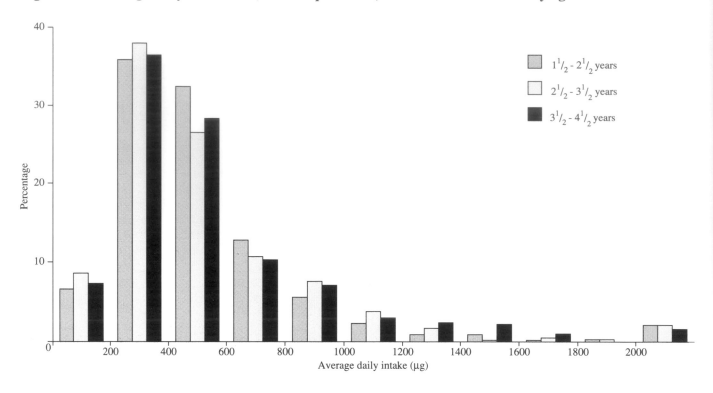

Figure 8.4b Average daily vitamin A (retinol equivalents) intake from food sources by age of child

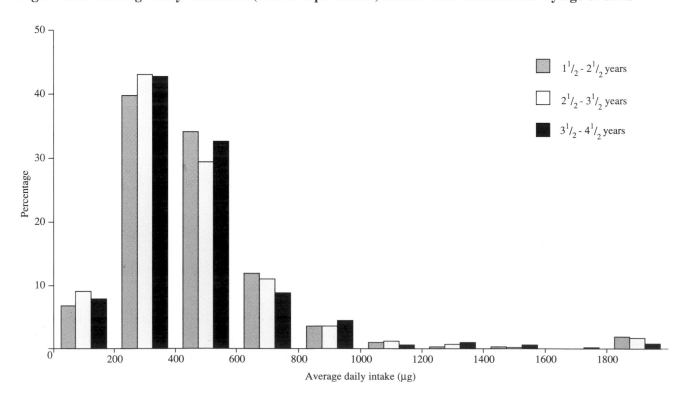

Figure 8.5a Average daily vitamin C intake from all sources by sex of child

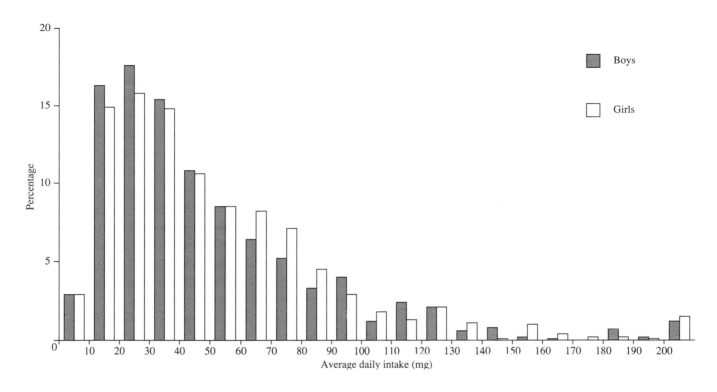

Figure 8.5b Average daily vitamin C intake from food sources by sex of child

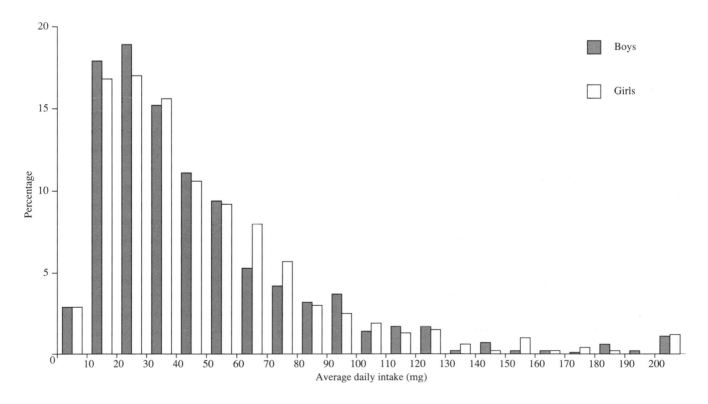

Figure 8.6a Average daily vitamin C intake from all sources by age of child

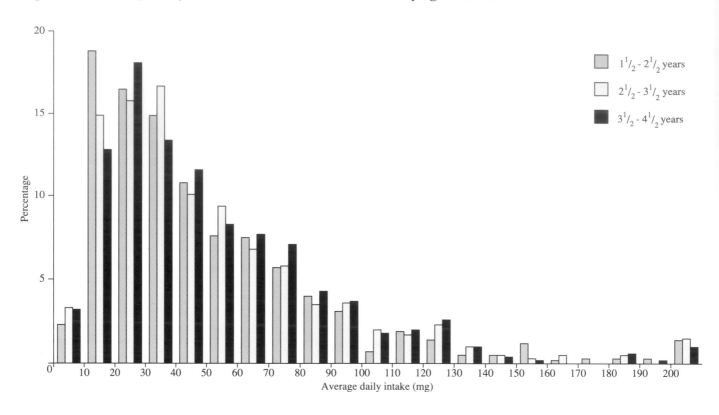

Figure 8.6b Average daily vitamin C intake from food sources by age of child

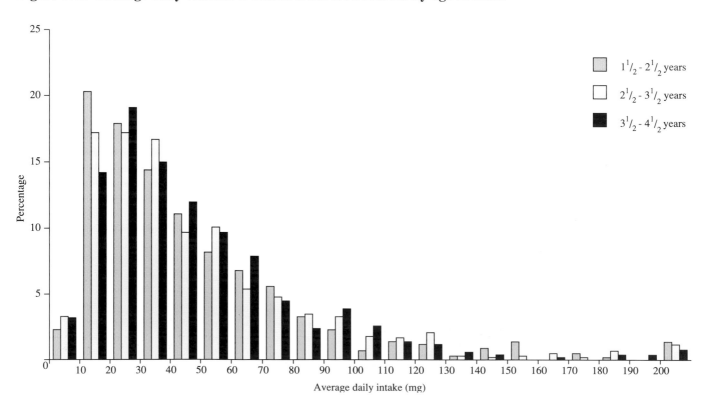

Figure 8.7a Average daily vitamin D intake from all sources by sex of child

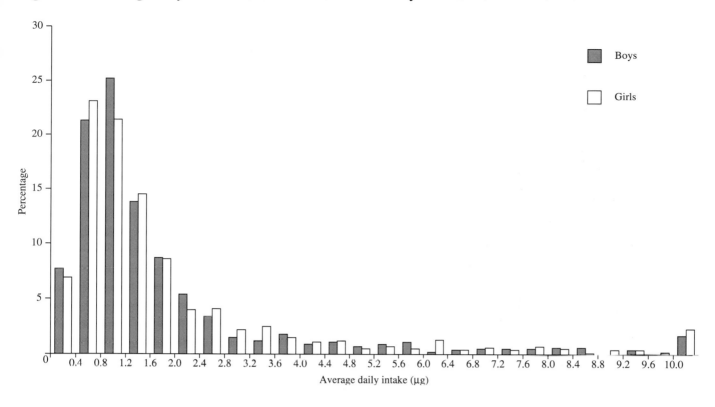

Figure 8.7b Average daily vitamin D intake from food sources by sex of child

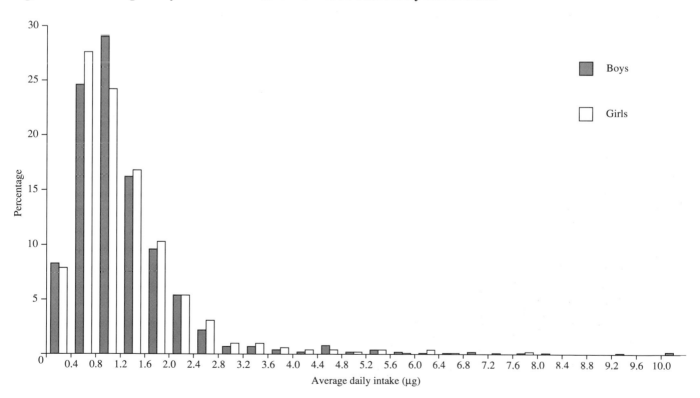

Figure 8.8a Average daily vitamin D intake from all sources by age of child

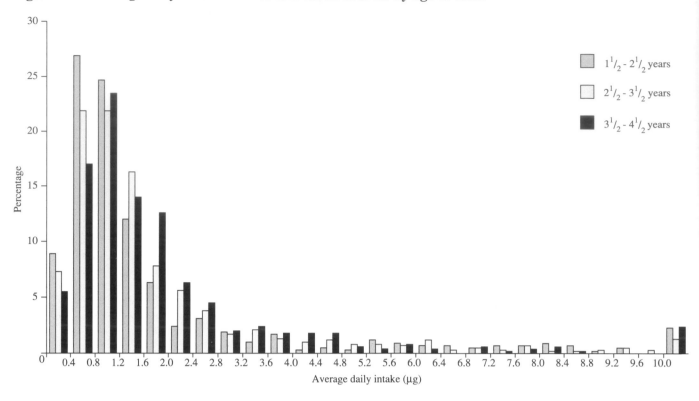

Figure 8.8b Average daily vitamin D intake from food sources by age of child

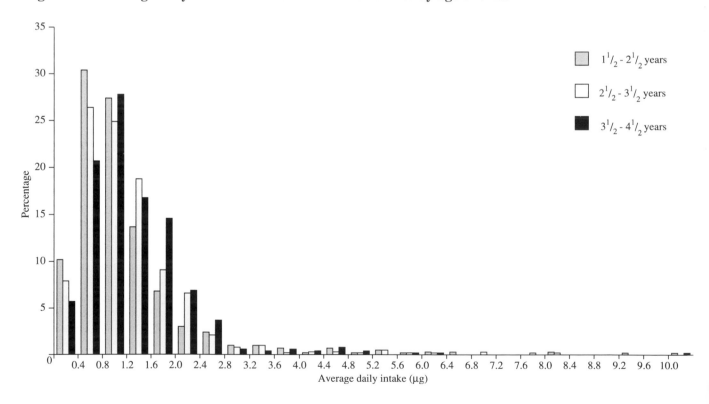

Table 8.1 Reference Nutrient Intakes (RNI) and Lower Reference Nutrient Intakes (LRNI) for vitamins*

Vitamin	RNI		LRNI	
	1–3 years	4–6 years	1–3 years	4–6 years
Vitamin A µg/d	400	400	200	200
Thiamin mg/d	0.5	0.7	0.3†	0.4†
Riboflavin mg/d	0.6	0.8	0.3	0.4
Niacin mg/d	8	11	5.3†	7.3†
Vitamin B_6 mg/d**	0.7	0.9	0.5††	0.7††
Vitamin B_{12} µg/d	0.5	0.8	0.3	0.5
Folate µg/d	70	100	35	50
Vitamin C mg/d	30	30	8	8
Vitamin D µg/d	7	–	–	–

*Source: Department of Health. Report on Health and Social Subjects 41. *Dietary Reference Values for Food Energy and Nutrients for the United Kingdom.* HMSO (London 1991).
**Based on protein providing 14.7% of the Estimated Average Requirement (EAR).
†Calculated values based on quoted LRNIs mg/1000kcal.
††Calculated values based on quoted LRNIs µg/g protein.

Table 8.2 Average daily intake of pre-formed retinol (µg) by age and sex of child

Pre-formed retinol (µg)	Age and sex of child						
	All aged 1½ – 2½ years	All aged 2½ – 3½ years	All aged 3½ – 4½ years		All boys	All girls	All
			Boys	Girls			
	cum %	cum %	cum %	cum %	cum %	cum %	cum %
(a) Intakes from *all sources*							
Less than 150	12	14	12	14	12	13	13
Less than 225	29	37	31	37	32	34	33
Less than 300	47	56	56	58	53	54	53
Less than 450	75	78	78	81	77	78	77
Less than 600	88	86	84	86	86	86	86
Less than 750	92	90	88	90	90	91	90
All	100	100	100	100	100	100	100
Base	*576*	*606*	*250*	*243*	*848*	*827*	*1675*
Mean (average value)	456	433	396	414	452	413	433
Median value	317	277	277	269	285	286	286
Lower 2.5 percentile	76.5	79.2	89.7	67.3	86.4	69.6	79.1
Upper 2.5 percentile	997	1056	1144	1388	1112	1083	1093
Standard error of the mean	46.3	29.9	25.0	44.1	35.2	21.0	20.6
	cum %	cum %	cum %	cum %	cum %	cum %	cum %
(b) Intakes from *food sources*							
Less than 150	13	15	13	15	13	15	14
Less than 225	31	41	34	42	35	38	37
Less than 300	51	63	64	68	59	62	60
Less than 450	84	87	90	93	86	89	87
Less than 600	93	94	96	98	94	95	95
Less than 750	96	97	98	98	97	97	97
All	100	100	100	100	100	100	100
Base	*576*	*606*	*250*	*243*	*848*	*827*	*1675*
Mean (average value)	409	361	312	314	390	336	363
Median value	291	252	267	242	273	261	268
Lower 2.5 percentile	76.5	78.7	72.1	67.3	85.7	69.2	75.2
Upper 2.5 percentile	697	648	565	501	654	624	637
Standard error of the mean	45.7	28.1	20.4	40.5	34.6	18.8	19.8

Table 8.3   Average daily intake of β-carotene (μg) by by age and sex of child

β-carotene (μg)	Age and sex of child						
	All aged 1½ – 2½ years	All aged 2½ – 3½ years	All aged 3½ – 4½ years		All boys	All girls	All
			Boys	Girls			
	cum %	cum %	cum %	cum %	cum %	cum %	cum %
Intakes from *food sources*							
Less than 200	6	5	7	6	5	7	6
Less than 400	28	29	29	29	27	30	29
Less than 600	49	50	48	51	48	52	50
Less than 800	68	65	60	68	64	68	66
Less than 1600	93	90	86	92	90	92	91
Less than 2000	97	95	91	95	94	96	95
All	100	100	100	100	100	100	100
Base	*576*	*606*	*250*	*243*	*848*	*827*	*1675*
Mean (average value)	727	794	921	797	822	758	790
Median value	609	594	630	586	628	578	600
Lower 2.5 percentile	130	163	134	158	151	134	150
Upper 2.5 percentile	2071	2609	3335	2793	2785	2443	2616
Standard error of the mean	20.9	26.7	55.3	44.0	23.8	21.3	16.0

*None of the dietary supplements taken by children in this survey provided any β-carotene.

Table 8.4   Average daily intake of α-carotene (μg) by age and sex of child

α-carotene (μg)	Age and sex of child						
	All aged 1½ – 2½ years	All aged 2½ – 3½ years	All aged 3½ – 4½ years		All boys	All girls	All
			Boys	Girls			
	cum %	cum %	cum %	cum %	cum %	cum %	cum %
Intakes from *food sources*							
Less than 25	32	37	35	36	35	35	35
Less than 50	42	45	42	47	42	45	44
Less than 75	51	51	48	53	50	52	51
Less than 150	71	68	65	70	67	70	69
Less than 300	88	84	78	85	83	86	85
Less than 400	94	90	87	91	90	92	91
All	100	100	100	100	100	100	100
Base	*576*	*606*	*250*	*243*	*848*	*827*	*1675*
Mean (average value)	124	144	199	155	156	137	147
Median value	71.4	66.7	89.1	63.5	77.1	64.4	70.8
Lower 2.5 percentile	0.0	0.0	0.0	0.0	0.0	0.0	0.0
Upper 2.5 percentile	521	758	1081	1107	828	685	739
Standard error of the mean	6.5	8.5	23.1	16.7	8.8	7.2	5.7

*None of the dietary supplements taken by children in this survey provided any α-carotene.

Table 8.5 Average daily intake of β-cryptoxanthin (µg) by age and sex of child

β-cryptoxanthin (µg)	Age and sex of child						
	All aged 1½ – 2½ years	All aged 2½ – 3½ years	All aged 3½ – 4½ years		All boys	All girls	All
			Boys	Girls			
	cum %	cum %	cum %	cum %	cum %	cum %	cum %
Intakes from *food sources*							
Less than 5	40	36	36	29	38	32	35
Less than 10	57	55	53	43	56	51	53
Less than 15	67	65	67	57	66	63	65
Less than 30	85	82	84	79	84	82	83
Less than 60	96	96	96	95	96	96	96
All	100	100	100	100	100	100	100
Base	*576*	*606*	*250*	*243*	*848*	*827*	*1675*
Mean (average value)	15.3	16.5	16.3	19.4	15.7	17.2	16.5
Median value	7.7	8.4	9.0	11.4	8.0	9.9	8.9
Lower 2.5 percentile	0.0	0.0	0.0	0.0	0.0	0.0	0.0
Upper 2.5 percentile	73.6	83.4	77.0	82.1	73.4	78.9	75.6
Standard error of the mean	0.9	1.0	1.4	1.5	0.7	0.8	0.6

*None of the dietary supplements taken by children in this survey provided any β-cryptoxanthin.

Table 8.6 Average daily intake of total carotene (β-carotene equivalents) (µg) by age and sex of child

Total carotene (β-carotene equivalents) (µg)	Age and sex of child						
	All aged 1½ – 2½ years	All aged 2½ – 3½ years	All aged 3½ – 4½ years		All boys	All girls	All
			Boys	Girls			
	cum %	cum %	cum %	cum %	cum %	cum %	cum %
Intakes from *food sources*							
Less than 300	15	15	16	16	15	16	15
Less than 600	45	47	44	49	44	49	46
Less than 900	70	67	61	69	65	70	67
Less than 1200	82	78	73	76	78	79	78
Less than 1500	88	86	80	85	85	86	86
Less than 1800	93	90	86	91	90	91	91
All	100	100	100	100	100	100	100
Base	*576*	*606*	*250*	*243*	*848*	*827*	*1675*
Mean (average value)	796	874	1029	884	908	835	872
Median value	659	640	700	621	682	618	648
Lower 2.5 percentile	133	164	144	162	159	139	155
Upper 2.5 percentile	2324	2997	3881	3382	3163	2828	3002
Standard error of the mean	23.9	30.8	66.0	52.0	27.9	24.7	18.7

*None of the dietary supplements taken by children in this survey provided any carotene.

Table 8.7(a) Average daily intake of vitamins from food sources per 1000 kcal food energy by age of child

Nutrient	Age of child											
	All aged 1½–2½ years			All aged 2½–3½ years			All aged 3½–4½ years					
							Boys			Girls		
Intake per 1000 kcal energy:	Mean	Median	se	Mean	Median	se	Mean	Median	se	Mean	Median	se
Total carotene (β-carotene equivalents) (µg)	773	620	22.9	757	564	25.1	801	533	48.1	754	573	42.3
Vitamin A (retinol equivalents) (µg)	521	405	45.6	432	333	22.7	376	327	16.0	392	315	36.7
Thiamin (mg)	0.7	0.7	0.01	0.7	0.6	0.01	0.7	0.6	0.01	0.7	0.7	0.01
Riboflavin (mg)	1.1	1.1	0.01	1.0	1.0	0.01	0.9	0.9	0.02	1.0	1.0	0.02
Niacin equivalents (mg)	14.2	13.8	0.1	14.0	13.6	0.1	14.2	13.9	0.2	14.5	14.1	0.2
Vitamin B_6 (mg)	1.1	1.0	0.01	1.0	1.0	0.01	1.0	1.0	0.02	1.1	1.0	0.02
Vitamin B_{12} (µg)	2.7	2.5	0.09	2.4	2.1	0.05	2.2	2.0	0.06	2.3	2.1	0.08
Folate (µg)	116	112	1.5	115	111	1.5	113	108	2.1	118	115	2.4
Vitamin C (mg)	46.7	35.1	1.6	42.7	32.5	1.4	40.2	31.2	2.1	38.9	32.1	1.6
Vitamin D (µg)	1.2	0.9	0.05	1.0	0.9	0.03	1.1	0.9	0.05	1.1	0.9	0.04
Vitamin E (α–tocopherol equivalents) (mg)	3.7	3.4	0.06	3.8	3.5	0.05	3.9	3.6	0.09	3.8	3.6	0.09
Base		*576*			*606*			*250*			*243*	

Table 8.7(b) Average daily intake of vitamins from food sources per 1000 kcal food energy by sex of child

Nutrient	Sex of child								
	Boys			Girls			All		
Intake per 1000 kcal energy:	*Mean*	*Median*	*se*	*Mean*	*Median*	*se*	*Mean*	*Median*	*se*
Total carotene (β–carotene equivalents) (µg)	781	569	22.5	756	578	20.7	768	571	15.3
Vitamin A (retinol equivalents) (µg)	465	351	32.7	430	356	17.5	448	355	18.7
Thiamin (mg)	0.7	0.7	0.01	0.7	0.7	0.01	0.7	0.7	0.00
Riboflavin (mg)	1.0	1.0	0.01	1.0	1.0	0.01	1.0	1.0	0.01
Niacin equivalents (mg)	14.1	13.7	0.1	14.3	13.9	0.1	14.2	13.8	0.08
Vitamin B$_6$ (mg)	1.1	1.0	0.01	1.1	1.0	0.01	1.1	1.0	0.01
Vitamin B$_{12}$ (µg)	2.4	2.2	0.06	2.5	2.3	0.05	2.5	2.2	0.04
Folate (µg)	114	109	1.2	117	114	1.3	116	111	0.9
Vitamin C (mg)	41.3	31.4	1.1	45.0	35.6	1.2	43.1	33.0	0.8
Vitamin D (µg)	1.1	0.9	0.03	1.1	0.9	0.03	1.1	0.9	0.02
Vitamin E (α–tocopherol equivalents) (mg)	3.7	3.4	0.05	3.8	3.6	0.05	3.8	3.5	0.03
Base		848			827			1675	

Table 8.8(a) Average daily intake of vitamins from all sources per kilogram child's body weight by age of child

Nutrient	Age of child											
	All aged 1½–2½ years			All aged 2½–3½ years			All aged 3½–4½ years					
							Boys			Girls		
Intake per kilogram child's body weight:	*Mean*	*Median*	*se*	*Mean*	*Median*	*se*	*Mean*	*Median*	*se*	*Mean*	*Median*	*se*
Total carotene (β–carotene equivalents) (µg)*	66.4	54.6	2.1	59.8	44.1	2,1	62.3	43.2	4.2	54.3	38.0	3.2
Vitamin A (retinol equivalents) (µg)	48.9	36.0	3.9	40.1	28.5	2.2	34.9	26.7	1.7	35.3	25.0	3.5
Thiamin (mg)	0.06	0.06	0.00	0.06	0.05	0.00	0.05	0.05	0.00	0.05	0.05	0.00
Riboflavin (mg)	0.10	0.10	0.00	0.08	0.08	0.00	0.07	0.07	0.00	0.07	0.07	0.00
Niacin equivalents (mg)	1.2	1.2	0.02	1.1	1.1	0.01	1.1	1.1	0.02	1.1	1.0	0.02
Vitamin B$_6$ (mg)	0.09	0.09	0.00	0.09	0.08	0.00	0.08	0.08	0.00	0.08	0.08	0.00
Vitamin B$_{12}$ (µg)	0.2	0.2	0.01	0.2	0.2	0.00	0.2	0.2	0.00	0.2	0.1	0.01
Folate (µg)	9.9	9.4	0.1	9.2	8.7	0.1	8.8	8.5	0.2	8.6	8.3	0.2
Vitamin C (mg)	4.3	3.2	0.1	3.6	2.9	0.1	3.4	2.6	0.2	3.0	2.5	0.1
Vitamin D (µg)	0.1	0.1	0.01	0.1	0.1	0.01	0.1	0.1	0.01	0.1	0.1	0.01
Vitamin E (α–tocopherol equivalents) (mg)	0.3	0.3	0.01	0.3	0.3	0.01	0.3	0.3	0.01	0.3	0.2	0.01
*Base**		538			578			237			239	

*None of the dietary supplements taken by children on this survey provided any carotene.
**Includes only children for whom a valid weight measurement was obtained.

Table 8.8(b) Average daily intake of vitamins from all sources per kilogram child's body weight by sex of child

Nutrient	Sex of child								
	Boys			Girls			All		
Intake per kilogram child's body weight:	*Mean*	*Median*	*se*	*Mean*	*Median*	*se*	*Mean*	*Median*	*se*
Total carotene (β–carotene equivalents) (µg)*	63.3	46.9	2.0	59.9	46.2	1.7	61.6	46.2	1.3
Vitamin A (retinol equivalents) (µg)	42.8	29.7	2.9	40.3	30.0	1.7	41.6	29.9	1.7
Thiamin (mg)	0.06	0.05	0.00	0.06	0.05	0.00	0.06	0.05	0.00
Riboflavin (mg)	0.09	0.08	0.00	0.09	0.08	0.00	0.09	0.08	0.00
Niacin equivalents (mg)	1.1	1.1	0.01	1.1	1.1	0.01	1.1	1.1	0.01
Vitamin B$_6$ (mg)	0.09	0.08	0.00	0.09	0.08	0.00	0.09	0.08	0.00
Vitamin B$_{12}$ (µg)	0.2	0.2	0.00	0.2	0.2	0.00	0.2	0.2	0.00
Folate (µg)	9.2	8.9	0.1	9.4	8.8	0.1	9.3	8.9	0.1
Vitamin C (mg)	3.5	2.8	0.1	3.8	3.0	0.1	3.7	2.9	0.1
Vitamin D (µg)	0.1	0.1	0.01	0.1	0.1	0.01	0.1	0.1	0.00
Vitamin E (α–tocopherol equivalents) (mg)	0.3	0.3	0.00	0.3	0.3	0.00	0.3	0.3	0.00
*Base**		793			799			1592	

*None of the dietary supplements taken by children on this survey provided any carotene.
**Includes only children for whom a valid weight measurement was obtained.

Table 8.9(a) Contribution of food types to average daily total carotene (β−carotene equivalents) intake by age and sex of child

Food types	Age and sex of child						
	All aged 1½ – 2½ years	All aged 2½ – 3½ years	All aged 3½ – 4½ years		All boys	All girls	All
			Boys	Girls			
	µg	µg	µg	µg	µg	µg	µg
Cereals & cereal products	34.7	38.2	42.6	50.4	39.5	39.3	39.4
Milk & milk products	79.2	65.0	57.6	55.0	69.1	65.5	67.3
of which:							
milk (whole, semi-skimmed, skimmed)	64.8	51.9	43.2	41.3	55.6	51.4	53.5
other milk & products	14.3	13.0	14.4	13.7	13.5	14.1	13.8
Eggs & egg dishes	0.9	2.2	1.0	1.6	1.1	1.8	1.5
Fat spreads	23.7	29.0	36.8	31.6	29.4	28.0	28.7
Meat & meat products	58.0	75.7	59.3	56.3	65.8	62.9	64.4
Fish & fish dishes	1.9	1.1	1.1	6.2	1.4	2.9	2.1
Vegetables, potatoes & savoury snacks	413	482	650	521	516	461	489
of which:							
raw carrots	29.8	53.2	132	119	70.6	62.2	66.5
cooked carrots	280	319	391	258	333	280	307
Fruit & nuts	15.3	18.1	14.9	19.8	15.8	18.0	16.9
Sugars, preserves & confectionery	6.2	8.8	13.1	7.9	9.0	7.8	8.4
Beverages	127	124	126	108	131	115	123
of which:							
soft drinks, including low calorie drinks	123	120	122	104	127	110	119
Commercial infant foods & drinks	3.2	0.4	0.04	–	1.4	1.1	1.3
Miscellaneous	33.5	29.8	26.3	26.5	28.5	31.6	30.1
Average daily intake (µg)	**796**	**874**	**1029**	**884**	**908**	**835**	**872**
Total number of children	**576**	**606**	**250**	**243**	**848**	**827**	**1675**

Table 8.9(b) Percentage contribution of food types to average daily total carotene (β−carotene equivalents) intake by age and sex of child

Food types	Age and sex of child						
	All aged 1½ – 2½ years	All aged 2½ – 3½ years	All aged 3½ – 4½ years		All boys	All girls	All
			Boys	Girls			
	%	%	%	%	%	%	%
Cereals & cereal products	4	4	4	6	4	5	4
Milk & milk products	10	7	6	6	8	8	8
of which:							
milk (whole, semi-skimmed, skimmed)	8	6	4	5	6	6	6
other milk & products	2	2	1	2	2	2	2
Eggs & egg dishes	0	0	0	0	0	0	0
Fat spreads	3	3	4	4	3	3	3
Meat & meat products	7	9	6	6	7	8	8
Fish & fish dishes	0	0	0	1	0	0	0
Vegetables, potatoes & savoury snacks	52	55	63	59	57	55	56
of which:							
raw carrots	4	6	13	14	8	7	8
cooked carrots	35	36	38	29	37	34	35
Fruit & nuts	2	2	1	2	2	2	2
Sugars, preserves & confectionery	1	1	1	1	1	1	1
Beverages	16	14	12	12	14	14	14
of which:							
soft drinks, including low calorie drinks	15	14	12	12	14	13	14
Commercial infant foods & drinks	0	0	0	–	0	0	0
Miscellaneous	4	3	3	3	3	4	3
Average daily intake (µg)	**796**	**874**	**1029**	**884**	**908**	**835**	**872**
Total number of children	**576**	**606**	**250**	**243**	**848**	**827**	**1675**

Table 8.10 Average daily intake of vitamin A (retinol equivalents (µg)) by age and sex of child

Vitamin A (retinol equivalents) (µg)	All aged 1½ – 2½ years	All aged 2½ – 3½ years	All aged 3½ – 4½ years		All aged under 4 years	All aged 4 years and over	All boys	All girls	All
			Boys	Girls					
	cum %	cum %	cum %	cum %	cum %	cum %	cum %	cum %	cum %
(a) Intakes from *all sources*									
Less than 200	7	9	8	7	8	7	7	8	8
Less than 400	42	46	40	48	44	43	43	45	44
Less than 600	75	73	70	74	74	71	73	75	74
Less than 800	88	84	80	85	85	80	84	85	85
Less than 1000	93	91	89	90	92	88	91	92	92
All	100	100	100	100	100	100	100	100	100
Base	*576*	*606*	*250*	*243*	*1457*	*218*	*848*	*827*	*1675*
Mean (average value)	589	579	568	561	575	599	603	552	578
Median value	441	417	436	408	429	422	434	421	428
Lower 2.5 percentile	146	142	144	132	146	124	156	131	142
Upper 2.5 percentile	1837	1816	1632	1971	1701	1712	1708	1609	1695
Standard error of the mean	46.7	30.7	27.8	45.5	22.9	51.1	35.7	21.7	21.0
	cum %	cum %	cum %	cum %	cum %	cum %	cum %	cum %	cum %
(b) Intakes from *food sources*									
Less than 200	7	9	8	8	8	8	7	9	8
Less than 400	46	52	46	56	49	51	48	52	50
Less than 600	81	82	81	86	82	82	80	84	82
Less than 800	93	93	90	95	93	92	91	93	63
Less than 1000	96	96	97	97	96	98	96	97	96
All	100	100	100	100	100	100	100	100	100
Base	*576*	*606*	*250*	*243*	*1457*	*218*	*848*	*827*	*1675*
Mean (average value)	542	506	484	462	512	489	541	475	509
Median value	423	385	411	360	402	389	411	387	401
Lower 2.5 percentile	146	142	136	132	146	116	155	131	142
Upper 2.5 percentile	1313	1210	1391	1123	1241	1051	1402	1085	1225
Standard error of the mean	46.1	29.0	23.8	42.0	22.2	47.7	35.1	19.6	20.3

Table 8.11 Average daily intake of vitamin A (retinol equivalents) as percentage of the Reference Nutrient Intake (RNI) by age and sex of child

Age and sex of child	Average daily intake as % of RNI							
	(a) All sources				(b) Food sources			
	Mean	Median	se	Base	Mean	Median	se	Base
All aged 1½–2½ years	147	110	11.7	*576*	135	106	11.5	*576*
All aged 2½–3½ years	145	104	7.7	*606*	127	96	7.2	*606*
Aged 3½–4½ years*:								
Boys	142	109	6.9	*250*	121	103	5.9	*250*
Girls	140	102	11.4	*243*	115	89	10.5	*243*
All aged under 4 years	144	107	5.7	*1457*	128	100	5.5	*1457*
All aged 4 years and over	150	106	12.8	*218*	122	97	11.9	*218*
All boys	151	108	8.9	*848*	135	103	8.8	*848*
All girls	138	105	5.4	*827*	119	97	4.9	*827*
All	144	107	5.3	*1675*	127	100	5.1	*1675*

*Vitamin A intake as a percentage of the RNI was calculated for each child; thus in this age group RNI values for children under 4 years and 4 years and over were the same, 400µg/d.

Table 8.12(a)   Contribution of food types to average daily vitamin A (retinol equivalents) intake by age and sex of child

Food types	Age and sex of child						
	All aged 1½ – 2½ years	All aged 2½ – 3½ years	All aged 3½ – 4½ years		All boys	All girls	All
			Boys	Girls			
	µg	µg	µg	µg	µg	µg	µg
Cereals & cereal products	36.0	43.3	49.5	44.0	43.8	39.8	41.8
Milk & milk products	213	164	149	140	181	169	175
of which:							
milk (whole, semi-skimmed, skimmed)	*164*	*130*	*113*	*107*	*142*	*129*	*136*
other milk & products	*49.3*	*34.3*	*36.0*	*32.8*	*39.5*	*39.5*	*39.5*
Eggs & egg dishes	14.3	16.8	15.9	19.7	13.9	18.6	16.2
Fat spreads	38.5	48.5	57.6	52.1	47.5	46.4	47.0
Meat & meat products	124	107	59.4	75.9	124	78.6	101
of which:							
beef, veal & dishes	*7.0*	*8.5*	*7.2*	*6.4*	*7.9*	*7.0*	*7.5*
liver & liver dishes	*106*	*85.8*	*37.8*	*55.1*	*103*	*58.4*	*81.1*
meat pies etc.	*5.5*	*5.5*	*6.0*	*6.9*	*5.7*	*5.8*	*5.8*
Fish & fish dishes	5.0	5.6	5.0	7.8	4.5	6.7	5.6
Vegetables, potatoes & savoury snacks	72.9	84.0	112	91.8	90.0	81.0	85.5
of which:							
vegetables, excluding potatoes	*67.0*	*79.1*	*103*	*82.9*	*83.4*	*74.4*	*79.0*
all potatoes	*2.9*	*2.2*	*6.9*	*5.4*	*3.5*	*3.8*	*3.6*
savoury snacks	*3.0*	*2.7*	*2.7*	*3.5*	*3.0*	*2.8*	*2.9*
Fruit & nuts	2.6	3.0	2.5	3.3	2.6	3.0	2.8
Sugars, preserves & confectionery	2.1	3.3	4.3	3.3	3.2	2.9	3.0
Beverages	21.3	22.2	21.5	17.9	22.1	20.2	21.2
Commercial infant foods & drinks	2.5	0.5	0.5	0.1	1.1	1.1	1.1
Miscellaneous	8.8	7.8	6.0	6.0	7.3	7.9	7.6
Average daily intake (µg)	**542**	**506**	**484**	**462**	**541**	**475**	**509**
Total number of children	**576**	**606**	**250**	**243**	**848**	**827**	**1675**

Table 8.12(b)   Percentage contribution of food types to average daily vitamin A (retinol equivalents) intake by age and sex of child

Food types	Age and sex of child						
	All aged 1½ – 2½ years	All aged 2½ – 3½ years	All aged 3½ – 4½ years		All boys	All girls	All
			Boys	Girls			
	%	%	%	%	%	%	%
Cereals & cereal products	7	8	10	10	8	8	8
Milk & milk products	39	32	31	30	34	36	34
of which:							
milk (whole, semi-skimmed, skimmed)	*30*	*26*	*23*	*23*	*26*	*27*	*27*
other milk & products	*9*	*7*	*7*	*7*	*7*	*8*	*8*
Eggs & egg dishes	3	3	3	4	3	4	3
Fat spreads	7	9	12	11	9	10	9
Meat & meat products	23	21	12	16	23	16	20
of which:							
beef, veal & dishes	*1*	*2*	*2*	*1*	*1*	*2*	*2*
liver & liver dishes	*20*	*17*	*8*	*12*	*19*	*12*	*16*
meat pies etc.	*1*	*1*	*1*	*2*	*1*	*1*	*1*
Fish & fish dishes	1	1	1	2	1	1	1
Vegetables, potatoes & savoury snacks	14	17	23	20	17	17	17
of which:							
vegetable, excluding potatoes	*12*	*16*	*21*	*18*	*15*	*16*	*16*
all potatoes	*0*	*0*	*1*	*1*	*1*	*1*	*1*
savoury snacks	*1*	*0*	*1*	*1*	*1*	*1*	*1*
Fruit & nuts	0	1	0	1	0	1	0
Sugars, preserves & confectionery	0	1	1	1	1	1	1
Beverages	4	4	4	4	4	4	4
Commercial infant foods & drinks	0	0	0	0	0	0	0
Miscellaneous	2	2	1	1	1	2	2
Average daily intake (µg)	**542**	**506**	**484**	**462**	**541**	**475**	**509**
Total number of children	**576**	**606**	**250**	**243**	**848**	**827**	**1675**

Table 8.13 Average daily intake of thiamin (mg) by age and sex of child

Thiamin (mg)	Age and sex of child								
	All aged 1½ – 2½ years	All aged 2½ – 3½ years	All aged 3½ – 4½ years		All aged under 4 years	All aged 4 years and over	All boys	All girls	All
			Boys	Girls					
	cum %	cum %	cum %	cum %	cum %	cum %	cum %	cum %	cum %
(a) Intakes from *all sources*									
Less than 0.3	0	1	–	–	0	–	0	0	0
Less than 0.4	3	2	2	0	2	1	2	3	2
Less than 0.5	13	8	5	6	10	4	8	11	9
Less than 0.7	49	39	28	35	42	31	37	43	40
Less than 0.9	81	71	55	62	73	56	70	72	71
Less than 1.1	91	88	82	86	89	80	88	88	88
Less than 1.3	95	93	92	92	94	90	94	93	94
All	100	100	100	100	100	100	100	100	100
Base	*576*	*606*	*250*	*243*	*1457*	*218*	*848*	*827*	*1675*
Mean (average value)	0.8	0.8	0.9	0.9	0.8	0.9	0.8	0.8	0.8
Median value	0.7	0.8	0.9	0.8	0.7	0.8	0.8	0.7	0.7
Lower 2.5 percentile	0.4	0.4	0.4	0.4	0.4	0.5	0.4	0.4	0.4
Upper 2.5 percentile	1.6	1.7	1.7	1.8	1.7	1.9	1.7	1.7	1.7
Standard error of the mean	0.01	0.01	0.02	0.02	0.01	0.02	0.01	0.01	0.01
	cum %	cum %	cum %	cum %	cum %	cum %	cum %	cum %	cum %
(b) Intakes from *food sources*									
Less than 0.3	0	1	–	–	0	–	0	0	0
Less than 0.4	3	2	2	0	2	1	2	3	2
Less than 0.5	14	9	6	6	10	5	8	11	10
Less than 0.7	51	41	30	35	43	32	38	45	42
Less than 0.9	84	74	58	65	76	58	71	76	74
Less than 1.1	93	91	85	90	92	84	90	92	91
Less than 1.3	97	96	95	97	96	94	96	96	96
All	100	100	100	100	100	100	100	100	100
Base	*576*	*606*	*250*	*243*	*1457*	*218*	*848*	*827*	*1675*
Mean (average value)	0.7	0.8	0.9	0.8	0.8	0.9	0.8	0.8	0.8
Median value	0.7	0.7	0.9	0.8	0.7	0.8	0.8	0.7	0.7
Lower 2.5 percentile	0.4	0.4	0.4	0.4	0.4	0.5	0.4	0.4	0.4
Upper 2.5 percentile	1.3	1.5	1.4	1.3	1.4	1.4	1.4	1.4	1.4
Standard error of the mean	0.01	0.01	0.02	0.02	0.01	0.02	0.01	0.01	0.01

Table 8.14 Average daily intake of thiamin as a percentage of the Reference Nutrient Intake (RNI) by age and sex of child

Age and sex of child	Average daily intake as % of RNI							
	(a) All sources				(b) Food sources			
	Mean	*Median*	*se*	*Base*	*Mean*	*Median*	*se*	*Base*
All aged 1½–2½ years	152	141	2.5	*576*	146	139	2.2	*576*
All aged 2½–3½ years	162	151	2.5	*606*	156	150	2.1	*606*
Aged 3½–4½ years*:								
Boys	157	148	3.5	*250*	151	145	3.1	*250*
Girls	148	136	4.2	*243*	141	133	3.6	*243*
All aged under 4 years	160	149	1.6	*1457*	154	147	1.4	*1457*
All aged 4 years and over	128	121	3.2	*218*	123	120	2.6	*218*
All boys	158	148	2.0	*848*	153	146	1.7	*848*
All girls	154	142	2.3	*827*	147	139	2.0	*827*
All	156	146	1.5	*1675*	150	143	1.3	*1675*

*Thiamin intake as a percentage of the RNI was calculated for each child; thus in this age group values for children under 4 years of age used 0.5mg/d as the RNI and for children aged 4 and over 0.7mg/d was taken as the RNI. The values for all children aged 3½ to 4½ years were then pooled to give a mean, median and standard error (se) for the age group.

Table 8.15 Average daily intake of riboflavin (mg) by age and sex of child

Riboflavin (mg)	Age and sex of child								
	All aged 1½ – 2½ years	All aged 2½ – 3½ years	All aged 3½ – 4½ years		All aged under 4 years	All aged 4 years and over	All boys	All girls	All
			Boys	Girls					
	cum %	cum %	cum %	cum %	cum %	cum %	cum %	cum %	cum %
(a) Intakes from *all sources*									
Less than 0.3	0	0	–	–	0	–	0	0	0
Less than 0.4	1	1	1	1	1	0	1	1	1
Less than 0.6	6	7	4	9	6	8	4	8	7
Less than 0.8	17	19	17	23	18	21	16	21	18
Less than 1.2	50	55	50	56	53	52	50	55	53
Less than 1.6	82	83	81	83	83	79	81	84	83
Less than 2.0	95	94	96	96	95	95	95	94	95
All	100	100	100	100	100	100	100	100	100
Base	*576*	*606*	*250*	*243*	*1457*	*218*	*848*	*827*	*1675*
Mean (average value)	1.2	1.2	1.2	1.2	1.2	1.2	1.2	1.2	1.2
Median value	1.2	1.1	1.2	1.1	1.2	1.2	1.2	1.1	1.2
Lower 2.5 percentile	0.5	0.4	0.5	0.5	0.5	0.5	0.5	0.5	0.5
Upper 2.5 percentile	2.2	2.5	2.1	2.2	2.3	2.1	2.1	2.3	2.2
Standard error of the mean	0.02	0.02	0.03	0.03	0.01	0.03	0.01	0.02	0.01
	cum %	cum %	cum %	cum %	cum %	cum %	cum %	cum %	cum %
(b) Intakes from *food sources*									
Less than 0.3	0	0	–	–	0	–	0	0	0
Less than 0.4	1	1	1	1	1	0	1	1	1
Less than 0.6	6	7	4	9	6	8	5	9	7
Less than 0.8	18	19	17	23	18	21	16	21	19
Less than 1.2	52	57	52	58	55	53	52	57	55
Less than 1.6	84	85	85	85	85	83	83	86	85
Less than 2.0	95	95	98	98	96	98	96	96	96
All	100	100	100	100	100	100	100	100	100
Base	*576*	*606*	*250*	*243*	*1457*	*218*	*848*	*827*	*1675*
Mean (average value)	1.2	1.2	1.2	1.1	1.2	1.2	1.2	1.1	1.2
Median value	1.2	1.1	1.2	1.1	1.1	1.2	1.2	1.1	1.1
Lower 2.5 percentile	0.5	0.4	0.5	0.5	0.5	0.5	0.5	0.5	0.5
Upper 2.5 percentile	2.2	2.3	2.0	2.0	2.1	2.0	2.1	2.1	2.1
Standard error of the mean	0.02	0.02	0.02	0.02	0.01	0.03	0.01	0.01	0.01

Table 8.16 Average daily intake of riboflavin as a percentage of the Reference Nutrient Intake (RNI) by age and sex of child

Age and sex of child	Average daily intake as % of RNI							
	(a) All sources				(b) Food sources			
	Mean	Median	se	Base	Mean	Median	se	Base
All aged 1½–2½ years	204	200	3.2	*576*	200	198	3.1	*576*
All aged 2½–3½ years	201	190	3.3	*606*	196	186	3.0	*606*
Aged 3½–4½ years*:								
Boys	183	179	4.2	*250*	178	175	3.8	*250*
Girls	171	159	4.6	*243*	166	158	4.1	*243*
All aged under 4 years	202	195	2.0	*1457*	197	191	1.9	*1457*
All aged 4 years and over	151	145	3.9	*218*	147	144	3.4	*218*
All boys	199	192	2.6	*848*	195	187	2.4	*848*
All girls	191	181	2.7	*827*	185	179	2.5	*827*
All	195	187	1.9	*1675*	191	184	1.7	*1675*

*Riboflavin intake as a percentage of the RNI was calculated for each child; thus in this age group values for children under 4 years of age used 0.6mg/d as the RNI and for children aged 4 and over 0.8mg/d was taken as the RNI. The values for all children aged 3½ to 4½ years were then pooled to give a mean, median and standard error (se) for the age group.

151

Table 8.17(a)   Contribution of food types to average daily riboflavin intake by age and sex of child

Food types	Age and sex of child						
	All aged 1½ – 2½ years	All aged 2½ – 3½ years	All aged 3½ – 4½ years		All boys	All girls	All
			Boys	Girls			
	mg	mg	mg	mg	mg	mg	mg
Cereals & cereal products	0.25	0.30	0.35	0.32	0.31	0.28	0.29
of which:							
breakfast cereals	*0.16*	*0.19*	*0.22*	*0.19*	*0.20*	*0.17*	*0.19*
Milk & milk products	0.68	0.58	0.53	0.51	0.61	0.59	0.60
of which:							
milk (whole, semi-skimmed, skimmed)	*0.55*	*0.47*	*0.43*	*0.41*	*0.50*	*0.47*	*0.48*
other milk & products	*0.14*	*0.11*	*0.10*	*0.10*	*0.12*	*0.12*	*0.12*
Eggs & egg dishes	0.03	0.03	0.03	0.04	0.03	0.03	0.03
Fat spreads	0.00	0.00	0.00	0.00	0.00	0.00	0.00
Meat & meat products	0.08	0.09	0.10	0.10	0.09	0.09	0.09
Fish & fish dishes	0.01	0.01	0.01	0.01	0.01	0.01	0.01
Vegetables, potatoes & savoury snacks	0.04	0.04	0.04	0.04	0.04	0.04	0.04
Fruit & nuts	0.02	0.02	0.02	0.02	0.02	0.02	0.02
Sugars, preserves & confectionery	0.04	0.05	0.05	0.05	0.05	0.05	0.05
Beverages	0.02	0.03	0.03	0.03	0.02	0.03	0.02
Commercial infant foods & drinks	0.01	0.00	0.00	0.00	0.00	0.00	0.00
Miscellaneous	0.03	0.02	0.02	0.02	0.03	0.02	0.03
Average daily intake (mg)	**1.2**	**1.2**	**1.2**	**1.1**	**1.2**	**1.1**	**1.2**
Total number of children	**576**	**606**	**250**	**243**	**848**	**827**	**1675**

Table 8.17(b)   Percentage contribution of food types to average daily riboflavin intake by age and sex of child

Food types	Age and sex of child						
	All aged 1½ – 2½ years	All aged 2½ – 3½ years	All aged 3½ – 4½ years		All boys	All girls	All
			Boys	Girls			
	%	%	%	%	%	%	%
Cereals & cereal products	21	25	29	28	26	24	24
of which:							
breakfast cereals	*13*	*16*	*18*	*17*	*16*	*15*	*16*
Milk & milk products	56	49	44	45	50	51	51
of which:							
milk (whole, semi-skimmed, skimmed)	*46*	*40*	*36*	*36*	*41*	*41*	*41*
other milk & products	*12*	*9*	*8*	*9*	*10*	*10*	*10*
Eggs & egg dishes	2	2	2	4	2	3	2
Fat spreads	0	0	0	0	0	0	0
Meat & meat products	7	8	8	9	7	8	8
Fish & fish dishes	1	1	1	1	1	1	1
Vegetables, potatoes & savoury snacks	3	3	3	4	3	3	3
Fruit & nuts	2	2	2	2	2	2	2
Sugars, preserves & confectionery	3	4	4	4	4	4	4
Beverages	2	2	2	3	2	3	2
Commercial infant foods & drinks	1	0	0	0	0	0	0
Miscellaneous	2	2	2	2	2	2	2
Average daily intake (mg)	**1.2**	**1.2**	**1.2**	**1.1**	**1.2**	**1.1**	**1.2**
Total number of children	**576**	**606**	**250**	**243**	**848**	**827**	**1675**

Table 8.18 Average daily intake of niacin equivalents (mg) by age and sex of child

Niacin equivalents (mg)	Age and sex of child								
	All aged 1½ – 2½ years	All aged 2½ – 3½ years	All aged 3½ – 4½ years		All aged under 4 years	All aged 4 years and over	All boys	All girls	All
			Boys	Girls					
	cum %	cum %	cum %	cum %	cum %	cum %	cum %	cum %	cum %
(a) Intakes from *all sources*									
Less than 8	–	–	–	–	–	–	–	–	–
Less than 11	17	11	7	9	13	6	10	14	12
Less than 14	29	34	20	28	37	23	33	38	35
Less than 17	73	60	43	52	63	43	60	62	61
Less than 20	88	80	68	74	82	68	79	82	80
Less than 23	95	92	83	85	92	81	90	91	91
Less than 26	98	96	92	92	96	90	96	96	96
All	100	100	100	100	100	100	100	100	100
Base	576	606	250	243	1457	218	848	827	1675
Mean (average value)	14.9	16.4	18.2	17.5	16.0	18.3	16.5	16.1	16.3
Median value	14.3	16.0	18.1	16.5	15.3	17.8	16.0	15.5	15.7
Lower 2.5 percentile	8.2	8.2	9.6	8.6	8.2	8.9	8.5	8.2	8.3
Upper 2.5 percentile	24.7	29.4	30.1	32.4	27.9	31.6	27.9	28.6	28.5
Standard error of the mean	0.2	0.2	0.3	0.3	0.1	0.4	0.2	0.2	0.1
	cum %	cum %	cum %	cum %	cum %	cum %	cum %	cum %	cum %
(b) Intakes from *food sources*									
Less than 8	–	–	–	–	–	–	–	–	–
Less than 11	18	11	8	9	13	6	10	15	12
Less than 14	30	35	20	28	38	23	33	40	36
Less than 17	76	61	45	53	65	44	61	65	63
Less than 20	90	82	70	76	84	70	80	84	82
Less than 23	96	92	84	88	93	84	91	93	92
Less than 26	99	97	93	95	97	93	96	97	97
All	100	100	100	100	100	100	100	100	100
Base	576	606	250	243	1457	218	848	827	1675
Mean (average value)	14.7	16.1	17.9	17.1	15.8	17.9	16.4	15.7	16.0
Median value	14.1	15.8	17.9	16.5	15.8	17.7	15.8	15.3	15.5
Lower 2.5 percentile	8.2	8.2	9.1	8.6	8.2	8.9	8.5	8.2	8.3
Upper 2.5 percentile	24.2	27.7	29.1	28.9	26.5	30.6	27.1	27.1	27.1
Standard error of the mean	0.2	0.2	0.3	0.3	0.1	0.3	0.2	0.2	0.1

Table 8.19 Average daily niacin intake as a percentage of the Reference Nutrient Intake (RNI) by age and sex of child

Age and sex of child	Average daily intake as % of RNI							
	(a) All sources				(b) Food sources			
	Mean	Median	se	Base	Mean	Median	se	Base
All aged 1½–2½ years	187	179	2.3	576	184	176	2.2	576
All aged 2½–3½ years	205	200	2.6	606	202	197	2.4	606
Aged 3½–4½ years*:								
Boys	201	190	3.8	250	198	189	3.7	250
Girls	190	177	4.3	243	186	175	4.0	243
All aged under 4 years	200	191	1.6	1457	197	190	1.5	1457
All aged 4 years and over	167	162	3.5	218	163	161	3.2	218
All boys	199	189	2.0	848	197	188	1.9	848
All girls	193	185	2.2	827	189	181	2.0	827
All	195	187	1.5	1675	193	185	1.4	1675

*Niacin intake as a percentage of the RNI was calculated for each child; thus in this age group values for children under 4 years of age used 8mg/d as the RNI and for children aged 4 and over 11mg/d was taken as the RNI. The values for all children aged 3½ to 4½ years were then pooled to give a mean, median and standard error (se) for the age group.

Table 8.20   Average daily intake of vitamin B$_6$ (mg) by age and sex of child

Vitamin B$_6$ (mg)	Age and sex of child								
	All aged 1½ – 2½ years	All aged 2½ – 3½ years	All aged 3½ – 4½ years		All aged under 4 years	All aged 4 years and over	All boys	All girls	All
			Boys	Girls					
	cum %	cum %	cum %	cum %	cum %	cum %	cum %	cum %	cum %
(a) Intakes from *all sources*									
Less than 0.5	2	1	2	–	1	2	1	1	1
Less than 0.7	11	8	4	4	8	5	7	10	8
Less than 0.9	31	21	14	18	24	17	21	25	23
Less than 1.1	53	40	30	37	44	31	40	45	43
Less than 1.3	69	62	52	54	50	52	61	63	62
Less than 1.5	82	80	64	72	77	65	75	77	76
Less than 1.7	91	87	79	84	88	77	86	87	87
Less than 1.9	97	92	90	89	94	88	94	93	93
All	100	100	100	100	100	100	100	100	100
Base	*576*	*606*	*250*	*243*	*1457*	*218*	*848*	*827*	*1675*
Mean (average value)	1.1	1.2	1.4	1.3	1.2	1.4	1.2	1.2	1.2
Median value	1.1	1.2	1.3	1.2	1.1	1.3	1.2	1.1	1.2
Lower 2.5 percentile	0.5	0.5	0.6	0.6	0.5	0.5	0.6	0.5	0.5
Upper 2.5 percentile	1.9	2.4	2.4	2.7	2.3	2.7	2.4	2.3	2.3
Standard error of the mean	0.02	0.02	0.03	0.03	0.01	0.04	0.02	0.02	0.01
	cum %	cum %	cum %	cum %	cum %	cum %	cum %	cum %	cum %
(b) Intakes from *food sources*									
Less than 0.5	2	1	2	–	1	2	2	1	1
Less than 0.7	11	8	4	4	9	5	7	10	8
Less than 0.9	32	22	14	19	25	17	22	26	24
Less than 1.1	55	42	31	38	46	32	41	47	44
Less than 1.3	72	63	53	56	65	52	62	65	64
Less than 1.5	84	78	67	74	79	67	77	79	78
Less than 1.7	93	89	82	86	90	80	88	89	89
Less than 1.9	97	94	92	91	95	90	94	94	94
All	100	100	100	100	100	100	100	100	100
Base	*576*	*606*	*250*	*243*	*1457*	*218*	*848*	*827*	*1675*
Mean (average value)	1.1	1.2	1.3	1.3	1.2	1.3	1.2	1.2	1.2
Median value	1.0	1.2	1.3	1.2	1.1	1.3	1.2	1.1	1.1
Lower 2.5 percentile	0.5	0.5	0.6	0.6	0.5	0.5	0.6	0.5	0.5
Upper 2.5 percentile	1.9	2.3	2.3	2.6	2.2	2.4	2.3	2.2	2.2
Standard error of the mean	0.02	0.02	0.03	0.03	0.01	0.04	0.01	0.02	0.01

Table 8.21   Average daily intake of vitamin B$_6$ as a percentage of the Reference Nutrient Intake (RNI) by age and sex of child

Age and sex of child	Average daily intake as % of RNI							
	(a) All sources				(b) Food sources			
	Mean	Median	se	Base	Mean	Median	se	Base
All aged 1½–2½ years	163	154	2.4	*576*	160	151	2.3	*576*
All aged 2½–3½ years	178	168	2.6	*606*	175	167	2.5	*606*
Aged 3½–4½ years*:								
Boys	175	166	4.1	*250*	172	165	3.9	*250*
Girls	168	155	4.4	*243*	164	150	4.2	*243*
All aged under 4 years	174	164	1.6	*1457*	170	163	1.6	*1457*
All aged 4 years and over	152	142	4.4	*218*	148	140	4.2	*218*
All boys	173	165	2.1	*848*	171	164	2.0	*848*
All girls	169	158	2.3	*827*	164	155	2.2	*827*
All	171	162	1.6	*1675*	167	159	1.5	*1675*

*Vitamin B$_6$ intake as a percentage of the RNI was calculated for each child; thus in this age group values for children under 4 years of age used 0.7mg/d as the RNI and for children aged 4 and over 0.9mg/d was taken as the RNI. The values for all children aged 3½ to 4½ years were then pooled to give a mean, median and standard error (se) for the age group.

Table 8.22(a)   Contribution of food types to average daily vitamin B$_6$ intake by age and sex of child

Food types	All aged 1½ – 2½ years	All aged 2½ – 3½ years	All aged 3½ – 4½ years		All boys	All girls	All
			Boys	Girls			
	mg	mg	mg	mg	mg	mg	mg
Cereals & cereal products	0.23	0.29	0.33	0.32	0.29	0.27	0.28
of which:							
breakfast cereals	*0.14*	*0.19*	*0.21*	*0.20*	*0.18*	*0.17*	*0.18*
Milk & milk products	0.35	0.29	0.27	0.25	0.31	0.29	0.30
of which:							
milk (whole, semi-skimmed, skimmed)	*0.31*	*0.27*	*0.24*	*0.23*	*0.28*	*0.27*	*0.27*
Eggs & egg dishes	0.01	0.01	0.01	0.01	0.01	0.01	0.01
Fat spreads	–	–	–	–	–	–	–
Meat & meat products	0.09	0.11	0.13	0.12	0.11	0.11	0.11
Fish & fish dishes	0.02	0.03	0.02	0.03	0.02	0.02	0.02
Vegetables, potatoes & savoury snacks	0.24	0.29	0.32	0.32	0.29	0.28	0.28
of which:							
vegetables, excluding potatoes	*0.04*	*0.04*	*0.04*	*0.04*	*0.04*	*0.04*	*0.04*
all potatoes	*0.16*	*0.19*	*0.22*	*0.22*	*0.19*	*0.18*	*0.19*
savoury snacks	*0.04*	*0.06*	*0.06*	*0.06*	*0.05*	*0.05*	*0.05*
Fruit & nuts	0.08	0.08	0.08	0.07	0.08	0.08	0.08
Sugars, preserves & confectionery	0.00	0.00	0.00	0.00	0.00	0.00	0.00
Beverages	0.08	0.12	0.16	0.14	0.11	0.11	0.11
of which:							
fruit juice	*0.03*	*0.03*	*0.02*	*0.02*	*0.02*	*0.03*	*0.03*
soft drinks, including low calorie drinks	*0.05*	*0.09*	*0.13*	*0.12*	*0.09*	*0.09*	*0.09*
Commercial infant foods & drinks	0.01	0.00	0.00	0.00	0.00	0.00	0.00
Miscellaneous	0.01	0.01	0.01	0.01	0.01	0.01	0.01
Average daily intake (mg)	**1.1**	**1.2**	**1.3**	**1.3**	**1.2**	**1.2**	**1.2**
Total number of children	**576**	**606**	**250**	**243**	**848**	**827**	**1675**

Table 8.22(b)   Percentage contribution of food types to average daily vitamin B$_6$ intake by age and sex of child

Food types	All aged 1½ – 2½ years	All aged 2½ – 3½ years	All aged 3½ – 4½ years		All boys	All girls	All
			Boys	Girls			
	%	%	%	%	%	%	%
Cereals & cereal products	20	24	25	25	24	23	23
of which:							
breakfast cereals	*12*	*16*	*16*	*16*	*15*	*14*	*15*
Milk & milk products	31	24	20	19	25	24	25
of which:							
milk (whole, semi-skimmed, skimmed)	*28*	*22*	*18*	*18*	*23*	*23*	*22*
Eggs & egg dishes	1	1	1	1	1	1	1
Fat spreads	–	–	–	–	–	–	–
Meat & meat products	8	9	10	9	9	9	9
Fish & fish dishes	2	2	2	2	2	2	2
Vegetables, potatoes & savoury snacks	21	24	24	25	24	24	23
of which:							
vegetables, excluding potatoes	*4*	*3*	*3*	*3*	*3*	*3*	*3*
all potatoes	*14*	*16*	*16*	*17*	*15*	*15*	*16*
savoury snacks	*4*	*5*	*4*	*5*	*4*	*4*	*4*
Fruit & nuts	7	6	6	5	6	7	7
Sugars, preserves & confectionery	0	0	0	0	0	0	0
Beverages	7	10	12	11	9	9	9
of which:							
fruit juice	*3*	*2*	*2*	*2*	*2*	*2*	*2*
soft drinks, including low calorie drinks	*4*	*7*	*10*	*9*	*7*	*8*	*7*
Commercial infant foods & drinks	1	0	0	0	0	0	0
Miscellaneous	1	1	1	1	1	1	1
Average daily intake (mg)	**1.1**	**1.2**	**1.3**	**1.3**	**1.2**	**1.2**	**1.2**
Total number of children	**576**	**606**	**250**	**243**	**848**	**827**	**1675**

Table 8.23 Average daily intake of vitamin B$_{12}$ (μg) by age and sex of child

Vitamin B$_{12}$ (μg)	Age and sex of child								
	All aged 1½ – 2½ years	All aged 2½ – 3½ years	All aged 3½ – 4½ years		All aged under 4 years	All aged 4 years and over	All boys	All girls	All
			Boys	Girls					
	cum %	cum %	cum %	cum %	cum %	cum %	cum %	cum %	cum %
(a) Intakes from *all sources*									
Less than 0.3	0	0	–	–	–	–	0	0	0
Less than 0.5	0	0	1	0	–	–	0	0	0
Less than 0.8	2	2	2	2	2	2	2	2	2
Less than 1.0	3	4	3	4	4	3	3	4	4
Less than 2.0	29	30	27	30	29	27	29	29	29
Less than 3.0	65	66	62	66	66	60	64	66	65
Less than 4.0	87	86	88	87	87	85	86	87	87
Less than 5.0	94	93	94	95	94	94	93	94	94
All	100	100	100	100	100	100	100	100	100
Base	*576*	*606*	*250*	*243*	*1457*	*218*	*848*	*827*	*1675*
Mean (average value)	2.9	2.8	2.8	2.8	2.8	2.9	2.9	2.8	2.8
Median value	2.5	2.4	2.6	2.5	2.5	2.6	2.5	2.5	2.5
Lower 2.5 percentile	0.9	0.9	0.8	0.9	0.9	0.8	0.9	0.9	0.9
Upper 2.5 percentile	6.7	7.2	6.3	6.2	6.7	6.7	6.8	6.6	6.6
Standard error of the mean	0.09	0.06	0.09	0.10	0.05	0.12	0.07	0.06	0.04
	cum %	cum %	cum %	cum %	cum %	cum %	cum %	cum %	cum %
(b) Intakes from *food sources*									
Less than 0.3	0	0	–	–	–	–	0	0	0
Less than 0.5	0	0	1	0	–	–	0	0	0
Less than 0.8	2	2	2	2	2	2	2	2	2
Less than 1.0	4	4	3	4	4	3	3	4	4
Less than 2.0	29	30	28	30	30	27	29	30	30
Less than 3.0	66	67	62	67	67	60	64	67	66
Less than 4.0	87	86	89	88	87	87	86	87	87
Less than 5.0	94	93	94	95	94	95	94	94	94
All	100	100	100	100	100	100	100	100	100
Base	*576*	*606*	*250*	*243*	*1457*	*218*	*848*	*827*	*1675*
Mean (average value)	2.9	2.8	2.8	2.8	2.8	2.9	2.8	2.8	2.8
Median value	2.5	2.4	2.6	2.4	2.5	2.6	2.5	2.5	2.5
Lower 2.5 percentile	0.8	0.9	0.8	0.9	0.9	0.8	0.9	0.9	0.9
Upper 2.5 percentile	6.7	7.2	6.2	6.2	6.4	6.5	6.8	6.3	6.4
Standard error of the mean	0.09	0.06	0.09	0.10	0.05	0.11	0.07	0.06	0.04

Table 8.24 Average daily intake of vitamin B$_{12}$ as a percentage of the Reference Nutrient Intake (RNI) by age and sex of child

Age and sex of child	Average daily intake as % of RNI							
	(a) All sources				(b) Food sources			
	Mean	Median	se	Base	Mean	Median	se	Base
All aged 1½–2½ years	576	510	19.0	*576*	574	509	19.0	*576*
All aged 2½–3½ years	560	489	12.4	*606*	556	486	12.3	*606*
Aged 3½–4½ years*:								
Boys	470	427	14.8	*250*	465	423	14.7	*250*
Girls	460	398	17.4	*243*	454	397	17.1	*243*
All aged under 4 years	563	502	9.5	*1457*	560	496	9.5	*1457*
All aged 4 years and over	365	325	15.0	*218*	360	325	14.8	*218*
All boys	547	478	13.4	*848*	544	476	13.4	*848*
All girls	528	471	10.9	*827*	523	469	10.8	*827*
All	538	474	8.6	*1675*	534	471	8.6	*1675*

*Vitamin B$_{12}$ intake as a percentage of the RNI was calculated for each child; thus in this age group values for children under 4 years of age used 0.5μg/d as the RNI and for children aged 4 and over 0.8μg/d was taken as the RNI. The values for all children aged 3½ to 4½ years were then pooled to give a mean, median and standard error (se) for the age group.

Table 8.25(a) Contribution of food types to average daily vitamin B$_{12}$ intake by age and sex of child

Food types	All aged 1½ – 2½ years	All aged 2½ – 3½ years	All aged 3½ – 4½ years Boys	All aged 3½ – 4½ years Girls	All boys	All girls	All
	µg	µg	µg	µg	µg	µg	µg
Cereals & cereal products	0.2	0.3	0.4	0.4	0.4	0.3	0.3
Milk & milk products	1.5	1.3	1.2	1.1	1.4	1.3	1.3
of which:							
milk (whole, semi-skimmed, skimmed)	*1.3*	*1.1*	*1.0*	*0.9*	*1.1*	*1.1*	*1.1*
other milk & products	*0.3*	*0.2*	*0.2*	*0.2*	*0.2*	*0.2*	*0.2*
Eggs & egg dishes	0.1	0.1	0.1	0.2	0.1	0.2	0.1
Fat spreads	–	–	–	–	–	–	–
Meat & meat products	0.6	0.6	0.6	0.6	0.6	0.5	0.6
of which:							
beef, veal & dishes	*0.1*	*0.1*	*0.1*	*0.1*	*0.1*	*0.1*	*0.1*
liver & liver dishes	*0.2*	*0.1*	*0.05*	*0.1*	*0.1*	*0.1*	*0.1*
Fish & fish dishes	0.2	0.2	0.2	0.2	0.2	0.2	0.2
Vegetables, potatoes & savoury snacks	0.00	0.00	0.03	0.02	0.02	0.02	0.02
Fruit & nuts	0.00	–	–	–	–	0.00	0.00
Sugars, preserves & confectionery	0.02	0.04	0.04	0.04	0.03	0.03	0.03
Beverages	0.1	0.2	0.2	0.2	0.2	0.2	0.2
of which:							
soft drinks, including low calorie drinks	*0.1*	*0.2*	*0.2*	*0.2*	*0.2*	*0.2*	*0.2*
Commercial infant foods & drinks	0.01	0.00	–	0.00	0.00	0.00	0.00
Miscellaneous	0.02	0.01	0.01	0.01	0.01	0.01	0.01
Average daily intake (µg)	**2.9**	**2.8**	**2.8**	**2.8**	**2.8**	**2.8**	**2.8**
Total number of children	**576**	**606**	**250**	**243**	**848**	**827**	**1675**

Table 8.25(b) Percentage contribution of food types to average daily vitamin B$_{12}$ intake by age and sex of child

Food types	All aged 1½ – 2½ years	All aged 2½ – 3½ years	All aged 3½ – 4½ years Boys	All aged 3½ – 4½ years Girls	All boys	All girls	All
	%	%	%	%	%	%	%
Cereals & cereal products	9	12	14	14	12	11	11
Milk & milk products	53	47	42	41	48	47	47
of which:							
milk (whole, semi-skimmed, skimmed)	*44*	*39*	*35*	*34*	*40*	*39*	*39*
other milk & products	*9*	*8*	*8*	*8*	*8*	*8*	*8*
Eggs & egg dishes	4	5	5	6	4	6	5
Fat spreads	–	–	–	–	–	–	–
Meat & meat products	21	20	20	20	21	20	20
of which:							
beef, veal & dishes	*5*	*5*	*5*	*5*	*5*	*5*	*5*
liver & liver dishes	*6*	*4*	*2*	*2*	*5*	*2*	*4*
Fish & fish dishes	7	8	8	7	7	8	7
Vegetables, potatoes & savoury snacks	1	1	1	1	1	1	1
Fruit & nuts	0	–	–	–	–	0	0
Sugars, preserves & confectionery	1	1	1	1	1	1	1
Beverages	4	6	9	9	6	6	6
of which:							
soft drinks, including low calorie drinks	*4*	*6*	*9*	*9*	*6*	*6*	*6*
Commercial infant foods & drinks	0	0	–	0	0	0	0
Miscellaneous	1	0	0	0	0	0	0
Average daily intake (µg)	**2.9**	**2.8**	**2.8**	**2.8**	**2.8**	**2.8**	**2.8**
Total number of children	**576**	**606**	**250**	**243**	**848**	**827**	**1675**

Table 8.26 Average daily intake of folate (µg) by age and sex of child

Folate (µg)	Age and sex of child								
	All aged 1½–2½ years	All aged 2½–3½ years	All aged 3½–4½ years		All aged under 4 years	All aged 4 years and over	All boys	All girls	All
			Boys	Girls					
	cum %	cum %	cum %	cum %	cum %	cum %	cum %	cum %	cum %
(a) Intakes from *all sources*									
Less than 35	0	0	–	–	0	–	0	0	0
Less than 50	2	1	1	0	1	1	0	2	1
Less than 70	7	6	4	3	6	4	5	6	6
Less than 100	33	25	15	22	27	19	24	28	26
Less than 130	66	53	42	46	56	42	52	57	55
Less than 160	85	76	66	67	78	62	76	76	76
Less than 190	94	88	86	85	90	83	90	89	89
Less than 210	96	93	92	92	94	88	94	94	94
All	100	100	100	100	100	100	100	100	100
Base	*576*	*606*	*250*	*243*	*1457*	*218*	*848*	*827*	*1675*
Mean (average value)	120	134	145	140	130	145	133	130	132
Median value	114	127	140	135	122	140	126	122	124
Lower 2.5 percentile	59.6	60.7	58.8	62.7	60.8	54.8	63.3	55.5	60.7
Upper 2.5 percentile	225	254	256	251	241	257	253	242	246
Standard error of the mean	1.8	2.0	3.2	3.1	1.2	3.6	1.7	1.7	1.2
	cum %	cum %	cum %	cum %	cum %	cum %	cum %	cum %	cum %
(b) Intakes from *food sources*									
Less than 35	0	0	–	–	0	–	0	0	0
Less than 50	2	1	1	0	1	1	0	2	1
Less than 70	8	6	4	4	6	4	5	6	6
Less than 100	33	25	16	22	27	20	24	28	26
Less than 130	66	53	42	47	57	43	53	57	55
Less than 160	85	76	66	68	79	63	77	77	77
Less than 190	94	88	87	86	91	84	90	90	90
Less than 210	97	93	92	92	95	89	94	94	94
All	100	100	100	100	100	100	100	100	100
Base	*576*	*606*	*250*	*243*	*1457*	*218*	*848*	*827*	*1675*
Mean (average value)	120	133	143	138	129	143	132	129	131
Median value	114	126	138	134	122	137	125	122	123
Lower 2.5 percentile	59.6	60.7	58.8	62.7	60.8	54.8	63.3	55.5	60.7
Upper 2.5 percentile	222	252	244	248	237	250	245	238	241
Standard error of the mean	1.8	2.0	3.0	2.9	1.2	3.3	1.6	1.6	1.1

Table 8.27 Average daily intake of folate as a percentage of the Reference Nutrient Intake (RNI) by age and sex of child

Age and sex of child	Average daily intake as % of RNI							
	(a) All sources				(b) Food sources			
	Mean	*Median*	*se*	*Base*	*Mean*	*Median*	*se*	*Base*
All aged 1½–2½ years	172	162	2.6	*576*	171	162	2.5	*576*
All aged 2½–3½ years	191	181	2.9	*606*	190	180	2.8	*606*
Aged 3½–4½ years*:								
Boys	181	174	4.3	*250*	179	173	4.2	*250*
Girls	171	164	4.1	*243*	169	163	4.0	*243*
All aged under 4 years	185	174	1.8	*1457*	184	174	1.7	*1457*
All aged 4 years and over	145	140	3.6	*218*	143	137	3.3	*218*
All boys	183	172	2.3	*848*	182	172	2.3	*848*
All girls	177	167	2.3	*827*	176	167	2.3	*827*
All	180	170	1.6	*1675*	179	170	1.6	*1675*

*Folate intake as a percentage of the RNI was calculated for each child; thus in this age group values for children under 4 years of age used 70µg/d as the RNI and for children aged 4 and over 100µg/d was taken as the RNI. The values for all children aged 3½ to 4½ years were then pooled to give a mean, median and standard error (se) for the age group.

Table 8.28(a)   Contribution of food types to average daily folate intake by age and sex of child

Food types	Age and sex of child						
	All aged 1½ – 2½ years	All aged 2½ – 3½ years	All aged 3½ – 4½ years		All boys	All girls	All
			Boys	Girls			
	µg	µg	µg	µg	µg	µg	µg
Cereals & cereal products	38.8	49.6	57.4	55.0	49.5	46.1	47.8
of which:							
white bread	4.2	5.6	7.1	6.6	5.5	5.4	5.5
wholemeal bread	2.5	2.4	2.9	2.6	2.6	2.5	2.5
high fibre breakfast cereals	6.7	8.3	9.6	7.9	8.2	7.6	7.9
other breakfast cereals	15.9	21.3	24.3	24.8	21.2	19.6	20.4
Milk & milk products	25.0	21.0	19.3	18.3	22.0	21.5	21.7
of which:							
milk (whole, semi-skimmed, skimmed)	17.1	14.8	13.5	12.9	15.4	14.8	15.1
other milk & products	8.0	6.2	5.8	5.4	6.6	6.7	6.6
Eggs & egg dishes	2.4	2.8	2.9	3.3	2.4	3.1	2.8
Fat spreads	–	–	–	–	–	–	–
Meat & meat products	5.7	6.2	6.6	6.2	6.2	5.9	6.1
Fish & fish dishes	1.5	1.8	1.6	1.9	1.7	1.7	1.7
Vegetables, potatoes & savoury snacks	24.5	28.4	30.8	31.5	28.1	27.7	27.9
of which:							
vegetables, excluding potatoes	10.5	11.9	12.0	12.6	11.4	11.7	11.6
fried potatoes	6.3	7.8	9.1	9.3	8.1	7.3	7.7
other potatoes	4.9	4.9	5.6	5.7	5.0	5.3	5.1
savoury snacks	2.8	3.7	4.0	3.9	3.6	3.4	3.5
Fruit & nuts	5.6	5.5	5.0	5.2	5.2	5.7	5.4
of which:							
fruit, excluding nuts	5.3	5.2	4.5	4.7	4.8	5.3	5.0
all nuts	0.3	0.4	0.5	0.5	0.4	0.4	0.4
Sugars, preserves & confectionery	0.9	1.1	1.3	1.3	1.1	1.1	1.1
Beverages	9.1	10.9	13.1	10.5	10.3	10.8	10.6
of which:							
fruit juice	4.8	5.0	4.5	4.2	4.4	5.1	4.7
soft drinks, including low calorie drinks	3.7	5.5	8.1	5.9	5.6	5.1	5.3
Commercial infant foods & drinks	0.4	0.1	0.03	0.02	0.2	0.2	0.2
Miscellaneous	6.1	5.5	5.0	5.0	5.8	5.3	5.6
Average daily intake (µg)	**120**	**133**	**143**	**138**	**132**	**129**	**131**
Total number of children	**576**	**606**	**250**	**243**	**848**	**827**	**1675**

Table 8.28(b)   Percentage contribution of food types to average daily folate intake by age and sex of child

Food types	Age and sex of child						
	All aged 1½ – 2½ years	All aged 2½ – 3½ years	All aged 3½ – 4½ years		All boys	All girls	All
			Boys	Girls			
	%	%	%	%	%	%	%
Cereals & cereal products	32	37	40	40	37	36	36
of which:							
white bread	*4*	*4*	*5*	*5*	*4*	*4*	*4*
wholemeal bread	*2*	*2*	*2*	*2*	*2*	*2*	*2*
high fibre breakfast cereals	*6*	*6*	*7*	*6*	*6*	*6*	*6*
other breakfast cereals	*13*	*16*	*17*	*18*	*16*	*15*	*15*
Milk & milk products	21	16	13	13	16	17	17
of which:							
milk (whole, semi-skimmed, skimmed)	*14*	*11*	*9*	*9*	*12*	*12*	*12*
other milk & products	*7*	*5*	*4*	*4*	*5*	*5*	*5*
Eggs & egg dishes	2	2	2	2	2	2	2
Fat spreads	–	–	–	–	–	–	–
Meat & meat products	5	5	5	4	5	4	5
Fish & fish dishes	1	1	1	1	1	1	1
Vegetables, potatoes & savoury snacks	20	21	22	23	21	21	21
of which:							
vegetables, excluding potatoes	*9*	*9*	*8*	*9*	*9*	*9*	*9*
fried potatoes	*5*	*6*	*6*	*7*	*6*	*6*	*6*
other potatoes	*4*	*4*	*4*	*4*	*4*	*4*	*4*
savoury snacks	*2*	*3*	*3*	*3*	*3*	*3*	*3*
Fruit & nuts	5	4	4	4	4	4	4
of which:							
fruit, excluding nuts	*4*	*4*	*3*	*3*	*4*	*4*	*4*
all nuts	*0*	*0*	*0*	*0*	*0*	*0*	*0*
Sugars, preserves & confectionery	1	1	1	1	1	1	1
Beverages	8	8	9	8	8	8	8
of which:							
fruit juice	*4*	*4*	*3*	*3*	*3*	*4*	*4*
soft drinks, including low calorie drinks	*3*	*4*	*6*	*4*	*4*	*4*	*4*
Commercial infant foods & drinks	0	0	0	0	0	0	0
Miscellaneous	5	4	3	4	4	4	4
Average daily intake (µg)	**120**	**133**	**143**	**138**	**132**	**129**	**131**
Total number of children	**576**	**606**	**250**	**243**	**848**	**827**	**1675**

Table 8.29 Average daily intake of biotin (µg) by age and sex of child

Biotin (µg)	Age and sex of child						
	All aged 1½ – 2½ years	All aged 2½ – 3½ years	All aged 3½ – 4½ years		All boys	All girls	All
			Boys	Girls			
	cum %	cum %	cum %	cum %	cum %	cum %	cum %
Intakes from *food sources**							
Less than 10	12	12	8	10	9	13	11
Less than 15	41	43	38	42	40	42	42
Less than 20	75	73	70	74	71	76	73
Less than 25	90	90	89	91	90	91	90
Less than 30	96	96	94	96	96	96	96
All	100	100	100	100	100	100	100
Base	*576*	*606*	*250*	*243*	*848*	*827*	*1675*
Mean (average value)	17.1	17.0	17.7	16.8	17.4	16.8	17.1
Median value	16.0	15.9	17.2	15.9	16.3	15.9	16.1
Lower 2.5 percentile	6.3	7.3	7.5	7.0	7.2	6.5	6.9
Upper 2.5 percentile	33.3	32.5	33.2	32.7	31.7	33.3	32.6
Standard error of the mean	0.3	0.3	0.4	0.4	0.3	0.2	0.2

*None of the dietary supplements taken by children in this survey provided any biotin.

Table 8.30 Average daily intake of pantothenic acid (mg) by age and sex of child

Pantothenic acid (mg)	Age and sex of child						
	All aged 1½ – 2½ years	All aged 2½ – 3½ years	All aged 3½ – 4½ years		All boys	All girls	All
			Boys	Girls			
	cum %	cum %	cum %	cum %	cum %	cum %	cum %
(a) Intakes from *all sources*							
Less than 1.5	6	5	3	4	3	6	5
Less than 2.0	21	19	15	20	18	20	19
Less than 2.5	46	64	36	46	42	46	44
Less than 3.0	69	70	62	66	67	69	68
Less than 3.5	84	83	79	85	82	84	83
Less than 4.0	91	91	88	92	91	91	91
All	100	100	100	100	100	100	100
Base	*576*	*606*	*250*	*243*	*848*	*827*	*1675*
Mean (average value)	2.7	2.7	2.9	2.7	2.8	2.7	2.8
Median value	2.6	2.6	2.7	2.6	2.6	2.6	2.6
Lower 2.5 percentile	1.2	1.4	1.4	1.4	1.4	1.2	1.3
Upper 2.5 percentile	5.3	5.3	4.9	4.8	4.9	5.3	5.0
Standard error of the mean	0.04	0.04	0.06	0.06	0.03	0.03	0.02
	cum %	cum %	cum %	cum %	cum %	cum %	cum %
(b) Intakes from *food sources*							
Less than 1.5	6	5	3	4	3	6	5
Less than 2.0	22	19	15	20	18	21	20
Less than 2.5	48	46	36	46	43	47	45
Less than 3.0	71	71	63	67	68	71	69
Less than 3.5	86	84	80	86	83	86	84
Less than 4.0	93	92	90	93	92	93	92
All	100	100	100	100	100	100	100
Base	*576*	*606*	*250*	*243*	*848*	*827*	*1675*
Mean (average value)	2.7	2.7	2.8	2.7	2.7	2.7	2.7
Median value	2.6	2.6	2.7	2.6	2.6	2.6	2.6
Lower 2.5 percentile	1.2	1.4	1.4	1.4	1.4	1.2	1.3
Upper 2.5 percentile	4.8	4.8	4.6	4.5	4.6	4.7	4.7
Standard error of the mean	0.04	0.04	0.05	0.05	0.03	0.03	0.02

Table 8.31 Average daily intake of vitamin C (mg) by age and sex of child

Vitamin C (mg)	Age and sex of child								
	All aged 1½ – 2½ years	All aged 2½ – 3½ years	All aged 3½ – 4½ years		All aged under 4 years	All aged 4 years and over	All boys	All girls	All
			Boys	Girls					
	cum %	cum %	cum %	cum %	cum %	cum %	cum %	cum %	cum %
(a) Intakes from *all sources*									
Less than 8	1	2	2	0	1	1	1	1	1
Less than 20	21	18	16	16	19	16	19	18	18
Less than 30	37	34	33	35	35	34	37	34	35
Less than 45	57	54	54	55	56	52	53	53	55
Less than 60	71	70	67	68	70	63	71	67	70
Less than 75	80	80	77	81	81	74	80	79	80
Less than 90	88	86	84	89	87	83	86	87	87
Less than 105	91	91	88	94	97	89	91	91	91
All	100	100	100	100	100	100	100	100	100
Base	576	606	250	243	1457	218	848	827	1675
Mean (average value)	50.7	52.2	54.6	50.0	51.1	56.4	50.7	52.9	51.8
Median value	38.4	39.7	41.6	41.4	39.5	42.3	38.5	41.8	39.8
Lower 2.5 percentile	10.2	8.9	9.0	9.6	9.4	9.9	9.4	9.5	9.5
Upper 2.5 percentile	169	160	187	132	156	187	153	160	157
Standard error of the mean	1.8	1.8	2.7	2.2	1.1	3.1	1.4	1.5	1.0
	cum %	cum %	cum %	cum %	cum %	cum %	cum %	cum %	cum %
(b) Intakes from *food sources*									
Less than 8	1	2	2	0	1	1	1	1	1
Less than 20	22	20	17	18	21	17	21	20	20
Less than 30	40	38	36	37	39	36	40	37	38
Less than 45	60	58	59	59	59	57	60	57	59
Less than 60	74	74	73	74	75	69	75	72	74
Less than 75	83	83	81	88	84	81	82	84	83
Less than 90	90	88	86	90	89	85	88	89	88
Less than 105	92	92	91	96	93	92	93	93	93
All	100	100	100	100	100	100	100	100	100
Base	576	606	250	243	1457	218	848	827	1675
Mean (average value)	48.2	49.2	50.8	45.9	48.1	52.2	48.0	49.2	48.6
Median value	36.9	37.6	38.4	38.7	37.2	39.9	37.1	37.9	37.7
Lower 2.5 percentile	10.2	8.9	9.0	9.6	9.4	9.9	9.4	9.5	9.5
Upper 2.5 percentile	158	160	183	113	154	187	150	157	154
Standard error of the mean	1.7	1.7	2.6	2.0	1.0	2.8	1.4	1.4	1.0

Table 8.32 Average daily intake of vitamin C as a percentage of the Reference Nutrient Intake (RNI) by age and sex of child

Age and sex of child	Average daily intake as % of RNI							
	(a) All sources				(b) Food sources			
	Mean	Median	se	Base	Mean	Median	se	Base
All aged 1½–2½ years	169	128	6.0	576	160	123	5.7	576
All aged 2½–3½ years	174	132	5.9	606	164	125	5.7	606
Aged 3½–4½ years*:								
Boys	182	139	9.1	250	169	128	8.6	250
Girls	167	138	7.4	243	153	129	6.7	243
All aged under 4 years	170	132	3.6	1457	160	124	3.5	1457
All aged 4 years and over	188	141	10.3	218	174	133	9.5	218
All boys	169	128	4.8	848	160	124	4.6	848
All girls	176	139	5.0	827	164	126	4.7	827
All	172	133	3.4	1675	162	126	3.3	1675

*Vitamin C intake as a percentage of the RNI was calculated for each child; thus in this age group RNI values for children under 4 years and 4 years and over were the same, 30mg/d.

Table 8.33(a) Contribution of food types to average daily vitamin C intake by age and sex of child

Food types	Age and sex of child						
	All aged 1½ – 2½ years	All aged 2½ – 3½ years	All aged 3½ – 4½ years		All boys	All girls	All
			Boys	Girls			
	mg	mg	mg	mg	mg	mg	mg
Cereals & cereal products	0.9	1.1	1.4	1.1	1.1	1.0	1.1
Milk & milk products	5.0	3.1	3.0	2.5	3.8	3.5	3.7
of which:							
milk (whole, semi-skimmed, skimmed)	*3.1*	*2.7*	*2.4*	*2.3*	*2.8*	*2.6*	*2.7*
other milk & products	*1.9*	*0.5*	*0.6*	*0.2*	*1.0*	*0.9*	*0.9*
Eggs & egg dishes	0.01	0.02	0.01	0.01	0.0	0.01	0.01
Fat spreads	–	–	–	–	–	–	–
Meat & meat products	0.9	1.1	1.1	1.1	1.1	1.0	1.0
Fish & fish dishes	0.04	0.05	0.1	0.03	0.1	0.03	0.05
Vegetables, potatoes & savoury snacks	8.1	9.3	10.3	11.2	9.1	9.5	9.3
of which:							
vegetables, excluding potatoes	*2.9*	*3.4*	*3.5*	*4.2*	*3.1*	*3.7*	*3.4*
fried potatoes	*3.0*	*3.8*	*4.5*	*4.5*	*4.0*	*3.5*	*3.7*
other potatoes	*1.8*	*1.7*	*1.8*	*2.1*	*1.7*	*1.9*	*1.8*
savoury snacks	*0.3*	*0.4*	*0.5*	*0.5*	*0.4*	*0.4*	*0.4*
Fruit & nuts	7.3	7.5	6.7	7.7	6.7	8.0	7.3
Sugars, preserves & confectionery	0.2	0.2	0.3	0.3	0.3	0.2	0.2
Beverages	22.5	25.2	27.8	21.9	24.5	23.8	24.2
of which:							
fruit juice	*9.6*	*10.1*	*8.9*	*8.4*	*8.6*	*10.4*	*9.5*
soft drinks, including low calorie drinks	*12.9*	*15.1*	*18.9*	*13.5*	*15.9*	*13.4*	*14.7*
Commercial infant foods & drinks	3.0	1.5	0.01	0.01	1.2	2.0	1.6
Miscellaneous	0.1	0.1	0.1	0.1	0.1	0.1	0.1
Average daily intake (mg)	**48.2**	**49.2**	**50.8**	**45.9**	**48.0**	**49.2**	**48.6**
Total number of children	**576**	**606**	**250**	**243**	**848**	**827**	**1675**

Table 8.33(b) Percentage contribution of food types to average daily vitamin C intake by age and sex of child

Food types	Age and sex of child						
	All aged 1½ – 2½ years	All aged 2½ – 3½ years	All aged 3½ – 4½ years		All boys	All girls	All
			Boys	Girls			
	%	%	%	%	%	%	%
Cereals & cereal products	2	2	3	2	2	2	2
Milk & milk products	10	6	6	5	8	7	8
of which:							
milk (whole, semi-skimmed, skimmed)	*6*	*5*	*5*	*5*	*6*	*5*	*6*
other milk & products	*4*	*1*	*1*	*0*	*2*	*2*	*2*
Eggs & egg dishes	0	0	0	0	0	0	0
Fat spreads	–	–	–	–	–	–	–
Meat & meat products	2	2	2	2	2	2	2
Fish & fish dishes	0	0	0	0	0	0	0
Vegetables, potatoes & savoury snacks	17	19	20	24	19	19	19
of which:							
vegetables, excluding potatoes	*6*	*7*	*7*	*9*	*6*	*7*	*7*
fried potatoes	*6*	*8*	*9*	*10*	*8*	*7*	*8*
other potatoes	*4*	*3*	*3*	*4*	*4*	*4*	*4*
savoury snacks	*1*	*1*	*1*	*1*	*1*	*1*	*1*
Fruit & nuts	15	15	13	17	14	16	15
Sugars, preserves & confectionery	0	0	1	1	0	0	0
Beverages	47	51	55	48	51	48	50
of which:							
fruit juice	*20*	*20*	*17*	*18*	*18*	*21*	*20*
soft drinks, including low calorie drinks	*27*	*30*	*37*	*29*	*33*	*27*	*30*
Commercial infant foods & drinks	6	3	0	0	2	4	3
Miscellaneous	0	0	0	0	0	0	0
Average daily intake (mg)	**48.2**	**49.2**	**50.8**	**45.9**	**48.0**	**49.2**	**48.6**
Total number of children	**576**	**606**	**250**	**243**	**848**	**827**	**1675**

Table 8.34   Average daily intake of vitamin D (µg) by age and sex of child

Vitamin D (µg)	Age and sex of child								
	All aged 1½ – 2½ years	All aged 2½ – 3½ years	All aged 3½ – 4½ years		All aged under 4 years	All aged 4 years and over	All boys	All girls	All
			Boys	Girls					
	cum %	cum %	cum %	cum %	cum %	cum %	cum %	cum %	cum %
(a) Intakes from *all sources*									
Less than 0.5	15	13	8	9	13	10	12	12	12
Less than 1.0	49	41	34	37	43	36	42	41	42
Less than 1.5	70	64	54	59	65	55	65	63	64
Less than 2.0	79	75	72	73	76	71	77	74	76
Less than 2.5	82	82	80	81	82	79	83	80	82
Less than 7.0	93	96	96	96	95	95	96	94	95
All	100	100	100	100	100	100	100	100	100
Base	*576*	*606*	*250*	*243*	*1457*	*218*	*848*	*827*	*1675*
Mean (average value)	1.8	1.8	2.0	1.9	1.9	2.0	1.8	2.0	1.9
Median value	1.0	1.2	1.3	1.3	1.1	1.3	1.1	1.2	1.1
Lower 2.5 percentile	0.2	0.2	0.3	0.3	0.2	0.3	0.2	0.3	0.3
Upper 2.5 percentile	9.4	8.9	8.5	10.4	9.1	10.9	8.5	9.7	9.2
Standard error of the mean	0.10	0.09	0.14	0.13	0.06	0.16	0.07	0.08	0.05
	cum %	cum %	cum %	cum %	cum %	cum %	cum %	cum %	cum %
(b) Intakes from *food sources*									
Less than 0.4	10	8	6	6	8	7	8	8	8
Less than 0.8	41	34	24	29	35	28	33	35	34
Less than 1.2	68	59	54	54	61	56	62	60	61
Less than 1.6	82	78	69	73	78	71	78	76	77
Less than 2.0	88	87	85	86	87	85	88	87	87
Less than 2.4	91	94	92	93	93	92	93	92	93
All	100	100	100	100	100	100	100	100	100
Base	*576*	*606*	*250*	*243*	*1457*	*218*	*848*	*827*	*1675*
Mean (average value)	1.2	1.2	1.4	1.3	1.2	1.3	1.3	1.2	1.3
Median value	0.9	1.0	1.1	1.1	1.0	1.1	1.0	1.0	1.0
Lower 2.5 percentile	0.2	0.2	0.3	0.3	0.2	0.3	0.2	0.3	0.2
Upper 2.5 percentile	4.8	3.5	4.6	2.9	4.0	4.2	4.5	3.7	4.1
Standard error of the mean	0.05	0.04	0.07	0.05	0.03	0.07	0.04	0.03	0.02

Table 8.35   Average daily intake of vitamin D as a percentage of the Reference Nutrient Intake (RNI) by age and sex of child

Age and sex of child	Average daily intake as % of RNI							
	(a) All sources				(b) Food sources			
	Mean	Median	se	Base	Mean	Median	se	Base
All aged 1½–2½ years	26	14	1.4	*576*	17	13	0.7	*576*
All aged 2½–3½ years	26	17	1.2	*606*	18	15	0.5	*606*
Aged 3½–4½ years*:								
Boys	28	17	2.6	*147*	19	16	1.0	*147*
Girls	26	19	2.1	*128*	19	17	0.9	*128*
All boys	25	16	1.1	*745*	18	14	0.6	*745*
All girls	28	17	1.2	*712*	18	15	0.5	*712*
All aged under 4 years	27	16	0.8	*1457*	18	14	0.4	*1457*

*There are no Dietary Reference Values specified for vitamin D intake for children aged 4 years and over.

Table 8.36(a) Contribution of food types to average daily vitamin D intake by age and sex of child

Food types	Age and sex of child						
	All aged 1½ – 2½ years	All aged 2½ – 3½ years	All aged 3½ – 4½ years		All boys	All girls	All
			Boys	Girls			
	µg	µg	µg	µg	µg	µg	µg
Cereals & cereal products	0.3	0.4	0.4	0.4	0.4	0.4	0.4
of which:							
breakfast cereals	*0.2*	*0.2*	*0.3*	*0.3*	*0.2*	*0.2*	*0.2*
Milk & milk products	0.3	0.1	0.1	0.1	0.2	0.2	0.2
of which:							
milk (whole, semi-skimmed, skimmed)	*0.1*	*0.1*	*0.1*	*0.1*	*0.1*	*0.1*	*0.1*
other milk & products	*0.21*	*0.06*	*0.07*	*0.03*	*0.12*	*0.10*	*0.11*
Eggs & egg dishes	0.1	0.1	0.1	0.2	0.1	0.2	0.1
Fat spreads	0.3	0.3	0.4	0.4	0.3	0.3	0.3
Meat & meat products	0.04	0.04	0.05	0.05	0.05	0.04	0.05
Fish & fish dishes	0.1	0.1	0.1	0.1	0.1	0.1	0.1
Vegetables, potatoes & savoury snacks	0.02	0.02	0.02	0.02	0.02	0.02	0.02
Fruit & nuts	0.00	–	–	–	–	0.00	0.00
Sugars, preserves & confectionery	0.00	0.00	0.00	0.00	0.00	0.00	0.00
Beverages	0.00	0.00	0.00	0.00	0.00	0.00	0.00
Commercial infant foods & drinks	0.07	0.01	0.02	0.02	0.03	0.03	0.03
Miscellaneous	0.02	0.01	0.01	0.01	0.01	0.01	0.01
Average daily intake (µg)	**1.2**	**1.2**	**1.4**	**1.3**	**1.3**	**1.2**	**1.3**
Total number of children	**576**	**606**	**250**	**243**	**848**	**827**	**1675**

Table 8.36(b) Percentage contribution of food types to average daily vitamin D intake by age and sex of child

Food types	Age and sex of child						
	All aged 1½ – 2½ years	All aged 2½ – 3½ years	All aged 3½ – 4½ years		All boys	All girls	All
			Boys	Girls			
	%	%	%	%	%	%	%
Cereals & cereal products	23	32	32	34	30	29	29
of which:							
breakfast cereals	*14*	*19*	*18*	*20*	*18*	*17*	*17*
Milk & milk products	24	10	9	7	16	13	14
of which:							
milk (whole, semi-skimmed, skimmed)	*7*	*6*	*4*	*5*	*5*	*5*	*5*
other milk & products	*17*	*5*	*5*	*2*	*9*	*8*	*9*
Eggs & egg dishes	10	11	10	13	9	13	11
Fat spreads	23	28	30	28	26	26	26
Meat & meat products	3	3	4	4	4	3	4
Fish & fish dishes	8	11	11	9	10	10	10
Vegetables, potatoes & savoury snacks	2	2	1	2	2	2	2
Fruit & nuts	0	–	–	–	–	0	0
Sugars, preserves & confectionery	0	0	0	0	0	0	0
Beverages	0	0	0	0	0	0	0
Commercial infant foods & drinks	6	1	1	1	2	2	2
Miscellaneous	2	1	1	1	1	1	1
Average daily intake (µg)	**1.2**	**1.2**	**1.4**	**1.3**	**1.3**	**1.2**	**1.3**
Total number of children	**576**	**606**	**250**	**243**	**848**	**827**	**1675**

Table 8.37 Average daily intake of vitamin E (α–tocopherol equivalents) (mg) by age and sex of child

Vitamin E (α–tocopherol equivalents) (mg)	Age and sex of child						
	All aged 1½ – 2½ years	All aged 2½ – 3½ years	All aged 3½ – 4½ years		All boys	All girls	All
			Boys	Girls			
	cum %	cum %	cum %	cum %	cum %	cum %	cum %
(a) Intakes from all sources							
Less than 2.0	9	4	2	3	5	5	5
Less than 3.0	36	21	14	20	24	26	25
Less than 4.0	60	47	35	46	48	51	50
Less than 5.0	79	67	58	67	70	70	70
Less than 6.0	89	83	74	79	83	84	83
Less than 7.0	94	89	86	86	90	90	90
All	100	100	100	100	100	100	100
Base	576	606	250	243	848	827	1675
Mean (average value)	3.9	4.5	5.1	4.6	4.4	4.4	4.4
Median value	3.6	4.1	4.6	4.3	4.1	4.0	4.0
Lower 2.5 percentile	1.4	1.8	2.1	2.0	1.7	1.7	1.7
Upper 2.5 percentile	9.0	9.6	10.7	10.6	9.6	9.9	9.7
Standard error of the mean	0.08	0.08	0.15	0.13	0.07	0.07	0.05
	cum %	cum %	cum %	cum %	cum %	cum %	cum %
(b) Intakes from food sources							
Less than 2.0	9	4	2	3	5	6	5
Less than 3.0	37	22	14	20	25	27	26
Less than 4.0	61	49	36	47	49	53	51
Less than 5.0	81	69	60	69	71	72	72
Less than 6.0	90	85	76	82	84	86	85
Less than 7.0	94	91	87	89	91	92	91
All	100	100	100	100	100	100	100
Base	576	606	250	243	848	827	1675
Mean (average value)	3.8	4.4	5.0	4.5	4.3	4.3	4.3
Median value	3.5	4.1	4.5	4.1	4.0	3.9	4.0
Lower 2.5 percentile	1.4	1.8	2.1	2.0	1.7	1.7	1.7
Upper 2.5 percentile	8.5	8.5	10.0	9.2	8.7	9.2	9.0
Standard error of the mean	0.07	0.07	0.13	0.12	0.06	0.06	0.04

Table 8.38(a) Contribution of food types to average daily vitamin E (α–tocopherol equivalents) intakes by age and sex of child

Food types	Age and sex of child						
	All aged 1½ – 2½ years	All aged 2½ – 3½ years	All aged 3½ – 4½ years		All boys	All girls	All
			Boys	Girls			
	mg	mg	mg	mg	mg	mg	mg
Cereals & cereal products	0.6	0.8	0.9	0.8	0.8	0.7	0.8
of which:							
breakfast cereals	0.1	0.1	0.2	0.2	0.2	0.1	0.1
biscuits	0.2	0.3	0.3	0.2	0.3	0.2	0.3
Milk & milk products	0.5	0.3	0.3	0.2	0.3	0.3	0.3
of which:							
milk (whole, semi-skimmed, skimmed)	0.3	0.2	0.2	0.2	0.2	0.2	0.2
other milk & products	0.21	0.06	0.09	0.04	0.12	0.11	0.11
Eggs & egg dishes	0.1	0.1	0.1	0.2	0.1	0.1	0.1
Fat spreads	0.8	1.0	1.2	1.0	1.0	1.0	1.0
Meat & meat products	0.3	0.3	0.4	0.3	0.3	0.3	0.3
Fish & fish dishes	0.1	0.1	0.1	0.1	0.1	0.1	0.1
Vegetables, potatoes & savoury snacks	1.0	1.2	1.3	1.2	1.1	1.1	1.1
of which:							
vegetables, excluding potatoes	0.2	0.2	0.3	0.3	0.2	0.2	0.2
fried potatoes	0.3	0.3	0.4	0.4	0.3	0.3	0.3
savoury snacks	0.4	0.6	0.6	0.5	0.5	0.5	0.5
Fruit & nuts	0.2	0.2	0.2	0.2	0.2	0.2	0.2
Sugars, preserves & confectionery	0.1	0.2	0.2	0.2	0.2	0.2	0.2
Beverages	0.05	0.06	0.05	0.05	0.05	0.06	0.06
Commercial infant foods & drinks	0.02	0.00	0.00	0.00	0.01	0.01	0.01
Miscellaneous	0.1	0.1	0.1	0.1	0.1	0.1	0.1
Average daily intake (mg)	**3.8**	**4.4**	**5.0**	**4.5**	**4.3**	**4.3**	**4.3**
Total number of children	**576**	**606**	**250**	**243**	**848**	**827**	**1675**

166

Table 8.38(b)   Percentage contribution of food types to average daily vitamin E (α−tocopherol equivalents) intake by age and sex of child

Food types	Age and sex of child						
	All aged 1½ – 2½ years	All aged 2½ – 3½ years	All aged 3½ – 4½ years		All boys	All girls	All
			Boys	Girls			
	%	%	%	%	%	%	%
Cereals & cereal products	17	18	18	18	18	17	18
of which:							
breakfast cereals	*4*	*3*	*3*	*4*	*4*	*3*	*3*
biscuits	*6*	*6*	*7*	*5*	*6*	*6*	*6*
Milk & milk products	13	6	5	5	8	8	8
of which:							
milk (whole, semi-skimmed, skimmed)	*7*	*5*	*4*	*4*	*5*	*5*	*5*
other milk & products	*5*	*1*	*2*	*1*	*3*	*2*	*2*
Eggs & egg dishes	3	3	3	4	2	3	3
Fat spreads	21	23	24	23	22	23	23
Meat & meat products	7	8	8	8	8	7	8
Fish & fish dishes	3	3	3	3	3	3	3
Vegetables, potatoes & savoury snacks	25	26	26	28	26	26	26
of which:							
vegetables, excluding potatoes	*5*	*5*	*5*	*6*	*5*	*5*	*5*
fried potatoes	*7*	*7*	*8*	*8*	*7*	*7*	*7*
savoury snacks	*11*	*13*	*12*	*12*	*12*	*12*	*12*
Fruit & nuts	4	4	4	4	4	4	4
Sugars, preserves & confectionery	3	4	4	4	4	4	4
Beverages	1	1	1	1	1	1	1
Commercial infant foods & drinks	0	0	0	0	0	0	0
Miscellaneous	2	2	3	2	2	2	2
Average daily intake (mg)	**3.8**	**4.4**	**5.0**	**4.5**	**4.3**	**4.3**	**4.3**
Total number of children	**576**	**606**	**250**	**243**	**848**	**827**	**1675**

Table 8.39   Average daily vitamin intakes by whether child was reported to be taking dietary supplements

Vitamins	Whether child reported to be taking any dietary supplements								
	(a) Not taking supplements			(b) Taking dietary supplements					
	Intake from all sources			Intake from all sources			Intake from food sources		
	Mean	Median	so	Mean	Median	se	Mean	Median	se
Pre-formed retinol (μg)	357	258	23.8	713	564	37.4	387	289	31.6
Vitamin A (retinol equivalents) (μg)	500	391	24.2	867	741	38.8	541	426	33.2
Thiamin (mg)	0.8	0.7	0.01	0.9	0.8	0.02	0.8	0.8	0.01
Riboflavin (mg)	1.2	1.1	0.01	1.4	1.3	0.03	1.2	1.2	0.02
Niacin equivalents (mg)	15.8	15.2	0.1	18.3	17.3	0.3	17.0	16.2	0.3
Vitamin B$_6$ (mg)	1.2	1.1	0.01	1.4	1.3	0.03	1.3	1.2	0.03
Vitamin B$_{12}$ (μg)	2.7	2.4	0.05	3.2	2.9	0.10	3.1	2.7	0.11
Folate (μg)	130	123	1.3	137	125	2.8	133	123	2.5
Pantothenic acid (mg)	2.7	2.5	0.02	3.1	2.8	0.06	2.8	2.8	0.04
Vitamin C (mg)	45.3	35.9	0.9	75.5	62.2	3.1	60.8	46.1	3.0
Vitamin D (μg)	1.2	1.0	0.03	4.3	3.4	0.18	1.3	1.1	0.06
Vitamin E (α-tocopherol equivalents) (mg)	4.2	3.9	0.05	5.0	4.5	0.13	4.5	4.1	0.10
Base		*1316*			*357*			*357*	

Table 8.40 Average daily vitamin intakes by whether child was reported as being unwell during four-day dietary recording period

| Vitamins | Whether child reported as being unwell during four-day period | | | | | | | | |
| | Unwell, eating affected | | | Unwell, eating not affected | | | Not unwell | | |
	Mean	Median	se	Mean	Median	se	Mean	Median	se
(a) Intakes from *all sources*									
Pre-formed retinol (μg)	361	271	26.0	455	288	54.9	445	289	26.4
Total carotene (β–carotene equivalents) (μg)*	789	588	40.2	831	593	54.6	897	673	22.5
Vitamin A (retinol equivalents) (μg)	493	414	27.0	594	409	56.1	594	434	26.9
Thiamin (mg)	0.7	0.7	0.02	0.8	0.7	0.02	0.8	0.8	0.01
Riboflavin (mg)	1.2	1.1	0.03	1.2	1.1	0.03	1.2	1.2	0.01
Niacin equivalents (mg)	14.7	14.0	0.3	15.7	15.1	0.3	16.8	16.2	0.1
Vitamin B_6 (mg)	1.1	1.1	0.03	1.2	1.1	0.03	1.3	1.2	0.01
Vitamin B_{12} (μg)	2.5	2.3	0.07	2.7	2.5	1.11	2.9	2.6	0.06
Folate (μg)	117	112	2.7	128	119	3.4	135	129	1.4
Biotin (μg)*	16.1	14.5	0.6	17.1	15.9	0.5	17.4	16.5	0.2
Pantothenic acid (mg)	2.5	2.4	0.05	2.7	2.6	0.07	2.8	2.6	0.03
Vitamin C (mg)	49.9	37.0	2.8	52.4	40.9	3.5	52.0	40.6	1.2
Vitamin D (μg)	1.7	1.0	0.1	2.1	1.1	0.2	1.9	1.2	0.1
Vitamin E (α–tocopherol equivalents) (mg)	4.0	3.5	0.1	4.3	3.8	0.1	4.5	4.1	0.6
Base		266			190			1219	
(b) Intakes from *food sources*									
Pre-formed retinol (μg)	299	237	20.4	387	272	50.6	374	272	25.7
Total carotene (β–carotene equivalents) (μg)	789	588	40.2	831	593	54.6	897	673	22.5
Vitamin A (retinol equivalents) (μg)	431	380	21.7	526	395	52.2	523	407	26.2
Thiamin (mg)	0.7	0.7	0.01	0.7	0.7	0.02	0.8	0.8	0.01
Riboflavin (mg)	1.1	1.1	0.02	1.2	1.1	0.03	1.2	1.2	0.01
Niacin equivalents (mg)	14.4	13.9	0.3	15.4	14.9	0.3	16.5	16.0	0.1
Vitamin B_6 (mg)	1.1	1.0	0.02	1.2	1.1	0.03	1.2	1.2	0.01
Vitamin B_{12} (μg)	2.5	2.3	0.07	2.7	2.4	0.11	2.9	2.5	0.06
Folate (μg)	116	112	2.5	127	119	3.4	135	128	1.4
Biotin (μg)	16.1	14.5	0.6	17.1	15.9	0.5	17.3	16.5	0.2
Pantothenic acid (mg)	2.5	2.4	0.05	2.6	2.5	0.06	2.8	2.6	0.02
Vitamin C (mg)	47.2	34.5	2.7	48.9	38.4	3.2	48.9	38.1	1.1
Vitamin D (μg)	1.2	0.9	0.07	1.3	1.0	0.08	1.3	1.0	0.03
Vitamin E (α–tocopherol equivalents) (mg)	3.9	3.4	0.1	4.2	3.8	0.1	4.4	4.1	0.05
Base		266			190			1219	

* None of the dietary supplements taken by children in this survey provided any carotene or biotin.

Table 8.41 Average daily intakes of vitamins from food sources per 1000 kcal food energy by whether child was reported as being unwell during four-day dietary recording period

| Nutrient | Whether child reported as being unwell during four-day period | | | | | | | | |
| | Unwell and eating affected | | | Unwell, eating not affected | | | Not unwell | | |
Intake per 1000 kcal energy:	Mean	Median	se	Mean	Median	se	Mean	Median	se
Total carotene (β–carotene equivalents) (μg)	783	571	37.8	748	564	44.4	769	573	18.1
Vitamin A (retinol equivalents) (μg)	421	375	20.4	467	356	40.8	451	349	24.5
Thiamin (mg)	0.7	0.7	0.01	0.7	0.7	0.02	0.7	0.7	0.00
Riboflavin (mg)	1.1	1.0	0.02	1.1	1.0	0.03	1.0	1.0	0.01
Niacin equivalents (mg)	14.2	13.8	0.2	14.0	13.7	0.2	14.2	13.8	0.1
Vitamin B_6 (mg)	1.1	1.1	0.02	1.0	1.0	0.02	1.1	1.0	0.01
Vitamin B_{12} (μg)	2.4	2.3	0.06	2.5	2.2	0.09	2.5	2.2	0.05
Folate (μg)	116	110	2.2	116	112	2.7	116	111	1.0
Vitamin C (mg)	46.8	33.6	2.5	44.9	35.9	2.9	42.1	32.4	0.9
Vitamin D (μg)	1.1	0.9	0.07	1.2	0.9	0.07	1.1	0.9	0.02
Vitamin E (α–tocopherol equivalents) (mg)	3.8	3.4	0.09	3.8	3.6	0.10	3.7	3.5	0.04
Base		266			190			1219	

Table 8.42   Average daily vitamin intakes by region

Vitamins	Region											
	Scotland			Northern			Central, South West and Wales			London and South East		
	Mean	Median	se	Mean	Median	se	Mean	Median	se	Mean	Median	se
(a) Intakes from *all sources*												
Pre-formed retinol (μg)	479	261	145	395	276	33.2	440	289	29.5	441	314	23.4
Total carotene (β–carotene equivalents) (μg)*	690	510	44.6	858	623	38.1	925	684	32.4	884	675	34.5
Vitamin A (retinol equivalents) (μg)	594	358	145	538	403	34.2	594	434	30.5	588	460	24.3
Thiamin (mg)	0.8	0.8	0.02	0.8	0.7	0.01	0.8	0.8	0.01	0.8	0.8	0.01
Riboflavin (mg)	1.2	1.2	0.04	1.2	1.1	0.02	1.2	1.2	0.02	1.2	1.2	0.02
Niacin equivalents (mg)	16.1	15.3	0.4	16.0	15.3	0.2	16.3	16.0	0.2	16.7	16.0	0.2
Vitamin B$_6$ (mg)	1.3	1.2	0.04	1.2	1.2	0.02	1.2	1.2	0.02	1.2	1.1	0.02
Vitamin B$_{12}$ (μg)	2.9	2.6	0.2	2.8	2.5	0.1	2.8	2.4	0.1	2.9	2.6	0.1
Folate (μg)	143	137	4.3	128	122	2.3	135	129	2.0	128	119	2.1
Biotin (μg)*	17.0	15.8	0.5	16.5	15.9	0.3	17.3	16.0	0.4	17.5	16.7	0.3
Pantothenic acid (mg)	2.7	2.6	0.07	2.7	2.6	0.04	2.8	2.6	0.04	2.8	2.6	0.04
Vitamin C (mg)	46.0	34.5	3.1	50.0	37.6	1.9	48.4	37.5	1.6	58.6	46.4	2.1
Vitamin D (μg)	1.4	1.1	0.1	1.7	1.1	0.1	1.9	1.2	0.1	0.8	1.2	0.1
Vitamin E (α–tocopherol equivalents) (mg)	4.3	3.9	0.1	4.3	3.9	0.1	4.5	4.1	0.1	4.4	4.0	0.1
Base		165			427			563			520	
(b) Intakes from *food sources*												
Pre-formed retinol (μg)	435	254	144	352	262	31.3	377	272	28.3	335	274	20.0
Total carotene (β–carotene equivalents) (μg)	690	510	44.6	858	623	38.1	925	684	32.4	883	675	34.5
Vitamin A (retinol equivalents) (μg)	550	345	145	495	385	32.3	531	410	29.3	482	420	21.0
Thiamin (mg)	0.8	0.7	0.02	0.8	0.7	0.01	0.8	0.7	0.01	0.8	0.7	0.01
Riboflavin (mg)	1.2	1.2	0.03	1.1	1.1	0.02	1.2	1.1	0.02	1.2	1.2	0.02
Niacin equivalents (mg)	15.9	15.3	0.4	15.8	15.2	0.2	16.0	15.7	0.2	16.3	15.7	0.2
Vitamin B$_6$ (mg)	1.3	1.2	0.04	1.2	1.1	0.02	1.2	1.2	0.02	1.2	1.1	0.02
Vitamin B$_{12}$ (μg)	2.9	2.6	0.2	2.7	2.5	0.1	2.8	2.4	0.1	2.9	2.6	0.1
Folate (μg)	142	137	4.0	127	121	2.3	134	128	1.9	127	118	2.0
Biotin (μg)	17.0	15.8	0.5	16.5	15.9	0.3	17.3	16.0	0.4	17.5	16.6	0.3
Pantothenic acid (mg)	2.7	2.6	0.07	2.7	2.6	0.04	2.7	2.6	0.04	2.7	2.6	0.04
Vitamin C (mg)	44.0	33.8	3.0	47.8	35.9	1.8	45.5	34.4	1.5	54.1	43.0	2.0
Vitamin D (μg)	1.2	1.1	0.05	1.2	1.0	0.05	1.3	1.0	0.05	1.2	1.0	0.05
Vitamin E (α–tocopherol equivalents) (mg)	4.2	3.9	0.1	4.2	3.9	0.1	4.4	4.0	0.1	4.3	3.9	0.1
Base		165			427			563			520	

*None of the dietary supplements taken by children in this survey provided any carotene or biotin.

Table 8.43   Average daily intake of vitamins from food sources per 1000 kcal food energy by region

Nutrient	Region											
	Scotland			Northern			Central, South West and Wales			London and South East		
Intake per 1000 kcal energy:	Mean	Median	se	Mean	Median	se	Mean	Median	se	Mean	Median	se
Total carotene (β–carotene equivalents) (μg)	622	442	41.1	740	561	30.1	811	599	27.5	792	586	27.3
Vitamin A (retinol equivalents) (μg)	495	304	145	432	336	28.9	462	362	24.5	431	375	15.5
Thiamin (mg)	0.7	0.7	0.01	0.7	0.6	0.01	0.7	0.7	0.01	0.7	0.7	0.01
Riboflavin (mg)	1.0	1.0	0.03	1.0	1.0	0.02	1.0	1.0	0.01	1.1	1.0	0.01
Niacin equivalents (mg)	14.0	13.9	0.2	13.8	13.4	0.1	14.0	14.0	0.1	14.7	14.4	0.1
Vitamin B$_6$ (mg)	1.1	1.1	0.03	1.0	1.0	0.01	1.0	1.0	0.01	1.1	1.0	0.02
Vitamin B$_{12}$ (μg)	2.6	2.3	0.22	2.4	2.1	0.08	2.4	2.2	0.06	2.5	2.4	0.05
Folate (μg)	125	120	3.0	111	106	1.8	117	114	1.5	115	111	1.5
Vitamin C (mg)	38.9	30.2	2.5	41.8	31.8	1.6	40.4	30.1	1.4	48.5	40.0	1.6
Vitamin D (μg)	1.0	0.9	0.04	1.0	0.9	0.04	1.2	0.9	0.05	1.1	0.9	0.04
Vitamin E (α–tocopherol equivalents) (mg)	3.7	3.6	0.1	3.6	3.4	0.1	3.8	3.5	0.1	3.8	3.5	0.1
Base		165			427			563			520	

Table 8.44 Average daily vitamin intakes by social class of head of household

Vitamins	Social class of head of household								
	Non-manual			Manual			All**		
(a) Intakes from *all sources*	Mean	Median	se	Mean	Median	se	Mean	Median	se
Pre-formed retinol (μg)	473	317	23.0	403	272	34.4	433	286	20.6
Total carotene (β–carotene equivalents) (μg)*	943	692	29.9	816	601	24.5	872	648	18.7
Vitamin A (retinol equivalents) (μg)	630	481	23.8	539	401	34.9	578	428	21.0
Thiamin (mg)	0.8	0.8	0.01	0.8	0.7	0.01	0.8	0.7	0.01
Riboflavin (mg)	1.2	1.1	0.02	1.2	1.1	0.01	1.2	1.2	0.01
Niacin equivalents (mg)	16.9	16.2	0.2	15.8	15.2	0.2	16.3	15.7	0.1
Vitamin B_6 (mg)	1.3	1.2	0.02	1.2	1.1	0.01	1.2	1.2	0.01
Vitamin B_{12} (μg)	3.0	2.6	0.06	2.7	2.4	0.06	2.8	2.5	0.04
Folate (μg)	134	126	1.7	130	122	1.6	132	124	1.2
Biotin (μg)*	17.9	17.0	0.2	16.5	15.3	0.2	17.1	16.1	0.2
Pantothenic acid (mg)	2.9	2.7	0.04	2.7	2.5	0.03	2.8	2.6	0.02
Vitamin C (mg)	60.0	48.2	1.7	45.1	33.8	1.3	51.8	39.8	1.0
Vitamin D (μg)	2.2	1.2	0.09	1.7	1.1	0.07	1.9	1.4	0.05
Vitamin E (α–tocopherol equivalents) (mg)	4.6	4.2	0.08	4.3	3.9	0.07	4.4	4.0	0.05
Base		748			867			1675	
(b) Vitamin intakes from *food sources*									
Pre-formed retinol (μg)	396	277	20.8	363	258	33.8	363	268	19.8
Total carotene (β–carotene equivalents) (μg)	943	692	29.9	816	601	24.5	872	648	18.7
Vitamin A (retinol equivalents) (μg)	526	426	21.7	499	381	34.2	509	401	20.6
Thiamin (mg)	0.8	0.7	0.01	0.8	0.7	0.01	0.8	0.7	0.01
Riboflavin (mg)	1.2	1.2	0.02	1.2	1.1	0.01	1.2	1.1	0.01
Niacin equivalents (mg)	16.5	16.0	0.2	15.7	15.1	0.2	16.0	15.5	0.1
Vitamin B_6 (mg)	1.2	1.2	0.02	1.2	1.1	0.01	1.2	1.1	0.01
Vitamin B_{12} (μg)	2.9	2.6	0.06	2.7	2.4	0.06	2.8	2.5	0.04
Folate (μg)	132	125	1.6	129	122	1.6	131	123	1.1
Biotin (μg)	17.9	17.1	0.2	16.5	15.3	0.3	17.1	16.1	0.2
Pantothenic acid (mg)	2.8	2.7	0.03	2.6	2.5	0.03	2.7	2.6	0.02
Vitamin C (mg)	55.4	44.6	1.6	43.2	32.1	1.3	48.6	37.7	1.0
Vitamin D (μg)	1.3	1.0	0.04	1.3	1.0	0.04	1.3	1.0	0.02
Vitamin E (α–tocopherol equivalents) (mg)	4.4	4.1	0.07	4.2	3.9	0.06	4.3	4.0	0.04
Base		748			867			1675	

* None of the dietary supplements taken by children in this survey provided any carotene or biotin.

** Includes those who could not be allocated a social class either because their job was inadequately described, they were a member of the Armed Forces or had never worked.

Table 8.45 Average daily intake of vitamins from food sources per 1000 kcal food energy by social class of head of household

Nutrients	Social class of head of household								
	Non-manual			Manual			All*		
Intake per 1000 kcal energy	Mean	Median	se	Mean	Median	se	Mean	Median	se
Total carotene β–carotene equivalents) (μg)	834	609	24.9	714	547	19.6	768	571	15.3
Vitamin A (retinol equivalents) (μg)	466	379	18.8	438	333	32.2	448	355	18.7
Thiamin (mg)	0.7	0.7	0.01	0.7	0.6	0.01	0.7	0.7	0.00
Riboflavin (mg)	1.1	1.0	0.01	1.0	1.0	0.01	1.0	1.0	0.01
Niacin equivalents (mg)	14.7	14.3	0.1	13.7	13.4	0.1	14.2	13.8	0.1
Vitamin B_6 (mg)	1.1	1.0	0.01	1.0	1.0	0.01	1.1	1.0	0.01
Vitamin B_{12} (μg)	2.6	2.3	0.05	2.4	2.2	0.06	2.5	2.2	0.04
Folate (μg)	118	113	1.3	114	110	1.2	116	111	0.9
Vitamin C (mg)	49.9	40.3	1.4	37.7	29.4	1.0	43.1	33.0	0.8
Vitamin D (μg)	1.1	0.9	0.03	1.1	0.9	0.03	1.1	0.9	0.02
Vitamin E (α–tocopherol equivalents) (mg)	3.9	3.6	0.05	3.7	3.4	0.04	3.8	3.5	0.03
Base		748			867			1675	

*Includes those who could not be allocated a social class either because their job was inadequately described, they were a member of the Armed Forces or had never worked.

Table 8.46 Average daily vitamin intakes by employment status of head of household

Vitamins	Working			Unemployed			Economically inactive		
	Mean	Median	se	Mean	Median	se	Mean	Median	se
(a) Intakes from *all sources*									
Pre-formed retinol (μg)	412	287	16.4	490	293	74.8	493	277	96.1
Total carotene (β–carotene equivalents) (μg)*	903	681	22.5	789	551	54.1	777	592	39.7
Vitamin A (retinol equivalents) (μg)	563	432	16.9	621	403	76.9	623	411	96.8
Thiamin (mg)	0.8	0.7	0.01	0.8	0.7	0.02	0.8	0.8	0.02
Riboflavin (mg)	1.2	1.2	0.01	1.2	1.1	0.04	1.2	1.2	0.03
Niacin equivalents (mg)	16.4	15.8	0.1	15.7	15.6	0.4	16.3	15.9	0.3
Vitamin B_6 (mg)	1.2	1.2	0.01	1.2	1.1	0.03	1.3	1.2	0.03
Vitamin B_{12} (μg)	2.8	2.5	0.04	2.7	2.4	0.12	2.9	2.6	0.17
Folate (μg)	131	123	1.3	127	120	3.9	138	132	3.2
Biotin (μg)*	17.1	16.1	0.2	18.2	16.2	1.0	16.6	15.8	0.4
Pantothenic acid (mg)	2.8	2.6	0.03	2.7	2.5	0.07	2.8	2.6	0.06
Vitamin C (mg)	54.9	43.4	1.2	41.1	31.4	2.5	43.5	31.2	2.6
Vitamin D (μg)	1.9	1.1	0.1	2.0	1.1	0.2	1.9	1.2	0.1
Vitamin E (α–tocopherol equivalents) (mg)	4.4	4.0	0.1	4.3	3.9	0.1	4.6	4.2	0.1
Base		*1249*			*167*			*259*	
(b) Intakes from *food sources*									
Pre-formed retinol (μg)	340	267	15.1	434	278	71.8	429	264	95.0
Total carotene (β–carotene equivalents) (μg)	903	681	22.5	789	551	54.1	777	592	39.7
Vitamin A (retinol equivalents) (μg)	491	402	15.7	565	391	73.9	558	392	95.8
Thiamin (mg)	0.8	0.7	0.08	0.8	0.7	0.02	0.8	0.8	0.01
Riboflavin (mg)	1.2	1.1	0.01	1.2	1.1	0.04	1.2	1.1	0.03
Niacin equivalents (mg)	16.1	15.5	0.1	15.5	15.1	0.4	16.1	15.7	0.3
Vitamin B_6 (mg)	1.2	1.1	0.01	1.2	1.1	0.03	1.2	1.2	0.03
Vitamin B_{12} (μg)	2.8	2.5	0.04	2.7	2.4	0.12	2.9	2.5	0.17
Folate (μg)	130	123	1.3	127	120	3.9	138	132	3.1
Biotin (μg)	17.1	16.1	0.2	18.2	16.2	1.0	16.6	15.7	0.4
Pantothenic acid (mg)	2.7	2.6	0.02	2.7	2.5	0.07	2.7	2.6	0.06
Vitamin C (mg)	51.6	41.0	1.2	38.4	31.1	2.3	40.9	30.4	2.5
Vitamin D (μg)	1.2	1.0	0.03	1.4	1.0	0.11	1.4	1.1	0.07
Vitamin E (α–tocopherol equivalents) (mg)	4.3	3.9	0.05	4.3	3.9	0.15	4.5	4.1	0.12
Base		*1249*			*167*			*259*	

*None of the dietary supplements taken by children in this survey provided any carotene or biotin.

Table 8.47 Average daily intake from food sources of vitamins per 1000 kcal food energy by employment status of head of household

Nutrient	Working			Unemployed			Economically inactive		
Intake per 1000 kcal energy	Mean	Median	se	Mean	Median	se	Mean	Median	se
Total carotene (β–carotene equivalents) (μg)	796	600	18.2	712	487	48.4	671	527	33.0
Vitamin A (retinol equivalents) (μg)	435	357	13.6	480	332	50.6	491	340	96.1
Thiamin (mg)	0.7	0.7	0.01	0.7	0.6	0.01	0.7	0.7	0.01
Riboflavin (mg)	1.0	1.0	0.01	1.0	1.0	0.03	1.0	1.0	0.02
Niacin equivalents (mg)	14.3	14.0	0.1	13.6	13.2	0.2	13.9	13.4	0.2
Vitamin B_6 (mg)	1.1	1.0	0.01	1.0	1.0	0.02	1.1	1.0	0.02
Vitamin B_{12} (μg)	2.5	2.3	0.04	2.4	2.2	0.08	2.5	2.1	0.17
Folate (μg)	115	111	1.0	111	109	2.7	120	114	2.6
Vitamin C (mg)	45.8	37.0	1.0	35.0	26.7	2.2	35.5	25.9	2.0
Vitamin D (μg)	1.1	0.9	0.02	1.3	0.9	0.12	1.2	0.9	0.06
Vitamin E (α–tocopherol equivalents) (mg)	3.7	3.5	0.04	3.8	3.5	0.12	3.8	3.5	0.09
Base		*1249*			*167*			*259*	

Table 8.48 Average daily vitamin intakes by whether child's parents were receiving Income Support or Family Credit

| Vitamins | Whether receiving benefit(s) | | | | | |
| | Receiving benefit(s) | | | Not receiving benefits | | |
	Mean	Median	se	Mean	Median	se
(a) Intakes from *all sources*						
Pre-formed retinol (μg)	441	277	29.8	443	292	26.9
Total carotene (β–carotene equivalents) (μg)*	770	581	27.5	920	690	24.1
Vitamin A (retinol equivalents) (μg)	540	398	30.8	596	440	27.3
Thiamin (mg)	0.8	0.7	0.01	0.8	0.7	0.01
Riboflavin (mg)	1.2	1.1	0.02	1.2	1.2	0.01
Niacin equivalents (mg)	16	16	0.2	16	16	0.1
Vitamin B$_6$ (mg)	1.2	1.2	0.02	1.2	1.2	0.01
Vitamin B$_{12}$ (μg)	2.7	2.4	0.07	2.9	2.5	0.06
Folate (μg)	133	123	2.8	131	124	1.4
Biotin (μg)*	17.0	15.4	0.4	17.2	16.5	0.2
Pantothenic acid (mg)	2.7	2.5	0.04	2.8	2.6	0.03
Vitamin C (mg)	42.7	31.9	1.6	56.0	45.3	1.3
Vitamin D (μg)	1.9	1.1	0.10	1.9	1.2	0.06
Vitamin E (α–tocopherol equivalents) (mg)	4.4	4.0	0.09	4.4	4.0	0.06
Base		534			1140	
(b) Intakes from *food sources*						
Pre-formed retinol (μg)	352	263	27.2	369	270	26.2
Total carotene (β–carotene equivalents) (μg)	770	581	27.5	920	690	24.1
Vitamin A (retinol equivalents) (μg)	480	380	28.2	522	409	26.7
Thiamin (mg)	0.8	0.7	0.01	0.8	0.7	0.01
Riboflavin (mg)	1.2	1.1	0.02	1.2	1.1	0.01
Niacin equivalents (mg)	15.9	15.4	0.2	16.1	15.5	0.1
Vitamin B$_6$ (mg)	1.2	1.1	0.02	1.2	1.1	0.01
Vitamin B$_{12}$ (μg)	2.7	2.4	0.07	2.9	2.5	0.06
Folate (μg)	133	123	2.2	130	123	1.3
Biotin μg)	17	15	0.4	17	16	0.2
Pantothenic acid (mg)	2.7	2.5	0.04	2.7	2.6	0.02
Vitamin C (mg)	40.3	2.0	31.4	52.5	42.1	1.2
Vitamin D (μg)	1.3	1.1	0.05	1.2	1.0	0.03
Vitamin E (α–tocopherol equivalents) (mg)	4.3	4.0	0.08	4.3	3.9	0.05
Base		534			1140	

*None of the dietary supplements taken by children in this survey provided any carotene or biotin.

Table 8.49 Average daily intake of vitamins from food sources per 1000 kcal food energy by whether child's parents were receiving Income Support or Family Credit

| Nutrients | Whether receiving benefit(s) | | | | | |
| | Receiving benefit(s) | | | Not receiving benefits | | |
	Mean	Median	se	Mean	Median	se
Intake per 1000 kcal energy:						
Total carotene (β–carotene equivalents) (μg)	676	525	23.1	812	607	19.6
Vitamin A (retinol equivalents) (μg)	414	334	22.6	464	361	25.3
Thiamin (mg)	0.7	0.6	0.01	0.7	0.7	0.01
Riboflavin (mg)	1.0	1.0	0.01	1.0	1.0	0.01
Niacin equivalents (mg)	13.8	13.4	0.1	14.3	14.0	0.1
Vitamin B$_6$ (mg)	1.0	1.0	0.01	1.1	1.0	0.01
Vitamin B$_{12}$ (μg)	2.4	2.1	0.06	2.5	2.3	0.05
Folate (μg)	116	109	1.7	116	112	1.0
Vitamin C (mg)	35.4	27.4	1.3	46.7	38.2	1.1
Vitamin D (μg)	1.2	0.9	0.05	1.1	0.9	0.03
Vitamin E (α–tocopherol equivalents) (mg)	3.7	3.5	0.06	3.8	3.5	0.04
Base		534			1140	

Table 8.50 Average daily vitamin intakes by mother's highest educational qualification

Vitamins	Mother's highest educational qualification level														
	Above GCE 'A' level			GCE 'A' level and equivalents			GCE 'O' level and equivalents			CSE and equivalents			None		
	Mean	Median	se	Mean	Median	se	Mean	Median	se	Mean	Median	se	Mean	Median	se
(a) Intakes from *all sources*															
Pre-formed retinol (μg)	476	327	30.1	430	309	29.9	395	276	25.5	377	271	47.9	497	275	75.1
Total carotene (β–carotene equivalents) (μg)*	965	717	44.9	953	694	64.6	845	625	31.8	835	586	46.8	822	612	36.9
Vitamin A (retinol equivalents) (μg)	637	505	30.8	588	465	32.8	536	417	26.4	516	385	49.5	637	404	75.7
Thiamin (mg)	0.9	0.8	0.02	0.9	0.8	0.03	0.8	0.7	0.01	0.8	0.7	0.02	0.8	0.7	0.02
Riboflavin (mg)	1.3	1.2	0.02	1.3	1.2	0.04	1.2	1.1	0.02	1.1	1.1	0.03	1.2	1.1	0.03
Niacin equivalents (mg)	17.3	16.8	0.3	17.6	17.3	0.4	16.0	15.2	0.2	15.5	14.9	0.3	16.0	15.2	0.3
Vitamin B₆ (mg)	1.3	1.2	0.03	1.3	1.2	0.04	1.2	1.2	0.02	1.2	1.1	0.03	1.2	1.1	0.02
Vitamin B₁₂ (μg)	3.1	2.8	0.1	3.0	2.6	0.1	2.7	2.4	0.1	2.6	2.4	0.1	2.9	2.4	0.1
Folate (μg)	139	131	2.7	132	124	3.5	129	122	1.9	126	117	3.3	133	127	2.7
Biotin (μg)*	18.9	18.2	0.4	18.1	16.7	0.5	16.4	15.6	0.3	16.7	14.9	0.7	16.5	15.4	0.4
Pantothenic acid (mg)	2.9	2.8	0.05	3.0	2.7	0.09	2.7	2.5	0.04	2.6	2.5	0.05	2.7	2.6	0.05
Vitamin C (mg)	71.4	61.1	2.9	61.2	52.8	3.3	51.4	39.0	1.8	40.4	33.6	1.9	38.5	28.9	1.6
Vitamin D (μg)	2.4	1.3	0.1	2.3	1.3	0.2	1.8	1.1	0.1	1.4	1.0	0.08	1.7	1.1	0.1
Vitamin E (α–tocopherol equivalents) (mg)	4.6	4.2	0.1	4.8	4.1	0.2	4.3	4.0	0.1	4.2	3.9	0.1	4.3	3.9	0.1
Base		305			183			590			236			358	
(b) Intakes from *food sources*															
Pre-formed retinol (μg)	356	289	26.5	330	274	21.8	333	254	23.3	357	258	47.6	441	259	74.3
Total carotene (β–carotene equivalents) (μg)	965	717	44.9	953	694	64.6	845	625	31.8	835	586	46.8	822	612	36.9
Vitamin A (retinol equivalents) (μg)	517	434	27.7	489	412	24.7	474	387	24.3	496	378	49.2	578	388	75.0
Thiamin (mg)	0.8	0.8	0.02	0.8	0.8	0.02	0.8	0.7	0.01	0.7	0.7	0.02	0.8	0.7	0.01
Riboflavin (mg)	1.2	1.2	0.02	1.2	1.2	0.03	1.2	1.1	0.02	1.1	1.1	0.03	1.2	1.1	0.02
Niacin equivalents (mg)	16.9	16.5	0.3	17.0	16.2	0.4	15.7	15.1	0.2	15.4	14.8	0.3	15.8	15.0	0.2
Vitamin B₆ (mg)	1.3	1.2	0.02	1.2	1.2	0.04	1.2	1.1	0.02	1.2	1.1	0.03	1.2	1.1	0.02
Vitamin B₁₂ (μg)	3.0	2.7	0.1	2.9	2.6	0.1	2.7	2.4	0.1	2.6	2.4	0.1	2.9	2.4	0.1
Folate (μg)	137	128	2.6	132	124	3.5	128	122	1.8	125	117	3.2	133	127	2.7
Biotin (μg)	18.9	18.2	0.4	18.1	16.7	0.5	16.4	15.6	0.3	16.7	14.9	0.7	16.5	15.4	0.4
Pantothenic acid (mg)	2.8	2.7	0.04	2.9	2.7	0.07	2.6	2.5	0.03	2.6	2.5	0.05	2.7	2.6	0.05
Vitamin C (mg)	66.1	54.9	2.8	56.8	50.8	3.1	48.4	36.6	1.7	39.4	33.2	1.8	36.2	28.3	1.5
Vitamin D (μg)	1.3	1.1	0.05	1.4	1.1	0.10	1.2	1.0	0.04	1.2	1.0	0.06	1.2	1.0	0.04
Vitamin E (α–tocopherol equivalents) (mg)	4.4	4.1	0.1	4.5	4.0	0.1	4.2	4.0	0.1	4.2	3.9	0.1	4.3	3.9	0.1
Base		305			183			590			236			358	

*None of the dietary supplements taken by children in this survey provided any carotene or biotin.

Table 8.51 Average daily intake of vitamins from food sources per 1000 kcal food energy by mother's highest educational qualification

Nutrients	Mother's highest educational qualification level														
	Above GCE 'A' level			GCE 'A' level and equivalents			GCE 'O' level and equivalents			CSE and equivalents			None		
Intakes per 1000 kcal energy:	Mean	Median	se	Mean	Median	se	Mean	Median	se	Mean	Median	se	Mean	Median	se
Total carotene (β–carotene equivalents) (μg)	852	638	37.3	837	599	53.1	746	565	25.1	732	541	37.8	724	544	31.8
Vitamin A (retinol equivalents) (μg)	464	389	28.0	434	363	21.5	417	342	20.4	427	334	34.7	507	340	72.8
Thiamin (mg)	0.7	0.7	0.01	0.7	0.7	0.01	0.7	0.7	0.01	0.7	0.6	0.01	0.7	0.6	0.01
Riboflavin (mg)	1.1	1.1	0.02	1.1	1.0	0.03	1.0	1.0	0.01	1.0	1.0	0.02	1.0	1.0	0.02
Niacin equivalents (mg)	15.0	14.8	0.2	15.0	14.8	0.2	13.9	13.7	0.1	13.7	13.3	0.2	13.7	13.3	0.2
Vitamin B₆ (mg)	1.1	1.1	0.02	1.1	1.0	0.03	1.0	1.0	0.01	1.0	1.0	0.02	1.0	1.0	0.02
Vitamin B₁₂ (μg)	2.7	2.5	0.07	2.6	2.3	0.12	2.4	2.2	0.05	2.3	2.1	0.07	2.5	2.2	0.1
Folate (μg)	122	119	2.0	118	112	2.8	114	111	1.3	111	106	2.2	116	109	2.2
Vitamin C (mg)	59.5	49.8	2.5	50.7	44.1	2.8	42.7	32.6	1.4	35.0	30.0	1.5	31.7	24.5	1.3
Vitamin D (μg)	1.1	1.0	0.05	1.3	0.9	0.11	1.1	0.9	0.04	1.1	0.9	0.05	1.1	0.9	0.04
Vitamin E (α–tocopherol equivalents) (mg)	3.9	3.7	0.07	3.9	3.5	0.12	3.7	3.5	0.05	3.7	3.4	0.09	3.7	3.4	0.07
Base		305			183			590			236			358	

Table 8.52   Average daily vitamin intakes by family type

Vitamins	Family type											
	Married or cohabiting couple						Lone parent					
	One child			More than one child			One child			More than one child		
	Mean	Median	se	Mean	Median	se	Mean	Median	se	Mean	Median	se
(a) Intakes from all sources												
Pre-formed retinol (μg)	414	309	23.0	447	282	31.5	442	285	55.3	381	267	43.6
Total carotene (β–carotene equivalents) (μg)*	892	659	41.6	883	664	24.2	850	567	68.9	781	601	49.2
Vitamin A (retinol equivalents) (μg)	562	450	24.1	595	428	32.0	584	435	57.2	511	388	46.3
Thiamin (mg)	0.8	0.7	0.02	0.8	0.8	0.01	0.9	0.8	0.03	0.8	0.8	0.02
Riboflavin (mg)	1.2	1.2	0.02	1.2	1.2	0.01	1.2	1.2	0.05	1.2	1.1	0.03
Niacin equivalents (mg)	16.1	15.3	0.3	16.3	15.7	0.2	17.4	16.5	0.5	16.3	15.9	0.4
Vitamin B_6 (mg)	1.2	1.2	0.02	1.2	1.1	0.01	1.3	1.3	0.04	1.3	1.2	0.04
Vitamin B_{12} (μg)	2.9	2.7	0.1	2.8	2.5	0.1	2.8	2.5	0.1	2.8	2.4	0.1
Folate (μg)*	129	120	2.4	131	124	1.5	137	135	4.0	138	128	4.1
Biotin (μg)*	17.9	17.1	0.5	17.0	16.0	0.2	17.3	15.7	0.6	16.1	14.8	0.5
Pantothenic acid (mg)	2.8	2.7	0.05	2.7	2.6	0.03	2.8	2.7	0.10	2.7	2.5	0.07
Vitamin C (mg)	50.0	8.25	2.3	50.8	39.3	1.3	56.1	36.5	5.4	39.1	30.3	2.3
Vitamin D (μg)	2.1	1.1	0.1	1.8	1.1	0.06	2.5	1.4	0.3	1.5	1.1	0.1
Vitamin E (α–tocopherol equivalents) (mg)	4.2	3.8	0.1	4.4	4.0	0.1	4.8	4.4	0.2	4.4	4.2	0.1
Base		366			1011			121			177	
(b) Intakes from food sources												
Pre-formed retinol (μg)	340	286	20.2	381	263	30.9	336	268	38.8	332	257	41.3
Total carotene (β–carotene equivalents) (μg)	892	659	41.6	883	664	24.2	850	567	68.9	781	601	49.2
Vitamin A (retinol equivalents) (μg)	488	411	21.5	528	398	31.3	478	424	40.9	462	374	44.2
Thiamin (mg)	0.8	0.7	0.01	0.8	0.7	0.01	0.8	0.7	0.02	0.8	0.8	0.02
Riboflavin (mg)	1.2	1.2	0.02	1.2	1.1	0.01	1.2	1.1	0.04	1.2	1.1	0.03
Niacin equivalents (mg)	15.8	15.2	0.2	16.0	15.5	0.1	16.9	16.1	0.5	16.1	15.8	0.4
Vitamin B_6 (mg)	1.2	1.2	0.02	1.2	1.1	0.01	1.2	1.2	0.04	1.3	1.2	0.03
Vitamin B_{12} (μg)	2.8	2.6	0.1	2.8	2.4	0.1	2.8	2.5	0.1	2.7	2.4	0.1
Folate (μg)	128	118	2.4	130	124	1.5	136	134	4.0	138	128	4.1
Biotin (μg)	17.9	17.1	0.5	17.0	16.0	0.2	17.3	15.7	0.6	16.1	14.8	0.5
Pantothenic acid (mg)	2.8	2.7	0.04	2.7	2.6	0.03	2.8	2.7	0.08	2.7	2.5	0.07
Vitamin C (mg)	55.7	46.4	2.2	47.6	36.9	1.2	51.2	32.9	5.3	37.6	28.5	2.1
Vitamin D (μg)	1.2	0.9	0.06	1.2	1.0	0.03	1.6	1.2	0.12	1.3	1.1	0.06
Vitamin E (α–tocopherol equivalents) (mg)	4.1	3.8	0.1	4.3	4.0	0.1	4.6	4.3	0.2	4.4	4.2	0.1
Base		366			1011			121			177	

*None of the dietary supplements taken by children in this survey provided any carotene or biotin.

Table 8.53   Average daily intake of vitamins from food sources per 1000 kcal food energy by family type

Nutrients	Family type											
	Married or cohabiting couple						Lone parent					
	One child			More than one child			One child			More than one child		
Intakes per 1000 kcal energy:	Mean	Median	se	Mean	Median	se	Mean	Median	se	Mean	Median	se
Total carotene (β–carotene equivalents) (μg)	804	579	34.6	777	587	19.7	739	518	59.4	665	534	37.5
Vitamin A (retinol equivalents) (μg)	444	383	19.1	463	345	28.9	409	367	39.8	399	334	41.4
Thiamin (mg)	0.7	0.7	0.01	0.7	0.7	0.01	0.7	0.7	0.01	0.7	0.7	0.01
Riboflavin (mg)	1.1	1.0	0.02	1.0	1.0	0.01	1.0	0.9	0.03	1.0	1.0	0.02
Niacin equivalents (mg)	14.3	14.0	0.1	14.1	13.8	0.1	14.5	13.9	0.3	13.9	13.4	0.2
Vitamin B_6 (mg)	1.1	1.0	0.02	1.0	1.0	0.01	1.1	1.0	0.03	1.1	1.0	0.02
Vitamin B_{12} (μg)	2.6	2.4	0.06	2.5	2.2	0.05	2.4	2.1	0.11	2.4	2.2	0.14
Folate (μg)	116	111	1.8	115	111	1.1	119	114	3.3	119	113	2.9
Vitamin C (mg)	51.5	41.5	2.1	42.1	32.8	1.0	42.1	28.6	3.6	32.7	25.6	1.8
Vitamin D (μg)	1.1	0.8	0.06	1.1	0.9	0.03	1.4	1.0	0.10	1.1	0.9	0.06
Vitamin E (α–tocopherol equivalents) (mg)	3.7	3.4	0.07	3.8	3.5	0.04	3.9	3.6	0.13	3.7	3.5	0.10
Base		366			1011			121			177	

9 Minerals

Minerals are inorganic elements. Essential minerals are required for the body's normal function and are therefore required in the diet; they include iron, calcium, phosphorus, potassium, magnesium, sodium and chloride. Trace elements are required in minute amounts, and include zinc, copper, iodine and manganese.

Data are presented in this chapter for average daily intakes of the above minerals, which were derived from weighting to seven days the intakes for the 1675 children for whom complete four-day weighed intake records containing two weekend days and two weekdays were obtained[1].

Iron was the only mineral to which dietary supplements made a noticeable contribution to intake and so for iron data are presented for intakes from all sources, including dietary supplements and for intakes from food sources alone. For the remaining minerals intakes are presented for food sources only.

Some foods are fortified with minerals, for example white flour is fortified with iron and calcium, and many breakfast cereals are fortified with iron. Thus food groups such as cereals and cereal products were found to be major sources of minerals such as iron and calcium for children in this survey.

For those minerals where UK Reference Nutrient Intakes (RNIs) and Lower Reference Nutrient Intakes (LRNIs) values have been published for children aged 1 to 3 years and 4 to 6 years, the proportion of children meeting the current RNIs and LRNIs are shown, and average daily intakes are compared with current RNIs, which are shown in Table 9.1.[2] A further explanation of RNIs and LRNIs can be found in Chapter 8, page 129. Intakes are also shown per 1000kcal energy intake and per kilogram body weight.

Food sources for iron and calcium are discussed in sections 9.1 and 9.2 respectively. Food sources for other minerals are discussed in section 9.8.

9.1 Total iron, haem and non-haem iron

Dietary iron occurs in two forms. About 90% of iron in the average British household diet is in the form of iron salts and is referred to as non-haem iron.[3] The extent to which this type of iron is absorbed is highly variable and depends both on the individual's iron status and on other components of the diet. The other 10% of dietary iron is in the form of haem iron, which comes mainly from the haemoglobin and myoglobin of meat. Haem iron is well absorbed, and its absorption is less strongly influenced by the individual's iron stores or other constituents of the diet.

Average daily intake of total iron for children aged between 1½ and 4½ years was 5.5mg (median 5.3mg). Haem iron contributed a mean of 0.3mg (median 0.2mg) and non-haem iron 5.3mg (median 5.0mg) to this total iron intake.   *(Tables 9.2 to 9.4 and Figs 9.1 to 9.6)*

Tables 9.2 and 9.4 show that average daily intake of total iron and non-haem iron increased with age. For example, mean total iron intake from all sources was lowest among those aged 1½ to 2½ years, 5.0mg, and highest among boys aged 3½ to 4½ years, 6.2mg (p<0.01). Overall, boys had significantly higher mean intakes of both total iron and non-haem iron from food sources than girls (p<0.05).

A survey of infants in 1986 found the average daily intake of total iron among infants aged 6 to 12 months was 8.1mg (median 7.0mg). The younger infants aged 6 to 9 months had significantly higher intakes of total iron than those aged 9 to 12 months (p<0.01). Iron intake in the older infants was only approximately 70% of the intake of the younger ones.[4] Evidence from the current and this previous survey suggests that average iron intakes decrease from age 6 to 9 months to 1½ to 2½ years, then increase.

Dietary supplements taken by children in the current survey provided 2% of the average daily intake of iron for children aged 1½ to 4½ years. This contribution is entirely in the form of non-haem iron. However the data suggest that dietary supplements providing iron were being taken predominantly by children whose average daily intake was already high. Among children aged 1½ to 4½ years, intakes for children at the upper 2.5 percentile of the distribution were 13% higher when intakes from supplements were taken into account. Virtually no increase was seen in average intakes for children at the lower 2.5 percentile or in median intakes.

The RNI for children aged under 4 years is 6.9mg/d which is higher than the RNI of 6.1mg/d for children aged 4 years and over. However daily intakes of total iron increased with age. As a result for children under 4 years of age the average intake of total iron from food sources was 77% of the RNI, while for those aged 4 years and over the average intake was 96% of the RNI.
(Table 9.5)

Table 9.2 shows that while 84% of children under 4 years of age had a mean total iron intake which was below the RNI, among those aged 4 years and over mean intake was below the RNI for 57% of the group. The proportions of children with total iron intakes below the

LRNIs were also greater among children aged under 4 years than those aged 4 years and over, 16% compared to 4%. *(Tables 9.2 to 9.5)*

After adjusting for variations in energy intake, differences in average intake by age and sex were no longer apparent. This suggests there were no differences between the groups of children in the iron density of their diet. Likewise after adjusting for variations in body weight there were no differences in average intake by age and sex. *(Tables 9.6 and 9.7)*

Ascorbic acid (vitamin C) enhances the absorption of non-haem iron, as does meat, fish and poultry. Bran, polyphenols, oxalates, phytates, the tannins in tea, and phosphates inhibit absorption. Haem iron itself promotes the absorption of non-haem iron. For example, adults absorb approximately four times as much non-haem iron when the principal protein source is meat, fish, or chicken than when it is milk, cheese, other dairy products or eggs. Beverages can improve or inhibit the absorption of iron depending on their type. Orange juice or soft drinks fortified with vitamin C can double the absorption of non-haem iron from an entire meal, where-as tea decreases it.[5] Data presented in Table 4.3 show that 37% of children consumed tea over the four-day dietary recording period.

The main source of haem iron was meat and meat products, providing 89% of the mean intake for children aged 1½ to 4½ years (*Table 9.9b*). Data presented in Table 4.3 show that meat consumption was low among children in this survey; sausages, chicken and turkey, and beef and veal (and dishes made from them), were consumed by about half the children during the four-day dietary recording period. Liver consumption was particularly low, with only 4% of children aged 1½ to 4½ years, consuming liver over the four-day recording period, and this is reflected in the low contribution of liver to haem iron intake for all children, 4%.

Non-haem iron intake accounted for 96% of total iron intake for children aged 1½ to 4½ years. The main source of non-haem iron in the diet of children aged 1½ to 4½ years was iron fortified cereals and cereal products, which provided half the average daily intake. Milk and milk products provided only 8% of the average daily intake (see *Table 9.10 b*). In a survey of infants aged 6 to 12 months, commercial infant foods including infant formula were found to be important sources of iron.[4] In this survey of children aged 1½ to 4½ years, only 2% had infant formula during the four-day recording period (see *Table 4.3*) resulting in a contribution to total iron intake for all children of 2%.[6] *(Table 9.8b)*

Vegetables, potatoes and savoury snacks were the other main source of non-haem iron, providing 15% of the mean intake among children aged 1½ to 4½ years. Seven per cent of the mean intake of non-haem iron came from vegetables alone. *(Table 9.10)*

9.2 Calcium

Calcium is the most abundant mineral in the body and is essential for growth. Among children aged 1½ to 4½

years the average daily intake of calcium was 637mg (median 606mg). Average intakes decreased with age; children aged 1½ to 2½ years had the highest intakes, 663mg, and girls aged 3½ to 4½ years the lowest, 595mg (p<0.05). Overall boys had higher average intakes than girls (NS). *(Table 9.11 and Figs 9.7 and 9.8)*

The majority of children had intakes in excess of the RNI, with those in the upper 2.5 percentile of the distribution having intakes between three and four times the RNI level (see *Table 9.1*). Eleven per cent of children aged under 4 years had mean intakes of calcium below the RNI, and 24% of children aged 4 years and over had intakes below the RNI.[7] One per cent of children aged under 4 years, and 2% of children aged 4 years and over, had intakes below the LRNIs. *(Table 9.11)*

Table 9.12 shows that among children aged under 4 years, mean intake of calcium from food sources was 183% of the RNI; for children aged 4 years and over mean intake was 138% of the RNI.

Average calcium intakes decreased markedly with age after controlling for variation in energy intake and body weight (see *Tables 9.6a and 9.7a*). This suggests that children's diets became lower in calcium density as they became older and heavier (p<0.01).

The main source of calcium in the diets of children aged 1½ to 4½ years was milk and milk products, which provided 64% of the mean intake of calcium. Milk alone (whole, semi-skimmed, and skimmed) provided 51% of the mean intake of calcium. However the contribution of milk to calcium intake decreased with age, from 56% among children aged 1½ to 2½ years to 46% for both boys and girls aged 3½ to 4½ years (NS). Cheese, and yogurt and fromage frais each provided a further 6% of the mean intake for all children.

Cereals and cereal products were the other main source of calcium for children aged 1½ to 4½ years, providing 19% of the mean intake. The contribution of calcium from cereals and cereal products increased with age, from 16% among children aged 1½ to 2½ years to 23% among boys aged 3½ to 4½ years (p<0.05).*(Table 9.13b)*

9.3 Phosphorus

Phosphorus is the second most abundant mineral in the body and has a variety of functions including being required for bone growth and in energy metabolism. Average daily intake by children aged 1½ to 4½ years was 742mg (median 716mg). Intakes did not vary significantly with age but boys had slightly higher mean intakes than girls, 757mg compared with 726mg (NS). *(Table 9.14)*

Phosphorus intake requirements are equivalent in molar terms to those for calcium, which means that RNI values expressed in weight are higher for calcium than for phosphorus.[2] The average daily intake of phosphorus by children aged 1½ to 4½ years was slightly higher than that of calcium, 742mg compared with 637mg. Differences in phosphorus intakes between age groups were not statistically significant. Overall, only 1% of children had intakes below the appropriate RNI values. Average intake of phosphorus for children aged under 4 years was 274% of the RNI and for children aged 4 years and over mean intake was 216% of the RNI.

(Tables 9.14 and 9.15)

After adjusting for differences in energy intake and body weight, average intakes of phosphorus decreased with age. For example, children in the youngest cohort had average intakes of 706mg per 1000kcal energy compared with 605mg for boys in the oldest cohort (p<0.01). (see *Tables 9.6a and 9.7a*)

9.4 Magnesium

Average daily intake of magnesium was 136mg (median 133mg). Intakes varied with age; children aged 1½ to 2½ years had the lowest, 132mg, and boys aged 3½ to 4½ years the highest, 146mg (p<0.01). *(Table 9.16)*

Table 9.17 shows that average intake among children aged under 4 years was 159% of the RNI and for children aged 4 years and over the mean intake was 119% of the RNI (see *Table 9.1*). Seven per cent of children aged under 4 years and 34% of children aged 4 years and over, had intakes below the RNI.[7] Less than 1% of children under 4 years of age, and only 2% of children aged 4 years and over, had intakes below the LRNI appropriate for their age. *(Tables 9.16 and 9.17)*

As with calcium and phosphorus intakes, when differences were considered relative to total energy intake and body weight, mean magnesium intakes decreased with age. For example, average intake of magnesium among children aged 1½ to 2½ years was 10.8mg/kg body weight compared with 8.4mg/kg among girls aged 3½ to 4½ years (p<0.01) (see *Tables 9.6a and 9.7a*.)

9.5 Sodium and chloride

Sodium chloride is present in all body fluids. Both sodium and chloride are required in small amounts in the diet and their concentrations are maintained by a variety of regulatory mechanisms.

Sodium and chloride are not generally found in high concentrations in unprocessed foods, but tend to be added to many foods during processing as well as by the addition of salt in the home. Although the average sodium and chloride content of foods was assessed, it was not possible to measure the amount of salt added to children's food during cooking or at the table. Thus intakes of sodium and chloride are based on average values attributed to foods eaten and do not allow for additions in cooking and at the table. These results are therefore underestimates of total sodium and chloride intake.

Questions on habitual use of salt in the cooking of the child's food and on the addition of salt to the child's food at the table were asked of parents in the interview questionnaire. These questions did not ask about how much salt was used, only about how often. Over half of parents reported using salt in cooking their child's food; no attempt was made to differentiate between practices for different types of food. A slightly higher proportion of parents of children in the oldest age cohort salted their child's food during cooking than did the parents of chil-

dren in the youngest age cohort, 58% compared with 53% (NS). As with the addition of salt during cooking, the use of salt at the table increased with age with children in the oldest age cohort being more likely 'usually' or 'occasionally' to have salt added at the table than children in the youngest age cohort (p<0.05).

(Tables 9.18 and 9.19)

Average daily intake of sodium for children aged between 1½ and 4½ years was 1506mg (median 1459mg) and mean intake of chloride for all children was 2261mg (median 2186mg). Both sodium and chloride intakes for children increased with age (p<0.01) and were slightly higher for boys than for girls (NS).

(Tables 9.20 and 9.21)

Intakes of both sodium and chloride were high, even after excluding additions during cooking and at the table, with the sodium intake of children under 4 years in the upper 2.5 percentile of the distribution being at least five times the RNI, and for children aged over 4 years in the upper 2.5 percentile intake was at least four times the RNI. Even children at the lower 2.5 percentile had intakes above the RNI. *(Table 9.20)*

Chloride intake for children in the upper 2.5 percentile was at least four and a half times the RNI for children aged under 4 years and at least three times the RNI for children aged 4 years and over (from *Table 9.21*). Among children aged under 4 years, mean sodium intake was 297% of the RNI, and for children aged 4 years and over mean intake was 233% of the RNI. Mean chloride intake for children under 4 years was 280% of the RNI and for children aged 4 years and over mean intake was 221%. *(Tables 9.22 and 9.23)*

Table 9.6 shows little variation in sodium intake by age and sex after adjusting for differences in energy intake. When intakes were adjusted for differences in body weight there was an apparent decline in intakes with increasing age. This would be accounted for by an associated reduction in energy intake per kilogram body weight with increasing age (see *Table 9.7a*).

9.6 Potassium

Among children aged between 1½ and 4½ years the average daily intake of potassium was 1508mg (median 1475mg). Intakes increased slightly with age, with children aged 1½ to 2½ years having the lowest intakes, 1476mg, and boys aged 3½ to 4½ years having the highest intakes, 1573mg (p<0.05). *(Table 9.24)*

Most children had intakes above the UK RNI for potassium. Table 9.25 shows that mean intake for children aged under 4 years was 187% of the RNI whereas for children aged 4 years and over mean intake was 143% of the RNI (from *Table 9.1*). As seen with calcium and magnesium, a higher proportion of children aged 4 years and over had intakes below the RNI, 11% compared with 3% of those under 4 years (p<0.05).[7] The average intake for children in the lower 2.5 percentile of the distribution was below the RNI, irrespective of age. However less than 1% of children aged under 4 years and only 1% of children aged 4 years and over had intakes below the LRNI (from *Table 9.1*). *(Table 9.24)*

Average intake of potassium decreased with age after adjusting for differences in energy intake and body weight (p<0.01) (see *Tables 9.6a and 9.7a*).

9.7 Trace elements

9.7.1 Zinc

Average daily intake of zinc for children aged between 1½ and 4½ years was 4.4mg (median 4.2mg). Average intakes increased slightly with age, being lowest for children aged 1½ to 2½ years, 4.3mg, and highest for boys aged 3½ to 4½ years, 4.7mg (NS). *(Table 9.26)*

RNI levels increase from 5.0mg/d for children under the age of 4, to 6.5mg/d for 4 to 6 year olds. The majority of children of both age groups had intakes below these levels. Seventy two per cent of children under 4, and 89% of children aged 4 years and over, had intakes below the RNIs. Moreover 14% of children under 4 years of age had intakes below the LRNI, compared with 37% of children aged 4 years and over (p<0.01). The average intake of zinc for children aged under 4 years was 87% of the RNI, whereas for children aged 4 years and over mean intake was 71% of the RNI. Thus, although zinc intakes increased slightly as children got older, for many children this increase was not sufficient to match the higher RNI[7]. *(Tables 9.26 and 9.27)*

As was found for a number of other minerals, zinc intakes decreased with age when differences in energy intake were taken into account, falling from 4.1mg/1000kcal for children aged 1½ to 2½ years to 3.7mg/1000kcal for boys aged 3½ to 4½ years (p<0.01). This suggests that the zinc content of the diet per 1000kcal energy reduced as the children got older. No age or sex related differences were found when intakes were expressed per kilogram body weight. (see *Tables 9.6 and 9.7*)

9.7.2 Copper

Average daily intake of copper by children aged between 1½ and 4½ years was 0.5mg (median 0.4mg). There were no differences in intakes between boys and girls or children of different ages. *(Table 9.28)*

Table 9.28 shows that around two thirds of children under the age of 4 years had intakes above the RNI for the age group of 0.4mg/d, but only around one third of the older children had intakes above their RNI of 0.6mg/d (p<0.01).[7] The average intake for children aged under 4 years was 119% of the RNI, but for children aged 4 years and over mean intake was 90% of the RNI. *(Table 9.29)*

No variation in intake between boys and girls or the different age cohorts was found after adjusting for differences in energy intake and body weight. (see *Tables 9.6 and 9.7*)

9.7.3 Iodine and manganese

Average daily intake of iodine by children aged between 1½ and 4½ years was 119μg (median 104μg). The range of intakes was large, with children in the lower 2.5 percentile having intakes only about a third of the median

intake whilst those in the top 2.5 percentile had intakes at least 120% higher than the median intake, irrespective of age. *(Table 9.30)*

Average intake of iodine for children aged under 4 years was 170% of the RNI whereas for children aged 4 years and over the mean intake was 119% of the RNI (see *Table 9.31*). As was seen for other minerals such as calcium and phosphorus, a greater proportion of children aged 4 years and over than children under 4 years, had intakes below the RNI, 46% compared with 24% (p<0.01).[7] Three per cent of children under 4 years of age and 5% of children aged 4 years and over had intakes below the LRNI. *(Table 9.30)*

After adjusting for differences in energy intake and body weight, average iodine intakes decreased with age. For example, children in the youngest age cohort had the highest intakes, 118μg/1000kcal, and boys in the oldest age cohort the lowest, 96μg/1000kcal (p<0.01) (see *Tables 9.6a and 9.7a*). This suggests that younger children had a diet richer in iodine than older children, due to higher milk consumption among this age group (see *Table 4.14*).

Average daily intake of manganese for children aged between 1½ and 4½ years was 1.2mg (median 1.1mg). Intakes increased with age from 1.1mg among children aged 1½ to 2½ years, to 1.4mg among boys aged 3½ to 4½ years (p<0.01). *(Table 9.32)*

There are no RNIs for manganese.

9.8 Main food sources of minerals

For children aged 1½ to 4½ years the main sources of most of the minerals measured were milk and milk products, cereals and cereal products, and meat and meat dishes. For some minerals, vegetables, potatoes and savoury snacks were also an important source. The contribution from food to intakes of haem iron, non-haem iron, total iron and calcium have already been discussed; this section looks at the main sources of the other minerals considered in this Chapter. *(Tables 9.33 to 9.38)*

There was an association between age and the contribution to mineral intake made by cereals and cereal products, and milk and milk products. The contribution from cereals and cereal products increased with age whereas that from milk and milk products decreased with age. Meat and meat products and vegetables, potatoes and savoury snacks all tended to contribute a greater proportion to total mineral intakes as the age of the child increased.

Although milk and milk products, and cereals and cereal products, were the main sources of most minerals there were substantial differences in the contribution these two food types made to mineral intakes. For example, milk and milk products provided 58% of the iodine intake of children aged 1½ to 4½ years but only 27% of the magnesium intake. Cereals and cereal products contributed 12% and 29% of the intakes of these two minerals respectively. *(Tables 9.34b and 9.38b)*

9.9 Variations in intakes

Children reported as being unwell
Children who were reported as being unwell and whose eating was affected, and to a lesser extent those whose eating was unaffected by being unwell, had lower intakes of most minerals than children who were not unwell during the four-day dietary recording period. For example, average daily calcium intake for children reported as being unwell and whose eating was affected was 593mg compared with 648mg for those children reported as not being unwell (p<0.05). However most of the differences in average daily mineral intakes were associated with differences in energy intake.

(Tables 9.39 and 9.40)

Region
Intakes of essential minerals tended to be highest among children living in London and the South East and lowest among children living in Scotland. For example, average calcium intakes were highest for children living in London and the South East, 651mg, and lowest among children living in Scotland, 614mg (NS), reflecting the higher mean intake of milk and cheese in London and the South East than in Scotland (see *Table 4.18*). However for sodium and chloride average intakes were highest among children living in Scotland and lowest among children living in London and the South East (p<0.01).

There was little variation in the average intakes of most trace elements by region, although iodine intakes were highest among children living in Scotland and lowest among children living in London and the South East (NS).

(Table 9.41)

Regional differences found in absolute intakes of essential minerals were less pronounced when differences in energy intake were controlled for. However sodium intakes were still highest among children living in Scotland and lowest among children living in London and the South East (p<0.01), and calcium intakes were still highest among children living in London and the South East.

(Table 9.42)

Socio-economic characteristics
Tables 9.43 to 9.50 show average daily intakes of minerals, and intakes adjusted for variations in energy intake, for different groups of children according to various socio-economic characteristics.

Children from a manual home background tended to have lower average intakes of most essential minerals than children from a non-manual background. However only intakes of iron, calcium, phosphorus and potassium were still lower among the manual group after adjusting for differences between groups in energy intake (p<0.01, except calcium, p<0.05). The exception was sodium, where intakes per 1000kcal energy for children from a manual home background were higher than the intakes of those from a non-manual home background (NS).

(Tables 9.43 and 9.44)

There was less variation in absolute intakes by whether the head of the household was in work. However there was clear evidence that sodium intakes were higher for children from homes where the head of household was either unemployed or economically inactive, even after controlling for differences in energy intake.

(Tables 9.45 and 9.46)

After controlling for differences in energy intake, children whose parents were receiving benefit or whose mothers highest qualifications were GCE 'O' levels or below had lower intakes of calcium, phosphorus, magnesium and potassium than other children (p<0.05).

(Tables 9.47 to 9.50)

Family type
Tables 9.51 and 9.52 compare absolute and adjusted intakes of minerals by children living in lone parent families with those of other children in the survey.

Average intakes of most minerals varied little according to family type, although for some minerals, calcium, phosphorus and magnesium, there was an apparent tendency for absolute intakes by children from lone parent families with brothers and sisters to be somewhat lower than those of other children (NS). Intakes of sodium were, in contrast, higher among children living with a lone parent (p <0.05). The data also suggest that intakes of some minerals, calcium, phosphorus, magnesium and potassium, by children who had brothers or sisters were likely to be lower than those of children who were only children; this applied whether the child was living in a one or two-parent family (NS). *(Table 9.51)*

After adjusting for variations in energy intake the differences seen in absolute intakes between children from lone and two-parent families, and between those with brothers and sisters and only children, became more marked. The relationship between family type and intakes of sodium and chloride were again different to those of other minerals; absolute intakes of both minerals tended to be higher for children in lone parent families and for children with siblings. After adjusting for variations in energy intake, children from lone parent families still had higher mean sodium intakes than other children.

(Table 9.52)

Notes and references

1 See *Chapter 5* and *Appendix J* for details of deriving average daily intakes.
2 Department of Health. Report on Health and Subjects: 41. *Dietary Reference Values for Food Energy and Nutrients for the United Kingdom*. HMSO (London, 1991).
3 Bull NL, Buss DH. Haem and Non-haem Iron in British Household Diets. *J Hum Nutr* 1980; **34**:141-145.
4 Mills A, Tyler H. *Food and Nutrient Intakes of British Infants Aged 6-12 Months*. HMSO (London, 1992).
5 Oski, FA. Iron deficiency in infancy and childhood. *N Engl J Med* 1993; **329**(3):190-3.
6 In Table 9.10 infant formula is included in the group 'other milk and milk products'.
7 See *footnote 6 of Chapter 8* for guidance on interpreting differences in the proportion of children meeting RNI values.

Figure 9.1a Average daily total iron intake from all sources by sex of child

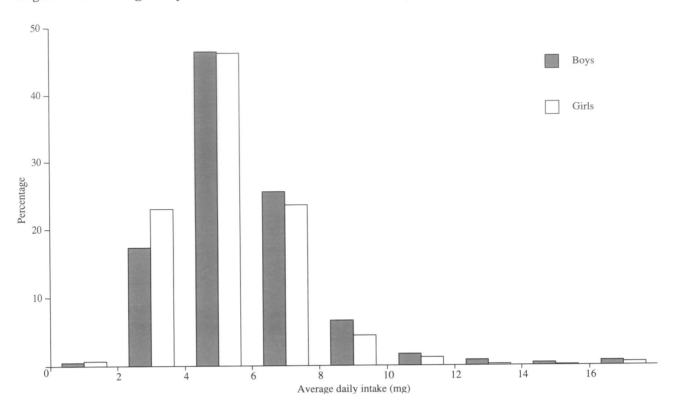

Figure 9.1b Average daily total iron intake from food sources by sex of child

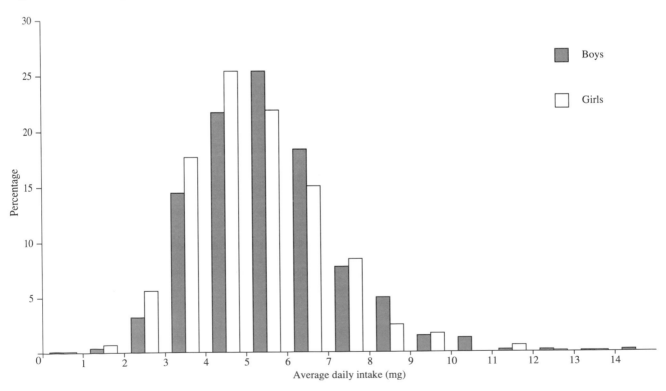

Figure 9.2a Average daily total iron intake from all sources by age of child

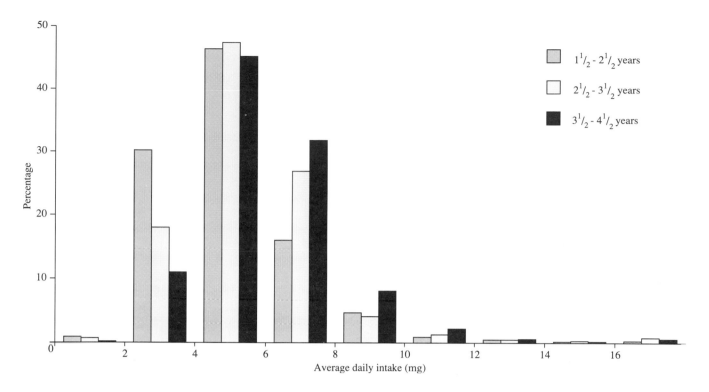

Figure 9.2b Average daily total iron intake from food sources by age of child

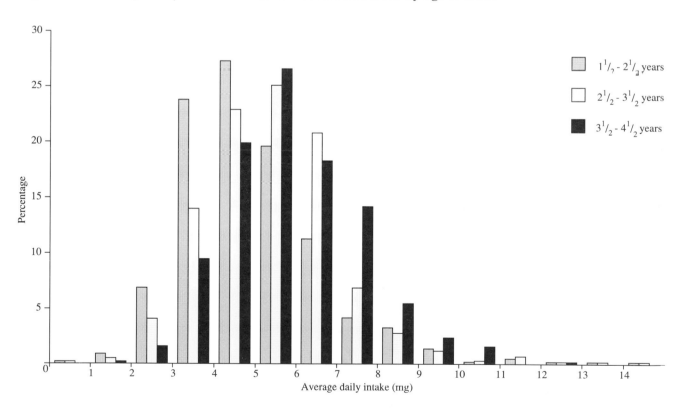

Figure 9.3 Average daily haem iron intake from food sources by sex of child

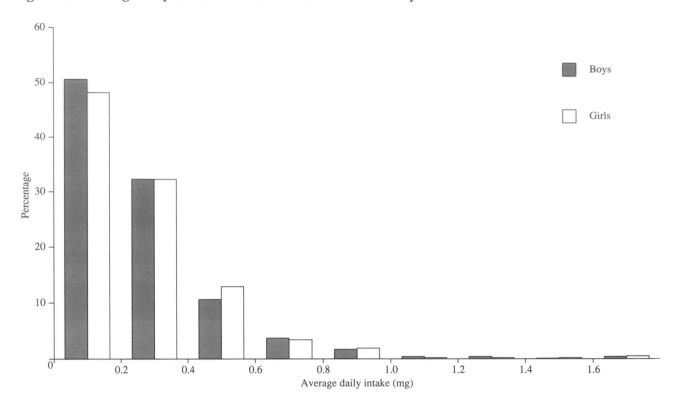

Figure 9.4 Average daily haem iron intake from food sources by age of child

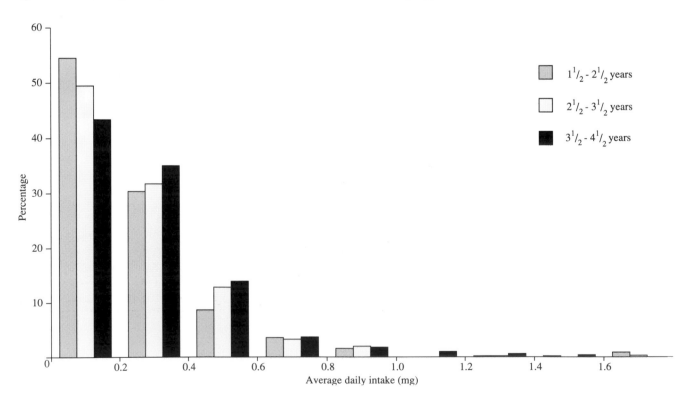

Figure 9.5 Average daily non-haem iron intake from all sources by sex of child

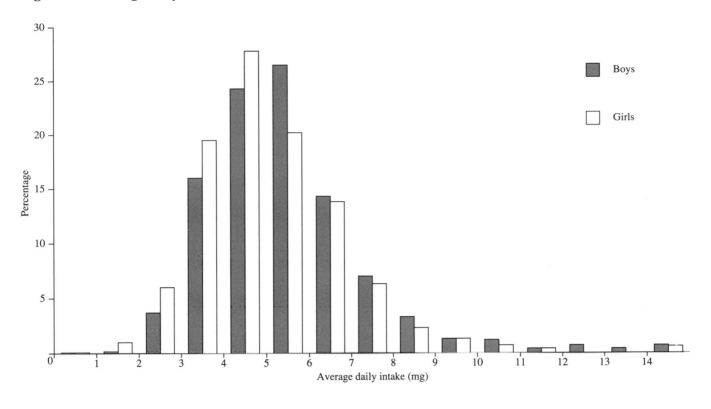

Figure 9.6 Average daily non-haem iron intake from all sources by age of child

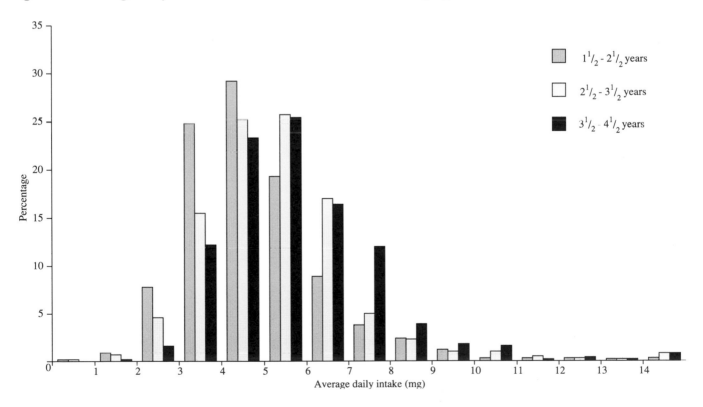

Figure 9.7 Average daily calcium intake from food sources by sex of child

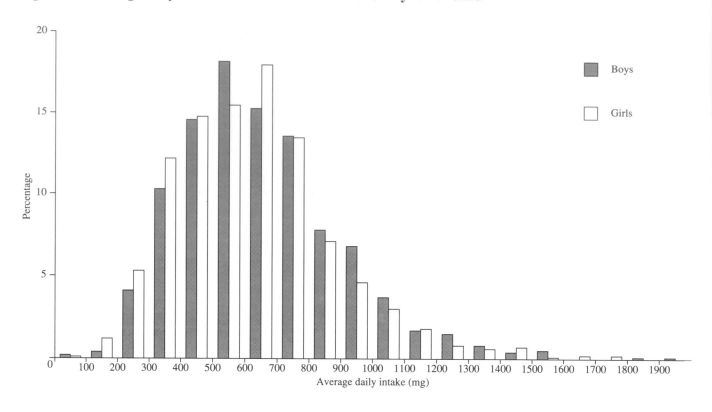

Figure 9.8 Average daily calcium intake from food sources by age of child

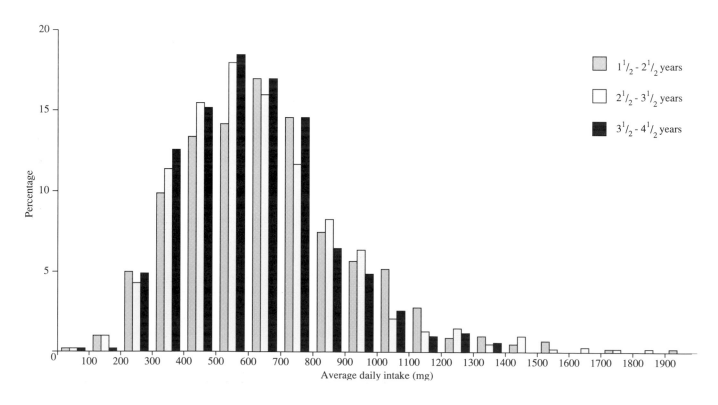

Table 9.1 Reference Nutrient Intakes (RNIs) and Lower Reference Nutrient Intakes (LRNIs) for minerals*

Minerals	RNI		LRNI	
	1–3 years	4–6 years	1–3 years	4–6 years
Iron (mg/d)	6.9	6.1	3.7	3.3
Calcium (mg/d)	350	450	200	275
Phosphorus (mg/d)	270	350	n/a	n/a
Magnesium (mg/d)	85	120	50	70
Sodium (mg/d)	500	700	200	280
Chloride (mg/d)	800	1100	n/a	n/a
Potassium (mg/d)	800	1100	450	600
Zinc (mg/d)	5.0	6.5	3.0	4.0
Copper (mg/d)	0.4	0.6	n/a	n/a
Iodine (μg/d)	70	100	40	50

*Source: Department of Health Report on Health and Social Subjects 41. *Dietary Reference Values for Food Energy and Nutrients for the United Kingdom.* HMSO (London, 1991).

n/a = no reference value set.

Table 9.2 Average daily intake of total iron (mg) by age and sex of child

Iron (mg)	Age and sex of child								
	All aged 1½ – 2½ years	All aged 2½ – 3½ years	All aged 3½ – 4½ years		All aged under 4 years	All aged 4 years and over	All boys	All girls	All
			Boys	Girls					
	cum %	cum %	cum %	cum %	cum %	cum %	cum %	cum %	cum %
(a) Intakes from *all sources*									
Less than 3.3	15	7	4	4	10	4	8	10	9
Less than 3.6	21	11	6	8	14	7	11	15	13
Less than 3.7	24	12	7	9	16	8	13	17	15
Less than 4.7	50	34	18	30	38	24	31	42	37
Less than 5.8	75	62	48	55	65	51	60	66	63
Less than 6.1	79	69	55	64	71	57	67	72	69
Less than 6.9	89	84	70	75	84	71	81	83	82
Less than 8.0	93	93	87	90	92	88	90	93	92
All	100	100	100	100	100	100	100	100	100
Base	576	606	250	243	1457	218	848	827	1675
Mean (average value)	5.0	5.6	6.2	5.9	5.5	6.1	5.7	5.4	5.5
Median value	4.7	5.4	5.9	5.5	5.1	5.8	5.4	5.0	5.3
Lower 2.5 percentile	2.5	2.6	3.1	3.0	2.6	3.1	2.8	2.5	2.6
Upper 2.5 percentile	9.6	11.0	10.7	10.0	10.5	10.5	10.7	9.5	10.4
Standard error of the mean	0.10	0.09	0.13	0.18	0.06	0.18	0.08	0.09	0.06
	cum %	cum %	cum %	cum %	cum %	cum %	cum %	cum %	cum %
(b) Intakes from *food sources*									
Less than 3.3	15	7	5	4	10	5	8	10	10
Less than 3.6	22	11	7	8	14	7	12	15	14
Less than 3.7	25	12	7	9	16	9	13	17	15
Less than 4.7	51	34	19	30	39	25	32	43	37
Less than 5.8	76	63	49	57	66	52	61	67	64
Less than 6.1	80	70	56	66	72	59	68	73	71
Less than 6.9	90	86	71	78	85	72	83	85	84
Less than 8.0	94	94	88	92	94	89	91	95	93
All	100	100	100	100	100	100	100	100	100
Base	576	606	250	243	1457	218	848	827	1675
Mean (average value)	4.9	5.4	6.1	5.6	5.3	5.9	5.5	5.2	5.4
Median value	4.7	5.3	5.9	5.5	5.1	5.7	5.4	5.0	5.2
Lower 2.5 percentile	2.4	2.6	3.1	3.0	2.6	3.1	2.8	2.5	2.6
Upper 2.5 percentile	9.2	9.1	10.4	9.1	9.2	9.1	9.6	9.0	9.2
Standard error of the mean	0.07	0.07	0.11	0.10	0.04	0.11	0.06	0.06	0.04

Table 9.3　Average daily intake of haem iron (mg) by age and sex of child

Haem iron (mg)	Age and sex of child						
	All aged 1½ – 2½ years	All aged 2½ – 3½ years	All aged 3½ – 4½ years		All boys	All girls	All
			Boys	Girls			
	cum %	cum %	cum %	cum %	cum %	cum %	cum %
Intakes from *food sources**							
Less than 0.1	27	22	17	21	23	23	23
Less than 0.2	54	49	45	42	50	48	49
Less than 0.3	74	68	65	66	69	70	70
Less than 0.4	85	81	81	76	83	80	82
Less than 0.5	91	89	87	87	89	89	89
All	100	100	100	100	100	100	100
Base	*576*	*606*	*250*	*243*	*848*	*827*	*1675*
Mean (average value)	0.2	0.2	0.3	0.3	0.2	0.3	0.3
Median value	0.2	0.2	0.2	0.2	0.2	0.2	0.2
Lower 2.5 percentile	0.0	0.0	0.0	0.0	0.0	0.0	0.0
Upper 2.5 percentile	0.8	0.8	1.0	0.9	0.8	0.8	0.8
Standard error of the mean	0.01	0.01	0.01	0.01	0.01	0.01	0.01

*None of the dietary supplements taken by children in this survey provided any haem iron.

Table 9.4　Average daily intake of non-haem iron (mg) by age and sex of child

Non-haem iron (mg)	Age and sex of child						
	All aged 1½ – 2½ years	All aged 2½ – 3½ years	All aged 3½ – 4½ years		All boys	All girls	All
			Boys	Girls			
	cum %	cum %	cum %	cum %	cum %	cum %	cum %
(a)　Intakes from *all sources*							
Less than 3.0	9	5	1	2	4	7	6
Less than 4.0	34	21	11	17	20	27	23
Less than 5.0	63	46	33	42	44	54	49
Less than 6.0	82	72	59	67	71	75	73
Less than 7.0	91	89	77	81	85	88	87
Less than 8.0	95	94	90	92	92	92	93
All	100	100	100	100	100	100	100
Base	*576*	*606*	*250*	*243*	*848*	*827*	*1675*
Mean (average value)	4.9	5.4	5.9	5.7	5.5	5.2	5.3
Median value	4.6	5.1	5.7	5.3	5.2	4.8	5.0
Lower 2.5 percentile	2.4	2.6	3.0	3.0	2.8	2.5	2.6
Upper 2.5 percentile	9.3	10.3	10.4	10.3	10.4	9.2	10.0
Standard error of the mean	0.09	0.09	0.12	0.18	0.08	0.09	0.06
	cum %	cum %	cum %	cum %	cum %	cum %	cum %
(b)　Intakes from *food sources*							
Less than 3.0	9	5	1	2	4	7	6
Less than 4.0	34	21	11	18	20	27	24
Less than 5.0	64	46	34	43	45	55	50
Less than 6.0	83	73	60	68	72	76	74
Less than 7.0	92	90	78	84	87	90	88
Less than 8.0	95	95	92	95	94	96	95
All	100	100	100	100	100	100	100
Base	*576*	*606*	*250*	*243*	*848*	*827*	*1675*
Mean (average value)	4.7	5.2	5.8	5.4	5.3	5.0	5.2
Median value	4.5	5.1	5.6	5.2	5.2	4.8	5.0
Lower 2.5 percentile	2.3	2.6	3.0	3.0	2.8	2.5	2.6
Upper 2.5 percentile	8.7	8.7	10.1	8.6	9.2	8.4	8.7
Standard error of the mean	0.07	0.06	0.10	0.09	0.06	0.05	0.04

Table 9.5 Average daily intake of iron as a percentage of the Reference Nutrient Intake (RNI) by age and sex of child

Age and sex of child	Average daily intake as % of RNI							
	(a) All sources				(b) Food sources			
	Mean	Median	se	Base	Mean	Median	se	Base
All aged 1½–2½ years	73	68	1.4	576	71	67	1.0	576
All aged 2½–3½ years	81	78	1.4	606	78	77	1.0	606
Aged 3½–4½ years:*								
Boys	95	90	1.9	250	93	89	1.7	250
Girls	92	86	2.9	243	87	85	1.6	243
All aged under 4 years	79	74	0.9	1457	77	74	0.6	1457
All aged 4 years and over	100	95	2.9	218	96	94	1.8	218
All boys	84	79	1.2	848	82	79	0.9	848
All girls	80	74	1.3	827	77	74	0.9	827
All	82	77	0.9	1675	79	77	0.6	1675

*Total iron intake as a percentage of the RNI was calculated for each child; thus in this age group values for children under 4 years of age used 6.9mg/d as the RNI and for children aged 4 years and over 6.1mg/d was taken as the RNI. The values for all children aged 3½ to 4½ years were then pooled to give a mean, median and standard error (se) for the age group.

Table 9.6(a) Average daily intake of minerals from food sources per 1000kcal food energy by age of child

Minerals	Age of child											
	All aged 1½–2½ years			All aged 2½–3½ years			All aged 3½–4½ years					
							Boys			Girls		
Intake per 1000kcal energy:	Mean	Median	se	Mean	Median	se	Mean	Median	se	Mean	Median	se
Iron (mg)	4.7	4.5	0.06	4.7	4.6	0.05	4.8	4.5	0.08	4.8	4.7	0.07
Haem iron (mg)	0.2	0.2	0.01	0.2	0.2	0.01	0.2	0.2	0.01	0.2	0.2	0.01
Non-haem iron (mg)	4.6	4.4	0.05	4.5	4.4	0.04	4.6	4.4	0.08	4.6	4.5	0.06
Calcium (mg)	637	618	9.2	547	516	7.7	492	472	9.7	504	488	9.7
Phosphorus (mg)	706	696	6.8	639	622	5.8	605	597	8.2	624	620	8.4
Magnesium (mg)	127	126	1.1	119	117	0.9	115	112	1.5	116	114	1.5
Sodium (mg)	1311	1294	12.3	1320	1294	12.0	1308	1275	16.6	1385	1367	21.2
Potassium (mg)	1422	1399	12.2	1309	1296	11.5	1241	1229	15.3	1277	1248	16.8
Zinc(mg)	4.1	4.0	0.04	3.8	3.7	0.04	3.7	3.5	0.06	3.8	3.6	0.06
Copper (mg)	0.4	0.4	0.01	0.4	0.4	0.01	0.4	0.4	0.01	0.4	0.4	0.01
Iodine (µg)	118	98	2.7	101	87	2.1	96	88	2.7	96	85	2.9
Base		576			606			250			243	

Table 9.6(b) Average daily intake of minerals from food sources per 1000kcal food energy by sex of child

Minerals	Sex of child								
	Boys			Girls			All		
Intake per 1000kcal energy:	Mean	Median	se	Mean	Median	se	Mean	Median	se
Iron (mg)	4.8	4.6	0.04	4.7	4.5	0.04	4.7	4.5	0.03
Haem iron (mg)	0.2	0.2	0.01	0.2	0.2	0.01	0.2	0.2	0.00
Non-haem iron (mg)	4.6	4.4	0.04	4.5	4.4	0.04	4.6	4.4	0.03
Calcium (mg)	561	529	6.8	566	536	7.0	563	532	4.9
Phosphorus (mg)	652	636	5.2	658	646	5.3	655	641	3.7
Magnesium (mg)	121	118	0.8	120	118	0.8	121	118	0.6
Sodium (mg)	1312	1291	10.0	1338	1316	10.5	1325	1302	7.2
Potassium (mg)	1323	1304	9.5	1343	1322	10.2	1333	1310	7.0
Zinc (mg)	3.9	3.7	0.03	3.9	3.8	0.03	3.9	3.8	0.02
Copper (mg)	0.4	0.4	0.00	0.4	0.4	0.01	0.4	0.4	0.00
Iodine (µg)	104	89	1.8	107	93	2.0	105	91	1.3
Base		848			827			1675	

Table 9.7(a)   Average daily intake of minerals from all sources per kilogram child's body weight by age of child

Minerals	Age of child											
	All aged 1½–2½ years			All aged 2½–3½ years			All aged 3½–4½ years					
							Boys			Girls		
Intake per kilogram child's body weight	*Mean*	*Median*	*se*	*Mean*	*Median*	*se*	*Mean*	*Median*	*se*	*Mean*	*Median*	*se*
Iron (mg)	0.4	0.4	0.01	0.4	0.4	0.01	0.4	0.4	0.01	0.4	0.3	0.01
Haem iron (mg)*	0.02	0.01	0.00	0.02	0.01	0.00	0.02	0.01	0.02	0.02	0.01	0.00
Non-haem irom (mg)	0.4	0.4	0.01	0.4	0.3	0.01	0.4	0.3	0.01	0.3	0.3	0.01
Calcium (mg)**	54.4	50.4	1.0	43.9	41.5	0.7	38.2	35.6	0.9	36.6	35.2	0.8
Phosphorus (mg)**	60.2	57.2	0.8	51.0	49.6	0.6	46.7	46.7	0.8	45.3	44.3	0.8
Magnesium (mg)*	10.8	10.5	0.1	9.5	9.2	0.1	8.9	8.7	0.2	8.4	8.3	0.1
Sodium (mg)*	112	107	1.5	105	100	1.3	101	101	1.8	100	95.4	2.0
Potassium (mg)*	122	117	1.5	104	102	1.2	95.7	94.2	1.7	92.4	91.4	1.5
Zinc (mg)**	0.3	0.3	0.00	0.3	0.3	0.00	0.3	0.3	0.01	0.3	0.3	0.01
Copper (mg)**	0.04	0.03	0.00	0.03	0.03	0.00	0.03	0.03	0.00	0.03	0.03	0.00
Iodine (μg)*	10.0	8.5	0.2	8.1	7.0	0.2	7.4	6.7	0.2	7.0	6.3	0.2
Base†		538			578			237			239	

*None of the dietary supplements taken by children in this survey provided any haem iron, magnesium, sodium, potassium or iodine.
**Dietary supplements provided negligible calcium, phosphorus, zinc and copper for children in this survey.
†Includes only those children for whom a valid weight measurement was obtained.

Table 9.7(b)   Average daily intake of minerals from all sources per kilogram child's body weight by sex of child

Minerals	Sex of child								
	Boys			Girls			All		
Intake per kilogram child's body weight	*Mean*	*Median*	*se*	*Mean*	*Median*	*se*	*Mean*	*Median*	*se*
Iron (mg)	0.4	0.4	0.01	0.4	0.4	0.01	0.4	0.4	0.00
Haem iron (mg)*	0.02	0.01	0.00	0.02	0.01	0.00	0.02	0.01	0.00
Non-haem iron (mg)	0.4	0.4	0.01	0.4	0.3	0.01	0.4	0.3	0.00
Calcium (mg)**	45.5	42.4	0.7	45.5	42.0	0.7	45.5	42.3	0.5
Phosphorus (mg)**	52.7	50.6	0.6	52.6	50.2	0.6	52.6	50.4	0.4
Magnesium (mg)*	9.7	9.4	0.1	9.6	9.3	0.1	9.7	9.4	0.07
Sodium (mg)*	106	102	1.1	106	101	1.2	106	102	0.8
Potassium (mg)*	107	104	1.1	107	103	1.2	107	104	0.8
Zinc (mg)**	0.3	0.3	0.00	0.3	0.3	0.00	0.3	0.3	0.00
Copper (mg)**	0.03	0.03	0.00	0.03	0.03	0.00	0.03	0.03	0.00
Iodine (μg)*	8.3	7.1	0.2	8.6	7.2	0.2	8.5	7.2	0.1
Base†		793			799			1592	

*None of the dietary supplements taken by children in this survey provided any haem iron, magnesium, sodium, potassium or iodine.
**Dietary supplements provided negligible calcium, phosphorus, zinc and copper for children in this survey.
†Includes only those children for whom a valid weight measurement was obtained.

Table 9.8(a)   Contribution of food types to average daily total iron intake by age and sex of child

Food types	Age and sex of child						
	All aged 1½ – 2½ years	All aged 2½ – 3½ years	All aged 3½ – 4½ years		All boys	All girls	All
			Boys	Girls			
	mg	mg	mg	mg	mg	mg	mg
Cereals & cereal products	2.2	2.6	3.1	2.7	2.7	2.4	2.6
of which:							
white bread	*0.3*	*0.5*	*0.6*	*0.5*	*0.4*	*0.4*	*0.4*
wholemeal bread	*0.2*	*0.2*	*0.2*	*0.2*	*0.2*	*0.2*	*0.2*
high fibre breakfast cereals	*0.5*	*0.6*	*0.7*	*0.5*	*0.6*	*0.5*	*0.6*
other breakfast cereals	*0.4*	*0.6*	*0.7*	*0.7*	*0.6*	*0.5*	*0.6*
biscuits	*0.2*	*0.3*	*0.3*	*0.3*	*0.3*	*0.2*	*0.3*
Milk & milk products	0.4	0.3	0.3	0.3	0.3	0.3	0.3
of which:							
milk (whole, semi-skimmed, skimmed)	*0.3*	*0.2*	*0.2*	*0.2*	*0.2*	*0.2*	*0.2*
other milk & products	*0.2*	*0.1*	*0.1*	*0.0*	*0.1*	*0.1*	*0.1*
Eggs & egg dishes	0.1	0.1	0.1	0.2	0.1	0.2	0.1
Fat spreads	0.0	0.0	0.0	0.0	0.0	0.0	0.0
Meat & meat products	0.7	0.8	0.9	0.8	0.8	0.7	0.8
of which:							
beef, veal & dishes	*0.2*	*0.2*	*0.2*	*0.2*	*0.2*	*0.2*	*0.2*
liver & liver dishes	*0.0*	*0.0*	*0.0*	*0.0*	*0.0*	*0.0*	*0.0*
Fish & fish dishes	0.1	0.1	0.1	0.1	0.1	0.1	0.1
Vegetables, potatoes & savoury snacks	0.7	0.8	0.8	0.8	0.8	0.8	0.8
of which:							
vegetables	*0.4*	*0.4*	*0.4*	*0.4*	*0.4*	*0.4*	*0.4*
potatoes, fried	*0.1*	*0.2*	*0.2*	*0.2*	*0.2*	*0.2*	*0.2*
other potatoes	*0.1*	*0.1*	*0.1*	*0.1*	*0.1*	*0.1*	*0.1*
savoury snacks	*0.1*	*0.1*	*0.1*	*0.1*	*0.1*	*0.1*	*0.1*
Fruit & nuts	0.1	0.1	0.1	0.1	0.1	0.1	0.1
of which:							
fruit	*0.1*	*0.1*	*0.1*	*0.1*	*0.1*	*0.1*	*0.1*
Sugars, preserves & confectionery	0.1	0.2	0.2	0.2	0.2	0.2	0.2
Beverages	0.1	0.1	0.1	0.1	0.1	0.1	0.1
Commercial infant foods & drinks	0.1	0.0	0.0	0.0	0.1	0.0	0.0
Miscellaneous	0.1	0.1	0.1	0.1	0.1	0.1	0.1
Average daily intake (mg)	**4.9**	**5.4**	**6.1**	**5.6**	**5.5**	**5.2**	**5.4**
Total number of children	**576**	**606**	**250**	**243**	**848**	**827**	**1675**

Table 9.8(b)   Percentage contribution of food types to average daily total iron intake by age and sex of child

Food types	Age and sex of child						
	All aged 1½ – 2½ years	All aged 2½ – 3½ years	All aged 3½ – 4½ years		All boys	All girls	All
			Boys	Girls			
	%	%	%	%	%	%	%
Cereals & cereal products	44	49	51	48	49	46	48
of which:							
white bread	7	8	9	9	8	8	8
wholemeal bread	4	3	3	3	3	3	3
high fibre breakfast cereals	11	11	11	8	11	10	10
other breakfast cereals	9	11	11	12	10	10	10
biscuits	5	5	6	5	5	5	5
Milk & milk products	9	6	5	5	6	6	6
of which:							
milk (whole, semi-skimmed, skimmed)	5	4	4	4	4	5	4
other milk & products	3	1	2	1	2	2	2
Eggs & egg dishes	3	3	2	3	2	3	3
Fat spreads	0	0	0	0	0	0	0
Meat & meat products	14	14	14	15	14	14	14
of which:							
beef, veal & dishes	5	4	4	4	4	4	4
liver & liver dishes	0	0	0	0	1	0	0
Fish & fish dishes	2	2	2	2	2	2	2
Vegetables, potatoes & savoury snacks	14	15	14	15	14	15	14
of which:							
vegetables	7	7	6	7	7	7	7
potatoes, fried	3	3	3	4	3	3	3
other potatoes	2	2	2	2	2	2	2
savoury snacks	2	2	2	2	2	2	2
Fruit & nuts	3	3	2	3	3	3	3
of which:							
fruit	3	3	2	2	2	3	3
Sugars, preserves & confectionery	3	4	4	4	4	3	3
Beverages	2	3	2	2	2	2	2
Commercial infant foods & drinks	2	0	0	0	1	1	1
Miscellaneous	3	2	2	2	2	2	2
Average daily intake (mg)	**4.9**	**5.4**	**6.1**	**5.6**	**5.5**	**5.2**	**5.4**
Total number of children	**576**	**606**	**250**	**243**	**848**	**827**	**1675**

Table 9.9(a)   Contribution of food types to average daily haem iron intake by age and sex of child

Food types	Age and sex of child						
	All aged 1½ – 2½ years	All aged 2½ – 3½ years	All aged 3½ – 4½ years		All boys	All girls	All
			Boys	Girls			
	mg	mg	mg	mg	mg	mg	mg
Meat & meat products	0.21	0.23	0.25	0.26	0.23	0.23	0.23
of which:							
beef, veal & dishes	0.07	0.07	0.08	0.07	0.08	0.07	0.07
liver & liver dishes	0.01	0.01	0.01	0.01	0.01	0.01	0.01
burgers & kebabs	0.02	0.02	0.03	0.02	0.02	0.02	0.02
sausages	0.03	0.03	0.03	0.04	0.03	0.03	0.03
Fish & fish dishes	0.02	0.02	0.02	0.02	0.02	0.02	0.02
Miscellaneous	0.01	0.01	0.00	0.01	0.01	0.01	0.01
Average daily intake (mg)	**0.2**	**0.2**	**0.3**	**0.3**	**0.2**	**0.3**	**0.3**
Total number of children	**576**	**606**	**250**	**243**	**848**	**827**	**1675**

Table 9.9(b)   Percentage contribution of food types to average daily haem iron intake by age and sex of child

Food types	All aged 1½ – 2½ years	All aged 2½ – 3½ years	All aged 3½ – 4½ years		All boys	All girls	All
			Boys	Girls			
	%	%	%	%	%	%	%
Meat & meat products	86	91	90	92	90	88	89
of which:							
beef, veal & dishes	*29*	*28*	*29*	*25*	*31*	*27*	*27*
liver & liver dishes	*4*	*4*	*4*	*3*	*4*	*4*	*4*
burgers & kebabs	*8*	*8*	*11*	*7*	*8*	*8*	*8*
sausages	*12*	*12*	*11*	*14*	*12*	*11*	*12*
Fish & fish dishes	8	8	7	7	8	8	8
Miscellaneous	4	4	0	3	4	4	4
Average daily intake (mg)	**0.2**	**0.2**	**0.3**	**0.3**	**0.2**	**0.3**	**0.3**
Total number of children	**576**	**606**	**250**	**243**	**848**	**827**	**1675**

Table 9.10(a)   Contribution of food types to average daily non-haem iron intake by age and sex of child

Food types	All aged 1½ – 2½ years	All aged 2½ – 3½ years	All aged 3½ – 4½ years		All boys	All girls	All
			Boys	Girls			
	mg	mg	mg	mg	mg	mg	mg
Cereals & cereal products	2.2	2.6	3.1	2.7	2.7	2.4	2.6
of which:							
white bread	*0.3*	*0.5*	*0.6*	*0.5*	*0.4*	*0.4*	*0.4*
wholemeal bread	*0.2*	*0.2*	*0.2*	*0.2*	*0.2*	*0.2*	*0.2*
high fibre breakfast cereals	*0.5*	*0.6*	*0.7*	*0.5*	*0.6*	*0.5*	*0.6*
other breakfast cereals	*0.4*	*0.6*	*0.7*	*0.7*	*0.6*	*0.5*	*0.6*
biscuits	*0.2*	*0.3*	*0.3*	*0.3*	*0.3*	*0.2*	*0.3*
Milk & milk products	0.5	0.4	0.4	0.3	0.4	0.4	0.4
of which:							
milk (whole, semi-skimmed, skimmed)	*0.3*	*0.3*	*0.3*	*0.3*	*0.3*	*0.3*	*0.3*
other milk & products	*0.2*	*0.1*	*0.1*	*0.0*	*0.1*	*0.1*	*0.1*
Eggs & egg dishes	0.1	0.1	0.1	0.2	0.1	0.2	0.1
Fat spreads	0.0	0.0	0.0	0.0	0.0	0.0	0.0
Meat & meat products	0.5	0.5	0.6	0.6	0.5	0.5	0.5
of which:							
beef, veal & dishes	*0.1*	*0.1*	*0.1*	*0.1*	*0.1*	*0.1*	*0.1*
liver & liver dishes	*0.0*	*0.0*	*0.0*	*0.0*	*0.0*	*0.0*	*0.0*
Fish & fish dishes	0.1	0.1	0.1	0.1	0.1	0.1	0.1
Vegetables, potatoes & savoury snacks	0.7	0.8	0.8	0.8	0.8	0.8	0.8
of which:							
vegetables	*0.4*	*0.4*	*0.4*	*0.4*	*0.4*	*0.4*	*0.4*
potatoes, fried	*0.1*	*0.2*	*0.2*	*0.2*	*0.2*	*0.2*	*0.2*
other potatoes	*0.1*	*0.1*	*0.1*	*0.1*	*0.1*	*0.1*	*0.1*
savoury snacks	*0.1*	*0.1*	*0.1*	*0.1*	*0.1*	*0.1*	*0.1*
Fruit & nuts	0.1	0.1	0.1	0.1	0.1	0.1	0.1
of which:							
fruit	*0.1*	*0.1*	*0.1*	*0.1*	*0.1*	*0.1*	*0.1*
Sugars, preserves & confectionery	0.1	0.2	0.2	0.2	0.2	0.2	0.2
Beverages	0.1	0.1	0.1	0.1	0.1	0.1	0.1
Commercial infant foods & drinks	0.1	0.0	0.0	0.0	0.1	0.0	0.0
Miscellaneous	0.1	0.1	0.1	0.1	0.1	0.1	0.1
Average daily intake (mg)	**4.7**	**5.2**	**5.8**	**5.4**	**5.3**	**5.0**	**5.2**
Total number of children	**576**	**606**	**250**	**243**	**848**	**827**	**1675**

Table 9.10(b) Percentage contribution of food types to average daily non-haem iron intake by age and sex of child

Food types	Age and sex of child						
	All aged 1½ – 2½ years	All aged 2½ – 3½ years	All aged 3½ – 4½ years		All boys	All girls	All
			Boys	Girls			
	%	%	%	%	%	%	%
Cereals & cereal products	46	51	53	51	51	48	49
of which:							
white bread	7	9	10	10	8	9	8
wholemeal bread	4	3	4	3	3	4	3
high fibre breakfast cereals	11	11	11	8	12	10	11
other breakfast cereals	9	11	11	13	11	11	11
biscuits	5	6	6	5	6	5	5
Milk & milk products	10	7	6	6	8	8	8
of which:							
milk (whole, semi-skimmed, skimmed)	7	6	4	5	6	6	6
other milk & products	4	1	2	1	2	2	2
Eggs & egg dishes	3	3	3	3	2	3	3
Fat spreads	0	0	0	0	0	0	0
Meat & meat products	10	10	10	11	10	10	10
of which:							
beef, veal & dishes	3	3	3	3	3	3	3
liver & liver dishes	0	0	0	0	0	0	0
Fish & fish dishes	2	2	2	2	2	2	2
Vegetables, potatoes & savoury snacks	15	15	14	16	15	15	15
of which:							
vegetables	8	7	6	7	7	7	7
potatoes, fried	3	3	4	4	3	3	3
other potatoes	2	2	2	2	2	2	2
savoury snacks	2	2	2	2	2	2	2
Fruit & nuts	3	3	3	3	3	3	3
of which:							
fruit	3	3	2	2	2	3	3
Sugars, preserves & confectionery	3	4	4	4	4	4	4
Beverages	2	3	3	2	2	3	2
Commercial infant foods & drinks	2	0	0	0	1	1	1
Miscellaneous	3	2	2	2	2	3	2
Average daily intake (mg)	**4.7**	**5.2**	**5.8**	**5.4**	**5.3**	**5.0**	**5.2**
Total number of children	**576**	**606**	**250**	**243**	**848**	**827**	**1675**

Table 9.11 Average daily intake of calcium (mg) by age and sex of child

Calcium (mg)	Age and sex of child								
	All aged 1½ – 2½ years	All aged 2½ – 3½ years	All aged 3½ – 4½ years		All aged under 4 years	All aged 4 years and over	All boys	All girls	All
			Boys	Girls					
	cum %	cum %	cum %	cum %	cum %	cum %	cum %	cum %	cum %
Intakes from *food sources**									
Less than 200	1	1	0	0	1	0	1	1	1
Less than 275	4	4	2	3	4	2	3	4	4
Less than 350	11	11	10	10	11	10	10	12	11
Less than 450	21	23	24	26	23	24	21	26	23
Less than 550	36	41	42	44	39	42	38	41	40
Less than 650	52	59	58	64	57	60	55	59	57
Less than 750	68	73	71	80	72	73	70	74	72
Less than 1000	88	93	94	95	91	93	91	92	92
All	100	100	100	100	100	100	100	100	100
Base	*576*	*606*	*250*	*243*	*1457*	*218*	*848*	*827*	*1675*
Mean (average value)	663	635	625	595	640	620	650	624	637
Median value	639	598	598	584	609	602	616	602	606
Lower 2.5 percentile	244	237	281	247	245	262	265	233	246
Upper 2.5 percentile	1305	1294	1198	1099	1260	1216	1260	1232	1255
Standard error of the mean	11.4	10.5	14.3	13.6	6.8	15.5	8.7	8.8	6.2

*Dietary supplements provided negligible calcium for children in this survey.

Table 9.12 Average daily intake of calcium as a percentage of the Reference Nutrient Intake (RNI) by age and sex of child

Age and sex of child	Average daily intake from food sources* as % of RNI			
	Mean	*Median*	*se*	*Base*
All aged 1½–2½ years	189	182	3.2	*576*
All aged 2½–3½ years	181	171	3.0	*606*
Aged 3½–4½ years:**				
Boys	161	155	3.7	*250*
Girls	152	147	3.8	*243*
All aged under 4 years	183	174	1.9	*1457*
All aged 4 years and over	138	134	3.4	*218*
All boys	181	170	2.5	*848*
All girls	173	166	2.5	*827*
All	177	168	1.8	*1675*

*Dietary supplements provided negligible calcium for children in this survey.

**Calcium intake as a percentage of the RNI was calculated for each child; thus in this age group values for children under 4 years of age used 350mg/d as the RNI and for children aged 4 and over 450mg/d was taken as the RNI. The values for all children aged 3½ to 4½ years were then pooled to give a mean, median and standard error (se) for the age group.

Table 9.13(a) Contribution of food types to average daily calcium intake by age and sex of child

Food types	Age and sex of child						
	All aged 1½ – 2½ years	All aged 2½ – 3½ years	All aged 3½ – 4½ years		All boys	All girls	All
			Boys	Girls			
	mg	mg	mg	mg	mg	mg	mg
Cereals & cereal products	104	125	141	129	127	115	121
of which:							
all bread	*34*	*43*	*52*	*46*	*43*	*40*	*41*
breakfast cereals	*18*	*18*	*17*	*10*	*19*	*15*	*17*
Milk & milk products	462	400	368	354	416	403	410
of which:							
milk (whole, semi-skimmed, skimmed)	*371*	*320*	*289*	*277*	*335*	*318*	*327*
other milk & cream	*14*	*7*	*7*	*5*	*9*	*9*	*9*
cheese	*36*	*37*	*41*	*42*	*37*	*39*	*38*
yogurt & fromage frais	*41*	*36*	*30*	*30*	*35*	*37*	*36*
Eggs & egg dishes	5	7	6	7	5	7	6
Fat spreads	1	1	1	1	1	1	1
Meat & meat products	16	18	22	21	19	17	18
Fish & fish dishes	8	8	9	9	9	8	8
Vegetables, potatoes & savoury snacks	20	22	23	23	21	21	21
Fruit & nuts	6	6	6	6	6	7	6
of which:							
fruit	*6*	*6*	*5*	*6*	*6*	*6*	*6*
Sugars, preserves & confectionery	17	22	25	24	21	21	21
Beverages	13	17	19	16	17	15	16
Commercial infant foods & drinks	4	1	1	1	2	2	2
Miscellaneous	7	7	5	6	6	7	6
Average daily intake (mg)	**663**	**635**	**625**	**595**	**650**	**624**	**637**
Total number of children	**576**	**606**	**250**	**243**	**848**	**827**	**1675**

Table 9.13(b) Percentage contribution of food types to average daily calcium intake by age and sex of child

Food types	All aged 1½ – 2½ years	All aged 2½ – 3½ years	All aged 3½ – 4½ years Boys	All aged 3½ – 4½ years Girls	All boys	All girls	All
	%	%	%	%	%	%	%
Cereals & cereal products	16	20	23	22	19	18	19
of which:							
all bread	5	7	8	8	7	6	6
breakfast cereals	3	3	3	2	3	2	3
Milk & milk products	70	63	59	59	64	65	64
of which:							
milk (whole, semi-skimmed, skimmed)	56	50	46	46	51	51	51
other milk & cream	2	1	1	1	1	1	1
cheese	5	6	7	7	6	6	6
yogurt & fromage frais	6	6	5	5	5	6	6
Eggs & egg dishes	1	1	1	1	1	1	1
Fat spreads	0	0	0	0	0	0	0
Meat & meat products	2	3	3	3	3	3	3
Fish & fish dishes	1	1	1	1	1	1	1
Vegetables, potatoes & savoury snacks	3	3	4	4	3	3	3
Fruit & nuts	1	1	1	1	1	1	1
of which:							
fruit	1	1	1	1	1	1	1
Sugars, preserves & confectionery	3	3	4	4	3	3	3
Beverages	2	3	3	3	3	2	2
Commercial infant foods & drinks	1	0	0	0	0	0	0
Miscellaneous	1	1	1	1	1	1	1
Average daily intake (mg)	**663**	**635**	**625**	**595**	**650**	**624**	**637**
Total number of children	**576**	**606**	**250**	**243**	**848**	**827**	**1675**

Table 9.14 Average daily intake of phosphorus (mg) by age and sex of child

Phosphorus (mg)	All aged 1½ – 2½ years	All aged 2½ – 3½ years	All aged 3½ – 4½ years Boys	All aged 3½ – 4½ years Girls	All aged under 4 years	All aged 4 years and over	All boys	All girls	All
	cum %	cum %	cum %	cum %	cum %	cum %	cum %	cum %	cum %
Intakes from *food sources*									
Less than 270	1	0	0	0	1	0	0	1	0
Less than 350	3	2	1	1	2	1	1	3	2
Less than 500	14	13	9	10	13	8	10	14	12
Less than 700	46	47	41	47	46	42	43	49	46
Less than 900	80	80	75	80	79	77	77	81	79
Less than 1100	93	92	94	94	93	94	93	93	93
Less than 1300	98	98	99	99	98	99	98	98	98
All	100	100	100	100	100	100	100	100	100
Base	*576*	*606*	*250*	*243*	*1457*	*218*	*848*	*827*	*1675*
Mean (average value)	735	740	767	736	739	758	757	726	742
Median value	712	714	750	711	714	744	731	706	716
Lower 2.5 percentile	346	358	384	385	358	372	382	345	360
Upper 2.5 percentile	1246	1270	1207	1195	1245	1244	1254	1243	1244
Standard error of the mean	9.8	9.2	13.4	13.3	5.9	14.2	7.6	7.8	5.5

*Dietary supplements provided negligible phosphorus for children in this survey.

Table 9.15 Average daily intake of phosphorus as a percentage of the Reference Nutrient Intake (RNI) by age and sex of child

Age and sex of child	Average daily intake from food sources* as % of RNI			
	Mean	*Median*	*se*	*Base*
All aged 1½–2½ years	272	264	3.6	*576*
All aged 2½–3½ years	274	264	3.4	*606*
Aged 3½–4½ years:**				
Boys	257	248	4.8	*250*
Girls	243	232	4.9	*243*
All aged under 4 years	274	264	2.2	*1457*
All aged 4 years and over	216	213	4.1	*218*
All boys	272	263	2.8	*848*
All girls	260	254	2.9	*827*
All	266	259	2.0	*1675*

*Dietary supplements provided negligible phosphorus for children in this survey.

**Phosphorus intake as a percentage of the RNI was calculated for each child; thus in this age group values for children under 4 years of age used 270mg/d as the RNI and for children aged 4 and over 350mg/d was taken as the RNI. The values for all children aged 3½ to 4½ years were then pooled to give a mean, median and standard error (se) for the age group.

Table 9.16 Average daily intake of magnesium (mg) by age and sex of child

Magnesium (mg)	Age and sex of child								
	All aged 1½ – 2½ years	All aged 2½ – 3½ years	All aged 3½ – 4½ years		All aged under 4 years	All aged 4 years and over	All boys	All girls	All
			Boys	Girls					
	cum %	cum %	cum %	cum %	cum %	cum %	cum %	cum %	cum %
Intakes from *food sources*									
Less than 50	1	0	–	–	0	–	0	1	0
Less than 70	4	2	1	2	2	2	1	3	2
Less than 85	10	6	3	5	7	4	5	8	7
Less than 90	12	8	5	6	9	4	6	11	9
Less than 120	39	34	30	37	36	34	32	40	36
Less than 150	73	65	58	66	68	59	64	69	67
Less than 180	92	89	79	87	89	82	86	90	88
Less than 210	97	96	95	98	97	95	96	97	97
All	100	100	100	100	100	100	100	100	100
Base	*576*	*606*	*250*	*243*	*1457*	*218*	*848*	*827*	*1675*
Mean (average value)	132	137	146	137	136	143	140	133	136
Median value	130	133	141	134	132	139	135	130	133
Lower 2.5 percentile	62	73	81	77	71	75	76	65	71
Upper 2.5 percentile	221	223	228	207	200	225	224	214	221
Standard error of the mean	1.6	1.5	2.4	2.3	1.0	2.6	1.3	1.3	0.9

*None of the dietary supplements taken by children in this survey provided any magnesium.

Table 9.17 Average daily intake of magnesium as a percentage of the Reference Nutrient Intake (RNI) by age and sex of child

Age and sex of child	Average daily intake from food sources* as % of RNI			
	Mean	*Median*	*se*	*Base*
All aged 1½–2½ years	155	153	1.9	*576*
All aged 2½–3½ years	162	157	1.8	*606*
Aged 3½–4½ years:**				
Boys	150	145	2.8	*250*
Girls	138	135	2.8	*243*
All aged under 4 years	159	155	1.2	*1457*
All aged 4 years and over	119	116	2.1	*218*
All boys	159	154	1.5	*848*
All girls	150	146	1.6	*827*
All	154	151	1.1	*1675*

*None of the dietary supplements taken by children in this survey provided any magnesium.

**Magnesium intake as a percentage of the RNI was calculated for each child; thus in this age group values for children under 4 years of age used 85mg/d as the RNI and for children aged 4 and over 120mg/d was taken as the RNI. The values for all children aged 3½ to 4½ years were then pooled to give a mean, median and standard error (se) for the age group.

Table 9.18 Use of salt in cooking and at the table by sex of child

Use of salt at the table	Use of salt in cooking and sex of child					
	Salt added*		No salt used		All**	
	Boys	Girls	Boys	Girls	Boys	Girls
	%	%	%	%	%	%
Usually adds salt	6	7	6	6	6	7
Occasionally adds salt	12	13	11	10	12	12
Rarely or never adds salt	82	80	83	83	82	81
Base = 100%	*534*	*494*	*390*	*413*	*943*	*916*

*Includes 2% of cases where a salt alternative was used in cooking.
**Includes no answers and 16 cases where use of salt in cooking was variable.

Table 9.19 Use of salt in cooking and at the table by age of child

Use of salt at the table	Use of salt in cooking and age of child (years)								
	Salt added*			No salt used			All**		
	1½–2½	2½–3½	3½–4½	1½–2½	2½–3½	3½–4½	1½–2½	2½–3½	3½–4½
	%	%	%	%	%	%	%	%	%
Usually adds salt	5	8	6	3	6	9	4	8	7
Occasionally adds salt	8	12	18	6	14	14	7	13	16
Rarely or never adds salt	88	79	76	92	80	77	88	79	76
Base = 100%	*345*	*366*	*317*	*293*	*287*	*223*	*648*	*668*	*543*

*Includes 2% of cases where a salt alternative was used in cooking.
**Includes no answers and 16 cases where use of salt in cooking was variable.

Table 9.20 Average daily intake of sodium (mg) by age and sex of child

Sodium (mg)	Age and sex of child								
	All aged 1½ – 2½ years	All aged 2½ – 3½ years	All aged 3½ – 4½ years		All aged under 4 years	All aged 4 years and over	All boys	All girls	All
			Boys	Girls					
	cum %	cum %	cum %	cum %	cum %	cum %	cum %	cum %	cum %
Intakes from *food sources*									
Less than 200	–	–	–	–	–	–	–	–	–
Less than 280	0	0	–	–	0	–	0	0	0
Less than 500	0	0	0	–	0	0	0	0	0
Less than 700	4	1	0	1	2	0	2	2	2
Less than 1000	18	8	4	7	12	6	9	12	11
Less than 1300	48	33	23	23	37	25	33	38	35
Less than 1600	76	60	47	56	64	54	60	66	63
Less than 1900	90	82	74	76	84	75	82	83	83
Less than 2200	96	92	88	86	92	88	92	92	92
All	100	100	100	100	100	100	100	100	100
Base	*576*	*606*	*250*	*243*	*1457*	*218*	*848*	*827*	*1675*
Mean (average value)	1365	1528	1658	1632	1487	1633	1532	1480	1506
Median value	1323	1490	1645	1508	1441	1562	1497	1426	1459
Lower 2.5 percentile	655	751	914	877	733	903	737	746	742
Upper 2.5 percentile	2414	2662	2711	2802	2613	2820	2545	2661	2626
Standard error of the mean	18.4	18.7	28.6	31.9	12.3	32.3	16.0	16.5	11.5

*None of the dietary supplements taken by children in this survey provided any sodium.

Table 9.21 Average daily intake of chloride (mg) by age and sex of child

Chloride (mg)	Age and sex of child								
	All aged 1½ – 2½ years	All aged 2½ – 3½ years	All aged 3½ – 4½ years		All aged under 4 years	All aged 4 years and over	All boys	All girls	All
			Boys	Girls					
	cum %	cum %	cum %	cum %	cum %	cum %	cum %	cum %	cum %
Intakes from *food sources*									
Less than 800	1	0	0	–	0	0	0	1	0
Less than 1100	3	1	0	1	2	0	2	1	2
Less than 1500	18	9	7	7	12	7	10	13	11
Less than 1750	32	21	14	13	24	15	20	25	23
Less than 2000	49	35	27	26	39	28	35	40	37
Less than 2250	67	52	37	46	55	45	51	57	54
Less than 2500	81	67	54	62	71	59	66	72	69
Less than 3000	92	86	82	81	88	81	87	87	87
Less than 3250	96	92	88	86	92	88	91	92	92
All	100	100	100	100	100	100	100	100	100
Base	*576*	*606*	*250*	*243*	*1457*	*218*	*848*	*827*	*1675*
Mean (average value)	2069	2291	2464	2436	2237	2427	2299	2223	2261
Median value	2013	2231	2444	2287	2168	2339	2238	2154	2186
Lower 2.5 percentile	1053	1187	1341	1281	1141	1336	1146	1152	1153
Upper 2.5 percentile	3664	3978	4138	4087	3919	4044	3921	3900	3916
Standard error of the mean	27.5	27.7	42.8	47.0	18.2	47.4	23.8	24.4	17.1

*Dietary supplements provided negligible chloride for children in this survey.

Table 9.22 Average daily intake of sodium as a percentage of the Reference Nutrient Intake (RNI) by age and sex of child

Age and sex of child	Average daily intake from food sources* as % of RNI			
	Mean	*Median*	*se*	*Base*
All aged 1½–2½ years	273	265	3.7	*576*
All aged 2½–3½ years	305	298	3.7	*606*
Aged 3½–4½ years:**				
Boys	292	284	5.7	*250*
Girls	283	270	6.6	*243*
All aged under 4 years	297	288	2.4	*1457*
All aged 4 years and over	233	223	4.6	*218*
All boys	295	286	3.1	*848*
All girls	283	271	3.3	*827*
All	289	278	2.3	*1675*

*None of the dietary supplements taken by children in this survey provided any sodium.

**Sodium intake as a percentage of the RNI was calculated for each child; thus in this age group values for children under 4 years of age used 500mg/d as the RNI and for children aged 4 and over 700mg/d was taken as the RNI. The values for all children aged 3½ to 4½ years were then pooled to give a mean, median and standard error (se) for the age group.

Table 9.23 Average daily intake of chloride as a percentage of the Reference Nutrient Intake (RNI) by age and sex of child

Age and sex of child	Average daily intake from food sources* as % of RNI			
	Mean	*Median*	*se*	*Base*
All aged 1½–2½ years	258	252	3.4	*576*
All aged 2½–3½ years	286	279	3.5	*606*
Aged 3½–4½ years:**				
Boys	273	268	5.3	*250*
Girls	266	252	6.1	*243*
All aged under 4 years	280	271	2.3	*1457*
All aged 4 years and over	221	213	4.3	*218*
All boys	277	269	2.9	*848*
All girls	266	257	3.0	*827*
All	272	264	2.1	*1675*

*Dietary supplements provided negligible chloride for children in this survey.

**Chloride intake as a percentage of the RNI was calculated for each child; thus in this age group values for children under 4 years of age used 800mg/d as the RNI and for children aged 4 and over 1100mg/d was taken as the RNI. The values for all children aged 3½ to 4½ years were then pooled to give a mean, median and standard error (se) for the age group.

Table 9.24 Average daily intake of potassium (mg) by age and sex of child

Potassium (mg)	Age and sex of child								
	All aged 1½ – 2½ years	All aged 2½ – 3½ years	All aged 3½ – 4½ years		All aged under 4 years	All aged 4 years and over	All boys	All girls	All
			Boys	Girls					
	cum %	cum %	cum %	cum %	cum %	cum %	cum %	cum %	cum %
Intakes from *food sources**									
Less than 450	0	0	–	–	0	–	0	0	0
Less than 600	1	1	1	–	1	1	1	1	1
Less than 800	3	3	4	2	3	3	2	4	3
Less than 1100	17	16	10	16	16	11	12	19	15
Less than 1400	46	43	34	43	43	38	40	45	43
Less than 1700	74	71	68	72	72	66	71	73	72
Less than 2000	91	87	83	86	88	83	87	88	88
Less than 2300	96	85	95	98	96	95	96	96	96
All	100	100	100	100	100	100	100	100	100
Base	*576*	*606*	*250*	*243*	*1457*	*218*	*848*	*827*	*1675*
Mean (average value)	1476	1513	1573	1501	1498	1571	1534	1480	1508
Median value	1431	1486	1531	1459	1464	1543	1493	1454	1475
Lower 2.5 percentile	716	760	784	807	761	794	809	721	762
Upper 2.5 percentile	2466	2538	2555	2268	2473	2519	2513	2461	2478
Standard error of the mean	17.7	17.9	26.6	25.3	11.2	28.3	14.3	15.2	10.4

*None of the dietary supplements taken by children in this survey provided any potassium.

Table 9.25   Average daily intake of potassium as a percentage of the Reference Nutrient Intake (RNI) by age and sex of child

Age and sex of child	Average daily intake from food sources* as % of RNI			
	Mean	*Median*	*se*	*Base*
All aged 1½–2½ years	184	179	2.2	*576*
All aged 2½–3½ years	189	186	2.2	*606*
Aged 3½–4½ years:**				
Boys	174	171	3.2	*250*
Girls	163	156	3.2	*243*
All aged under 4 years	187	183	1.4	*1457*
All aged 4 years and over	143	140	2.6	*218*
All boys	185	180	1.8	*848*
All girls	178	174	1.9	*827*
All	181	178	1.3	*1675*

  *None of the dietary supplements taken by children in this survey provided any potassium.

 **Potassium intake as a percentage of the RNI was calculated for each child; thus in this age group values for children under 4 years of age used 800mg/d as the RNI and for children aged 4 and over 1100mg/d was taken as the RNI. The values for all children aged 3½ to 4½ years were then pooled to give a mean, median and standard error (se) for the age group.

Table 9.26   Average daily intake of zinc (mg) by age and sex of child

Zinc (mg)	Age and sex of child								
	All aged 1½–2½ years	All aged 2½–3½ years	All aged 3½–4½ years		All aged under 4 years	All aged 4 years and over	All boys	All girls	All
			Boys	Girls					
	cum %	cum %	cum %	cum %	cum %	cum %	cum %	cum %	cum %
Intakes from *food sources*									
Less than 3.0	15	14	10	14	14	11	11	17	14
Less than 4.0	45	43	37	42	44	37	41	44	43
Less than 5.0	76	72	64	69	72	65	70	73	71
Less than 6.0	90	88	82	86	88	82	85	89	87
Less than 6.5	93	92	90	92	93	89	91	93	92
Less than 7.0	96	95	94	94	95	93	95	95	95
All	100	100	100	100	100	100	100	100	100
Base	*576*	*606*	*250*	*243*	*1457*	*218*	*848*	*827*	*1675*
Mean (average value)	4.3	4.4	4.7	4.4	4.4	4.6	4.5	4.3	4.4
Median value	4.1	4.2	4.6	4.2	4.2	4.4	4.2	4.2	4.2
Lower 2.5 percentile	2.0	2.2	2.2	2.2	2.2	2.2	2.2	2.0	2.2
Upper 2.5 percentile	7.7	7.6	8.1	8.4	7.8	8.0	7.9	7.7	7.8
Standard error of the mean	0.06	0.06	0.09	0.09	0.04	0.10	0.05	0.05	0.03

*Dietary supplements provided negligible zinc for children in this survey.

Table 9.27 Average daily intake of zinc as a percentage of the Reference Nutrient Intake (RNI) by age and sex of child

Age and sex of child	Average daily intake from food sources* as % of RNI			
	Mean	*Median*	*se*	*Base*
All aged 1½–2½ years	86	83	1.1	576
All aged 2½–3½ years	87	84	1.1	606
Aged 3½–4½ years:**				
Boys	84	79	1.7	250
Girls	79	74	1.8	243
All aged under 4 years	87	84	0.7	1457
All aged 4 years and over	71	68	1.5	218
All boys	87	83	0.9	848
All girls	83	80	1.0	827
All	85	82	0.7	1675

*Dietary supplements provided negligible zinc for children in this survey.

**Zinc intake as a percentage of the RNI was calculated for each child; thus in this age group values for children under 4 years of age used 5.0mg/d as the RNI and for children aged 4 and over 6.5mg/d was taken as the RNI. The values for all children aged 3½ to 4½ years were then pooled to give a mean, median and standard error (se) for the age group.

Table 9.28 Average daily intake of copper (mg) by age and sex of child

Copper (mg)	Age and sex of child								
	All aged 1½–2½ years	All aged 2½–3½ years	All aged 3½–4½ years		All aged under 4 years	All aged 4 years and over	All boys	All girls	All
			Boys	Girls					
	cum %	cum %	cum %	cum %	cum %	cum %	cum %	cum %	cum %
Intakes from *food sources*									
Less than 0.3	20	9	5	7	13	5	10	13	12
Less than 0.4	47	32	21	25	36	22	31	38	34
Less than 0.5	72	59	42	53	63	44	56	64	60
Less than 0.6	85	80	68	76	81	68	77	82	79
Less than 0.7	92	90	84	90	91	85	88	91	90
All	100	100	100	100	100	100	100	100	100
Base	576	606	250	243	1457	218	848	827	1675
Mean (average value)	0.4	0.5	0.5	0.5	0.5	0.5	0.5	0.5	0.5
Median value	0.4	0.5	0.5	0.5	0.4	0.5	0.5	0.4	0.4
Lower 2.5 percentile	0.2	0.2	0.2	0.2	0.2	0.2	0.2	0.2	0.2
Upper 2.5 percentile	0.9	0.9	1.1	0.9	0.9	1.0	0.9	0.9	0.9
Standard error of the mean	0.01	0.01	0.01	0.01	0.00	0.01	0.01	0.01	0.00

*Dietary supplements provided negligible copper for children in this survey.

Table 9.29 Average daily intake of copper as a percentage of the Reference Nutrient Intake (RNI) by age and sex of child

Age and sex of child	Average daily intake from food sources*, as % of RNI			
	Mean	*Median*	*se*	*Base*
All aged 1½–2½ years	110	102	1.8	*576*
All aged 2½–3½ years	124	117	2.0	*606*
Aged 3½–4½ years:**				
Boys	117	110	2.8	*250*
Girls	107	101	2.6	*243*
All aged under 4 years	119	112	1.2	*1457*
All aged 4 years and over	90	87	2.2	*218*
All boys	119	112	1.5	*848*
All girls	112	104	1.7	*827*
All	116	109	1.1	*1675*

*Dietary supplements provided negligible copper for children in this survey.

**Copper intake as a percentage of the RNI was calculated for each child; thus in this age group values for children under 4 years of age used 0.4mg/d as the RNI and for children aged 4 and over 0.6mg/d was taken as the RNI. The values for all children aged 3½ to 4½ years were then pooled to give a mean, median and standard error (se) for the age group.

Table 9.30 Average daily intake of iodine (µg) by age and sex of child

Iodine (µg)	Age and sex of child								
	All aged 1½ – 2½ years	All aged 2½ – 3½ years	All aged 3½ – 4½ years		All aged under 4 years	All aged 4 years and over	All boys	All girls	All
			Boys	Girls					
	cum %	cum %	cum %	cum %	cum %	cum %	cum %	cum %	cum %
Intakes from *food sources*									
Less than 40	3	3	2	2	3	1	2	3	3
Less than 50	8	8	6	6	8	5	7	8	7
Less than 70	24	24	18	27	24	21	21	26	23
Less than 100	49	50	41	50	48	46	46	50	48
Less than 130	67	69	64	69	68	65	66	69	68
Less than 160	76	80	79	80	79	77	78	79	78
Less than 190	83	87	88	88	86	87	86	86	86
Less than 210	88	91	93	93	90	93	91	90	90
All	100	100	100	100	100	100	100	100	100
Base	*576*	*606*	*250*	*243*	*1457*	*218*	*848*	*827*	*1675*
Mean (average value)	123	117	121	113	119	119	120	118	119
Median value	101	101	111	102	103	108	106	100	104
Lower 2.5 percentile	38	36	40	40	37	45	41	37	38
Upper 2.5 percentile	322	296	246	246	297	265	288	297	290
Standard error of the mean	3.0	2.6	3.6	3.6	1.7	4.0	2.2	2.3	1.6

*None of the dietary supplements taken by children in this survey provided any iodine.

Table 9.31 Average daily intake of iodine as a percentage of the Reference Nutrient Intake (RNI) by age and sex of child

Age and sex of child	Average daily intake from food sources* as % of RNI			
	Mean	Median	se	Base
All aged 1½–2½ years	175	145	4.3	576
All aged 2½–3½ years	168	145	3.8	606
Aged 3½–4½ years:**				
Boys	151	138	4.6	250
Girls	139	126	4.8	243
All aged under 4 years	170	147	2.5	1457
All aged 4 years and over	119	108	4.0	218
All boys	165	143	3.1	848
All girls	162	139	3.3	827
All	164	141	2.3	1675

*None of the dietary supplements taken by children in this survey provided any iodine.

**Iodine intake as a percentage of the RNI was calculated for each child; thus in this age group values for children under 4 years of age used 70µg/d as the RNI and for children aged 4 and over 100µg/d was taken as the RNI. The values for all children aged 3½ to 4½ years were then pooled to give a mean, median and standard error (se) for the age group.

Table 9.32 Average daily intake of manganese (mg) by age and sex of child

Manganese (mg)	Age and sex of child						
	All aged 1½ – 2½ years	All aged 2½ – 3½ years	All aged 3½ – 4½ years		All boys	All girls	All
			Boys	Girls			
	cum %	cum %	cum %	cum %	cum %	cum %	cum %
Intakes from *food sources*							
Less than 0.4	2	1	–	–	1	1	1
Less than 0.8	26	19	12	15	17	22	20
Less than 1.2	63	55	44	52	52	60	56
Less than 1.6	85	78	70	77	77	81	79
Less than 2.0	93	90	84	90	88	92	90
All	100	100	100	100	100	100	100
Base	576	606	250	243	848	827	1675
Mean (average value)	1.1	1.2	1.4	1.3	1.3	1.2	1.2
Median value	1.0	1.1	1.3	1.1	1.2	1.1	1.1
Lower 2.5 percentile	0.4	0.5	0.6	0.5	0.5	0.5	0.5
Upper 2.5 percentile	2.5	2.4	2.7	2.7	2.5	2.5	2.5
Standard error of the mean	0.02	0.02	0.03	0.03	0.02	0.02	0.01

*Dietary supplements provided negligible manganese for children in this survey.

Table 9.33(a)   Contribution of food types to average daily phosphorus intake by age and sex of child

Food types	Age and sex of child						
	All aged 1½ – 2½ years	All aged 2½ – 3½ years	All aged 3½ – 4½ years		All boys	All girls	All
			Boys	Girls			
	mg	mg	mg	mg	mg	mg	mg
Cereals & cereal products	138	164	187	170	167	151	159
of which:							
white & wholemeal bread	*40*	*48*	*57*	*51*	*49*	*45*	*47*
breakfast cereals	*35*	*38*	*42*	*32*	*41*	*33*	*37*
Milk & milk products	374	323	299	287	338	325	332
of which:							
milk (whole, semi-skimmed, skimmed)	*296*	*255*	*230*	*220*	*267*	*253*	*260*
other milk & products	*78*	*68*	*68*	*67*	*71*	*72*	*71*
Eggs & egg dishes	15	17	17	20	15	19	17
Fat spreads	1	2	2	2	2	2	2
Meat & meat products	76	87	106	101	89	87	88
Fish & fish dishes	19	20	22	21	20	20	20
Vegetables, potatoes & savoury snacks	56	64	68	69	64	61	62
Fruit & nuts	11	12	13	12	12	12	12
Sugars, preserves & confectionery	17	22	24	24	21	21	21
Beverages	12	18	21	19	18	16	17
Commercial infant foods & drinks	3	1	0	0	1	1	1
Miscellaneous	12	11	8	10	10	11	11
Average daily intake (mg)	**735**	**740**	**767**	**736**	**757**	**726**	**742**
Total number of children	**576**	**606**	**250**	**243**	**848**	**827**	**1675**

Table 9.33(b)   Percentage contribution of food types to average daily phosphorus intake by age and sex of child

Food types	Age and sex of child						
	All aged 1½ – 2½ years	All aged 2½ – 3½ years	All aged 3½ – 4½ years		All boys	All girls	All
			Boys	Girls			
	%	%	%	%	%	%	%
Cereals & cereal products	19	22	24	23	22	21	21
of which:							
white & wholemeal bread	*5*	*6*	*7*	*7*	*6*	*6*	*6*
breakfast cereals	*5*	*5*	*5*	*4*	*5*	*4*	*5*
Milk & milk products	51	44	39	39	45	45	45
of which:							
milk (whole, semi-skimmed, skimmed)	*40*	*34*	*30*	*30*	*35*	*35*	*35*
other milk & products	*11*	*9*	*9*	*9*	*9*	*10*	*10*
Eggs & egg dishes	2	2	2	3	2	3	2
Fat spreads	0	0	0	0	0	0	0
Meat & meat products	10	12	14	14	12	12	12
Fish & fish dishes	3	3	3	3	3	3	3
Vegetables, potatoes & savoury snacks	8	9	9	9	8	8	8
Fruit & nuts	1	2	2	2	2	2	2
Sugars, preserves & confectionery	2	3	3	3	3	3	3
Beverages	2	2	2	3	2	2	2
Commercial infant foods & drinks	0	0	0	0	0	0	0
Miscellaneous	2	1	1	1	1	1	1
Average daily intake (mg)	**735**	**740**	**767**	**736**	**757**	**726**	**742**
Total number of children	**576**	**606**	**250**	**243**	**848**	**827**	**1675**

Table 9.34(a)   Contribution of food types to average daily magnesium intake by age and sex of child

Food types	Age and sex of child						
	All aged 1½ – 2½ years	All aged 2½ – 3½ years	All aged 3½ – 4½ years		All boys	All girls	All
			Boys	Girls			
	mg	mg	mg	mg	mg	mg	mg
Cereals & cereal products	36	41	46	41	42	38	40
of which:							
white & wholemeal bread	*10*	*11*	*13*	*13*	*11*	*11*	*11*
breakfast cereals	*12*	*13*	*14*	*10*	*14*	*11*	*12*
Milk & milk products	42	36	33	32	38	36	37
of which:							
milk (whole, semi-skimmed, skimmed)	*35*	*30*	*28*	*26*	*32*	*30*	*31*
other milk & products	*7*	*6*	*5*	*5*	*6*	*6*	*6*
Eggs & egg dishes	1	1	1	1	1	1	1
Fat spreads	0	0	0	0	0	0	0
Meat & meat products	8	9	11	10	10	9	9
Fish & fish dishes	2	2	2	3	2	2	2
Vegetables, potatoes & savoury snacks	18	20	22	22	20	20	20
Fruit & nuts	9	9	9	8	9	9	9
Sugars, preserves & confectionery	4	6	6	6	5	5	5
Beverages	8	9	11	9	9	9	9
Commercial infant foods & drinks	1	0	0	0	0	0	0
Miscellaneous	3	2	2	3	2	3	3
Average daily intake (mg)	**132**	**137**	**146**	**137**	**140**	**133**	**136**
Total number of children	**576**	**606**	**250**	**243**	**848**	**827**	**1675**

Table 9.34(b)   Percentage contribution of food types to average daily magnesium intake by age and sex of child

Food types	Age and sex of child						
	All aged 1½ – 2½ years	All aged 2½ – 3½ years	All aged 3½ – 4½ years		All boys	All girls	All
			Boys	Girls			
	%	%	%	%	%	%	%
Cereals & cereal products	27	30	32	30	30	28	29
of which:							
white & wholemeal bread	*7*	*8*	*9*	*9*	*8*	*8*	*8*
breakfast cereals	*9*	*9*	*9*	*8*	*10*	*8*	*9*
Milk & milk products	32	26	23	23	27	27	27
of which:							
milk (whole, semi-skimmed, skimmed)	*27*	*22*	*19*	*19*	*23*	*23*	*23*
other milk & products	*5*	*4*	*4*	*4*	*4*	*4*	*4*
Eggs & egg dishes	1	1	1	1	1	1	1
Fat spreads	0	0	0	0	0	0	0
Meat & meat products	6	7	8	8	7	7	7
Fish & fish dishes	2	2	2	2	2	2	2
Vegetables, potatoes & savoury snacks	14	15	15	16	15	15	15
Fruit & nuts	7	6	6	6	6	6	6
Sugars, preserves & confectionery	3	4	4	4	4	4	4
Beverages	6	7	8	7	7	7	7
Commercial infant foods & drinks	1	0	0	0	0	0	0
Miscellaneous	2	2	1	2	2	2	2
Average daily intake (mg)	**131**	**137**	**146**	**137**	**140**	**133**	**136**
Total number of children	**576**	**606**	**250**	**243**	**848**	**827**	**1675**

Table 9.35(a)   Contribution of food types to average daily potassium intake by age and sex of child

Food types	Age and sex of child						
	All aged 1½ – 2½ years	All aged 2½ – 3½ years	All aged 3½ – 4½ years		All boys	All girls	All
			Boys	Girls			
	mg	mg	mg	mg	mg	mg	mg
Cereals & cereal products	184	219	249	230	223	203	213
Milk & milk products	533	457	413	395	477	458	467
of which:							
milk (whole, semi-skimmed, skimmed)	*453*	*393*	*355*	*341*	*411*	*390*	*400*
other milk & products	*80*	*64*	*57*	*54*	*66*	*68*	*67*
Eggs & egg dishes	10	12	12	13	10	13	12
Fat spreads	2	2	3	3	3	2	2
Meat & meat products	104	120	144	133	123	118	120
Fish & fish dishes	27	28	29	29	29	27	28
Vegetables, potatoes & savoury snacks	305	360	396	405	357	349	353
of which:							
vegetables	*79*	*86*	*85*	*91*	*84*	*84*	*84*
potatoes, fried	*113*	*139*	*165*	*168*	*145*	*131*	*138*
other potatoes	*66*	*65*	*70*	*77*	*64*	*71*	*68*
savoury snacks	*46*	*70*	*75*	*68*	*63*	*62*	*62*
Fruit & nuts	121	120	120	109	119	118	118
Sugars, preserves & confectionery	32	42	48	46	41	39	40
Beverages	113	117	129	104	117	114	115
Commercial infant foods & drinks	13	5	1	0	5	8	7
Miscellaneous	31	30	28	33	29	32	30
Average daily intake (mg)	**1476**	**1513**	**1573**	**1501**	**1534**	**1480**	**1508**
Total number of children	**576**	**606**	**250**	**243**	**848**	**827**	**1675**

Table 9.35(b)   Percentage contribution of food types to average daily potassium intake by age and sex of child

Food types	Age and sex of child						
	All aged 1½ – 2½ years	All aged 2½ – 3½ years	All aged 3½ – 4½ years		All boys	All girls	All
			Boys	Girls			
	%	%	%	%	%	%	%
Cereals & cereal products	12	14	16	15	15	14	14
Milk & milk products	37	30	26	26	31	31	31
of which:							
milk (whole, semi-skimmed, skimmed)	*31*	*26*	*23*	*23*	*27*	*26*	*27*
other milk & products	*5*	*4*	*4*	*4*	*4*	*5*	*4*
Eggs & egg dishes	1	1	1	1	1	1	1
Fat spreads	0	0	0	0	0	0	0
Meat & meat products	7	8	9	9	8	8	8
Fish & fish dishes	2	2	2	2	2	2	2
Vegetables, potatoes & savoury snacks	21	24	25	27	23	24	23
of which:							
vegetables	*5*	*6*	*5*	*6*	*5*	*6*	*6*
potatoes, fried	*8*	*9*	*10*	*11*	*9*	*9*	*9*
other potatoes	*4*	*4*	*4*	*5*	*4*	*5*	*4*
savoury snacks	*3*	*5*	*5*	*5*	*4*	*4*	*4*
Fruit & nuts	8	8	8	7	8	8	8
Sugars, preserves & confectionery	2	3	3	3	3	3	3
Beverages	8	8	8	7	8	8	8
Commercial infant foods & drinks	1	0	0	0	0	0	0
Miscellaneous	2	2	2	2	2	2	2
Average daily intake (mg)	**1476**	**1513**	**1573**	**1501**	**1534**	**1480**	**1508**
Total number of children	**576**	**606**	**250**	**243**	**848**	**827**	**1675**

205

Table 9.36(a) Contribution of food types to average daily zinc intake by age and sex of child

Food types	Age and sex of child						
	All aged 1½ – 2½ years	All aged 2½ – 3½ years	All aged 3½ – 4½ years		All boys	All girls	All
			Boys	Girls			
	mg	mg	mg	mg	mg	mg	mg
Cereals & cereal products	0.9	1.0	1.2	1.1	1.1	1.0	1.0
of which:							
white & wholemeal bread	*0.2*	*0.3*	*0.3*	*0,3*	*0,3*	*0,3*	*0.3*
breakfast cereals	*0.2*	*0.3*	*0.3*	*0.3*	*0.3*	*0.2*	*0.3*
biscuits	*0.1*	*0.1*	*0.1*	*0.1*	*0.1*	*0.1*	*0.1*
Milk & milk products	1.6	1.4	1.3	1.2	1.5	1.4	1.4
of which:							
milk (whole, semi-skimmed, skimmed)	*1.3*	*1.1*	*1.0*	*0.9*	*1.1*	*1.1*	*1.1*
other milk & products	*0.4*	*0.3*	*0.3*	*0.3*	*0.3*	*0.3*	*0.3*
Eggs & egg dishes	0.1	0.1	0.1	0.1	0.1	0.1	0.1
Fat spreads	0.0	0.0	0.0	0.0	0.0	0.0	0.0
Meat & meat products	1.0	1.1	1.3	1.2	1.1	1.1	1.1
of which:							
beef, veal & dishes	*0.4*	*0.4*	*0,4*	*0.4*	*0.4*	*0.4*	*0.4*
all chicken	*0.1*	*0.1*	*0.1*	*0.1*	*0.1*	*0.1*	*0.1*
burgers & kebabs	*0.1*	*0.1*	*0.2*	*0.1*	*0.1*	*0.1*	*0.1*
sausages	*0.1*	*0.1*	*0.1*	*0.1*	*0.1*	*0.1*	*0.1*
Vegetables, potatoes & savoury snacks	0.3	0.4	0.4	0.4	0.4	0.4	0.4
Fruit & nuts	0.1	0.1	0.1	0.1	0.1	0.1	0.1
Sugars, preserves & confectionery	0.1	0.1	0.1	0.1	0.1	0.1	0.1
Beverages	0.0	0.0	0.0	0.0	0.0	0.0	0.0
Commercial infant foods & drinks	0.0	0.0	0.0	0.0	0.0	0.0	0.0
Miscellaneous	0.1	0.0	0.0	0.0	0.0	0.1	0.0
Average daily intake (mg)	**4.3**	**4.4**	**4.7**	**4.4**	**4.5**	**4.3**	**4.4**
Total number of children	**576**	**606**	**250**	**243**	**848**	**827**	**1675**

Table 9.36(b) Percentage contribution of food types to average daily zinc intake by age and sex of child

Food types	Age and sex of child						
	All aged 1½ – 2½ years	All aged 2½ – 3½ years	All aged 3½ – 4½ years		All boys	All girls	All
			Boys	Girls			
	%	%	%	%	%	%	%
Cereals & cereal products	21	23	26	25	24	22	23
of which:							
white & wholemeal bread	*6*	*6*	*7*	*7*	*6*	*6*	*6*
breakfast cereals	*6*	*6*	*7*	*6*	*7*	*6*	*6*
biscuits	*2*	*2*	*3*	*2*	*2*	*2*	*2*
Milk & milk products	38	32	28	28	32	33	33
of which:							
milk (whole, semi-skimmed, skimmed)	*30*	*25*	*21*	*21*	*26*	*25*	*25*
other milk & products	*8*	*0*	*6*	*6*	*7*	*7*	*7*
Eggs & egg dishes	2	2	2	3	2	3	2
Fat spreads	0	0	0	0	0	0	0
Meat & meat products	23	25	28	27	25	25	25
of which:							
beef, veal & dishes	*9*	*9*	*8*	*8*	*8*	*9*	*9*
all chicken	*2*	*2*	*3*	*2*	*2*	*2*	*2*
burgers & kebabs	*2*	*2*	*4*	*3*	*3*	*2*	*3*
sausages	*3*	*3*	*3*	*3*	*3*	*3*	*3*
Vegetables, potatoes & savoury snacks	8	9	9	9	8	9	9
Fruit & nuts	2	2	2	2	2	2	2
Sugars, preserves & confectionery	2	2	3	3	2	2	2
Beverages	1	0	1	1	1	1	1
Commercial infant foods & drinks	0	0	0	0	0	0	0
Miscellaneous	1	1	1	1	1	1	1
Average daily intake (mg)	**4.3**	**4.4**	**4.7**	**4.4**	**4.5**	**4.3**	**4.4**
Total number of children	**576**	**606**	**250**	**243**	**848**	**827**	**1675**

Table 9.37(a) Contribution of food types to average daily copper intake by age and sex of child

Food types	Age and sex of child						
	All aged 1½ – 2½ years	All aged 2½ – 3½ years	All aged 3½ – 4½ years		All boys	All girls	All
			Boys	Girls			
	mg	mg	mg	mg	mg	mg	mg
Cereals & cereal products	0.17	0.20	0.22	0.20	0.20	0.18	0.19
of which:							
white & wholemeal bread	*0.05*	*0.06*	*0.07*	*0.06*	*0.06*	*0.05*	*0.06*
breakfast cereals	*0.05*	*0.05*	*0.05*	*0.04*	*0.05*	*0.04*	*0.05*
biscuits	*0.02*	*0.03*	*0.03*	*0.02*	*0.03*	*0.02*	*0.02*
Milk & milk products	0.02	0.01	0.01	0.01	0.01	0.01	0.01
Eggs & egg dishes	0.01	0.01	0.01	0.01	0.01	0.01	0.01
Fat spreads	0.00	0.00	0.00	0.00	0.00	0.00	0.00
Meat & meat products	0.08	0.09	0.10	0.09	0.09	0.09	0.09
of which:							
beef, veal & dishes	*0.02*	*0.02*	*0.02*	*0.02*	*0.02*	*0.02*	*0.02*
all chicken	*0.01*	*0.01*	*0.01*	*0.01*	*0.01*	*0.01*	*0.01*
burgers & kebabs	*0.01*	*0.01*	*0.01*	*0.01*	*0.01*	*0.01*	*0.01*
sausages	*0.01*	*0.01*	*0.01*	*0.02*	*0.01*	*0.01*	*0.01*
meat pies etc.	*0.01*	*0.01*	*0.01*	*0.01*	*0.01*	*0.01*	*0.01*
Fish & fish dishes	0.01	0.01	0.01	0.01	0.01	0.01	0.01
Vegetables, potatoes & savoury snacks	0.07	0.08	0.09	0.09	0.08	0.08	0.08
of which:							
all potatoes	*0.04*	*0.05*	*0.05*	*0.06*	*0.05*	*0.05*	*0.05*
Fruit & nuts	0.05	0.05	0.06	0.05	0.05	0.05	0.05
Sugars, preserves & confectionery	0.02	0.03	0.04	0.03	0.03	0.03	0.03
Beverages	0.00	0.00	0.00	0.00	0.00	0.00	0.00
Commercial infant foods & drinks	0.00	0.00	0.00	0.00	0.00	0.00	0.00
Miscellaneous	0.02	0.02	0.02	0.02	0.02	0.02	0.02
Average daily intake (mg)	**0.4**	**0.5**	**0.5**	**0.5**	**0.5**	**0.5**	**0.5**
Total number of children	**576**	**606**	**250**	**243**	**848**	**827**	**1675**

Table 9.37(b) Percentage contribution of food types to average daily copper intake by age and sex of child

Food types	Age and sex of child						
	All aged 1½ – 2½ years	All aged 2½ – 3½ years	All aged 3½ – 4½ years		All boys	All girls	All
			Boys	Girls			
	%	%	%	%	%	%	%
Cereals & cereal products	39	40	40	39	40	38	39
of which:							
white & wholemeal bread	*11*	*12*	*13*	*12*	*12*	*11*	*12*
breakfast cereals	*11*	*10*	*9*	*8*	*10*	*8*	*10*
biscuits	*4*	*6*	*5*	*4*	*6*	*4*	*4*
Milk & milk products	4	2	2	2	2	2	2
Eggs & egg dishes	2	2	2	2	2	2	2
Fat spreads	0	0	0	0	0	0	0
Meat & meat products	18	18	18	18	18	19	18
of which:							
beef, veal & dishes	*4*	*4*	*4*	*4*	*4*	*4*	*4*
all chicken	*2*	*2*	*2*	*2*	*2*	*2*	*2*
burgers & kebabs	*2*	*2*	*2*	*2*	*2*	*2*	*2*
sausages	*2*	*2*	*2*	*4*	*2*	*2*	*2*
meat pies etc.	*2*	*2*	*2*	*2*	*2*	*2*	*2*
Fish & fish dishes	2	2	2	2	2	2	2
Vegetables, potatoes & savoury snacks	16	16	16	18	16	17	16
of which:							
all potatoes	*9*	*10*	*9*	*12*	*10*	*11*	*10*
Fruit & nuts	11	12	11	10	10	11	10
Sugars, preserves & confectionery	4	6	7	6	6	6	6
Beverages	0	0	0	0	0	0	0
Commercial infant foods & drinks	0	0	0	0	0	2	0
Miscellaneous	4	4	4	4	4	4	4
Average daily intake (mg)	**0.4**	**0.5**	**0.5**	**0.5**	**0.5**	**0.5**	**0.5**
Total number of children	**576**	**606**	**250**	**243**	**848**	**827**	**1675**

Table 9.38(a) Contribution of food types to average daily iodine intake by age and sex of child

Food types	Age and sex of child						
	All aged 1½ – 2½ years	All aged 2½ – 3½ years	All aged 3½ – 4½ years		All boys	All girls	All
			Boys	Girls			
	µg	µg	µg	µg	µg	µg	µg
Cereals & cereal products	12	14	17	15	15	13	14
Milk & milk products	79	67	64	60	70	69	70
of which:							
milk (whole, semi-skimmed, skimmed)	*63*	*54*	*52*	*48*	*57*	*55*	*56*
other milk & products	*15*	*13*	*12*	*11*	*13*	*14*	*14*
Eggs & egg dishes	4	4	4	5	4	5	4
Fat spreads	1	2	2	2	2	2	2
Meat & meat products	4	4	5	5	5	4	4
Fish & fish dishes	9	9	10	10	10	9	9
Vegetables, potatoes & savoury snacks	3	3	4	4	3	3	3
Fruit & nuts	2	2	2	1	2	2	2
Sugars, preserves & confectionery	2	3	3	3	3	3	3
Beverages	4	5	7	6	5	5	5
Commercial infant foods & drinks	0	0	0	0	0	0	0
Miscellaneous	2	2	2	2	2	2	2
Average daily intake (µg)	**123**	**117**	**121**	**113**	**120**	**118**	**119**
Total number of children	**576**	**606**	**250**	**243**	**848**	**827**	**1675**

Table 9.38(b) Percentage contribution of food types to average daily iodine intake by age and sex of child

Food types	Age and sex of child						
	All aged 1½ – 2½ years	All aged 2½ – 3½ years	All aged 3½ – 4½ years		All boys	All girls	All
			Boys	Girls			
	%	%	%	%	%	%	%
Cereals & cereal products	10	12	14	13	12	11	12
Milk & milk products	64	57	53	53	58	59	58
of which:							
milk (whole, semi-skimmed, skimmed)	*51*	*46*	*43*	*43*	*47*	*47*	*47*
other milk & products	*13*	*11*	*10*	*10*	*11*	*12*	*11*
Eggs & egg dishes	3	4	4	4	3	4	3
Fat spreads	1	2	2	2	2	1	2
Meat & meat products	3	4	4	4	4	4	4
Fish & fish dishes	7	8	9	8	8	8	8
Vegetables, potatoes & savoury snacks	2	3	3	3	3	3	3
Fruit & nuts	1	1	1	1	1	1	1
Sugars, preserves & confectionery	2	2	2	3	2	2	2
Beverages	3	4	5	5	4	4	4
Commercial infant foods & drinks	0	0	0	0	0	0	0
Miscellaneous	2	2	1	2	2	2	2
Average daily intake (µg)	**123**	**117**	**121**	**113**	**120**	**118**	**119**
Total number of children	**576**	**606**	**250**	**243**	**848**	**827**	**1675**

Table 9.39 Average daily mineral intakes by whether child was reported as being unwell during four-day dietary recording period

| Minerals | Whether child reported as being unwell during four–day period | | | | | | | | |
| | Unwell, eating affected | | | Unwell, eating not affected | | | Not unwell | | |
	Mean	Median	se	Mean	Median	se	Mean	Median	se
Intakes from *all sources*									
Iron (mg)	5.2	4.8	0.18	5.2	5.0	0.14	5.7	5.4	0.07
Haem iron (mg)*	0.2	0.2	0.01	0.2	0.2	0.01	0.3	0.2	0.01
Non-haem iron (mg)	5.0	4.6	0.17	5.1	4.8	0.14	5.5	5.2	0.07
Calcium (mg)**	593	576	14.8	634	606	18.9	648	613	7.3
Phosphorus (mg)**	676	660	13.8	734	701	15.9	757	735	6.4
Magnesium (mg)*	125	122	2.3	137	131	2.7	139	135	1.1
Sodium (mg)*	1318	1285	26.7	1413	1389	28.9	1562	1505	13.7
Potassium (mg)*	1381	1352	27.4	1506	1431	31.8	1535	1508	11.9
Chloride (mg)**	1990	1955	40.2	2127	2091	42.8	2342	2266	20.2
Zinc (mg)**	4.2	4.0	0.10	4.2	4.1	0.09	4.5	4.3	0.04
Copper (mg)**	0.4	0.4	0.01	0.5	0.4	0.01	0.5	0.5	0.01
Iodine (µg)*	111	94	4.0	115	101	4.4	122	106	1.9
Manganese (mg)**	1.1	1.0	0.03	1.3	1.1	0.04	1.2	1.1	0.01
Base		266			190			1219	

*None of the dietary supplements taken by children in this survey provided any haem iron, magnesium, sodium, potassium or iodine.
**Dietary supplements provided negligible calcium, phosphorus, chloride, zinc, copper and manganese for children in this survey.

Table 9.40 Average daily intake of minerals from food sources per 1000kcal food energy by whether child was reported as being unwell during four-day dietary recording period

| Minerals | Whether child reported as being unwell during four–day period | | | | | | | | |
| | Unwell, eating affected | | | Unwell, eating not affected | | | Not unwell | | |
	Mean	Median	se	Mean	Median	se	Mean	Median	se
Intake per 1000kcal energy:									
Iron (mg)	4.8	4.5	0.08	4.7	4.6	0.09	4.7	4.5	0.03
Haem iron (mg)	0.2	0.2	0.01	0.2	0.2	0.01	0.2	0.2	0.01
Non-haem iron (mg)	4.6	4.4	0.08	4.5	4.3	0.08	4.6	4.4	0.03
Calcium (mg)	585	569	12.3	579	543	15.3	556	527	5.6
Phosphorus (mg)	667	655	9.6	670	650	11.3	650	636	4,3
Magnesium (mg)	124	121	1.6	125	123	1.8	119	117	0.7
Sodium (mg)	1298	1294	17.8	1291	1266	20.2	1336	1309	8.6
Potassium (mg)	1364	1342	18.6	1376	1356	23.2	1320	1300	7.9
Zinc (mg)	4.1	3.9	0.07	3.9	3.7	0.06	3.8	3.7	0.03
Copper (mg)	0.4	0.4	0.01	0.4	0.4	0.01	0.4	0.4	0.00
Iodine (µg)	109	95	3.6	105	90	3.8	104	90	1.6
Base		266			190			1219	

Table 9.41 Average daily mineral intakes by region

| Minerals | Region | | | | | | | | | | | |
| | Scotland | | | Northern | | | Central, South West and Wales | | | London and South East | | |
	Mean	Median	se	Mean	Median	se	Mean	Median	se	Mean	Median	se
Intakes from *all sources*												
Iron (mg)	5.4	5.1	0.15	5.5	5.3	0.12	5.5	5.4	0.08	5.6	5.1	0.13
Haem iron (mg)*	0.3	0.2	0.02	0.3	0.2	0.01	0.3	0.2	0.01	0.2	0.2	0.01
Non-haem iron (mg)	5.2	4.9	0.14	5.3	5.1	0.11	5.3	5.2	0.08	5.4	4.9	0.13
Calcium (mg)**	614	560	19.7	629	606	11.5	639	601	10.9	651	624	11.5
Phosphorus (mg)**	739	711	18.2	729	720	10.2	740	702	9.4	755	737	10.2
Magnesium (mg)*	131	125	3.0	136	132	1.8	137	133	1.5	138	134	1.8
Sodium (mg)*	1646	1555	39.6	1525	1462	22.9	1522	1498	19.4	1429	1377	20.1
Potassium (mg)*	1484	1491	35.6	1485	1454	19.9	1515	1472	17.2	1525	1485	19.7
Chloride (mg)**	2478	2350	58.3	2294	2192	34.1	2284	2240	28.8	2141	2083	29.5
Zinc (mg)**	4.4	4.2	0.12	4.4	4.2	0.07	4.4	4.2	0.06	4.4	4.2	0.06
Copper (mg)**	0.5	0.4	0.01	0.5	0.5	0.01	0.5	0.5	0.01	0.5	0.4	0.01
Iodine (µg)*	126	109	5.1	118	102	3.1	124	110	2.9	113	95	2.8
Manganese (mg)**	1.1	1.0	0.04	1.2	1.1	0.02	1.2	1.2	0.02	1.3	1.1	0.02
Base		165			427			563			520	

*None of the dietary supplements taken by children in this survey provided any haem iron, magnesium, sodium, potassium or iodine.
**Dietary supplements provided negligible calcium, phosphorus, chloride, zinc, copper and manganese for children in this survey.

209

Table 9.42 Average daily intake of minerals from food sources per 1000kcal food energy by region

Minerals	Region											
	Scotland			Northern			Central, South West and Wales			London and South East		
	Mean	Median	se	Mean	Median	se	Mean	Median	se	Mean	Median	se
Intakes per 1000kcal energy:												
Iron (mg)	4.7	4.6	0.09	4.7	4.5	0.06	4.8	4.6	0.05	4.7	4.5	0.06
Haem iron (mg)	0.3	0.2	0.02	0.2	0.2	0.01	0.2	0.2	0.01	0.2	0.2	0.01
Non-haem iron (mg)	4.5	4.4	0.08	4.5	4.4	0.05	4.6	4.4	0.05	4.6	4.4	0.05
Calcium (mg)	536	512	14.6	550	516	9.2	559	527	8.3	587	564	9.2
Phosphorus (mg)	648	642	11.5	637	623	7.1	647	634	6.2	680	663	7.0
Magnesium (mg)	116	114	1.9	119	117	1.2	120	118	1.0	125	123	1.1
Sodium (mg)	1457	1375	28.7	1324	1313	13.8	1328	1321	12.3	1279	1263	11.9
Potassium (mg)	1306	1293	23.8	1296	1294	13.0	1331	1304	11.6	1375	1351	13.2
Zinc (mg)	3.8	3.6	0.07	3.8	3.7	0.04	3.8	3.7	0.04	4.0	3.9	0.04
Copper (mg)	0.4	0.4	0.01	0.4	0.4	0.01	0.4	0.4	0.01	0.4	0.4	0.01
Iodine (μg)	110	94	4.1	104	90	2.7	109	94	2.3	101	86	2.4
Base		165			427			563			520	

Table 9.43 Average daily mineral intakes by social class of head of household

Minerals	Social class of head of household								
	Non-manual			Manual			All†		
	Mean	Median	se	Mean	Median	se	Mean	Median	se
Intakes from *all sources*									
Iron (mg)	5.7	5.3	0.10	5.4	5.1	0.07	5.5	5.3	0.06
Haem iron (mg)*	0.2	0.2	0.01	0.3	0.2	0.01	0.3	0.2	0.01
Non-haem iron (mg)	5.5	5.1	0.09	5.2	4.9	0.07	5.3	5.0	0.06
Calcium (mg)**	656	625	9.5	623	594	8.4	638	606	6.2
Phosphorus (mg)**	763	743	8.3	724	700	7.4	742	716	5.5
Magnesium (mg)*	141	138	1.4	133	130	1.2	136	133	0.9
Sodium (mg)*	1479	1441	16.4	1527	1474	16.4	1506	1459	11.5
Potassium (mg)*	1559	1538	15.8	1466	1425	14.1	1508	1475	10.4
Chloride (mg)**	2213	2167	24.1	2298	2214	24.5	2261	2186	17.1
Zinc (mg)**	4.5	4.3	0.05	4.3	4.1	0.05	4.4	4.2	0.03
Copper (mg)**	0.5	0.5	0.01	0.5	0.4	0.01	0.5	0.5	0.01
Iodine (μg)*	123	106	2.5	117	102	2.1	119	104	1.6
Manganese (mg)**	1.3	1.2	0.02	1.2	1.1	0.02	1.2	1.1	0.01
Base		748			867			1675	

*None of the dietary supplements taken by children in this survey provided any haem iron, magnesium, sodium, potassium or iodine.
**Dietary supplements provided negligible calcium, phosphorus, chloride, zinc, copper and manganese for children in this survey.
†Includes those who could not be allocated a social class either because their job was inadequately described, they were a member of the Armed Forces or had never worked.

Table 9.44 Average daily intake of minerals from food sources per 1000kcal food energy by social class of head of household

Minerals	Social class of head of household								
	Non-manual			Manual			All*		
	Mean	Median	se	Mean	Median	se	Mean	Median	se
Intake per 1000kcal energy:									
Iron (mg)	4.9	4.6	0.05	4.6	4.5	0.04	4.7	4.5	0.03
Haem iron (mg)	0.2	0.2	0.01	0.2	0.2	0.01	0.2	0.2	0.01
Non-haem iron (mg)	4.7	4.5	0.04	4.5	4.3	0.04	4.6	4.4	0.03
Calcium (mg)	580	549	7.2	548	520	6.7	563	532	4.9
Phosphorus (mg)	676	660	5.5	635	623	5.0	655	641	3.7
Magnesium (mg)	126	123	0.9	117	115	0.8	121	118	0.6
Sodium (mg)	1308	1290	10.2	1333	1315	10.1	1325	1302	7.2
Potassium (mg)	1386	1357	10.5	1289	1279	9.3	1333	1311	7.0
Zinc (mg)	4.0	3.9	0.03	3.8	3.7	0.03	3.9	3.8	0.02
Copper (mg)	0.4	0.4	0.01	0.4	0.4	0.00	0.4	0.4	0.00
Iodine (μg)	108	93	2.1	103	88	1.8	105	91	1.3
Base		748			867			1675	

*Includes those who could not be allocated a social class either because their job was inadequately described, they were a member of the Armed Forces or had never worked.

Table 9.45   Average daily mineral intakes by employment status of head of household

Minerals	Employment status of head of household								
	Working			Unemployed			Economically inactive		
	Mean	*Median*	*se*	*Mean*	*Median*	*se*	*Mean*	*Median*	*se*
Intakes from *all sources*									
Iron (mg)	5.5	5.2	0.07	5.5	5.1	0.20	5.7	5.5	0.14
Haem iron (mg)*	0.2	0.2	0.01	0.3	0.2	0.03	0.3	0.2	0.02
Non-haem iron (mg)	5.3	5.0	0.07	5.2	4.9	0.20	5.5	5.3	0.13
Calcium (mg)**	641	615	7.1	636	582	22.2	621	595	15.1
Phosphorus (mg)**	745	721	6.3	727	694	19.6	737	709	13.7
Magnesium (mg)*	137	134	1.0	133	127	3.4	134	127	2.3
Sodium (mg)*	1483	1436	12.7	1515	1471	42.2	1612	1576	31.7
Potassium (mg)*	1513	1487	11.9	1455	1406	36.3	1514	1468	26.8
Chloride (mg)**	2219	2161	18.6	2301	2205	64.4	2442	2389	47.7
Zinc (mg)**	4.4	4.2	0.04	4.4	4.2	0.13	4.5	4.2	0.09
Copper (mg)**	0.5	0.5	0.00	0.5	0.5	0.01	0.5	0.5	0.01
Iodine (μg)*	120	105	1.9	117	101	4.9	116	101	3.9
Manganese (mg)**	1.3	1.1	0.01	1.2	1.0	0.04	1.1	1.1	0.03
Base		1249			167			259	

*None of the dietary supplements taken by children in this survey provided any haem iron, magnesium, sodium, potassium or iodine.
**Dietary supplements provided negligible calcium, phosphorus, chloride, zinc, copper and manganese for children in this survey.

Table 9.46   Average daily intake of minerals from food sources per 1000kcal food energy by employment status of head of household

Minerals	Employment status of head of household								
	Working			Unemployed			Economically inactive		
	Mean	*Median*	*se*	*Mean*	*Median*	*se*	*Mean*	*Median*	*se*
Intake per 1000kcal energy:									
Iron (mg)	4.7	4.6	0.03	4.7	4.3	0.12	4.8	4.6	0.08
Haem iron (mg)	0.2	0.2	0.01	0.2	0.2	0.02	0.2	0.2	0.01
Non-haem iron (mg)	4.6	4.4	0.03	4.5	4.2	0.11	4.6	4.4	0.07
Calcium (mg)	570	537	5.7	557	531	14.8	533	513	11.5
Phosphorus (mg)	662	648	4.4	636	617	10.5	633	622	8.5
Magnesium (mg)	122	120	0.7	116	114	1.9	116	113	1.3
Sodium (mg)	1313	1291	8.2	1320	1308	21.6	1385	1361	20.9
Potassium (mg)	1346	1325	8.1	1280	1272	21.4	1308	1282	17.2
Zinc (mg)	3.9	3.8	0.03	3.9	3.7	0.08	3.9	3.7	0.06
Copper (mg)	0.4	0.4	0.00	0.4	0.4	0.01	0.4	0.4	0.01
Iodine (μg)	107	92	1.6	102	92	3.8	101	84	3.3
Base		1249			167			259	

Table 9.47   Average daily mineral intakes by whether child's parents were in receipt of Income Support or Family Credit

Minerals	Whether child's parents receiving Income Support or Family Credit					
	Receiving benefit(s)			Not receiving benefit(s)		
	Mean	*Median*	*se*	*Mean*	*Median*	*se*
Intakes from *all sources*						
Iron (mg)	5.5	5.3	0.10	5.6	5.2	0.07
Haem iron (mg)*	0.3	0.2	0.01	0.2	0.2	0.01
Non-haem iron (mg)	5.3	5.1	0.09	5.4	5.0	0.07
Calcium (mg)**	625	591	11.4	643	616	7.4
Phosphorus (mg)**	731	706	10.2	747	725	6.5
Magnesium (mg)*	133	128	1.7	138	135	1.1
Sodium (mg)*	1572	1521	22.6	1475	1429	13.1
Potassium (mg)*	1489	1436	19.8	1516	1494	12.2
Chloride (mg)**	2383	2296	34.2	2204	2149	19.0
Zinc (mg)**	4.4	4.2	0.07	4.4	4.2	0.04
Copper (mg)**	0.5	0.5	0.01	0.5	0.5	0.01
Iodine (μg)*	118	101	2.8	120	105	2.0
Manganese (mg)**	1.1	1.1	0.02	1.3	1.2	0.02
Base		534			1140	

*None of the dietary supplements taken by children in this survey provided any haem iron, magnesium, sodium, potassium or iodine.
**Dietary supplements provided negligible calcium, phosphorus, chloride, zinc, copper and manganese for children in this survey.

211

Table 9.48 Average daily intake of minerals from food sources per 1000kcal food energy by whether child's parents were receiving Income Support or Family Credit

Minerals	Whether child's parents receiving Income Support or Family Credit					
	Receiving benefit(s)			Not receiving benefits		
	Mean	Median	se	Mean	Median	se
Intake per 1000kcal energy:						
Iron (mg)	4.7	4.5	0.05	4.8	4.6	0.04
Haem iron (mg)	0.2	0.2	0.01	0.2	0.2	0.01
Non-haem iron (mg)	4.5	4.3	0.05	4.6	4.4	0.03
Calcium (mg)	543	515	8.3	573	539	6.0
Phosphorus (mg)	635	622	6.1	664	651	4.6
Magnesium (mg)	116	113	1.0	123	121	0.7
Sodium (mg)	1362	1347	13.6	1307	1283	8.5
Potassium (mg)	1295	1279	12.1	1351	1335	8.5
Zinc (mg)	3.8	3.7	0.04	3.9	3.8	0.03
Copper (mg)	0.4	0.4	0.01	0.4	0.4	0.00
Iodine (μg)	103	88	2.3	106	92	1.7
Base		*534*			*1140*	

Table 9.49 Average daily mineral intakes by mother's highest educational qualification

Minerals	Mother's highest educational qualification level														
	Above GCE 'A' level			GCE 'A' level and equivalents			GCE 'O' level and equivalents			CSE and equivalents			None		
	Mean	Median	se	Mean	Median	se	Mean	Median	se	Mean	Median	se	Mean	Median	se
Intakes from *all sources*															
Iron (mg)	5.7	5.4	0.12	5.9	5.6	0.22	5.4	5.1	0.08	5.5	5.0	0.19	5.5	5.1	0.14
Haem iron (mg)*	0.2	0.2	0.01	0.3	0.2	0.02	0.2	0.2	0.01	0.3	0.2	0.02	0.3	0.2	0.01
Non-haem iron (mg)	5.5	5.2	0.11	5.7	5.4	0.22	5.2	5.0	0.07	5.3	4.8	0.19	5.3	5.0	0.14
Calcium (mg)**	679	656	14.1	660	629	19.4	622	595	10.2	614	595	14.8	633	591	14.8
Phosphorus (mg)**	787	775	12.0	771	724	17.8	725	705	9.0	715	708	13.2	734	706	13.1
Magnesium (mg)*	149	147	2.1	143	138	2.7	134	131	1.5	131	128	2.3	131	125	2.0
Sodium (mg)*	1433	1413	23.4	1504	1443	37.8	1497	1458	17.6	1483	1454	29.1	1597	1523	29.8
Potassium (mg)*	1625	1603	23.7	1567	1535	31.0	1476	1431	17.2	1457	1410	27.4	1466	1425	23.3
Chloride (mg)**	2148	2125	34.8	2258	2177	55.8	2243	2186	25.7	2225	2194	43.3	2411	2287	44.4
Zinc (mg)**	4.6	4.4	0.08	4.6	4.5	0.1	4.3	4.1	0.06	4.2	4.1	0.09	4.4	4.1	0.08
Copper (mg)**	0.5	0.5	0.01	0.5	0.5	0.01	0.5	0.4	0.01	0.5	0.4	0.01	0.5	0.4	0.01
Iodine (μg)*	119	101	3.4	118	107	4.6	122	106	2.8	117	105	4.0	118	102	3.6
Maganese (mg)**	1.5	1.3	0.03	1.4	1.3	0.04	1.2	1.1	0.02	1.1	1.0	0.03	1.1	1.0	0.02
Base		*305*			*183*			*590*			*236*			*358*	

*None of the dietary supplements taken by children in this survey provided any haem iron, magnesium, sodium, potassium or iodine.
**Dietary supplements provided negligible calcium, phosphorus, chloride, zinc, copper and manganese for children in this survey.

Table 9.50 Average daily intake of minerals from food sources per 1000kcal food energy by mother's highest educational qualification

Minerals	Mother's highest educational qualification level														
	Above GCE 'A' level			GCE 'A' level and equivalents			GCE 'O' level and equivalents			CSE and equivalents			None		
	Mean	Median	se	Mean	Median	se	Mean	Median	se	Mean	Median	se	Mean	Median	se
Intake per 1000kcal energy:															
Iron (mg)	4.9	4.7	0.07	4.9	4.8	0.10	4.7	4.5	0.05	4.6	4.4	0.08	4.6	4.4	0.06
Haem iron (mg)	0.2	0.1	0.01	0.2	0.2	0.02	0.2	0.2	0.01	0.2	0.2	0.01	0.2	0.2	0.01
Non-haem iron (mg)	4.8	4.6	0.07	4.8	4.6	0.09	4.5	4.4	0.04	4.4	4.3	0.08	4.4	4.3	0.06
Calcium (mg)	606	578	11.4	581	548	15.0	552	520	8.0	552	511	13.0	545	518	10.6
Phosphorus (mg)	702	694	8.5	682	656	12.1	643	634	6.0	638	621	9.8	632	621	8.0
Magnesium (mg)	132	131	1.4	127	124	1.9	119	116	1.0	117	113	1.5	113	112	1.2
Sodium (mg)	1269	1268	14.8	1319	1301	24.4	1328	1306	11.3	1318	1311	19.2	1372	1335	17.7
Potassium (mg)	1448	1424	16.5	1393	1353	21.3	1310	1299	11.3	1296	1270	18.3	1270	1251	14.3
Zinc (mg)	4.1	4.0	0.05	4.0	4.0	0.07	3.8	3.7	0.04	3.7	3.6	0.06	3.8	3.7	0.05
Copper (mg)	0.4	0.4	0.01	0.4	0.4	0.01	0.4	0.4	0.00	0.4	0.4	0.01	0.4	0.4	0.01
Iodine (μg)	106	89	3.1	104	95	3.8	108	93	2.3	104	91	3.7	102	87	2.8
Base		*305*			*183*			*590*			*236*			*358*	

Table 9.51 Average daily mineral intakes by family type

Minerals	Family type											
	Married or cohabiting couple						Lone parent					
	One child			More than one child			One child			More than one child		
	Mean	Median	se	Mean	Median	se	Mean	Median	se	Mean	Median	se
Intakes from *all sources*												
Iron (mg)	5.5	5.0	0.16	5.5	5.2	0.07	6.0	5.5	0.27	5.5	5.4	0.14
Haem iron (mg)*	0.2	0.2	0.01	0.2	0.2	0.01	0.3	0.2	0.02	0.3	0.2	0.02
Non-haem iron (mg)	5.3	4.8	0.16	5.3	5.0	0.06	5.7	5.3	0.27	5.3	5.2	0.13
Calcium (mg)**	672	651	14.6	633	603	7.8	619	594	22.4	606	585	17.0
Phosphorus (mg)**	765	756	12.2	735	713	7.0	746	706	21.0	725	700	16.2
Magnesium (mg)*	139	135	2.0	136	134	1.2	137	129	3.9	132	127	2.7
Sodium (mg)*	1432	1393	23.9	1501	1462	14.3	1612	1541	48.2	1618	1571	39.4
Potassium (mg)*	1567	1533	22.6	1487	1459	13.1	1511	1431	43.0	1497	1451	32.8
Chloride (mg)**	2155	2095	35.0	2248	2185	21.2	2412	2297	69.4	2457	2389	59.8
Zinc (mg)**	4.5	4.4	0.08	4.3	4.2	0.04	4.5	4.2	0.15	4.5	4.1	9.11
Copper (mg)**	0.5	0.5	0.01	0.5	0.5	0.01	0.5	0.5	0.02	0.5	0.4	0.02
Iodine (μg)*	124	106	3.7	117	103	2.0	123	105	6.0	117	104	4.8
Manganese (mg)**	1.2	1.1	0.03	1.3	1.1	0.02	1.2	1.1	0.05	1.2	1.1	0.04
Base		366			1011			121			177	

*None of the dietary supplements taken by children in this survey provided any haem iron, magnesium, sodium, potassium or iodine.
**Dietary supplements provided negligible calcium, phosphorus, chloride, zinc, copper and manganese for children in this survey.

Table 9.52 Average daily intake of minerals from food sources per 1000kcal food energy by family type

Minerals	Family type											
	Married or cohabiting couple						Lone parent					
	One child			More than one child			One child			More than one child		
	Mean	Median	se	Mean	Median	se	Mean	Median	se	Mean	Median	se
Intakes per 1000kcal energy:												
Iron (mg)	4.7	4.5	0.07	4.8	4.5	0.04	4.8	4.8	0.10	4.7	4.6	0.09
Haem iron (mg)	0.2	0.2	0.01	0.2	0.2	0.01	0.2	0.2	0.02	0.2	0.2	0.02
Non-haem iron (mg)	4.5	4.4	0.06	4.6	4.4	0.04	4.6	4.5	0.10	4.5	4.4	0.08
Calcium (mg)	609	571	12.0	558	527	6.0	527	502	16.1	525	516	13.4
Phosphorus (mg)	693	674	8.7	648	640	4.7	640	619	12.4	624	620	10.1
Magnesium (mg)	126	126	1.3	120	118	0.8	117	113	2.1	114	112	1.5
Sodium (mg)	1289	1277	15.3	1319	1299	8.8	1386	1365	33.4	1389	1366	24.3
Potassium (mg)	1424	1406	16.4	1313	1308	8.7	1297	1274	26.1	1285	1264	18.1
Zinc (mg)	4.1	4.0	0.05	3.8	3.7	0.03	3.9	3.7	0.09	3.8	3.6	0.07
Copper (mg)	0.4	0.4	0.01	0.4	0.4	0.00	0.4	0.4	0.01	0.4	0.4	0.01
Iodine (μg)	113	96	3.3	103	91	1.6	107	86	5.2	102	86	4.3
Base		366			1011			121			177	

213

10 Blood and plasma analytes: results

10.1 Obtaining the blood sample

Chapters 1 and 2 of this Report described the purpose, methodology and other procedures associated with taking blood samples from children as part of this survey. This chapter reports on the results from the analyses of these blood samples. In Appendix L further information is given on the procedures for obtaining the samples and in Appendix N the assay techniques are described and quality assurance data are given.

During the preparation and testing of the protocol for this survey, expert advice was unanimous that for an adequate examination of diet and nutrition in this age group, blood analysis would be essential. These results would allow better evaluation of dietary data. For several nutrients there are no population data and the results from the children in this survey will provide reference ranges for the first time.

The analytes were ordered to take account of technical constraints and nutritional interest. Table 10.1 shows a list of blood analytes in order of analytical priority.

(Table 10.1)

Four millilitres blood was obtained from more than two thirds of the total of 1003 children from whom blood was obtained; the remaining children provided smaller amounts, with less than 1ml being obtained from 7% of children (see *Appendix L* for details). The first priority for blood analyses was providing 1ml of whole blood for haematology assays. It was hoped that once these were completed, residual plasma could be used to assay a number of minerals of nutritional and toxicological interest. In practice the level of incidental trace element contamination of the plasma sample during processing was too great to give reliable results from the residuum of the sample. Remaining blood, after the removal of this first 1ml, was used for the nutrient assays described below.

If less than 4ml was obtained, the sample of blood was exhausted during the assays accorded a high priority and thus less than the full total of analyses was done. For this reason, the bases for the tables of analyte results vary.

The lowest priority was given to the determination of immunoglobulin levels. The small number of children for whom these levels were measured, (just over 100) reflects the limited volume of blood taken from some children and mean levels are shown only for the total group of children. Residual bloods after all assays had been completed were stored.

A small number of samples were not analysed for reasons such as clotting, incorrect storage or undue delay in reaching the laboratory. Additionally there were 29 cases where although some analyses were carried out on the sample provided, on the advice of the laboratory, for quality control reasons, the results have been excluded from the tables presented in the Report.

Information was recorded at the time of the survey interview on any prescribed medication being taken by the child. For each drug identified, checks were subsequently made, in all cases with the pharmaceutical manufacturer, to establish whether the drug was likely to have an interaction that would affect the results of any of the full range of blood analyses being carried out. Although overall 11% of children were reported to be taking prescribed medication[1], none of the medicines was identified as having any interaction with the blood analytes being measured. Hence it has not been necessary to exclude any results from the tables in this Report for this reason.

Data are presented giving distributions for the blood analytes by sex and age cohorts[2]. For selected analytes, tables are given showing the variation in analyte levels for various subgroups in the sample based on demographic and socio-economic characteristics of the children and their households. Again for selected analytes, tables are also given showing correlation coefficients between the analyte and relevant dietary intakes[3]. Not all tables are commented upon in the text.

For convenience of reporting and discussion the analytes are divided into six main groups: haematology, including plasma ferritin and zinc protoporphyrin; water soluble vitamins and plasma zinc; carotenoids and fat soluble vitamins; blood lipids; acute phase proteins and immunoglobulins.

10.2 Haematology, including plasma ferritin and zinc protoporphyrin

10.2.1 The analytes

Haemoglobin concentration (g/dl)
Haemoglobin is the oxygen-carrying, iron-containing protein in red blood cells. Circulating levels are an indication of the oxygen-carrying capacity of the blood. Micro-nutrients essential for its production include iron, folic acid, and vitamin B_{12}. Low concentrations in the blood are termed anaemia which has been defined by the World Health Organisation for children aged 6 months to 6 years as values below 11.0g/dl[4].

Mean corpuscular volume (MCV) (fl)

This is a measure of the average size of the red blood cells, usually between about 70fl and 87fl. A low MCV (microcytosis) is usually an indication of iron deficiency. High MCV (macrocytosis) is rare in early childhood and may be due to certain haemolytic anaemias.

Haematocrit (packed cell volume—PCV) (l/l)

This is the proportion of the blood volume taken up by the red cells, and is determined by the cell size and number. A normal range for PCV in preschool children has been described as about 0.33 l/l to about 0.40 l/l (personal communication from Dr I Hann)[5].

Mean cell haemoglobin (MCH) (pg)

This is a measure of the mean weight of haemoglobin in each red blood cell. Cells with low values are termed hypochromic and haemoglobin production is impaired. A low MCH is a feature of iron deficiency, lead poisoning, inherited disorders of haemoglobin synthesis such as the thalassaemias and other rarer disorders.

Mean cell haemoglobin concentration (MCHC) (g/dl)

This is a measure of the mean haemoglobin concentration in each red blood cell. MCHC usually lies between about 30g/dl and 36g/dl.

Ferritin (µg/l)

Iron is stored in the reticulo-endothelial tissues in the protein complex ferritin. Plasma ferritin levels reflect the volume of iron stores except in certain circumstances, for example, inflammation (see *section 10.6* below). Concentrations of 10µg/l and of 5µg/l have both been used to assess the status of the iron stores in preschool children[6].

Zinc protoporphyrin (ZPP) (µmol/mol haem)

Protoporphyrin in the red blood cells binds with iron during the process of haemoglobin synthesis. Where iron is relatively unavailable, the protoporphyrin is progressively bound to zinc. Thus high levels of ZPP in the red blood cell are a functional indicator of an inadequate supply of iron.

10.2.2 The results

Tables 10.2 to 10.8 show the results for haematological analytes, including ferritin and ZPP, for boys and girls and children of different ages in the survey.

The mean *haemoglobin concentration* in all samples from children in this survey was 12.2g/dl; mean concentrations increased slightly with age, from 12.0g/dl for the youngest group to 12.4g/dl for the oldest group of boys (p<0.01). Overall about one in twelve children, and among the youngest group one in eight children, had a haemoglobin concentration below 11.0g/dl, the WHO level defining anaemia.

Similar age associations were found in respect of *MCH, MCHC, MCV, haematocrit and ferritin;* mean levels tended to increase with age and the youngest group of children were the most likely to have the lowest levels.

The overall *mean corpuscular volume* in samples from all children in the survey was 78.9fl. The proportions of children with levels below 75fl varied considerably by age, from 21% for the youngest group, to 5% for boys and girls in the oldest age group (p<0.01); across all age groups 33% of boys had levels below 75fl compared with only 11% of girls (p<0.01).

Haematocrit levels below 0.350 l/l were similarly more likely among the youngest children; just under half the samples from children aged 1½ to 2½ years had levels this low compared with less than one third of the samples from the oldest group of children (p<0.01).

Mean *ferritin* levels ranged from 21µg/l in samples from children aged 1½ to 2½ years to 26µg/l for girls aged 3½ to 4½ years (NS). Overall 20% of children had ferritin levels below 10µg/l, including 5% who had levels below 5µg/l. As with other haematological analytes the proportion of children with lower levels was highest among the youngest children.

As described above, high levels of ZPP may indicate low iron stores; as can be seen from Tables 10.7 and 10.8 the highest mean values for ZPP were for those groups with the lowest ferritin levels. Thus mean ZPP for the youngest children was 58µmol/mol haem, falling to 51µmol/mol haem for boys and girls aged 3½ to 4½ years (p<0.01).   *(Tables 10.2 to 10.8; Figs 10.1 and 10.2)*

Table 10.9 shows correlation coefficients between three measures of haematological status; haemoglobin concentration, ferritin and ZPP. Overall the correlations between the three analytes were marked for all children and for all girls (p<0.01), with ZPP levels falling as levels of haemoglobin and ferritin increased. Generally the correlations between ZPP and ferritin became weaker as the children got older; for the youngest group of children correlations between ZPP level and both ferritin and haemoglobin were marked (p<0.01), and were stronger than the correlations between haemoglobin and ferritin (p<0.05). For boys aged between 3½ and 4½ years, none of the correlations reached statistical significance (NS).

(Table 10.9)

10.2.3 Factors influencing the results of the haematological assays

Results for these analytes were examined in relation to various social and demographic characteristics of the child and their household, in the same way as variation in food and nutrient intakes has been considered.

Generally the associations were statistically weak, not reaching significance level, but there were a number of consistent patterns in the data.

There were no marked associations between the results for the haematology and *region.*   *(Table 10.10)*

Most haematological analytes showed no variation by *social class, employment status, or receipt of benefits.* There was an observed difference in mean levels of ferritin between samples from children whose head of household was working (24µg/l) and those from children where the head was economically inactive (21µg/l) and for the same two groups in mean ZPP levels (54µmol/mol haem and 57µmol/mol haem respectively).

The results for groups classified by the child's *mother's highest educational qualification level* showed some consistent patterns, although again the differences in mean analyte levels were small. Thus for all analytes except ZPP and haematocrit, mean levels in children were highest where the mother had educational qualifications above GCE 'A' level; these mean levels then fell as the mother's level of education got lower.

As might be expected, the trend was in the reverse direction for mean ZPP levels; thus children whose mothers had no formal educational qualifications had the highest mean ZPP levels, and those whose mothers were the most highly qualified had the lowest mean levels.

There was no observed difference in mean values for haematocrit. *(Tables 10.11 to 10.14)*

There were no clear associations between mean levels of the haematological analytes and whether the child was *living in a lone parent or two-parent family*, nor with whether the child was an only child or had siblings. *(Table 10.15)*

10.2.4 Correlation with dietary intakes

Table 10.16 gives correlation coefficients for haemoglobin, ferritin and ZPP with dietary intakes, from all sources, of total iron, haem and non-haem iron, and vitamin C.

In interpreting these and other correlations between blood analyte levels and dietary intakes, particularly when correlations appear not to reach levels of statistical significance, it should be remembered that blood samples could not be taken until the dietary record was completed, and while every effort was made to visit the child as soon as possible, in some cases a period of a week or longer elapsed before a blood sample could be taken.

Generally the correlations between these blood analytes and dietary intakes were weak. Only haemoglobin showed any significant correlation with intakes of total, haem and non-haem iron from all sources ($p < 0.05$). *(Table 10.16)*

10.3 Water soluble vitamins and plasma zinc

10.3.1 The analytes

Red blood cell folate and plasma folate (nmol/l)
The term folate includes several derivatives of the parent molecule folic acid. Folates are necessary for DNA synthesis. Tissue levels are better indicated by the concentration of folate in red blood cells while plasma levels are more likely to reflect the recent dietary intake of folates. A normal range of values for these analytes has not previously been defined for children in this age group.

Vitamin B$_{12}$ (pmol/l)
Circulating levels of vitamin B$_{12}$ are a good indicator of vitamin B$_{12}$ status. Vitamin B$_{12}$, with folate, is required for protein metabolism. It is also needed to maintain the integrity of the nervous system.

The *erythrocyte glutathione reductase activation coefficient (EGRAC)* is a measure of red cell biochemical saturation with riboflavin (vitamin B$_2$). The enzyme glutathione reductase requires riboflavin as a cofactor. Its activity in red blood cells is measured before and after the addition of flavin adenine dinucleotide. The coefficient is expressed as the ratio of the two activity measurements, and the higher the coefficient the lower the saturation. A coefficient of between 1.0 and 1.3 is generally regarded as normal.

Plasma ascorbate (µmol/l)
Plasma ascorbate (vitamin C) levels are sensitive to recent intake of vitamin C, with values of less than 11µmol/l indicating biochemical depletion[7].

10.3.2 The results

Tables 10.17 to 10.23 show the results of the assays for water soluble vitamins and plasma zinc for boys and girls and children of different ages in the survey.
(Tables 10.17 to 10.23; Figs 10.3 and 10.4)

The mean level of *red cell folate* in the samples taken from children in the survey was 914nmol/l *(Table 10.17)*. Children at the lower and upper 2.5 percentiles of the distribution had levels which were about half and about twice the median value (868nmol/l) respectively. Levels showed no clear variation by either age or sex.

Mean *plasma folate* levels ranged between 20.4nmol/l for girls aged 3½ to 4½ years to 22.0nmol/l for boys in the same age group *(Table 10.18 and Fig 10.3)*. Thus the variation was small and not clearly associated with either the age or the sex of the child.

The correlation between levels of red cell folate and plasma folate was significant ($p < 0.01$) for children in each age cohort and for boys and girls. Plasma folate levels increased as levels of red cell folate increased and correlation coefficients ranged between 0.34 and 0.51, increasing with age. *(Table 10.19)*

The lowest mean levels of *vitamin B$_{12}$* were from the samples from the youngest group of children, 620pmol/l, rising to 654pmol/l for boys aged 3½ to 4½ years *(Table 10.20)*. As was found for plasma folate, levels for the oldest group of girls were lower (627pmol/l) than for the comparable group of boys but none of the differences reached the level of statistical significance.

The mean value for the *EGRAC* for samples taken from children was 1.24 *(Table 10.21)*. Overall about one quarter of the children had an EGRAC above 1.30, but this proportion varied with age increasing as the children got older. For example, 14% of all children aged 1½ to 2½ years had an EGRAC of 1.30 or higher, compared with 29% and 38% of the oldest group of boys and girls respectively ($p < 0.05$ and $p < 0.01$). The difference in the EGRAC between boys and girls in the oldest group was not statistically significant (NS).

Overall the mean level of *plasma vitamin C* for children in the survey was 67.6µmol/l, with a wide range between the lower and upper 2.5 percentiles (8.8μmol/l to 124.5μmol/l) (*Table 10.22 and Fig 10.4*). There was almost no variation by age. However, boys had significantly lower mean levels than girls (p<0.05). Children at the lower 2.5 percentile of the distribution had plasma vitamin C levels which ranged from only 5.2μmol/l for the youngest cohort to 14.8μmol/l among girls aged 3½ to 4½ years. Overall 3% of children in the survey had levels below 10.0μmol/l.

Plasma zinc levels showed very little variation with either age or sex; the overall mean level was 13.0μmol/l (*Table 10.23*). About 5% of children had levels below 10.0μmol/l, and 10% had levels at or above 16.0μmol/l.

10.3.3 Factors influencing the levels of water soluble vitamins

Tables 10.10 to 10.15 show the variation in results from the assays for water soluble vitamins for children classified by various social and demographic characteristics of their households and families.

Region
Results of assays of samples from children living in the Northern region gave values for all water soluble vitamins apart from the EGRAC, which were generally lower than for children living elsewhere in Great Britain. Although not reaching the level of statistical significance, the most marked differences were in respect of levels of vitamins B₁₂ and C.

Socio-economic characteristics
The results for all water soluble vitamins, except the EGRAC, show a marked association with the various measures of socio-economic status examined, with a consistent trend for levels to be considerably lower in the samples from children from less advantaged backgrounds. Thus children from a manual home background, from households where the head was not working, where the parents were in receipt of Family Credit or Income Support and where the mother had qualifications below GCE 'O' level standard, all had markedly lower levels of red cell and plasma folate and vitamins B₁₂ and C than children in the other groups.

Considering, for example, levels of red cell folate and vitamin C, samples from children from a manual home background gave, respectively, levels of 869nmol/l and 60.9μmol/l compared with levels of 964nmol/l and 74.7μmol/l for the samples from children from a non-manual home background (p<0.01).

Family type
Levels of all water soluble vitamins assayed (except the EGRAC) were also generally lower for children from lone-parent families compared with those for other children. The variation was not generally as marked as for the other socio-economic characteristics, but levels of vitamin C again showed the largest relative differences, for example, comparing two-parent families with one child and lone parents with more than one child the mean vitamin C levels for the children in the survey were 75.2μmol/l and 58.4μmol/l respectively (p<0.01).
(Tables 10.9 to 10.15)

10.3.4 Correlation with dietary intakes

Correlation coefficients were calculated for blood levels of red cell folate and dietary intakes of vitamin B₁₂ and folate, from all sources (*Table 10.24*). For vitamin B₁₂ the correlations for groups of children in different age groups and for boys were generally weak and only significant between blood levels and dietary intake for all girls in the survey. Correlations with dietary intakes of folate were stronger, being significant for all children, girls and all children aged 2½ to 3½ years (p<0.01).

When dietary intakes of riboflavin were correlated with the EGRAC, significant negative correlations were found for boys and girls and children in each age group (p<0.01). The coefficients indicate that, as would be expected, the EGRAC increased as the dietary intake of riboflavin fell and, as can be seen from Table 10.25, the relationship was found when intakes from food sources alone, as well as from all sources, including dietary supplements, were correlated.

Blood levels of vitamin C and dietary intakes from all sources and from food sources alone also showed strong, positive correlations (p<0.01) for boys and girls and children in each age cohort, with blood levels increasing as dietary intakes increased. *(Tables 10.24 to 10.26)*

10.4 Fat soluble vitamins and carotenoids

Plasma retinol (vitamin A) (μmol/l)
Blood retinol levels are homeostatically controlled and the variation both within and between subjects is considerably lower than for carotenoids. As a result plasma retinol concentrations are sensitive indicators of vitamin A status. They fall below 0.7μmol/l only in the later stages of deficiency, when other signs appear. A very low level is suggestive of long-term dietary restriction.

Retinol (vitamin A) values varied little by age and there were no marked differences between the values for boys or girls overall or between age groups. The overall mean value for the samples taken from all children was 1.02μmol/l. About 12% of children had levels below 0.75μmol/l and children in the lower 2.5 percentile had levels of 0.54μmol/l or lower. *(Table 10.33)*

α- and β-carotene and α- and β-cryptoxanthin (μmol/l)
These are all carotenoids with vitamin A activity. Blood concentrations of carotenoids, tocopherol and ascorbate are markers of antioxidant status and are being used increasingly as biological markers for fruit and vegetable consumption. Blood levels of carotenoids may be influenced by conversion to vitamin A, the amount of conversion being dependent on vitamin A status and requirements. If the consumption of pre-formed vitamin A (retinol) is low, more ß-carotene and possibly more of these other carotenoids will be converted. This may confound comparison between the dietary and blood levels.

Although mean levels of both *α-carotene and β-carotene* tended to decrease slightly with age, none of the differences was statistically significant (*Tables 10.27 and*

10.28). However, at lower levels differences were more marked and boys aged 3½ to 4½ years appeared to be particularly likely to have low levels of carotenes, although differences did not reach significance levels. For example, 32% of boys aged 3½ to 4½ years had α-carotene levels below 0.050μmol/l compared with 24% of girls in the same age group and 23% of all children aged 1½ to 2½ years.

The mean level of *α-cryptoxanthin* in samples taken from children in the study was 0.088μmol/l with no marked variation in mean levels associated with either the age or the sex of the child (*Table 10.29*)[8]. Again however the data suggest that at lower levels there was some variation with younger children being more likely to have lower levels than older children, and the older boys being more likely to have lower levels than older girls (NS).

Overall the mean level of *β-cryptoxanthin* was 0.194μmol/l and the oldest group of boys tended to have lower levels than either younger children or girls in the same age group (*Table 10.30*)[8]. Levels of less than 0.100μmol/l were found in samples from 39% of boys aged 3½ to 4½ years, but in only 25% of the samples from girls in the same age group (NS).

Lycopene and lutein (μmol/l)
Lycopene and lutein are also carotenoids but with no pro-vitamin A activity. Tomato and tomato products are the main source of lycopene and so blood levels reflect intake of tomatoes and can show considerable seasonal variation.

The assay for *lycopene* in samples taken from all children in the survey gave a mean value of 0.523μmol/l (*Table 10.31*)[8]. There was no significant variation in mean level associated with either the age or sex of the child.

Plasma lutein concentrations may be a useful marker of green vegetable intake. The mean level of lutein in the samples from children aged between 1½ and 4½ years was 0.229μmol/l and between the lower and upper 2.5 percentiles ranged between 0.080μmol/l and 0.478μmol/l (*Table 10.32*)[8]. The proportion of children with lower levels tended to be somewhat higher among younger children, for example 8% of 1½ to 2½ year olds had levels below 0.100μmol/l compared with only 2% of children in the oldest age group (NS). The difference in mean level between boys and girls aged 3½ to 4½ years suggests a difference in vegetable consumption; however as food consumption data were not analysed separately for boys and girls in this age group this has not been confirmed.

Plasma 25-hydroxyvitamin D (nmol/l)
Vitamin D in humans is obtained as ergocalciferol and cholecalciferol from the diet and from the synthesis in the skin following ultraviolet irradiation as sunlight. The circulating form in plasma is 25-hydroxyvitamin D. Vit-

amin D is required to maintain blood calcium at optimum levels for bone mineralisation.

The assay for plasma *vitamin D* in the samples from all children in the survey gave a mean value of 68.1nmol/l (*Table 10.34* and *Fig 10.6*). There was no apparent association between mean values and either the age or sex of the child.

Most of the body's requirement for vitamin D can be synthesised by the skin in the presence of sunlight, and plasma levels of vitamin D are therefore likely to be higher during the summer months. Although it was not possible to measure the exposure of children in this survey to sunlight, most of them had the use of a garden or communal play area and therefore at least had the opportunity to play outdoors and be exposed to sunlight (see *Table 4.1*). Figure 10.7 shows that plasma vitamin D levels varied by fieldwork wave, with mean levels being highest among children who were included in the survey between July and September and lowest among children in the fieldwork wave covering January to March.

α- and γ-tocopherol (μmol/l)
Plasma tocopherol concentration can be used as a measure of vitamin E status, but increased concentrations of plasma lipids appear to cause tocopherols to partition out of cellular membranes into the circulation, thus increasing blood levels. For this reason plasma tocopherol concentrations can also be expressed as the tocopherol : cholesterol ratio.

In adults a plasma tocopherol concentration of less than 11.6μmol/l causes red blood cells to haemolyse after exposure to oxidising agents. This is sometimes taken as a biochemical deficiency but is not indicative of a clinical deficiency of vitamin E. The COMA Panel on Dietary Reference Values considered plasma tocopherol concentrations of 11.6μmol/l to be the lowest satisfactory value for adults[7].

Levels of both *α-tocopherol and γ-tocopherol* tended to increase as the children got older and overall girls had higher mean levels than boys, although none of the differences was statistically significant (*Tables 10.35* and *10.36*). As was found for carotenes, for both α- and γ-tocopherol differences were more marked among children with lower levels; for example, about one in five of the youngest group of children had α-tocopherol levels below 15μmol/l compared with one in ten children aged between 3½ and 4½ years ($p < 0.05$).
(*Tables 10.27 to 10.36; Figs 10.5 to 10.7*)

10.4.1 *Correlation with dietary intakes*

Correlation coefficients between blood levels of fat soluble vitamins and corresponding dietary intakes were generally lower than those for many of the water soluble vitamins assayed.

As can be seen from Table 10.37 the correlation coefficients between plasma retinol levels and dietary intakes from all sources of both pre-formed retinol and total carotene were low and only statistically significant between plasma retinol and intakes of pre-formed retinol for all children.

218

Overall α-tocopherol levels and intakes of vitamin E from both food sources alone and with the addition from dietary supplements were positively correlated, blood levels rising slightly as intakes rose. Correlations were strongest for all children (p<0.01), girls (p<0.01 and p<0.05 for intakes from all and food sources respectively) and for children aged 1½ to 2½ years (p<0.05 for intakes from all sources).

Although there was a clear seasonal variation in plasma vitamin D levels, associated with exposure to sunlight, plasma levels also correlated significantly with dietary intakes of vitamin D. In Chapter 8 intakes of vitamin D for children aged between 1½ and 4½ years were reported as being only 18% of the Reference Nutrient Intake (RNI) from food sources, and 27% of the RNI when the intake from dietary supplements was included (see *Table 8.35*) with little variation between the age groups.

Positive correlations between blood levels and dietary intakes of vitamin D were greatest for children aged between 2½ and 3½ and for all girls (p<0.01), and for these groups of children were still marked even when intakes of vitamin D from food sources alone were correlated with blood levels.   *(Tables 10.37 to 10.39)*

10.5 Blood lipids

Plasma total cholesterol (mmol/l)
Total cholesterol levels in the blood are influenced by a number of factors, in particular age and diet. High levels occur in some diseases, for example kidney, liver and thyroid disorders, or in diabetes. The specific genetic condition of familial hypercholesterolaemia, which occurs in homozygous form in about 1 in 500 children, results in very high levels. Other genetic conditions, including heterozygous familial hypercholesterolaemia, cause variable elevations in plasma total cholesterol. It is not clear whether, in children of preschool age who are not affected by these genetic and clinical disorders, cholesterol levels predict risk in adult life of cardiovascular disease[9].

Cholesterol is carried in the blood attached to proteins (lipoproteins). Most cholesterol is carried on low density lipoprotein (LDL), which is the component related directly to cardiovascular risk in adults. A smaller proportion is carried on high density lipoprotein (HDL).

High density lipoprotein (HDL) cholesterol (mmol/l)
In adults with high levels of total cholesterol, higher levels of this component have been associated with lower risk of cardiovascular disease. The implications for preschool children of different concentrations of HDL cholesterol are not known.

Plasma triglycerides (mmol/l)
Blood triglyceride levels are particularly influenced by the composition of recently consumed food. Values for individuals that are more stable over time are obtained if the sample is taken fasting, but this was regarded as an unreasonable requirement for such young children in the survey. This needs to be taken into account in interpreting the results of the blood lipid analyses. Because of

the uncertainty about the significance of these results they are presented in Table 10.42 without commentary.

Low density lipoprotein (LDL) cholesterol
Values for LDL cholesterol were not measured directly, but can be estimated from the measured values for total cholesterol, HDL cholesterol and triglycerides described above using standard formulas. Because of uncertainty about the significance of the lipid results, estimated LDL values have not been calculated.

The assays for both *plasma total and HDL cholesterol* for samples from children in this survey showed no marked variation in mean levels associated with either the age or sex of the child.

The overall mean plasma total cholesterol level was 4.28mmol/l; 3% of children had levels below 3.00mmol/l and 5% had levels of 5.50mmol/l or above. The mean HDL cholesterol value was 1.14mmol/l; 16% of children had levels of 1.40mmol/l or higher, and the data suggest that in the oldest age group boys were somewhat more likely to have levels this high than girls of the same age. This same group of boys was also less likely to have levels of HDL cholesterol of less than 0.80mmol/l.
                (Tables 10.40 and 10.41)

10.5.1 Correlation with dietary intakes

Table 10.43 gives coefficients of correlation between levels of plasma total and HDL cholesterol and intakes of fatty acids.

When identifying the apparent presence or absence of any relationships between plasma cholesterol levels and dietary intakes it should be remembered that the blood samples were not taken from children after a period of fasting.

Plasma levels of both total and HDL cholesterol generally correlated positively with intakes of total fat, saturated, *trans* unsaturated and *cis* monounsaturated fatty acids and with dietary cholesterol, blood levels increasing as dietary intakes increased. The relationships were however generally weak, particularly with respect to levels of plasma total cholesterol. Stronger relationships were found between HDL cholesterol level and intakes of total fat, saturated, *trans* unsaturated and *cis* monounsaturated fatty acids for children aged 2½ to 3½ years (p<0.01) and for all girls in the survey (p<0.05, except for saturated fatty acids where p<0.01). To a lesser extent significant positive correlations were found between levels of HDL cholesterol and dietary cholesterol for most groups (p<0.05).

Correlation coefficients between plasma cholesterol levels and dietary intakes of *cis* n-3 and n-6 polyunsaturated fatty acids were low and for all children in the survey did not reach statistical significance levels. The data did suggest however that plasma total cholesterol levels tended to fall as dietary intakes of n-6 polyunsaturated fatty acids increased; the association between plasma total cholesterol levels and intakes of n-3 polyunsaturated fatty acids was not clear. HDL cholesterol levels rose as intakes of n-3 and n-6 polyunsaturated fatty acids increased, except in the youngest age group. Other relationships between polyunsaturated fatty acids and dietary intakes were not consistent across the various age groups or between boys and girls.   *(Table 10.43)*

Levels of plasma HDL cholesterol also showed stronger relationships than plasma total cholesterol levels to measures of the percentage energy obtained from total fat and from saturated fatty acids for children in the survey. In respect of both dietary total and dietary saturated fatty acids, HDL cholesterol levels tended to increase as the percentage of energy derived from these sources increased. These relationships were strongest for the girls in the survey, and for energy from saturated fatty acids for children aged between 1½ and 2½ years ($p < 0.01$).   *(Table 10.44)*

10.6 Acute phase proteins

Caeruloplasmin (g/l) and α_1-antichymotrypsin (g/l)
These are known as 'acute phase reaction proteins'. They are produced in the liver in response to inflammation which, in this age group, is most likely to signify infection. Ferritin is also an acute phase reactant (see *section 10.2* above) and blood ferritin levels may be raised in response to infection. The measurement of acute phase proteins such as caeruloplasmin or α_1-antichymotrypsin could provide independent evidence of infection in addition to data from the questionnaire. This information could assist in the interpretation of the haematological assay results, especially plasma ferritin.

Mean levels of *caeruloplasmin and α_1-antichymotrypsin* measured in the samples did not vary significantly with either the age or sex of the child. In each age group about 10% of children had levels of α_1-antichymotrypsin above 0.650g/l.   *(Tables 10.45 and 10.46)*

Table 10.47 shows correlation coefficients for plasma ferritin with caeruloplasmin and α_1-antichymotrypsin. There was a highly significant correlation between plasma ferritin and α_1-antichymotrypsin but no correlation between plasma ferritin and caeruloplasmin.   *(Table 10.47)*

Albumin
Albumin is a major plasma protein which is synthesised in the liver. Blood levels do not reflect short-term dietary variations in protein intake and are maintained except in cases of extreme starvation or excessive protein loss as a result of disease. Plasma albumin levels rise in response to inflammation and in this respect are similar to other acute phase proteins. Table 10.48 shows plasma albumin levels for children in the survey.   *(Table 10.48)*

10.7 Immunoglobulins

IgA, IgG and IgM
Immunoglobins are plasma proteins derived from B-lymphocytes. They are produced in response to specific protein stimuli, for example viral protein antigens. Immunoglobulins take part in the immune response.

Table 10.49 shows the mean, median and percentile values for levels of these three immunoglobulins in the samples from all children for whom there was sufficient plasma remaining for these assays. As was noted in the introduction to this Chapter these analyses were designated of lowest priority. Thus the results are based on the smallest number of samples and hence should be interpreted with caution.   *(Table 10.49)*

References and notes

1   Relates to all children in the survey, including those who did not give a blood sample (but excluding those not answering the question).
2   The laboratory of the Dunn Nutrition Unit needed to know the child's age when the blood sample was taken, to allow results for individual children to be compared with known reference values. The parents of children with levels outside the reference values or ranges were notified of the result and the desirability of seeking medical advice. GPs were also informed. (See *Chapter 2, and Appendices L and N*). The age of the child on the date the sample was taken has been used in presenting the results in this chapter. In reporting on dietary aspects of the survey the child's age at the mid-point of the 3-month fieldwork period has been used for analysis purpose (see *Chapter 3*). Table 10.50 shows the age and sex distribution of the sample based on these two classifications.
3   Distributions for blood analytes and dietary intakes which were skewed were transformed to approximate more closely to normal before correlating, by taking the base$_{10}$ logarithmic value. Distributions where the skewness statistic was greater than or equal to 1 were defined, for this purpose, as being skewed, and requiring transformation.
4   World Health Organisation. WHO Technical Report Series No. 503 *Nutritional Anaemias*. WHO (Geneva, 1972).
5   Range established from analyses of samples from children attending the Hospital for Sick Children, Great Ormond Street, London.
6   Department of Health. Report on Health and Social Subjects: 45. *Weaning and the Weaning Diet*. HMSO (London, 1994).
7   Department of Health. Report on Health and Social Subjects: 41. *Dietary Reference Values for Food Energy and Nutrients for the United Kingdom*. HMSO (London, 1991).
8   Data from the results of sample analyses of cryptoxanthins, lutein and lycopene were adjusted to take account of the results of assays of quality control materials (*see Appendix N*).
9   Department of Health. Report on Health and Social Subjects: 46. *Nutritional Aspects of Cardiovascular Disease*. HMSO (London, 1994).

Table 10.1 Blood analytes in order of priority for analysis

Analyte	No of cases with reported results	Unit of measurement	Conversion from SI units (factor)	Resulting metric units
Haematology				
Haemoglobin concentration	951	g/dl	*	*
Mean corpuscular volume	951	fl	*	*
Haematocrit	951	l/l	*	*
Mean cell haemoglobin	951	pg	*	*
Mean cell haemoglobin concentration	951	g/dl	*	*
Ferritin	930	µg/l	*	*
Zinc protoporphyrin	950	µmol/mol haem	**	**
Water soluble vitamins and plasma zinc				
Plasma folate	819	nmol/l	× 0.441	µg/l
Vitamin B_{12}	817	pmol/l	× 1.357	ng/l
The erythrocyte glutathione reductase activation coefficient	828	ratio	***	***
Plasma zinc	602	µmol/l	× 0.065	mg/l
Fat soluble vitamins and carotenoids				
Plasma retinol	816	µmol/l	× 0.286	mg/l
α-carotene	807	µmol/l	× 0.537	mg/l
β-carotene	812	µmol/l	× 0.537	mg/l
α-cryptoxanthin	811	µmol/l	× 0.552	mg/l
β-cryptoxanthin	813	µmol/l	× 0.552	mg/l
Lycopene	807	µmol/l	× 0.537	mg/l
Lutein	812	µmol/l	× 0.569	mg/l
Plasma 25-hydroxyvitamin D	737	nmol/l	× 0.400	mg/l
α-tocopherol	816	µmol/l	× 0.552	mg/l
γ-tocopherol	816	µmol/l	× 0.417	mg/l
Blood lipids				
Plasma triglycerides	682	mmol/l	****	****
Plasma total cholesterol	683	mmol/l	× 0.387	g/l
High density lipoprotein cholesterol	683	mmol/l	× 0.387	g/l
Acute phase proteins				
Caeruloplasmin	763	g/l	*	*
α₁-antichymotrypsin	763	g/l	*	*
Albumin	754	g/l	*	*
Red cell folate	743	nmol/l	× 0.441	µg/l
Plasma ascorbate	744	µmol/l	× 0.176	mg/l
Immunoglobulins				
IgA	105	g/l	*	*
IgG	106	g/l	*	*
IgM	99	g/l	*	*

*   Analyte measured in metric units

**   The metabolite ratio µmol/mol haem is the expression of choice. Porphyrin concentration units found in the literature include:

         µg ZPP/dl whole blood

         µg ZPP/dl RBC

         µg ZPP/g haemoglobin

Direct, retrospective conversion to the ratio is not possible without haemoglobin concentration having been obtained at the time of the ZPP assay. Where this is available, the conversion becomes, for example,

$$(\mu g\ ZPP \times 64{,}500) \div (g\ Hb \times 562.27 \times 4)$$
$$= (\mu g\ ZPP/g\ haemoglobin) \times 28.68$$
$$= \mu mol\ ZPP/mol\ haem$$

***   Analyte measured as a ratio

****   Triglycerides are measured as glycerol; the molecular weight of a triglyceride molecule varies with different fatty acid constitutents; conversion from SI to metric units is not appropriate.

Figure 10.1 Haemoglobin concentration: all children aged 1¹/₂ - 4¹/₂ years

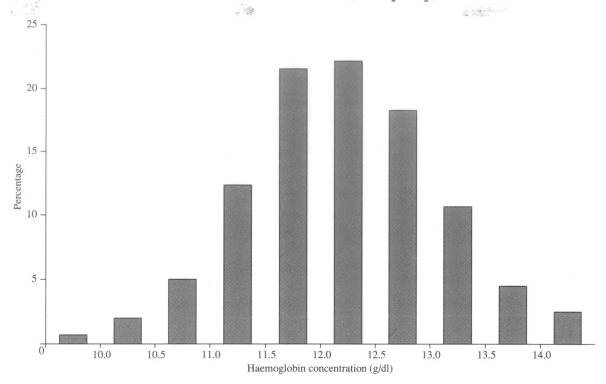

Figure 10.2 Ferritin: all children aged 1¹/₂ - 4¹/₂ years

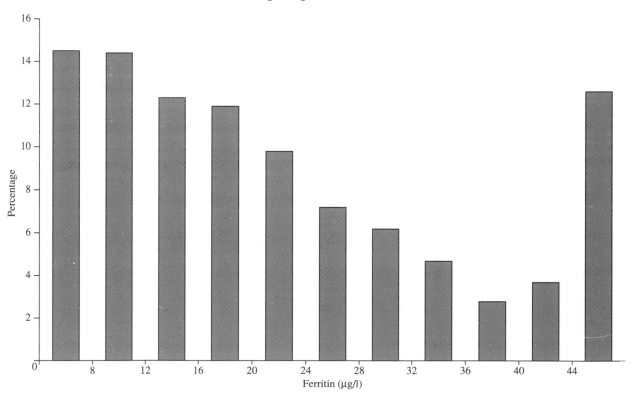

Figure 10.3 Plasma folate: all children aged 1¹/₂ - 4¹/₂ years

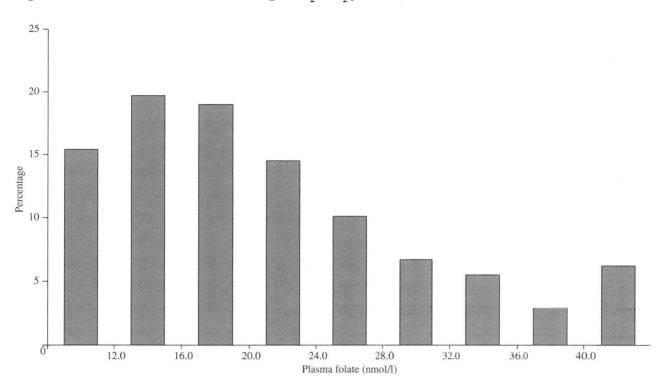

Plasma folate (nmol/l)

Figure 10.4 Plasma ascorbate (vitamin C): all children aged 1¹/₂ - 4¹/₂ years

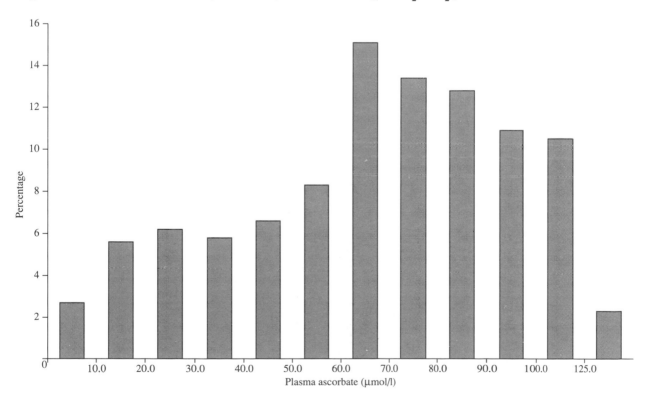

Plasma ascorbate (μmol/l)

Figure 10.5 Plasma retinol (vitamin A): all children aged $1^1/_2$ - $4^1/_2$ years

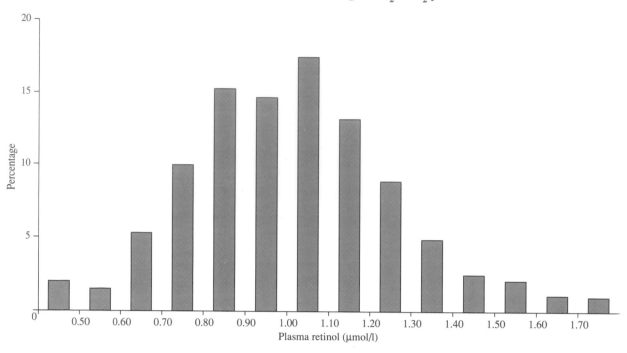

Figure 10.6 Plasma 25-hydroxyvitamin D: all children aged $1^1/_2$ - $4^1/_2$ years

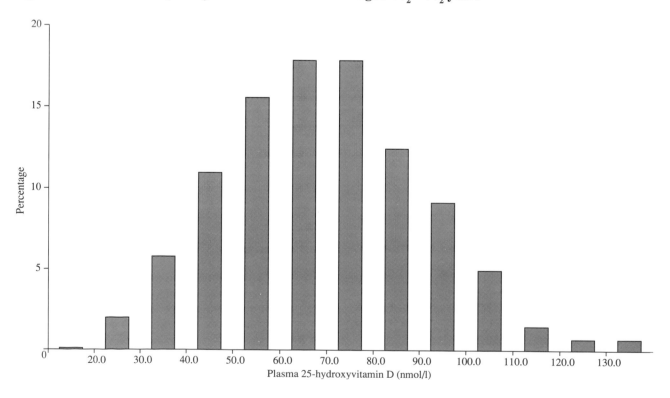

Figure 10.7 Variation in levels of plasma 25-hydroxyvitamin D by fieldwork wave: all children aged 1$^1/_2$ - 4$^1/_2$ years

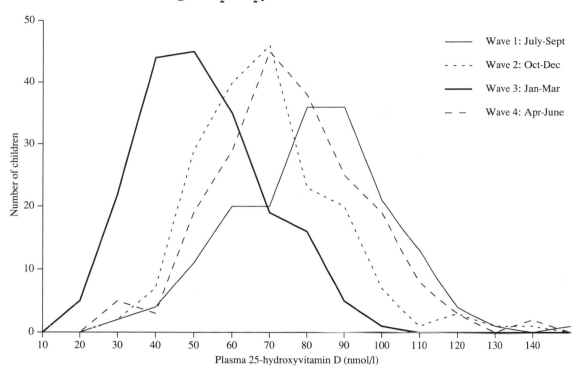

Table 10.2 Percentage distribution of haemoglobin concentration by age and sex of child

Haemoglobin concentration (g/dl)	Age and sex of child						
	All aged 1½ – 2½ years	All aged 2½ – 3½ years	All aged 3½ – 4½ years		All boys	All girls	All
			Boys	Girls			
	cum %	cum %	cum %	cum %	cum %	cum %	cum %
Less than 10.0	2	1	–	–	0	1	1
Less than 10.5	4	2	2	2	3	3	3
Less than 11.0	12	6	4	8	7	9	8
Less than 12.0	51	42	32	31	40	44	42
Less than 13.0	84	82	80	82	82	83	82
Less than 14.0	99	97	96	98	97	98	97
All	100	100	100	100	100	100	100
Base	310	351	137	153	475	476	951
Mean (average value)	12.0	12.2	12.4	12.3	12.2	12.1	12.2
Median value	11.9	12.1	12.4	12.2	12.2	12.1	12.1
Lower 2.5 percentile	10.2	10.6	10.6	10.5	10.4	10.3	10.4
Upper 2.5 percentile	13.7	14.1	15.0	13.9	14.2	13.9	14.0
Standard error of the mean	0.05	0.05	0.09	0.07	0.04	0.04	0.03
Standard deviation	0.92	0.88	1.0	0.83	0.94	0.89	0.91

Table 10.3 Percentage distribution of mean cell haemoglobin (MCH) by age and sex of child

Mean cell haemoglobin (pg)	Age and sex of child						
	All aged 1½ – 2½ years	All aged 2½ – 3½ years	All aged 3½ – 4½ years		All boys	All girls	All
			Boys	Girls			
	cum %	cum %	cum %	cum %	cum %	cum %	cum %
Less than 24.0	9	5	2	3	6	5	5
Less than 25.0	18	11	4	6	13	10	12
Less than 26.0	37	24	15	16	28	23	26
Less than 27.0	61	47	45	36	53	46	50
Less than 28.0	84	76	72	69	79	75	77
Less than 29.0	94	93	93	87	94	91	92
All	100	100	100	100	100	100	100
Base	310	351	137	153	475	476	951
Mean (average value)	26.2	26.9	27.2	27.3	26.7	26.9	26.8
Median value	26.5	27.0	27.2	27.4	26.8	27.0	27.0
Lower 2.5 percentile	21.5	23.3	23.8	23.9	22.3	22.9	22.7
Upper 2.5 percentile	29.3	29.7	29.6	29.9	29.5	29.7	29.6
Standard error of the mean	0.12	0.09	0.12	0.12	0.08	0.08	0.06
Standard deviation	2.0	1.7	1.4	1.4	1.8	1.8	1.8

Table 10.4 Percentage distribution of mean cell haemoglobin concentration (MCHC) by age and sex of child

Mean cell haemoglobin concentration (g/dl)	Age and sex of child						
	All aged 1½ – 2½ years	All aged 2½ – 3½ years	All aged 3½ – 4½ years		All boys	All girls	All
			Boys	Girls			
	cum %	cum %	cum %	cum %	cum %	cum %	cum %
Less than 32.5	8	5	7	3	5	6	6
Less than 33.5	35	32	23	32	27	36	32
Less than 34.5	73	72	68	65	71	71	71
Less than 35.5	92	93	91	94	92	93	93
All	100	100	100	100	100	100	100
Base	*310*	*351*	*137*	*153*	*475*	*476*	*951*
Mean (average value)	33.8	34.0	34.1	34.0	34.0	33.9	33.9
Median value	33.9	34.0	34.0	34.1	34.0	33.9	33.9
Lower 2.5 percentile	31.2	32.2	32.0	32.1	32.0	31.9	32.0
Upper 2.5 percentile	36.1	36.1	36.2	36.1	36.1	36.1	36.1
Standard error of the mean	0.08	0.05	0.09	0.08	0.05	0.05	0.04
Standard deviation	1.4	0.98	1.0	0.95	1.1	1.1	1.1

Table 10.5 Percentage distribution of mean corpuscular volume (MCV) by age and sex of child

Mean corpuscular volume (fl)	Age and sex of child						
	All aged 1½ – 2½ years	All aged 2½ – 3½ years	All aged 3½ – 4½ years		All boys	All girls	All
			Boys	Girls			
	cum %	cum %	cum %	cum %	cum %	cum %	cum %
Less than 70.0	5	2	1	–	3	2	2
Less than 75.0	21	12	5	5	33	11	13
Less than 80.0	75	56	53	48	84	56	61
Less than 85.0	96	95	93	92	96	93	95
All	100	100	100	100	100	100	100
Base	*310*	*351*	*137*	*153*	*475*	*476*	*951*
Mean (average value)	77.5	79.2	79.9	80.2	78.5	79.4	78.9
Median value	78.1	79.3	79.7	80.0	78.7	79.6	79.1
Lower 2.5 percentile	66.6	70.9	73.0	73.2	69.4	70.5	70.4
Upper 2.5 percentile	85.7	86.3	86.4	85.9	85.7	86.5	86.1
Standard error of the mean	0.26	0.21	0.31	0.26	0.18	0.19	0.13
Standard deviation	4.5	3.9	3.6	3.2	4.0	4.1	4.1

Table 10.6 Percentage distribution of haematocrit by age and sex of child

Haematocrit (l/l)	Age and sex of child						
	All aged 1½ – 2½ years	All aged 2½ – 3½ years	All aged 3½ – 4½ years		All boys	All girls	All
			Boys	Girls			
	cum %	cum %	cum %	cum %	cum %	cum %	cum %
Less than 0.325	9	5	2	8	6	6	6
Less than 0.350	47	38	30	31	38	40	39
Less than 0.375	79	78	72	76	76	78	77
Less than 0.400	97	95	94	96	95	96	96
All	100	100	100	100	100	100	100
Base	*310*	*351*	*137*	*153*	*475*	*476*	*951*
Mean (average value)	0.354	0.359	0.364	0.360	0.359	0.357	0.358
Median value	0.352	0.359	0.361	0.359	0.358	0.356	0.357
Lower 2.5 percentile	0.310	0.314	0.325	0.311	0.313	0.312	0.313
Upper 2.5 percentile	0.404	0.411	0.420	0.406	0.408	0.406	0.406
Standard error of the mean	0.001	0.001	0.002	0.002	0.001	0.001	0.001
Standard deviation	0.023	0.023	0.027	0.022	0.024	0.023	0.024

Table 10.7 Percentage distribution of ferritin by age and sex of child

| Ferritin (µg/l) | All aged 1½ – 2½ years | All aged 2½ – 3½ years | All aged 3½ – 4½ years | | All boys | All girls | All |
| | | | Boys | Girls | | | |
	cum %	cum %	cum %	cum %	cum %	cum %	cum %
Less than 5	9	3	4	3	6	4	5
Less than 10	28	18	16	14	24	17	20
Less than 20	60	51	56	41	58	48	53
Less than 30	77	72	70	67	74	71	73
All	100	100	100	100	100	100	100
Base	*300*	*345*	*135*	*150*	*467*	*463*	*930*
Mean (average value)	21	24	25	26	23	24	24
Median value	16	19	17	23	17	20	18
Lower 2.5 percentile*	4	4	4	4	4	4	4
Upper 2.5 percentile	78	70	80	76	71	76	71
Standard error of the mean	1.1	1.0	1.8	1.4	0.88	0.84	0.61
Standard deviation	18.7	18.1	21.0	16.7	19.0	18.2	18.6

*Below the precision of the analytic methodology.

Table 10.8 Percentage distribution of zinc protoporphyrin (ZPP) by age and sex of child

| Zinc protoporphyrin (ZPP) (µmol/mol haem) | All aged 1½ – 2½ years | All aged 2½ – 3½ years | All aged 3½ – 4½ years | | All boys | All girls | All |
| | | | Boys | Girls | | | |
	cum %	cum %	cum %	cum %	cum %	cum %	cum %
Less than 30	1	1	1	–	1	1	1
Less than 45	25	30	42	31	32	29	30
Less than 60	66	75	84	78	76	72	74
Less than 75	88	90	94	97	91	92	91
Less than 80	91	96	97	99	94	96	95
All	100	100	100	100	100	100	100
Base	*309*	*351*	*137*	*153*	*474*	*476*	*950*
Mean (average value)	58	54	51	51	54	54	54
Median value	54	50	46	50	50	52	50
Lower 2.5 percentile	32	32	30	33	32	32	32
Upper 2.5 percentile	126	92	91	75	113	93	102
Standard error of the mean	1.5	1.0	1.7	0.9	1.0	0.9	0.7
Standard deviation	26.5	19.0	19.7	11.2	22.0	20.2	21.1

Table 10.9 Correlation coefficients between haemoglobin concentration, ferritin and ZPP

Age and sex of child	Correlation coefficients for					
	Haemoglobin concentration with:				Ferritin with:	
	Ferritin	Base	ZPP	Base	ZPP	Base
All aged 1½–2½ years	0.12*	300	−0.39**	309	−0.24**	299
All aged 2½–3½ years	0.18**	345	−0.28**	351	−0.12*	345
Boys aged 3½–4½ years	0.04	135	−0.16	137	−0.09	135
Girls aged 3½–4½ years	0.18*	150	−0.22**	153	−0.13	150
All boys	0.08	467	−0.30**	474	−0.16**	466
All girls	0.25**	463	−0.32**	476	−0.18**	463
All children	0.15**	930	−0.31**	950	−0.17**	929

*p<0.05
**p<0.01

Table 10.10 Mean levels for haematology and water soluble vitamins by region

Blood analyte	Region									
	Scotland					Northern				
	Mean	Median	se	sd	Base	Mean	Median	se	sd	Base
Haemoglobin concentration (g/dl)	12.0	12.0	0.1	0.8	94	12.2	12.2	0.1	0.9	245
Mean cell haemoglobin (pg)	26.8	26.9	0.2	1.6	94	26.9	26.9	0.1	1.8	245
Mean cell haemoglobin concentration (g/dl)	33.9	33.9	0.1	1.0	94	33.9	33.9	0.1	1.1	245
Mean corpuscular volume (fl)	78.8	79.2	0.4	3.5	94	79.2	79.1	0.2	3.7	245
Haematocrit (l/l)	0.355	0.352	0.002	0.020	94	0.361	0.360	0.002	0.025	245
Ferritin (µg/l)	24	21	2	16	93	25	18	1	19	240
ZPP (µmol/mol haem)	51	46	2	18	94	53	51	1	17	245
Red cell folate (nmol/l)	967	926	38	359	87	887	822	25	334	179
Plasma folate (nmol/l)	21.4	19.4	1.0	10.0	92	20.3	18.1	0.7	10.0	207
Vitamin B$_{12}$ (pmol/l)	650	597	26	246	90	604	564	16	237	207
EGRAC	1.22	1.21	0.01	0.10	90	1.27	1.26	0.01	0.12	215
Plasma ascorbate (µmol/l)	65.2	64.9	3.0	27.9	88	63.0	65.9	2.4	32.4	182

Blood analyte	Region									
	Central, South West and Wales					London and South East				
	Mean	Median	se	sd	Base	Mean	Median	se	sd	Base
Haemoglobin concentration (g/dl)	12.1	12.0	0.0	0.9	325	12.2	12.2	0.1	0.9	287
Mean cell haemoglobin (pg)	26.7	26.9	0.1	1.8	325	26.9	27.1	0.1	1.9	287
Mean cell haemoglobin concentration (g/dl)	33.9	33.9	0.1	1.0	325	34.1	34.1	0.1	1.2	287
Mean corpuscular volume (fl)	78.6	79.0	0.2	4.2	325	78.9	79.2	0.3	4.4	287
Haematocrit (l/l)	0.356	0.356	0.001	0.023	325	0.359	0.359	0.001	0.024	287
Ferritin (µg/l)	23	18	1	18	316	23	18	1	19	281
ZPP (µmol/mol haem)	56	52	1	24	325	54	50	1	21	286
Red cell folate (nmol/l)	905	857	21	337	257	925	881	22	325	220
Plasma folate (nmol/l)	21.0	19.3	0.6	9.3	279	21.8	20.4	0.6	9.9	241
Vitamin B$_{12}$ (pmol/l)	628	563	16	268	279	666	608	18	283	241
EGRAC	1.23	1.22	0.01	0.10	282	1.25	1.23	0.01	0.11	241
Plasma ascorbate (µmol/l)	70.2	71.9	2.0	31.5	254	69.4	71.8	1.9	27.9	220

Table 10.11   Mean levels for haematology and water soluble vitamins by social class of head of household

| Blood analyte | Social class of head of household | | | | | | | | | |
| | Non-manual | | | | | Manual | | | | |
	Mean	*Median*	*se*	*sd*	*Base*	*Mean*	*Median*	*se*	*sd*	*Base*
Haemoglobin concentration (g/dl)	12.2	12.2	0.0	0.9	*448*	12.1	12.1	0.0	0.9	*467*
Mean cell haemoglobin (pg)	26.9	27.0	0.1	1.6	*448*	26.7	26.9	0.1	1.9	*467*
Mean cell haemoglobin concentration (g/dl)	34.0	34.0	0.0	1.1	*448*	33.9	33.9	0.0	1.2	*467*
Mean corpuscular volume (fl)	78.9	79.0	0.2	3.8	*448*	78.8	79.3	0.2	4.2	*467*
Haematocrit (l/l)	0.358	0.357	0.001	0.023	*448*	0.359	0.357	0.001	0.024	*467*
Ferritin (µg/l)	25	20	1	19	*441*	22	17	1	17	*453*
ZPP (µmol/mol haem)	54	51	1	19	*447*	54	50	1	23	*467*
Red cell folate (nmol/l)	964	901	19	353	*348*	869	823	16	314	363
Plasma folate (nmol/l)	21.9	19.6	0.5	10.0	*386*	20.3	18.7	0.5	9.5	*402*
Vitamin B$_{12}$ (pmol/l)	661	612	13	260	*384*	612	549	13	264	*402*
EGRAC	1.24	1.23	0.01	0.11	*389*	1.25	1.23	0.00	0.11	*405*
Plasma ascorbate (µmol/l)	74.7	76.7	1.5	28.2	*353*	60.9	63.5	1.7	31.4	*359*

Table 10.12   Mean levels for haematology and water soluble vitamins by employment status of head of household

| Blood analyte | Employment status of head of household | | | | | | | | | |
| | Working | | | | | Unemployed | | | | |
	Mean	*Median*	*se*	*sd*	*Base*	*Mean*	*Median*	*se*	*sd*	*Base*
Haemoglobin concentration (g/dl)	12.2	12.2	0.0	0.9	*711*	12.0	12.0	0.1	0.9	*94*
Mean cell haemoglobin (pg)	26.9	27.0	0.1	1.8	*711*	26.6	26.8	0.2	1.8	*94*
Mean cell haemoglobin concentration (g/dl)	34.0	34.0	0.0	1.2	*711*	33.8	33.8	0.1	1.0	*94*
Mean corpuscular volume (fl)	79.0	79.2	0.1	4.1	*711*	78.8	79.2	0.4	4.3	*94*
Haematocrit (l/l)	0.359	0.358	0.001	0.024	*711*	0.357	0.354	0.002	0.023	*94*
Ferritin (µg/l)	24	19	1	19	*694*	23	19	2	16	*94*
ZPP (µmol/mol haem)	54	50	1	21	*710*	52	49	1	13	*94*
Red cell folate (nmol/l)	928	883	14	342	*567*	891	811	41	334	*67*
Plasma folate (nmol/l)	21.5	19.7	0.4	9.8	*614*	19.6	16.6	1.0	9.0	*76*
Vitamin B$_{12}$ (pmol/l)	643	588	11	267	*612*	629	579	30	2642	*76*
EGRAC	1.24	1.23	0.00	0.11	*622*	1.25	1.25	0.01	0.10	*79*
Plasma ascorbate (µmol/l)	70.4	72.5	1.2	29.3	*569*	55.2	59.7	3.7	30.7	*67*

| Blood analyte | Employment status of head of household | | | | |
| | Economically inactive | | | | |
	Mean	*Median*	*se*	*sd*	*Base*
Haemoglobin concentration (g/dl)	12.0	12.0	0.1	0.8	*146*
Mean cell haemoglobin (pg)	26.6	26.6	0.2	1.9	*146*
Mean cell haemoglobin concentration (g/dl)	33.8	33.8	0.8	1.0	*146*
Mean corpuscular volume (fl)	78.6	78.7	0.3	3.9	*146*
Haematocrit (l/l)	0.355	0.356	0.002	0.021	*146*
Ferritin (µg/l)	21	17	1	15	*142*
ZPP (µmol/mol haem)	57	53	2	24	*146*
Red cell folate (nmol/l)	857	810	28	296	*109*
Plasma folate (nmol/l)	20.1	17.5	0.8	9.7	*129*
Vitamin B$_{12}$ (pmol/l)	607	550	22	246	*129*
EGRAC	1.26	1.24	0.01	0.12	*127*
Plasma ascorbate (µmol/l)	60.4	61.9	3.2	33.2	*108*

Table 10.13 Mean levels for haematology and water soluble vitamins by whether child's parents were receiving Income Support or Family Credit

Blood analyte	Whether receiving benefit(s)									
	Receiving benefits					Not receiving benefits				
	Mean	Median	se	sd	Base	Mean	Median	se	sd	Base
Haemoglobin concentration (g/dl)	12.1	12.1	0.5	0.9	304	12.2	12.2	0.0	0.9	647
Mean cell haemoglobin (pg)	26.6	26.7	0.1	1.9	304	26.9	27.0	0.1	1.7	647
Mean cell haemoglobin concentration (g/dl)	33.8	33.8	0.1	1.2	304	34.0	34.0	0.0	1.1	647
Mean corpuscular volume (fl)	78.7	78.8	0.2	4.0	304	79.0	79.2	0.2	4.1	647
Haematocrit (l/l)	0.358	0.359	0.001	0.023	304	0.359	0.357	0.001	0.024	647
Ferritin (μ/l)	23	18	1	19	300	24	19	1	19	630
ZPP (μmol/mol haem)	55	51	1	22	304	54	50	1	21	646
Red cell folate (nmol/l)	865	813	21	318	229	936	883	15	342	514
Plasma folate (nmol/l)	20.3	17.7	0.6	9.7	264	21.5	19.7	0.4	9.8	555
Vitamin B$_{12}$ (pmol/l)	621	551	16	259	264	643	590	11	265	553
EGRAC	1.25	1.25	0.01	0.11	264	1.24	1.22	0.00	0.11	564
Plasma ascorbate (μmol/l)	58.7	63.1	2.1	30.9	224	71.4	73.1	1.3	29.4	520

Table 10.14 Mean levels for haematology and water soluble vitamins by mother's highest educational qualification level

Blood analyte	Mother's highest educational qualification level														
	Above GCE 'A' level					GCE 'A' level and equivalent					GCE 'O' level and equivalent				
	Mean	Median	se	sd	Base	Mean	Median	se	sd	Base	Mean	Median	se	sd	Base
Haemoglobin concentration (g/dl)	12.3	12.2	0.1	0.9	177	12.1	12.1	0.1	0.9	112	12.2	12.2	0.0	0.9	328
Mean cell haemoglobin (pg)	27.0	27.1	0.1	1.5	177	26.8	27.0	0.2	2.1	112	26.9	27.0	0.1	1.6	328
Mean cell haemoglobin concentration (g/dl)	34.1	34.0	0.1	1.1	177	34.0	34.0	0.1	1.6	112	34.0	34.0	0.1	1.0	328
Mean corpuscular volume (fl)	79.2	79.2	0.3	3.6	177	78.7	79.1	0.4	4.2	112	79.1	79.3	0.2	3.9	328
Haematocrit (l/l)	0.360	0.357	0.002	0.022	177	0.356	0.357	0.002	0.022	112	0.360	0.360	0.001	0.024	328
Ferritin (μ/l)	24	19	2	21	176	24	21	2	17	110	23	18	1	16	317
ZPP (μmol/mol haem)	53	50	1	18	176	54	50	2	27	112	54	51	1	19	328
Red cell folate (nmol/l)	1025	964	30	361	140	964	918	36	326	83	899	858	21	344	264
Plasma folate (nmol/l)	22.9	21.1	0.7	9.2	158	22.6	20.4	1.0	10.2	95	21.6	19.5	0.6	10.2	280
Vitamin B$_{12}$ (pmol/l)	684	629	21	263	157	663	583	30	290	95	614	561	15	255	280
EGRAC	1.24	1.24	0.01	0.12	156	1.22	1.22	0.01	0.08	92	1.25	1.23	0.01	0.11	290
Plasma ascorbate (μmol/l)	78.5	79.2	2.2	27.0	146	72.3	73.8	3.3	29.8	83	68.4	69.6	1.9	31.2	262

Blood analyte	Mother's highest educational qualification level									
	CSE and equivalent					None				
	Mean	Median	se	sd	Base	Mean	Median	se	sd	Base
Haemoglobin concentration (g/dl)	12.1	12.0	0.9	1.0	130	12.0	12.0	0.1	0.9	201
Mean cell haemoglobin (pg)	26.9	26.8	0.2	2.0	130	26.4	26.7	0.1	1.9	201
Mean cell haemoglobin concentration (g/dl)	33.9	33.9	1.1	1.2	130	33.7	33.8	0.1	0.9	201
Mean corpuscular volume (fl)	79.0	79.3	0.3	3.9	130	78.3	78.5	0.3	4.8	201
Haematocrit (l/l)	0.358	0.356	0.002	0.027	130	0.356	0.355	0.002	0.024	201
Ferritin (μ/l)	24	18	2	21	129	23	19	1	19	195
ZPP (μmol/mol haem)	54	50	2	20	130	57	53	2	24	201
Red cell folate (nmol/l)	842	797	31	301	97	859	811	24	298	157
Plasma folate (nmol/l)	19.4	16.8	0.9	9.5	112	19.0	17.2	0.7	8.9	171
Vitamin B$_{12}$ (pmol/l)	609	550	24	257	111	631	576	20	263	171
EGRAC	1.25	1.23	0.01	0.11	113	1.25	1.24	0.01	0.11	174
Plasma ascorbate (μmol/l)	60.6	62.7	2.8	27.8	95	57.4	60.7	2.4	30.0	156

231

Table 10.15   Mean levels for haematology and water soluble vitamins by family type

Blood analyte	Family type									
	Married or cohabiting couple									
	One child					More than one child				
	Mean	Median	se	sd	Base	Mean	Median	se	sd	Base
Haemoglobin concentration (g/dl)	12.2	12.1	0.1	0.9	189	12.1	12.1	0.0	0.9	592
Mean cell haemoglobin (pg)	26.6	26.9	0.1	1.9	189	26.9	27.0	0.1	1.8	592
Mean cell haemoglobin concentration (g/dl)	33.9	33.9	0.1	1.2	189	34.0	34.0	0.0	1.1	592
Mean corpuscular volume (fl)	78.5	79.0	0.3	4.2	189	79.0	79.2	0.2	4.1	592
Haematocrit (l/l)	0.360	0.357	0.002	0.024	189	0.357	0.357	0.001	0.023	592
Ferritin (μ/l)	24	18	1	21	183	23	18	1	18	580
ZPP (μmol/mol haem)	55	50	2	22	188	54	50	1	20	592
Red cell folate (nmol/l)	938	865	30	364	150	917	879	15	333	463
Plasma folate (nmol/l)	21.0	19.7	0.8	9.9	159	21.1	19.3	0.4	9.6	505
Vitamin B_{12} (pmol/l)	640	569	24	306	159	645	594	11	259	503
EGRAC	1.24	1.22	0.01	0.12	164	1.24	1.23	0.00	0.10	513
Plasma ascorbate (μmol/l)	75.2	78.5	2.5	31.4	151	67.1	69.1	1.4	29.7	463

Blood analyte	Family type									
	Lone parent									
	One child					More than one child				
	Mean	Median	se	sd	Base	Mean	Median	se	sd	Base
Haemoglobin concentration (g/dl)	12.3	12.2	0.1	0.8	70	12.1	12.0	0.1	1.1	100
Mean cell haemoglobin (pg)	27.2	27.3	0.2	1.8	70	26.5	26.6	0.2	1.8	100
Mean cell haemoglobin concentration (g/dl)	34.1	34.0	0.1	1.0	70	33.7	33.9	0.1	1.0	100
Mean corpuscular volume (fl)	79.6	79.7	0.3	2.9	70	78.8	78.7	0.4	4.2	100
Haematocrit (l/l)	0.361	0.360	0.003	0.022	70	0.359	0.358	0.003	0.029	100
Ferritin (μ/l)	27	22	2	20	70	21	17	1	15	97
ZPP (μmol/mol haem)	49	46	1	11	70	58	53	3	27	100
Red cell folate (nmol/l)	872	844	48	362	57	877	832	31	264	73
Plasma folate (nmol/l)	21.5	19.0	1.2	10.2	66	20.9	18.1	1.1	10.1	89
Vitamin B_{12} (pmol/l)	582	540	27	222	66	616	558	24	229	89
EGRAC	1.26	1.24	0.01	0.12	64	1.26	1.25	0.01	0.11	87
Plasma ascorbate (μmol/l)	63.7	66.0	3.84	28.1	56	58.4	57.9	3.6	31.4	74

Table 10.16 Correlation coefficients between blood analytes and dietary intakes: haemoglobin, ferritin and ZPP with dietary iron and vitamin C

Dietary intake	Blood analyte		
	Haemoglobin concentration	Ferritin	ZPP
Total iron (from all sources)			
All aged 1½ – 2½ years	0.00	0.02	0.10
All aged 2½ – 3½ years	0.02	0.04	−0.04
Boys aged 3½ – 4½ years	0.17*	−0.07	−0.11
Girls aged 3½ – 4½ years	0.08	0.13	−0.06
All boys	0.10	0.06	−0.09
All girls	0.04	0.05	0.02
All children	0.08*	0.05	−0.03
Haem iron (from all sources)†			
All aged 1½ – 2½ years	0.00	−0.04	0.06
All aged 2½ – 3½	0.06	0.13*	−0.05
Boys aged 3½ – 4½ years	0.08	−0.04	0.02
Girls aged 3½ – 4½ years	0.23	0.13	−0.00
All boys	0.04	0.02	0.02
All girls	0.14**	0.08	−0.04
All children	0.08*	0.05	−0.01
Non-haem iron (from all sources)			
All aged 1½ – 2½ years	0.01	0.02	0.09
All aged 2½ – 3½ years	0.02	0.02	−0.03
Boys aged 3½ – 4½ years	0.16	−0.07	−0.14
Girls aged 3½ – 4½ years	0.04	0.11	−0.07
All boys	0.10*	0.04	−0.09*
All girls	0.03	0.04	0.02
All children	0.07+	0.04	−0.03
Vitamin C			
All aged 1½ – 2½ years	0.06	0.08	−0.09
All aged 2½ – 3½ years	0.09	0.02	0.00
Boys aged 3½ – 4½ years	0.00	−0.02	−0.03
Girls aged 3½ – 4½ years	0.02	0.13	−0.05
All boys	0.07	0.01	−0.00
All girls	0.05	0.08	−0.06
All children	0.06	0.05	−0.03

*p<0.05
**p<0.01
†Excludes 13 children with nil haem iron intakes.

Table 10.16(a) Base numbers

Dietary intake	Blood analyte		
	Haemoglobin concentration	Ferritin	ZPP
	Base	Base	Base
Total iron, non-haem iron and vitamin C (from all sources)			
All aged 1½ – 2½ years	302	293	301
All aged 2½ – 3½ years	337	332	337
Boys aged 3½ – 4½ years	135	133	135
Girls aged 3½ – 4½ years	149	146	149
All boys	463	452	459
All girls	460	452	463
All children	923	904	922
Haem iron (from all sources)†			
All aged 1½ – 2½ years	300	291	299
All aged 2½ – 3½ years	331	326	331
Boys aged 3½ – 4½ years	135	141	135
Girls aged 3½ – 4½ years	144	133	144
All boys	453	445	452
All girls	457	446	457
All children	910	891	909

†Excludes 13 children with nil haem iron intakes.

Table 10.17 Percentage distribution of red cell folate by age and sex of child

Red cell folate (nmol/l)	Age and sex of child						
	All aged 1½ – 2½ years	All aged 2½ – 3½ years	All aged 3½ – 4½ years		All boys	All girls	All
			Boys	Girls			
	cum %	cum %	cum %	cum %	cum %	cum %	cum %
Less than 400	2	2	–	1	1	2	2
Less than 600	14	18	10	11	14	15	15
Less than 800	38	43	31	46	35	46	40
Less than 1000	67	70	63	67	66	69	68
Less than 1200	82	85	84	82	83	84	83
Less than 1400	90	92	91	90	91	92	91
All	100	100	100	100	100	100	100
Base	220	283	118	122	382	361	743
Mean (average value)	931	884	941	926	934	894	914
Median value	891	838	888	866	890	832	868
Lower 2.5 percentile	418	397	484	418	446	407	429
Upper 2.5 percentile	1859	1696	1637	1874	1847	1716	1749
Standard error of the mean	24	20	28	31	18	17	12
Standard deviation	357	328	305	341	344	326	336

233

Table 10.18 Percentage distribution of plasma folate by age and sex of child

Plasma folate (nmol/l)	Age and sex of child						
	All aged 1½ – 2½ years	All aged 2½ – 3½ years	All aged 3½ – 4½ years		All boys	All girls	All
			Boys	Girls			
	cum %	cum %	cum %	cum %	cum %	cum %	cum %
Less than 10.0	7	10	9	5	8	8	8
Less than 20.0	55	55	48	56	55	53	54
Less than 30.0	84	84	82	85	84	84	84
Less than 40.0	94	93	93	96	94	93	94
All	100	100	100	100	100	100	100
Base	*255*	*309*	*124*	*131*	*420*	*399*	*819*
Mean (average value)	21.0	21.1	22.0	20.4	20.9	21.3	21.1
Median value	18.6	19.3	20.9	19.0	19.0	19.3	19.3
Lower 2.5 percentile	7.9	6.1	7.9	8.8	7.3	6.8	7.0
Upper 2.5 percentile	47.6	47.6	47.4	42.5	47.6	47.6	47.6
Standard error of the mean	0.61	0.57	0.92	0.78	0.47	0.49	0.34
Standard deviation	9.7	10.0	10.2	8.9	9.7	9.8	9.8

Table 10.19 Correlation coefficients between red cell folate and plasma folate

Age and sex of child	Correlation coefficient	*Base*
All aged 1½ – 2½ years	0.34**	*204*
All aged 2½ – 3½ years	0.42**	*265*
Boys aged 3½ – 4½ years	0.51**	*107*
Girls aged 3½ – 4½ years	0.44**	*112*
All boys	0.42**	*355*
All girls	0.39**	*333*
All children	0.40**	*688*

**p < 0.01

Table 10.20 Percentage distribution of vitamin B$_{12}$ by age and sex of child

Vitamin B$_{12}$ (pmol/l)	Age and sex of child						
	All aged 1½ – 2½ years	All aged 2½ – 3½ years	All aged 3½ – 4½ years		All boys	All girls	All
			Boys	Girls			
	cum %	cum %	cum %	cum %	cum %	cum %	cum %
Less than 250	1	2	2	2	2	2	2
Less than 500	39	34	33	36	38	34	36
Less than 750	73	70	73	71	72	71	72
Less than 1000	93	90	88	91	91	90	90
Less than 1250	96	98	96	97	97	97	97
All	100	100	100	100	100	100	100
Base	*254*	*308*	*124*	*131*	*418*	*399*	*817*
Mean (average value)	620	645	654	627	632	639	636
Median value	557	605	597	558	578	580	578
Lower 2.5 percentile	262	251	276	279	254	271	263
Upper 2.5 percentile	1427	1238	1329	1395	1315	1367	1336
Standard error of the mean	17.0	14.8	24.1	22.4	12.8	13.3	9.2
Standard deviation	270	259	269	256	261	266	263

Table 10.21 Percentage distribution of the erythrocyte glutathione reductase activation coefficient (EGRAC) by age and sex of child

Erythrocyte glutathione reductase activation coefficient	Age and sex of child						
	All aged 1½ – 2½ years	All aged 2½ – 3½ years	All aged 3½ – 4½ years		All boys	All girls	All
			Boys	Girls			
	cum %	cum %	cum %	cum %	cum %	cum %	cum %
Less than 1.10	7	4	2	1	5	3	4
Less than 1.20	50	34	23	23	39	31	35
Less than 1.30	86	79	71	62	81	73	77
Less than 1.40	95	96	91	87	95	92	93
Less than 1.50	98	98	97	94	98	96	97
All	100	100	100	100	100	100	100
Base	249	316	127	136	421	407	828
Mean (average value)	1.22	1.24	1.26	1.29	1.23	1.26	1.24
Median value	1.20	1.24	1.22	1.27	1.22	1.24	1.23
Lower 2.5 percentile	1.02	1.05	1.08	1.10	1.03	1.07	1.06
Upper 2.5 percentile	1.46	1.45	1.50	1.62	1.44	1.55	1.50
Standard error of the mean	0.01	0.01	0.01	0.01	0.01	0.01	0.00
Standard deviation	0.11	0.095	0.10	0.13	0.10	0.11	0.11

Table 10.22 Percentage distribution of plasma ascorbate (vitamin C) by age and sex of child

Plasma ascorbate (vitamin C) (μmol/l)	Age and sex of child						
	All aged 1½ – 2½ years	All aged 2½ – 3½ years	All aged 3½ – 4½ years		All boys	All girls	All
			Boys	Girls			
	cum %	cum %	cum %	cum %	cum %	cum %	cum %
Less than 10.0	5	3	1	1	3	2	3
Less than 25.0	12	9	13	9	11	10	11
Less than 40.0	22	18	26	17	22	18	20
Less than 55.0	33	30	35	27	36	27	31
Less than 70.0	52	47	61	43	56	44	50
Less than 85.0	70	69	78	66	76	64	70
Less than 100.0	85	87	94	86	90	84	87
All	100	100	100	100	100	100	100
Base	218	284	117	125	380	364	744
Mean (average value)	66.7	69.0	62.0	71.4	64.1	71.3	67.6
Median value	69.0	71.9	64.1	73.8	66.0	74.0	69.8
Lower 2.5 percentile	5.2	7.1	10.1	14.8	8.2	9.2	8.8
Upper 2.5 percentile	122.9	129.8	103.3	124.7	115.5	127.0	124.5
Standard error of the mean	2.1	1.8	2.6	2.6	1.5	1.6	1.1
Standard deviation	31.6	30.6	28.2	29.3	30.1	30.4	30.4

Table 10.23 Percentage distribution of plasma zinc by age and sex of child

Plasma zinc (μmol/l)	Age and sex of child						
	All aged 1½ – 2½ years	All aged 2½ – 3½ years	All aged 3½ – 4½ years		All boys	All girls	All
			Boys	Girls			
	cum %	cum %	cum %	cum %	cum %	cum %	cum %
Less than 10.0	5	5	5	5	4	6	5
Less than 12.0	31	34	36	29	34	31	33
Less than 14.0	71	78	79	64	75	72	73
Less than 16.0	89	93	93	91	91	92	91
All	100	100	100	100	100	100	100
Base	170	221	100	111	300	302	602
Mean (average value)	13.2	12.7	12.9	13.2	13.0	12.9	13.0
Median value	13.0	12.6	12.9	13.0	13.0	12.8	12.9
Lower 2.5 percentile	9.4	9.4	9.1	9.1	9.7	9.2	9.4
Upper 2.5 percentile	18.8	16.8	19.1	18.0	18.7	17.5	18.1
Standard error of the mean	0.18	0.13	0.21	0.21	0.12	0.12	0.09
Standard deviation	2.3	2.0	2.1	2.2	2.1	2.1	2.1

Table 10.24 Correlation coefficients between red cell folate and dietary intakes of vitamin B₁₂ and folate

Blood analyte: red cell folate	Dietary intake, from all sources, of:		Base
	vitamin B_{12}	folate	
All children aged 1½ – 2½ years	0.07	0.02	215
All children aged 2½ – 3½ years	0.07	0.23**	272
All boys aged 3½ – 4½ years	0.02	0.08	116
All girls aged 3½ – 4½ years	−0.01	0.10	119
All boys	−0.02	0.06	371
All girls	0.12*	0.19**	351
All children	0.05	0.12**	722

*p<0.05
**p<0.01

Table 10.25 Correlation coefficients between the erythrocyte glutathione reductase activation coefficient (EGRAC) and dietary intakes of riboflavin

Blood analyte: erythrocyte glutathione reductase activation coefficient (EGRAC)	Dietary intake of riboflavin from:		Base
	all sources	food sources	
All aged 1½ – 2½ years	−0.34**	−0.34**	243
All aged 2½ – 3½ years	−0.29**	−0.28**	303
Boys aged 3½ – 4½ years	−0.31**	−0.24**	125
Girls aged 3½ – 4½ years	−0.32**	−0.33**	133
All boys	−0.30**	−0.29**	408
All girls	−0.31**	−0.31**	396
All children	−0.31**	−0.31**	804

**p<0.01

Table 10.26 Correlation coefficients between plasma ascorbate and dietary intakes of vitamin C

Blood analyte: plasma ascorbate	Dietary intake of vitamin C from:		
	all sources	food sources	Base
All aged 1½ – 2½ years	0.47**	0.43**	213
All aged 2½ – 3½ years	0.47**	0.42**	273
Boys aged 3½ – 4½ years	0.57**	0.54**	115
Girls aged 3½ – 4½ years	0.29**	0.29**	122
All boys	0.48**	0.43**	369
All girls	0.41**	0.39**	354
All children	0.45**	0.42**	723

**p<0.01

Table 10.27 Percentage distribution of α-carotene by age and sex of child

α-carotene (μmol/l)	All aged 1½ – 2½ years	All aged 2½ – 3½ years	All aged 3½ – 4½ years		All boys	All girls	All
			Boys	Girls			
	cum %	cum %	cum %	cum %	cum %	cum %	cum %
Less than 0.020	4	5	2	2	4	3	4
Less than 0.050	23	30	32	24	28	27	27
Less than 0.080	45	54	52	50	51	49	50
Less than 0.110	62	73	68	70	68	70	69
Less than 0.140	75	83	77	82	78	81	79
Less than 0.170	83	89	85	87	85	87	86
All	100	100	100	100	100	100	100
Base	238	310	124	135	407	400	807
Mean (average value)	0.111	0.097	0.096	0.100	0.101	0.103	0.102
Median value	0.089	0.077	0.077	0.076	0.079	0.081	0.079
Lower 2.5 percentile	0.017	0.018	0.021	0.020	0.018	0.018	0.018
Upper 2.5 percentile	0.334	0.347	0.254	0.341	0.324	0.342	0.327
Standard error of the mean	0.006	0.005	0.006	0.007	0.004	0.005	0.003
Standard deviation	0.094	0.094	0.071	0.083	0.081	0.096	0.089

Table 10.28 Percentage distribution of ß-carotene by age and sex of child

ß-carotene (μmol/l)	Age and sex of child						
	All aged 1½ – 2½ years	All aged 2½ – 3½ years	All aged 3½ – 4½ years		All boys	All girls	All
			Boys	Girls			
	cum %	cum %	cum %	cum %	cum %	cum %	cum %
Less than 0.250	12	17	18	11	15	14	14
Less than 0.500	42	55	60	52	51	52	52
Less than 0.750	66	81	78	80	75	77	76
Less than 1.000	83	90	89	91	86	89	88
Less than 1.250	91	94	95	95	92	94	93
Less than 1.500	93	96	96	98	94	97	95
All	100	100	100	100	100	100	100
Base	240	312	125	135	410	402	812
Mean (average value)	0.702	0.562	0.564	0.561	0.626	0.581	0.603
Median value	0.546	0.466	0.444	0.476	0.492	0.479	0.488
Lower 2.5 percentile	0.153	0.117	0.099	0.164	0.120	0.141	0.133
Upper 2.5 percentile	2.224	1.827	1.731	1.539	2.013	1.762	1.856
Standard error of the mean	0.036	0.023	0.040	0.036	0.025	0.021	0.016
Standard deviation	0.551	0.413	0.446	0.417	0.507	0.422	0.467

Table 10.29 Percentage distribution of α-cryptoxanthin by age and sex of child

α-cryptoxanthin (μmol/l)	Age and sex of child						
	All aged 1½ – 2½ years	All aged 2½ – 3½ years	All aged 3½ – 4½ years		All boys	All girls	All
			Boys	Girls			
	cum %	cum %	cum %	cum %	cum %	cum %	cum %
Less than 0.020	5	1	1	–	2	2	2
Less than 0.040	16	13	12	7	14	11	13
Less than 0.060	40	35	34	21	36	32	34
Less than 0.080	60	58	57	47	59	54	56
Less than 0.100	72	70	74	69	72	70	71
Less than 0.120	81	80	85	79	82	80	81
Less than 0.140	89	88	89	86	89	86	88
All	100	100	100	100	100	100	100
Base	240	311	124	136	408	403	811
Mean (average value)	0.084	0.087	0.087	0.096	0.084	0.091	0.088
Median value	0.072	0.075	0.073	0.083	0.074	0.076	0.075
Lower 2.5 percentile	0.016	0.024	0.027	0.034	0.022	0.024	0.023
Upper 2.5 percentile	0.210	0.253	0.262	0.245	0.208	0.264	0.240
Standard error of the mean	0.004	0.003	0.005	0.005	0.002	0.003	0.002
Standard deviation	0.056	0.052	0.055	0.058	0.048	0.060	0.055

Table 10.30   Percentage distribution of ß-cryptoxanthin by age and sex of child

ß-cryptoxanthin (μmol/l)	Age and sex of child						
	All aged 1½ – 2½ years	All aged 2½ – 3½ years	All aged 3½ – 4½ years		All boys	All girls	All
			Boys	Girls			
	cum %	cum %	cum %	cum %	cum %	cum %	cum %
Less than 0.100	35	31	39	25	35	30	32
Less than 0.200	67	66	73	66	70	64	67
Less than 0.300	81	83	88	87	86	82	84
Less than 0.400	90	90	96	92	92	90	91
Less than 0.500	95	94	97	94	96	94	95
All	100	100	100	100	100	100	100
Base	240	312	125	136	410	403	813
Mean (average value)	0.298	0.190	0.168	0.219	0.178	0.210	0.194
Median value	0.140	0.144	0.120	0.151	0.125	0.154	0.143
Lower 2.5 percentile	0.031	0.034	0.029	0.045	0.032	0.038	0.033
Upper 2.5 percentile	0.757	0.597	0.686	1.015	0.590	0.757	0.681
Standard error of the mean	0.012	0.008	0.014	0.022	0.008	0.010	0.006
Standard deviation	0.192	0.144	0.152	0.257	0.154	0.208	0.183

Table 10.31   Percentage distribution of lycopene by age and sex of child

Lycopene (μmol/l)	Age and sex of child						
	All aged 1½ – 2½ years	All aged 2½ – 3½ years	All aged 3½ – 4½ years		All boys	All girls	All
			Boys	Girls			
	cum %	cum %	cum %	cum %	cum %	cum %	cum %
Less than 0.300	32	30	27	21	29	28	29
Less than 0.600	65	69	70	56	69	63	66
Less than 0.900	84	90	89	82	88	86	87
Less than 1.200	93	95	98	95	95	95	95
All	100	100	100	100	100	100	100
Base	238	310	124	135	407	400	807
Mean (average value)	0.532	0.502	0.489	0.587	0.503	0.543	0.523
Median value	0.436	0.424	0.425	0.563	0.430	0.482	0.444
Lower 2.5 percentile	0.036	0.039	0.046	0.096	0.034	0.071	0.049
Upper 2.5 percentile	1.616	1.475	1.210	1.421	1.372	1.476	1.426
Standard error of the mean	0.026	0.021	0.026	0.028	0.017	0.019	0.013
Standard deviation	0.400	0.373	0.295	0.325	0.439	0.377	0.363

Table 10.32 Percentage distribution of lutein by age and sex of child

Lutein (μmol/l)	All aged 1½ – 2½ years	All aged 2½ – 3½ years	All aged 3½ – 4½ years		All boys	All girls	All
			Boys	Girls			
	cum %	cum %	cum %	cum %	cum %	cum %	cum %
Less than 0.100	8	6	2	2	5	5	5
Less than 0.200	50	45	43	36	45	44	45
Less than 0.300	80	81	81	74	81	78	79
Less than 0.400	96	94	93	90	95	92	94
All	100	100	100	100	100	100	100
Base	*240*	*312*	*124*	*136*	*409*	*403*	*812*
Mean (average value)	0.217	0.228	0.227	0.255	0.224	0.235	0.229
Median value	0.199	0.213	0.208	0.236	0.206	0.213	0.210
Lower 2.5 percentile	0.077	0.076	0.103	0.100	0.084	0.077	0.080
Upper 2.5 percentile	0.424	0.475	0.513	0.549	0.436	0.517	0.478
Standard error of the mean	0.006	0.006	0.009	0.009	0.005	0.005	0.004
Standard deviation	0.101	0.111	0.097	0.109	0.103	0.109	0.106

Table 10.33 Percentage distribution of plasma retinol (vitamin A) by age and sex of child

Plasma retinol (μmol/l)	All aged 1½ – 2½ years	All aged 2½ – 3½ years	All aged 3½ – 4½ years		All boys	All girls	All
			Boys	Girls			
	cum %	cum %	cum %	cum %	cum %	cum %	cum %
Less than 0.50	2	1	2	2	2	2	2
Less than 0.75	12	11	15	14	13	12	12
Less than 1.00	47	49	58	43	53	44	49
Less than 1.25	81	85	88	85	86	83	84
Less than 1.50	95	96	97	95	97	95	96
Less than 1.75	99	99	100	100	99	99	99
All	100	100			100	100	100
Base	*242*	*313*	*125*	*136*	*411*	*405*	*816*
Mean (average value)	1.03	1.02	0.98	1.02	1.00	1.03	1.02
Median value	1.02	1.00	0.96	1.02	0.98	1.02	1.00
Lower 2.5 percentile	0.45	0.58	0.50	0.50	0.57	0.53	0.54
Upper 2.5 percentile	1.61	1.56	1.54	1.60	1.53	1.60	1.56
Standard error of the mean	0.02	0.02	0.02	0.02	0.02	0.01	0.01
Standard deviation	0.26	0.32	0.24	0.26	0.30	0.26	0.28

Table 10.34 Percentage distribution of plasma 25-hydroxyvitamin D by age and sex of child

Plasma 25-hydroxyvitamin D (nmol/l)	Age and sex of child						
	All aged 1½ – 2½ years	All aged 2½ – 3½ years	All aged 3½ – 4½ years		All boys	All girls	All
			Boys	Girls			
	cum %	cum %	cum %	cum %	cum %	cum %	cum %
Less than 25.0	1	1	–	–	–	1	1
Less than 50.0	17	23	12	22	17	21	19
Less than 75.0	64	62	58	58	59	63	61
Less than 100.0	93	92	92	90	91	94	92
Less than 125.0	99	99	99	99	99	99	99
Less than 150.0	99	100	100	100	100	99	99
All	100					100	100
Base	213	274	120	130	377	360	737*
Mean (average value)	67.4	66.6	70.1	70.3	69.0	67.1	68.1
Median value	67.5	67.5	70.0	70.0	67.5	67.5	67.5
Lower 2.5 percentile	27.5	27.5	32.5	35.7	31.1	27.5	30.0
Upper 2.5 percentile	155	108	110	121	113	110	110
Standard error of the mean	1.50	1.30	1.77	1.90	1.09	1.13	0.79
Standard deviation	21.8	21.6	19.4	21.6	21.2	21.5	21.3

*Excludes 41 children for whom results were not available in time for inclusion in this table.

Table 10.35 Percentage distribution of α-tocopherol by age and sex of child

α-tocopherol (μmol/l)	Age and sex of child						
	All aged 1½ – 2½ years	All aged 2½ – 3½ years	All aged 3½ – 4½ years		All boys	All girls	All
			Boys	Girls			
	cum %	cum %	cum %	cum %	cum %	cum %	cum %
Less than 10.0	4	1	–	1	1	2	2
Less than 15.0	21	14	10	11	16	14	15
Less than 20.0	69	66	67	53	71	60	65
Less than 25.0	92	94	95	89	94	91	93
All	100	100	100	100	100	100	100
Base	242	313	125	136	411	405	816
Mean (average value)	18.2	18.8	18.9	19.8	18.5	19.1	18.8
Median value	17.8	18.2	18.7	19.4	18.1	18.7	18.3
Lower 2.5 percentile	8.4	11.5	12.1	12.6	11.3	10.4	10.9
Upper 2.5 percentile	27.7	27.3	27.0	30.8	27.4	29.0	28.1
Standard error of the mean	0.3	0.2	0.3	0.4	0.2	0.2	0.2
Standard deviation	4.5	4.4	3.4	4.4	4.3	4.3	4.3

Table 10.36   Percentage distribution of γ-tocopherol by age and sex of child

γ-tocopherol (μmol/l)	Age and sex of child						
	All aged 1½ – 2½ years	All aged 2½ – 3½ years	All aged 3½ – 4½ years		All boys	All girls	All
			Boys	Girls			
	cum %	cum %	cum %	cum %	cum %	cum %	cum %
Less than 0.5	3	1	1	1	1	2	1
Less than 1.0	28	19	8	16	24	18	21
Less than 1.5	60	44	54	40	53	46	50
Less than 2.0	81	71	70	62	75	70	72
Less than 2.5	93	89	86	82	89	88	89
All	100	100	100	100	100	100	100
Base	*242*	*313*	*125*	*136*	*411*	*405*	*816*
Mean (average value)	1.4	1.6	1.6	1.8	1.5	1.6	1.6
Median value	1.2	1.5	1.4	1.7	1.4	1.5	1.5
Lower 2.5 percentile	0.4	0.5	0.6	0.6	0.5	0.5	0.5
Upper 2.5 percentile	3.1	3.4	3.3	4.5	3.3	3.5	3.4
Standard error of the mean	0.04	0.05	0.07	0.08	0.04	0.04	0.03
Standard deviation	0.67	0.86	0.74	0.87	0.80	0.79	0.80

Table 10.37   Correlation coefficients between plasma retinol and dietary intakes of pre-formed retinol and total carotene

Blood analyte: plasma retinol	Dietary intake, from all sources, of:		*Base*
	pre-formed retinol	total carotene**	
All aged 1½ – 2½ years	0.10	−0.01	*237*
All aged 2½ – 3½ years	0.11	0.07	*300*
Boys aged 3½ – 4½ years	−0.02	0.11	*123*
Girls aged 3½ – 4½ years	0.07	0.04	*133*
All boys	0.06	0.06	*398*
All girls	0.10	0.03	*395*
All children	0.08*	0.04	*793*

*p<0.05
**correlation coefficients were identical for intakes of carotene from food sources (that is, excluding dietary supplements).

Table 10.38   Correlation coefficients between α-tocopherol and dietary intakes of vitamin E

Blood analyte: α-tocopherol	Dietary intake of vitamin E from:		*Base*
	all sources	food sources	
All aged 1½ – 2½ years	0.15*	0.12	*237*
All aged 2½ – 3½ years	0.08	0.06	*300*
Boys aged 3½ – 4½ years	0.00	0.02	*123*
Girls aged 3½ – 4½ years	0.04	0.02	*133*
All boys	0.05	0.06	*398*
All girls	0.14**	0.13*	*395*
All children	0.10**	0.08**	*793*

*p<0.05
**p<0.01

Table 10.39   Correlation coefficients between plasma 25-hydroxyvitamin D and dietary intakes of vitamin D

Blood analyte: plasma 25-hydroxyvitamin D	Dietary intake of vitamin D from:		*Base*
	all sources	food sources	
All aged 1½ – 2½ years	0.10	0.04	*208*
All aged 2½ – 3½ years	0.23**	0.18**	*267*
Boys aged 3½ – 4½ years	0.17	0.12	*118*
Girls aged 3½ – 4½ years	0.01	0.06	*127*
All boys	0.12*	0.06	*365*
All girls	0.18**	0.18**	*350*
All children	0.15**	0.11**	*715*

*p<0.05
**p<0.01

Table 10.40 Percentage distribution of plasma total cholesterol by age and sex of child

Plasma total cholesterol (mmol/l)	Age and sex of child						
	All aged 1½ – 2½ years	All aged 2½ – 3½ years	All aged 3½ – 4½ years		All boys	All girls	All
			Boys	Girls			
	cum %	cum %	cum %	cum %	cum %	cum %	cum %
Less than 3.00	5	3	2	3	2	4	3
Less than 3.50	14	14	11	11	12	13	13
Less than 4.00	34	34	39	33	35	34	35
Less than 4.50	65	64	71	59	65	64	65
Less than 5.00	85	85	85	85	86	85	85
Less than 5.50	93	95	95	95	94	95	95
Less than 6.00	97	98	98	97	98	97	98
All	100	100	100	100	100	100	100
Base	195	256	111	121	341	342	683
Mean (average value)	4.26	4.29	4.23	4.32	4.27	4.38	4.28
Median value	4.24	4.30	4.22	4.24	4.27	4.24	4.25
Lower 2.5 percentile	2.48	2.90	3.00	2.78	2.99	2.74	2.84
Upper 2.5 percentile	6.04	5.97	5.82	6.21	5.79	6.04	5.96
Standard error of the mean	0.06	0.05	0.06	0.07	0.04	0.04	0.03
Standard deviation	0.80	0.74	0.66	0.77	0.70	0.80	0.75

Table 10.41 Percentage distribution of plasma high density lipoprotein cholesterol by age and sex of child

Plasma high density lipoprotein cholesterol (mmol/l)	Age and sex of child						
	All aged 1½ – 2½ years	All aged 2½ – 3½ years	All aged 3½ – 4½ years		All boys	All girls	All
			Boys	Girls			
	cum %	cum %	cum %	cum %	cum %	cum %	cum %
Less than 0.60	3	3	–	2	2	3	2
Less than 0.80	11	10	7	17	7	15	11
Less than 1.00	35	26	26	40	25	37	31
Less than 1.20	59	52	59	65	53	62	58
Less than 1.40	85	83	79	88	79	88	84
Less than 1.60	94	94	92	97	92	97	94
All	100	100	100	100	100	100	100
Base	195	256	111	121	341	342	683
Mean (average value)	1.13	1.16	1.17	1.09	1.19	1.10	1.14
Median value	1.13	1.18	1.12	1.09	1.17	1.10	1.15
Lower 2.5 percentile	0.59	0.53	0.65	0.63	0.63	0.59	0.60
Upper 2.5 percentile	1.80	1.78	1.74	1.67	1.81	1.64	1.76
Standard error of the mean	0.02	0.02	0.03	0.02	0.02	0.02	0.01
Standard deviation	0.28	0.28	0.28	0.27	0.29	0.27	0.28

Table 10.42 Percentage distribution of triglycerides by age and sex of child

Triglycerides (mmol/l)	Age and sex of child						
	All aged 1½ – 2½ years	All aged 2½ – 3½ years	All aged 3½ – 4½ years		All boys	All girls	All
			Boys	Girls			
	cum %	cum %	cum %	cum %	cum %	cum %	cum %
Less than 0.50	–	2	2	2	2	1	1
Less than 1.00	28	30	29	25	31	25	28
Less than 1.50	57	62	65	59	65	56	61
Less than 2.00	82	83	82	76	84	79	81
Less than 2.50	94	91	93	88	94	90	92
All	100	100	100	100	100	100	100
Base	195	255	111	121	341	341	682
Mean (average value)	1.47	1.44	1.40	1.54	1.38	1.53	1.46
Median value	1.39	1.34	1.26	1.37	1.28	1.41	1.34
Lower 2.5 percentile	0.57	0.50	0.51	0.51	0.50	0.57	0.53
Upper 2.5 percentile	3.43	2.94	2.99	3.26	2.78	3.60	2.98
Standard error of the mean	0.05	0.04	0.06	0.08	0.03	0.04	0.03
Standard deviation	0.69	0.67	0.64	0.82	0.61	0.77	0.70

Table 10.43 Correlation coefficients between plasma cholesterol and dietary intakes of total fat and fatty acids

Blood analyte	Dietary intakes							
	Total fat	Saturated fatty acids	trans unsaturated fatty acids	cis monounsaturated fatty acids	cis polyunsaturated fatty acids		Cholesterol	Base
					n-3	n-6		
Plasma total cholesterol								
All aged 1½ – 2½ years	−0.06	−0.03	0.03	−0.07	−0.06	−0.07	0.05	190
All aged 2½ – 3½ years	0.06	0.10	−0.00	0.06	0.02	−0.05	0.07	248
Boys aged 3½ – 4½ years	0.09	0.10	0.06	0.08	−0.03	0.02	0.30**	110
Girls aged 3½ – 4½ years	0.07	0.08	−0.01	0.09	0.04	−0.00	0.06	118
All boys	−0.01	0.03	0.00	−0.02	−0.08	−0.07	0.12*	333
All girls	0.06	0.06	0.02	0.07	0.05	−0.02	0.03	333
All children	0.03	0.05	0.01	0.02	−0.01	−0.04	0.06*	666
HDL cholesterol								
All aged 1½ – 2½ years	0.05	0.12	0.02	0.02	−0.05	−0.14*	0.03	190
All aged 2½ – 3½ years	0.21**	0.20**	0.18**	0.20**	0.16*	0.10	0.16*	248
Boys aged 3½ – 4½ years	0.12	0.13	0.06	0.12	0.02	0.02	0.10	110
Girls aged 3½ – 4½ years	0.12	0.14	0.01	0.14	0.05	0.11	0.19*	118
All boys	0.11	0.14*	0.07	0.10	0.03	0.02	0.12*	333
All girls	0.13*	0.15**	0.09	0.14*	0.08	−0.07	0.12*	333
All children	0.13**	0.16**	0.09*	0.13**	0.06	−0.01	0.12*	666

*p<0.05
**p<0.01

243

Table 10.44 Correlation coefficients between plasma cholesterol and percentage energy from total fat and saturated fatty acids

Blood analyte	Dietary intake		Base
	Percentage energy from:		
	total fat	saturated fatty acids	
Plasma total cholesterol			
All children aged 1½ – 2½ years	−0.05	0.00	190
All children aged 2½ – 3½ years	−0.00	0.07	248
All boys aged 3½ – 4½ years	0.02	0.03	110
All girls aged 3½ – 4½ years	0.06	0.09	118
All boys	−0.03	0.04	333
All girls	0.02	0.05	333
All children	−0.00	0.05	666
HDL cholesterol			
All children aged 1½ – 2½ years	0.08	0.19**	190
All children aged 2½ – 3½ years	0.11	0.12*	248
All boys aged 3½ – 4½ years	0.16	0.17	110
All girls aged 3½ – 4½ years	0.15	0.17	118
All boys	0.09	0.13*	333
All girls	0.15**	0.18**	333
All children	0.11**	0.15**	666

*$p < 0.05$
**$p < 0.01$

Table 10.45 Percentage distribution of caeruloplasmin by age and sex of child

Caeruloplasmin (g/l)	Age and sex of child						
	All aged 1½ – 2½ years	All aged 2½ – 3½ years	All aged 3½ – 4½ years		All boys	All girls	All
			Boys	Girls			
	cum %	cum %	cum %	cum %	cum %	cum %	cum %
Less than 0.200	7	4	4	5	4	6	5
Less than 0.250	25	25	21	25	22	27	24
Less than 0.300	60	58	59	61	56	62	59
Less than 0.350	80	83	75	79	79	81	80
Less than 0.400	88	89	87	87	88	88	88
All	100	100	100	100	100	100	100
Base	227	297	112	127	391	372	763
Mean (average value)	0.30	0.30	0.30	0.29	0.30	0.29	0.30
Median value	0.28	0.28	0.28	0.28	0.28	0.28	0.28
Lower 2.5 percentile	0.17	0.18	0.18	0.15	0.18	0.17	0.18
Upper 2.5 percentile	0.49	0.49	0.48	0.45	0.49	0.47	0.48
Standard error of the mean	0.005	0.004	0.007	0.007	0.004	0.004	0.003
Standard deviation	0.076	0.076	0.074	0.077	0.074	0.077	0.076

Table 10.46 Percentage distribution of α_1-antichymotrypsin by age and sex of child

α_1-antichymotrypsin (g/l)	Age and sex of child						
	All aged 1½ – 2½ years	All aged 2½ – 3½ years	All aged 3½ – 4½ years		All boys	All girls	All
			Boys	Girls			
	cum %	cum %	cum %	cum %	cum %	cum %	cum %
Less than 0.250	2	1	3	1	2	1	2
Less than 0.350	24	15	10	20	15	21	18
Less than 0.450	58	50	43	55	51	54	52
Less than 0.550	79	74	75	81	77	76	77
Less than 0.650	90	87	91	92	90	89	89
All	100	100	100	100	100	100	100
Base	226	298	113	126	393	370	763
Mean (average value)	0.46	0.49	0.49	0.46	0.48	0.48	0.48
Median value	0.43	0.46	0.47	0.44	0.45	0.44	0.45
Lower 2.5 percentile	0.24	0.27	0.21	0.27	0.25	0.27	0.27
Upper 2.5 percentile	0.87	1.0	0.81	0.78	0.86	0.95	0.87
Standard error of the mean	0.010	0.009	0.013	0.011	0.007	0.008	0.005
Standard deviation	0.16	0.16	0.14	0.13	0.14	0.16	0.15

Table 10.47 Correlation coefficients between plasma ferritin and caeruloplasmin and α_1-antichymotrypsin

	Caeruloplasmin	Base	α_1-antichymotrypsin	Base
Plasma ferritin				
All aged 1½ – 2½ years	0.01	220	0.28**	219
All aged 2½ – 3½ years	0.06	287	0.28**	288
Boys aged 3½ – 4½ years	−0.14	108	0.30**	109
Girls aged 3½ – 4½ years	0.11	124	0.33**	123
All boys	−0.04	378	0.28**	380
All girls	0.09	361	0.31**	359
All children	0.02	739	0.29**	739

**$p<0.01$

Table 10.48 Percentage distribution of albumin by age and sex of child

Albumin (g/l)	Age and sex of child						
	All aged 1½ – 2½ years	All aged 2½ – 3½ years	All aged 3½ – 4½ years		All boys	All girls	All
			Boys	Girls			
	cum %	cum %	cum %	cum %	cum %	cum %	cum %
Less than 40.0	12	13	21	10	15	12	13
Less than 45.0	60	54	56	56	55	58	56
Less than 50.0	87	79	79	86	81	85	83
Less than 55.0	96	92	96	96	93	96	95
All	100	100	100	100	100	100	100
Base	225	290	112	127	384	370	754
Mean (average value)	44.3	45.3	44.5	44.4	44.9	44.6	44.7
Median value	43.0	44.0	43.5	44.0	44.0	44.0	44.0
Lower 2.5 percentile	35.0	36.0	36.8	36.2	36.0	36.0	36.0
Upper 2.5 percentile	58.4	61.0	57.0	57.0	60.0	58.7	59.0
Standard error of the mean	0.34	0.35	0.52	0.44	0.29	0.27	0.20
Standard deviation	5.1	5.9	5.5	5.0	5.8	5.2	5.5

Table 10.49   Immunoglobulin levels for all children

Immunoglobulin	Levels in all children (g/l)						No of children
	Mean	Median	Percentiles		Standard error of the mean	Standard deviation	
			Lower 2.5	Upper 2.5			
IgA	0.88	0.79	0.43	1.9	0.045	0.46	105
IgG	9.3	9.2	4.5	14.3	0.26	2.6	106
IgM	0.91	0.82	0.41	1.7	0.032	0.32	99

Table 10.50   Age and sex distribution of children: comparisons between those for whom dietary information was available and those from whom a blood sample was obtained

Age and sex of child	Four-day dietary record kept*	Sufficient blood obtained for assay for:		
		haemoglobin	plasma folate	plasma total cholesterol
	%	%	%	%
All aged 1½ – 2½ years	34	32	31	28
All aged 2½ – 3½ years	36	37	38	37
Boys aged 3½ – 4½ years	15	14	15	16
Girls aged 3½ – 4½ years	15	16	16	18
All boys	51	50	51	50
All girls	49	50	49	50
All children	1675	951	819	683

*Diary containing both weekend days and two weekdays.

11 Anthropometric measurements: results

11.1 Introduction

Chapter 2 described the purpose of making each of the body measurements, weight, height, head and mid upper-arm circumference and supine length, and the equipment and methodologies used; further information on these aspects is given in Appendix O.

This chapter gives results of the anthropometric measurements, presenting descriptive statistics[1] for boys and girls separately in each of three age groups, 1½ to 2½ years, 2½ to 3½ years and 3½ to 4½ years[2]. Not all children would co-operate with every measurement and for this reason the bases of the tables of results vary; for a total of 63 children none of the anthropometric measurements were made. Chapter 3 gave information on the proportions of children who were willing or able to co-operate with the different measurements.

Some measurements have been excluded from the analysis because, from information recorded by the interviewer, they were regarded as unreliable. Table 11.1 shows for each type of measurement, the number of children measured and the number of measurements available for analysis after these exclusions. More information on the reasons for excluding measurements from the tables of results is given in the relevant sections below. *(Table 11.1)*

In addition to the descriptive statistics, for each measurement, except (mid upper-)arm circumference and supine length, where the number of children measured was relatively small, tables are presented giving results from an analysis of variance. These show the combined effects of a number of characteristics of the child and their households and families on that measurement.

11.1.1 The relationship between age and anthropometric measurements in children

A particular problem in presenting and interpreting results of anthropometric measurements taken from preschool children is that, being at a developmental stage of rapid growth, there is a strong correlation between the age of the child and the measurement. Therefore when considering apparent differences between subgroups the effect of age needs to be considered.

Analysis of variance methods allow for the effect of age to be controlled independent of other effects and associations, and in later tables which show correlation coefficients between the various anthropometric measurements, the effect of age has again been controlled for

in each measure. However in interpreting the data presented for groups of children classified by 12-month age cohort, where no standardisation has been applied, this correlation between age and measurement should be remembered.

11.2 Reference curves of stature and weight for children in the UK

At the time this survey was commissioned the standard reference curves of stature and weight being used for children in the UK, the 'Tanner/Whitehouse Standards'[3], were based on data collected prior to 1966. There was concern that these did not adequately describe the growth in stature and weight of the current population of children in this country, firstly because of a trend towards earlier maturity and greater achieved size and second because the original data were not nationally representative. In 1991 a project was begun to produce new reference curves of stature and weight for the UK, using up-to-date data that were, if possible, nationally representative. The results of this project have been reported (Freeman, Cole *et al*, 1995)[4]. Seven data sources were used and most were nationally representative, and it has been proposed that the reference curves should be adopted as the new UK reference curves. Data from this NDNS of children aged 1½ to 4½ years were not available in time to contribute to the construction of the new curves; however, the results from this survey are presented as centiles of the distribution which correspond closely to those used in the new published charts[5] to facilitate comparison.

11.3 Body weight

Interviewers attempted to weigh all children who took part in the survey, and after excluding cases where the measurement was considered to be unreliable results were available for 1707 children.

The main reason for excluding weight measurements was that the children were not sufficiently undressed; this included wearing a dry terry nappy or any type of wet nappy. Measurements for children who could not remain still for long enough for the scales accurately to register their weight were also excluded as were those where a sufficiently firm, level surface on which to place the scales could not be found. In total, measurements for 74 children were excluded for such quality control reasons.

There are a number of other difficulties in measuring weight, not least that it can vary for the same individual at different times of the same day, and controlling for this variation is not easily attained within the constraints imposed by a general population household-based survey. Additionally there are problems associated with the interpretation of weight measurements, in that for adults and children it is highly correlated with height. Moreover weight alone is not a measure of fat, since body weight includes, as well as body fat, the weight of bone, non-fat tissue and body fluids. The association between weight and height may be partly overcome by standardising the two measures to produce an index; for adults, the most widely used of the various indices which standardise weight for height is the Quetelet, or Body Mass Index (weight(kg)/height(m)^2), which is discussed in *section 11.7* below.

Table 11.2 shows descriptive statistics for weight for boys and girls in three 12-month age cohorts.

In the two youngest cohorts boys were on average over half a kilogram heavier than girls (p<0.01); by the age of 3½ years the average weight of girls was close to that of boys, 16.4kg compared to 16.6kg (NS). *(Table 11.2)*

The heights and weights of preschool children were measured in the 1967/8 national survey, and reported as measurements adjusted for age[6,7]. The mean weights for boys and girls in the three age cohorts from the 1967/8 survey are reproduced in Table 11.3. Due to the age-adjustment the standard deviations are slightly smaller than for the unadjusted data shown in Table 11.2. Comparison of the age-adjusted mean weights for children in the 1967/8 survey with unadjusted mean weights for children in this survey nevertheless suggests that there has been a slight reduction in mean weight for both boys and girls in the youngest age group, almost no change for boys aged 2½ to 4½ years and a slight increase in mean weight for girls aged 2½ to 4½ years.

(Table 11.3 and Fig 11.1)

11.4 Height and supine length

A child's height or supine length provides a useful index of their development, reflecting the various influences on growth, including nutrition. Indeed the monitoring of a child's rate of gain in height with age against height growth charts is widely used to identify failure to thrive.

Interviewers were asked to attempt to measure the standing height of all children in the survey and additionally to attempt to measure the supine length of children aged under 2 years on the day the measurement was taken. As was noted in Chapter 2 these were technically the most difficult measurements to make and measurements with which the children were the least likely to co-operate.

The height of a total of 1709 children was measured by interviewers, but from these, results for 103 children were subsequently excluded from the analyses as likely to be unreliable. The main reasons for exclusion were that the child would not stand sufficiently still, or would or could not maintain the correct posture. A very small number of measurements were excluded because the

child had her or his hair dressed in a 'permanent' style which increased their height, or because the measurement was taken by someone other than the interviewer — usually the child's mother. After exclusions, a total of 1606 measurements of standing height was available for analysis.

A measure of supine length was obtained for 226 of the total of 317 children under 2 years of age in the survey. Again a number of these were subsequently rejected as being unreliable, for the same reasons as given above, leaving 191 measurements of supine length available for analysis.

11.4.1 Comparison of measures of supine length and standing height

Acceptable measures of both standing height and supine length were obtained for 162 children under age 2 years, 75 boys and 87 girls, and hence it was possible to compare the two measures for these children.

For boys supine length was on average, 1.60cm greater than standing height (standard deviation = 1.04cm); for girls the difference was similar, a mean difference of 1.63cm (standard deviation = 1.20cm)[8]. These differences are slightly larger than the mean difference of 1.3cm reported by Roche and Davila (1974)[9] and should be borne in mind when considering the tables that follow which show descriptive statistics for the measures of height of boys and girls, in tables showing the body mass index (BMI) of children and in the results of the analysis of variance for height and BMI. In all these tables the measure of standing height has been used for all children, *including those aged under 2 years.*

The difference in the mean height between boys and girls reduced as the children got older; in the youngest cohort the difference was 1.6cm (p<0.01), but in the 3½ to 4½ years age group boys were less than 1cm taller, on average, than girls (NS). The increase in mean height between the two youngest cohorts for both boys and girls was greater than that between the middle and oldest age cohorts. Between 1½ to 2½ years and 2½ to 3½ years, the increase was slightly greater for girls than boys, 9.4cm compared with 8.7cm. *(Table 11.4)*

In the 1967/8 survey all children were measured supine[7]. Comparison of the age-adjusted supine measurements (Table 11.3) with measures of standing height, before allowing for the differences in technique, suggests that there has been an increase of between about 0.5cm and 2cm in the average over the period since 1967/8, depending on age and sex. If the differences in technique are assumed to account for a mean difference of +1.6cm between the supine and standing measures then the increase in mean height between 1967/8 and the time of this survey could be as much as between 2cm and 3.5cm.

(Fig 11.2)

11.5 Head circumference

Interviewers were asked to attempt to measure the head circumference of all children in the survey. Measurements were obtained for 1776 children, but 56 were subsequently excluded as likely to be unreliable, leaving measurements from 1720 children available for analysis.

Measurements of head circumference made by someone other than the interviewer and measures affected by the child's hairstyle were excluded as were those taken from a child who would not sit sufficiently still for an accurate measurement to be taken.

Mean head circumferences for children in the survey are shown in Table 11.5. Differences in mean circumferences between boys and girls ranged from 1.3cm for children in the youngest age cohort ($p<0.01$) to 0.9cm for those in the oldest group ($p<0.01$), boys consistently having the larger circumference. As was observed for measures of weight and height the absolute increase in mean circumference reduced, for both boys and girls, as they got older. *(Table 11.5)*

11.6 Mid upper-arm circumference

Interviewers were asked to attempt to measure the (mid upper-) arm circumference of all children in the survey. A total of 1760 measurements was recorded, but from these 41 have been excluded either because the measurement was not taken by the interviewer or because the child was unco-operative and in the interviewer's opinion this affected the reliability of the measure. Thus arm circumferences from 1719 children are available for analysis.

For children in the two oldest cohorts there was almost no difference in mean arm circumference between girls and boys but in the youngest group boys had on average a circumference about 0.4cm larger than girls ($p<0.05$). For boys the absolute increase in mean circumference between each of the three age cohorts was about 0.5cm, but for girls the increase was about 0.9cm between the two youngest groups, and then reduced to about 0.6cm difference between the middle and oldest age groups. *(Table 11.6)*

11.7 Body mass index (BMI)

As noted above the Quetelet, or Body Mass Index is the most widely used of the indices which standardise weight for height. In adults it has the advantage, compared with other indices, of having a relatively low correlation with height, but is correlated with the percentage of body weight that is fat. It is therefore often used as a measure of obesity. It is, however, known to give a misleading measure of fatness in lean adults with a muscular physique, and for the elderly[10].

The index is calculated as $weight(kg)/height(m)^2$. For this survey the standing height measurement has been used for all children, including those under age 2 years, and the age groups are based on the age of the child at the time height was measured. Measurements of height and weight which were excluded for reasons described above were also excluded from the calculation of BMI and thus these children are excluded from the analyses based on BMI calculations.

Mean BMI for boys and girls in the three age cohorts is shown in Table 11.7. Except in the oldest age group, where mean BMI was the same for boys and girls (15.9),

boys had mean BMI greater than that of girls (age 1½ to 2½ years: $p<0.05$; age 2½ to 3½ years: $p<0.01$). For boys there was a reduction in mean BMI as they got older, but for girls there was no significant difference in mean BMI between the middle and oldest age groups (all other differences $p<0.05$). *(Table 11.7)*

It was noted above that since 1967/8 there have been slight changes in mean weight for children aged between 1½ and 4½ years (lower for the youngest cohort and higher for girls aged 2½ to 4½ years) and an increase in mean height. The effect of these changes in mean weight and height on the BMI for children in the 1967/8 survey[6] (see *Table 11.3*) and this NDNS have apparently resulted in there being no change in BMI for children aged 2½ to 4½ years and a slight reduction in mean BMI for children aged between 1½ and 2½ years. However as noted earlier the 1967/8 survey used age-adjusted measurements in calculating BMI and the 'heights' of all children were taken from a supine measurement.

A longitudinal study of growth in normal French children[11] reports body mass index for children at single year ages (except for children aged 1½ years)[12]. As was found for children in this survey, at each age from 1½ to 5 years the index was slightly lower for the French girls than boys and for both sexes BMI decreased with increasing age. The values are very close to those found for this NDNS study of children in Great Britain. *(Table 11.8)*

11.8 Correlations between measurements

Table 11.9 is a correlation matrix for the various anthropometric measurements made; coefficients above and below the 'diagonal' are for boys and girls respectively.

Because, as also noted earlier, individual anthropometric measures tend to be highly correlated with age, *partial correlation coefficients* were calculated which allow for the effect of age to be controlled. The matrix thus gives partial correlation coefficients and identifies those which were statistically significant ($p<0.05$ or $p<0.01$).

It was noted above that in adults the BMI has been shown to have relatively low correlation with height. Partial correlation coefficients between each pair of measurements for both boys and girls in this survey were significant at $p<0.01$, except in the case of BMI with height, where for the girls the coefficient (0.03) did not reach the level of statistical significance and for boys (0.06) was significant only at $p<0.05$ level.

The highest partial correlation coefficients were between BMI and body weight, BMI and arm circumference, and body weight and arm circumference, all greater than 0.72. Height and weight were also strongly positively correlated (0.67 and 0.66 for boys and girls), and although the coefficients for the remaining pairs of measurements were all below 0.50, they were all nevertheless significant at $p<0.01$ level. Correlations between circumference measurements of both head and arm and other measurements and between these two circumferences were generally slightly greater for girls than boys. *(Table 11.9)*

11.9 Correlations with dietary intakes

Partial correlation coefficients were also calculated between both the BMI and arm circumference and the child's average daily intake of food energy and the average daily percentage of energy from total fat and total carbohydrates. The calculation again controlled for the effect of age (see *section 11.8* above) and Table 11.10 shows the partial coefficients for boys and girls separately.

The only statistically significant correlations were with food energy, where, particularly for boys, intakes showed quite strong positive correlations with the BMI and arm circumference, each measure increasing as food energy intake increased ($p < 0.01$).

Partial correlation coefficients for the percentage of energy from total carbohydrates and the percentage of energy derived from total fat intake with BMI and with arm circumference were low and not statistically significant. *(Table 11.10)*

These findings are similar to those from the 1967/8 survey where an analysis of the nutrient intakes and measurements of the heights and weights of preschool children found evidence of a direct relationship between energy intake and the Quetelet index. Any relationship with the percentage of energy from either fat or total carbohydrate is not reported but the authors do report that intakes of carbohydrates and 'added sugars' showed no association with the BMI of the children in that survey[6].

11.10 Variation in measurements

Tables 11.11 to 11.19 show the combined effects of a number of characteristics of the children, their households and families on the measurements of height, weight, head circumference and body mass index.

11.10.1 Statistical methods

The technique of analysis of variance[13] was used to identify which of the characteristics (the independent variables) was most important in explaining variation in each of the measurements (the dependent variable), and the technique of multiple regression was used to produce standardised regression coefficients for a number of variables independently associated with variation in standing height and body weight.

The analysis of variance for the individual anthropometric measures was carried out as a single step, for boys and girls separately, therefore all the independent variables that were considered are shown in the tables.

The tables of results identify those characteristics where there was a significant difference ($p < 0.01$ or $p < 0.05$) between the means for the subgroups after allowing for the effects of the other characteristics included in the analysis. Deviations of the means for the various groups within the sample from the grand mean (overall sample mean) are shown, again adjusted for the effects of other independent variables in the analysis.

As noted above, for children there is a strong association

between age and the measurement. To control for this effect, the age of the child was included in the analysis as a *covariate*; thus differences in measurements have been tested for significance after taking account of any age variation between groups.

The independent variables considered in explaining variation in body measurements using analysis of variance related to characteristics of the child, or the child's household or family, such as whether the parents were receiving Income Support or Family Credit, the mother's highest educational qualification level, and in which region the child was living. Although effects of smoking during pregnancy on the growth and development of the fetus have been reported[14], information on whether the mother had smoked during her pregnancy was not collected during the survey interview. However the mother's reported smoking behaviour *at the time of the survey* has been considered in examining variation between children. Table 11.11 shows for all children in the survey the proportion whose mothers smoked more than 20 cigarettes a day, smoked 20 or fewer a day and who were non-smokers. *(Table 11.11)*

The technique of analysis of variance cannot be used if any of the independent variables being considered is continuous in nature. Information was collected during the survey interview on the height of the child's parents and on the child's birth weight, all of which are continuous, rather than discrete, variables. To investigate the relationship between these measures and the child's own body measurements the technique of backwards stepwise *multiple regression analysis* was therefore used.

Therefore, as well as age, variables for parents' reported height were introduced into the analysis for height, and the child's reported birth weight, into the analysis for body weight (*see below*). Other independent, socioeconomic variables which were used in the analysis of variance were transformed, where possible, into dichotomous variables as required by the multiple regression technique, before being included in the analysis. For example, the information on the employment status of the head of the child's household was transformed to a dichotomous variable to indicate whether the head was working or not working, and data on mother's smoking behaviour at the time of the survey into a variable indicating whether she did or did not smoke.

11.10.2 Parents' reported height and child's birth weight

The association between parental height and body weight and the achieved height and body weight of their children is widely reported[15]. Parental height was therefore included in the analysis which considered variation in the height of the children in this sample. The section below describes how the information was collected and tables are given showing descriptive statistics for these measures. Information on the parents' body weight was not collected.

After all the measurements of the child had been made or attempted, the interviewer asked the child's mother for her own height and that of the child's father. These measurements were only recorded where the parent was the biological parent of the child and was living in the household at the time of the interview, although proxy information was often collected about the father's height from the child's mother. The measurement was recorded in either imperial or metric units, with imperial measurements subsequently being converted. Interviewers were not asked to take measurements of the parents, although this was reported as having happened quite frequently.

Information on the child's weight at birth was also collected during the interview. Weights were recorded as either pounds and ounces or in grams, with the imperial units subsequently being converted to a metric weight. Data are also available on number of weeks premature for premature births although this has not been used in the analysis[16]. *(Tables 11.12 and 11.13)*

11.10.3 Results

Variation in weight
The results from the analysis of variance (*Table 11.14*) showed almost none of the characteristics examined had a significant relationship with body weight, after adjusting for the effect of age. Only for girls was a significant association ($p<0.05$) found between their weight and their mother's level of education, girls whose mothers were qualified at or above GCE 'A' level being heavier than those whose mothers had lower level or no formal educational qualifications. Not only were none of the other characteristics significantly associated with variation in body weight, but the direction of any association was often not the same for boys as for girls.

Thus although overall the characteristics considered accounted for 50% of the variation in the measurements of boys' weight and 56% for girls, in each case about 50% of the total variation was accounted for by age.

In the multiple regression analysis (*Table 11.15*), where the child's birth weight was introduced, it was found to be significantly correlated with present body weight for both boys and girls ($p<0.01$). Associations with none of the other characteristics reached the level of statistical significance ($p<0.05$) for boys. Among girls those whose parents were receiving benefits were significantly lighter than average, while those whose mothers had educational qualifications at or above GCE 'A' level were heavier than the average ($p<0.05$).

Overall the factors included in the regression analysis accounted for 54% of the variation in boys' weight and 60% of that among the girls in the survey; for both sexes age accounted for 50% of the variation.
(Tables 11.14 and 11.15)

Variation in height
Table 11.16 shows that although the characteristics included in the analysis to examine variation in height accounted for nearly 80% of the overall variance, almost none, apart from age which alone accounted for about 75% of the total variation, were significantly correlated with height. For girls the only significant independent association ($p<0.05$) was for the daughters of mothers who reported being non-smokers who were taller than average; boys from a non-manual home background were taller than average ($p<0.05$).

Multiple regression analysis showed the reported height of the child's father and mother both being independently associated with the height of the child ($p<0.01$). Boys living in households where the head was working were taller than those where the head was either unemployed or economically inactive ($p<0.05$).
(Tables 11.16 and 11.17)

The 1967/8 survey[6] considered a number of socio-economic factors which might have affected the height of preschool children in that survey — number of children under 15 in the household, social class, income of the head of household and age at which the child's mother left school. The distribution of the children according to their age-standardised height for each of the factors was calculated and few significant associations were found, generally more for girls than boys. It was reported for example that girls' height tended to fall significantly with increasing family size ($p=0.05$), and that the oldest girls in non-manual social classes and whose fathers had earnings of £19 a week or more were significantly taller than other girls ($p=0.02$ and $p=0.05$ respectively). A positive association between the age at which the mother had left school and height was reported for the oldest group of boys ($p=0.10$).

Variation in head circumference
Variation in head circumference was examined in relation to differences in social class and mother's reported smoking behaviour, controlling for significant age effects. Of these only the current smoking behaviour had any significant association, daughters of mothers who reported being non-smokers having a larger than average head circumference. The characteristics included in the analysis accounted for 21% and 28% of the variance in the measurement for boys and girls respectively, but age alone accounted for 20% and 25% of the total variation for boys and girls respectively.
(Table 11.18)

Variation in BMI
Significant associations, independent of the effect of age, were found between the body mass index and region for boys in the sample ($p<0.01$) and with the social class of the head of household and the mother's highest level of educational qualification for girls ($p<0.05$). Overall, however, the characteristics examined only accounted for 10% of the variation in the BMI of boys and 5% of that of girls, of which about 6% and 3% respectively were accounted for by age.

As Table 11.19 shows, boys living in Scotland and the Northern region of England had a BMI above the average; girls in the sample from a non-manual home background and with mothers with no formal educational qualifications had a lower than average BMI.
(Table 11.19)

References and notes

1 The tables of descriptive statistics show values for the mean and standard deviation and a range of percentiles. The percentiles were selected as being regular multiples of standard deviation (sd) scores. The centiles are equivalent to two thirds of the standard deviation score increments. For example:

    two thirds of sd score below the mean = 25th percentile
    2 × two thirds of sd score below the mean = 9th percentile
    3 × two thirds of sd score below the mean = 2.3rd percentile

2 The date on which each body measurement was made was recorded by the interviewer and this has been used to calculate the age of the child. It is this information which is used in this Chapter, rather than the child's age calculated from the mid-point of the 3-month fieldwork period. Because the measurements were not usually all made on the same day, theoretically children could be classified into two different 12-month age cohorts for different measurements.

3 Tanner JM, Whitehouse RH, Takaishi M. Standards from birth to maturity for height, weight, height velocity and weight velocity: British Children 1965. *Arch Dis Childh* 1966; **41:** 454–71 and 613–35.

4 Freeman JV, Cole TJ, Chinn S, Jones PRM, White EM, Preece M A. Cross-sectional stature and weight reference curves for the UK, 1990. *Arch Dis Childh*; in press.

5 The published charts are available from Harlow Printing Ltd, Maxwell Street, South Shields, NE33 4PX.

6 Department of Health and Social Security. Report on Health and Social Subjects: 10. *A Nutrition Survey of Pre-school Children, 1967–68.* HMSO (London, 1975).

7 See Appendix P for details of the equipment and methods used for measuring height and weight.

8 Differences were computed at the individual child level; mean difference = sum of all differences divided by total number of measurements made.

9 Roche AF and Davila NG (1974) Differences between recumbent length and stature within individuals. *Growth* **38** (3).

10 For a review and evaluation of the various indices see Knight I, *The heights and weights of adults in Great Britain*, HMSO (London, 1984).

11 Rolland-Cachera MF, Sempé M, Guilloud-Bataille M, Patois E, Péquignot-Guggenbuhl F, Fautrad V. Adiposity indices in children. *Am J Clin Nutr* July 1982; **36:** 178–184.

12 In this longitudinal study, started in 1953, 494 children were followed from age 1 month, of whom 117 were observed until the age of 16 years.

13 *Analysis of variance* operates by testing whether observed differences in the dependent variable—the anthropometric measure—between sub-groups are greater than those which might be attributed to sampling variation alone, and so are unlikely to have occurred by chance.

The ratio of the observed intra-group variability about the group mean to inter-group variability between the group means is calculated for each independent variable being considered, and this F-ratio is then tested for statistical significance. When, as in this case, a number of characteristics are being considered in the same analysis, the means are first adjusted for the effects of the other characteristics before being tested for significance. The technique thus identifies from a number of characteristics those which explain a significant amount of the total variation in the dependent variable (the anthropometric measure), after allowing for the effects of all the other variables being considered.

14 For example: Metcoff J. Association of fetal growth with maternal nutrition. In: *Human Growth*. eds. Falkner F and Tanner JM. 2nd edition. Plenum Press, 1986.

15 For example: Tanner JM Use and abuse of growth standards. In: *Human Growth*. eds. Falkner F and Tanner JM. 2nd edition. Plenum Press 1986.

Poskitt EME. Which children are at risk of obesity? *Nutrition Research* 1993; **13** Suppl 1: S83-S93.

Anonymous. Born to be fat? *Lancet* 1992; **340:** 881-882

16 This information forms part of the total dataset for the survey which is available to researchers for secondary analysis from the ESRC Data Archive at the University of Essex (see *Chapter 1* for details).

Figure 11.1 Mean weight of children, 1967/8* and 1992/3**: children aged $1^1/_2$ - $4^1/_2$ years

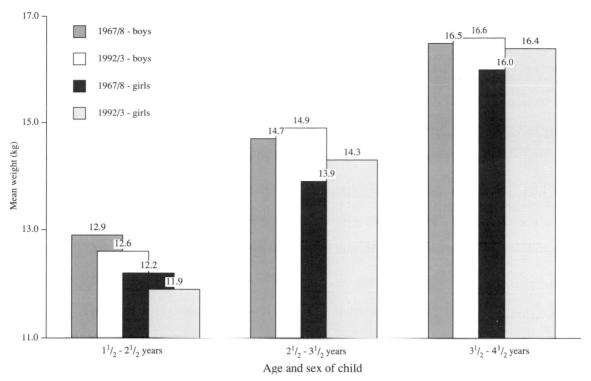

* Department of Health and Social Security (1975)

** NDNS 1992/3

Figure 11.2 Mean height of children, 1967/8* and 1992/3**: children aged $1^1/_2$ - $4^1/_2$ years

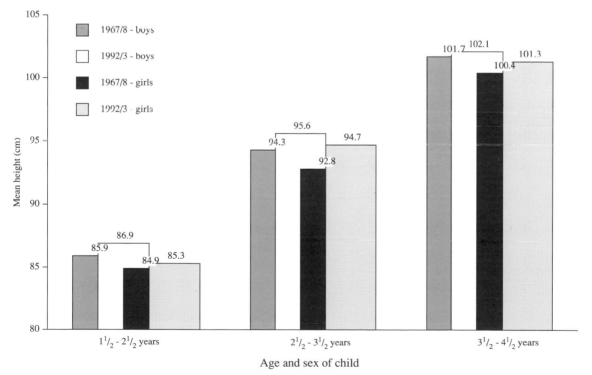

* Department of Health and Social Security (1975)

** NDNS 1992/3

Table 11.1 Numbers and percentages of children for whom measurements were available for analysis after exclusions

Response	Type of measurement									
	Body weight		Standing height		Supine length		Head circumference		Mid upper-arm circumference	
	No.	%	No.	%	No.	%	No.	%	No.	%
Total children eligible to be measured of whom:	1859	100	1859	100	317	100	1859	100	1859	100
all measurements refused	63	3	63	3	8	2	63	3	63	3
all measurements made	1781	96	1709	92	226	71	1776	96	1760	95
measurement made, but excluded	74	4	103	6	35	11	56	3	41	2
Total no of measurements available for analysis, after exclusions	1707	92	1606	86	191	60	1720	92	1719	92

Table 11.2 Body weight of child by age and sex

Body weight (kg)	Age and sex of child					
	1½ – 2½ years		2½ – 3½ years		3½ – 4½ years	
	Boys	Girls	Boys	Girls	Boys	Girls
Mean	12.6	11.9	14.9	14.3	16.6	16.4
Standard deviation	1.6	1.6	1.9	1.7	2.1	2.1
Percentiles						
2.3	9.4	8.8	11.6	11.2	13.1	12.7
9.0	10.4	10.1	12.6	12.0	13.9	13.4
25.0	11.6	10.8	13.7	13.1	15.1	15.0
50.0	12.6	11.7	14.8	14.3	16.8	16.3
75.0	13.6	12.8	15.9	15.3	17.8	17.8
91.0	14.8	13.9	17.6	16.5	19.3	19.3
97.7	15.9	15.2	19.3	17.9	21.0	20.1
Base	*294*	*283*	*307*	*314*	*251*	*258*

Table 11.3 Age adjusted weight, supine length and body mass index for children in the 1967/8 survey by age and sex*

Measurement	Age and sex of child					
	1½ – 2½ years		2½ – 3½ years		3½ – 4½ years	
	Boys	Girls	Boys	Girls	Boys	Girls
Weight (kg)						
Mean	12.9	12.2	14.7	13.9	16.5	16.0
Standard deviation	1.5	1.5	1.8	1.8	2.0	1.9
Base	*200*	*194*	*195*	*200*	*167*	*147*
Supine length (cm)						
Mean	85.9	84.9	94.3	92.8	101.7	100.4
Standard deviation	4.1	3.8	5.4	4.9	5.0	4.7
Base	*186*	*181*	*188*	*194*	*164*	*142*
Body mass index**						
Mean	18	17	17	16	16	16

* Department of Health and Social Security. Report on Health and Social Subjects 10. *A Nutrition Survey of Pre-school Children, 1967–8*. Report by the Committee on the Medical Aspects of Food Policy. HMSO (London, 1975).
**Base numbers not reported.

Table 11.4 Standing height of child by age and sex

Standing height (cm)	Age and sex of child					
	1½ – 2½ years		2½ – 3½ years		3½ – 4½ years	
	Boys	Girls	Boys	Girls	Boys	Girls
Mean	86.9	85.3	95.6	94.7	102.1	101.3
Standard deviation	3.9	4.2	4.0	4.3	4.6	4.3
Percentiles						
2.3	78.5	77.7	87.8	86.2	92.8	92.7
9.0	81.6	79.0	90.2	89.2	96.0	95.3
25.0	84.3	82.1	92.6	91.6	99.0	98.4
50.0	87.0	85.4	95.4	94.6	102.2	101.4
75.0	90.0	88.4	98.3	97.7	105.3	103.9
91.0	91.8	90.6	100.8	100.4	108.0	107.3
97.7	94.2	93.7	103.6	102.8	111.9	109.9
Base	*252*	*236*	*305*	*304*	*255*	*254*

Table 11.5   Head circumference of child by age and sex

Head circumference (cm)	Age and sex of child					
	1½ – 2½ years		2½ – 3½ years		3½ – 4½ years	
	Boys	Girls	Boys	Girls	Boys	Girls
Mean	50.1	48.8	51.3	50.2	51.9	51.0
Standard deviation	1.6	1.7	1.8	1.5	1.4	1.5
Percentiles						
2.3	46.5	45.4	47.8	47.0	48.8	48.0
9.0	48.0	46.7	49.2	48.1	50.0	49.0
25.0	49.0	47.7	50.3	49.1	51.2	50.0
50.0	50.1	49.0	51.2	50.1	52.0	51.0
75.0	51.1	50.0	52.3	51.1	53.0	52.0
91.0	52.0	51.0	53.5	52.0	53.8	53.0
97.7	53.5	52.1	54.9	53.9	54.5	54.0
Base	*298*	*285*	*316*	*309*	*257*	*255*

Table 11.6   Mid upper-arm circumference of child by age and sex

Mid upper-arm circumference (cm)	Age and sex of child					
	1½ – 2½ years		2½ – 3½ years		3½ – 4½ years	
	Boys	Girls	Boys	Girls	Boys	Girls
Mean	16.5	16.1	17.0	17.0	17.5	17.6
Standard deviation	1.2	1.4	1.3	1.3	1.6	1.4
Percentiles						
2.3	14.4	13.6	14.4	14.4	15.0	15.0
9.0	14.8	14.4	15.6	15.4	15.8	15.8
25.0	15.6	15.2	16.0	16.2	16.6	16.6
50.0	16.6	16.0	17.0	17.0	17.4	17.6
75.0	17.2	17.0	17.8	17.8	18.4	18.4
91.0	18.2	18.0	18.8	18.6	19.2	19.4
97.7	19.0	19.0	20.0	20.1	21.3	20.8
Base	*293*	*286*	*314*	*312*	*256*	*258*

Table 11.7   Body mass index of child by age and sex

Body mass index*	Age** and sex of child					
	1½ – 2½ years		2½ – 3½ years		3½ – 4½ years	
	Boys	Girls	Boys	Girls	Boys	Girls
Mean	16.8	16.4	16.4	15.9	15.9	15.9
Standard deviation	1.4	1.5	1.4	1.4	1.5	1.4
Percentiles						
2.3	13.8	13.6	13.7	13.6	13.6	13.3
9.0	14.8	14.4	14.6	14.2	14.3	14.1
25.0	15.9	15.4	15.3	14.9	15.1	15.0
50.0	16.8	16.2	16.4	15.9	15.8	15.8
75.0	17.7	17.4	17.0	16.7	16.8	16.8
91.0	18.5	18.4	18.3	17.5	17.5	17.9
97.7	19.7	19.5	19.6	18.9	20.0	18.8
Base	*240*	*229*	*289*	*297*	*244*	*250*

* For children aged under 2 years, measurement of standing height has been used in calculating BMI.
** Age at time of measuring height of child.

Table 11.8   Comparison of body mass index for French children* and children in NDNS

	Age	Boys		Girls	
		BMI	*Base*	BMI	*Base*
French children:					
	1½ years	17.1	*195*	16.8	*177*
	2 years	16.6	*183*	16.3	*170*
	3 years	16.1	*104*	16.0	*100*
	4 years	15.8	*145*	15.6	*132*
	5 years	15.6	*144*	15.3	*127*
NDNS children:					
	1½ – 2½ years	16.8	*240*	16.4	*229*
	2½ – 3½ years	16.4	*289*	15.9	*297*
	3½ – 4½ years	15.9	*244*	15.9	*250*

* Rolland-Cachera et al (1982)

255

Table 11.9 Partial correlation coefficient matrix for anthropometric measurements controlling for age of child by sex of child

Measurement and sex of child	Standing height		Body weight		Head circumference		Mid upper-arm circumference		Body mass index	
	Coefficient	Base	Coefficient	Base	Coefficient	Base	Coefficient	Base	Coefficient	Base
Boys										
Standing height	1.00	1606†	0.67**	770	0.32**	789	0.32**	790	0.06**	770
Girls										
Body weight	0.66**	773	1.00	1701†	0.44**	822	0.73**	813	0.79**	770
Head circumference	0.36**	775	0.49**	819	1.00	1720†	0.32**	845	0.31**	756
Mid upper-arm circumference	0.30**	781	0.76**	826	0.38**	833	1.00	1719†	0.73**	753
Body mass index	0.03 (NS)	773	0.78**	773	0.35**	757	0.76**	763	1.00	1549†

* $p < 0.05$
** $p < 0.01$
NS not significant – $p > 0.05$

†   All children

Table 11.10 Partial correlation coefficient matrix for body masss index and mid upper-arm circumference with dietary intakes controlling for age of child by sex of child

Measurement and sex of child	Dietary intake			Base: total number of children
	Average daily energy intake	Percentage energy from:		
		Total fat	Total carbohydrates	
	Correlation coefficients			
Boys				
Body mass index	0.15**	0.01 (NS)	–0.04 (NS)	717
Mid upper-arm circumference	0.12**	0.05 (NS)	–0.04 (NS)	800
Girls				
Body mass index	0.06*	–0.04 (NS)	–0.01 (NS)	717
Mid upper-arm circumference	0.07*	–0.04 (NS)	–0.01 (NS)	795

* $p < 0.05$
** $p < 0.01$
NS not significant – $p > 0.05$

Table 11.11 Mother's reported smoking behaviour at time of interview by age and sex of child

Mother's reported smoking behaviour at time of interview	Age of child			Sex of child		All children
	1½ – 2½ years	2½ – 3½ years	3½ – 4½ years	Boys	Girls	
	%	%	%	%	%	%
Does not smoke cigarettes	71	67	66	69	67	68
Smokes cigarettes:						
fewer than 20 a day	20	24	24	21	24	22
20 or more a day	8	9	10	9	9	9
number not known	–	1	1	1	0	0
Base = 100%	648	668	543	943	916	1859

Table 11.12 Reported height of child's parents*

Height (cm)	Mother	Father
Mean	163	177
Standard deviation	6.4	7.1
Percentiles:		
2.3	150	162
9.0	155	168
25.0	157	173
50.0	163	178
75.0	168	183
91.0	170	188
97.7	175	190
*Base***	*1764*	*1412*

* Based only on biological parents of the child who were living in the child's household at the time of interview.

** Excludes those for whom height was not known.

Table 11.13 Reported weight of child at birth by sex of child

Birth weight (g)	Sex of child		All children
	Boys	Girls	
Mean	3405	3276	3341
Standard deviation	579	553	570
Percentiles:			
2.3	2013	1928	2013
9.0	2722	2551	2608
25.0	3062	2977	3033
50.0	3459	3317	3374
75.0	3799	3629	3714
91.0	4111	3912	4026
97.7	4479	4196	4394
*Base**	*939*	*907*	*1846*

* Excludes 13 children for whom weight at birth not known.

Table 11.14 Analysis of variance for body weight for boys and girls

Characteristic	Adjusted deviations from grand mean and significance of F ratios for height for:		No of cases	
	Boys	Girls	Boys	Girls
Grand mean (kg)	14.64	14.11		
Covariate – age	**p<0.01**	**p<0.01**		
Correlation coefficient	0.696	0.737		
Region	NS	NS		
Scotland	–0.06	0.17	72	91
Northern	0.26	–0.05	195	202
Central, South West & Wales	–0.03	0.09	287	281
London & South East	–0.14	–0.13	266	240
Social class of HOH	NS	NS		
Non-manual	0.13	–0.09	381	389
Manual	–0.12	0.08	439	425
Employment status of HOH	NS	NS		
Working	0.05	0.0	622	605
Unemployed	–0.28	0.14	76	87
Economically inactive	–0.27	–0.26	122	122
Receipt of benefits	NS	NS		
Receiving	0.05	–0.11	243	262
Not receiving	0.02	0.07	577	552
Family type	NS	NS		
Married couple with:				
one child	–0.01	–0.01	169	192
two or more children	–0.02	–0.07	512	485
Lone parent with:				
one child	0.23	0.27	59	50
two or more children	0.00	0.25	80	87
Mother's qualification level	NS	**p<0.05**		
GCE 'A' level & above	0.12	0.26	230	240
Below GCE 'A' level	–0.03	–0.03	410	403
None	0.09	–0.30	180	171
Mother's smoking behaviour	NS	NS		
Non-smoker	–0.03	0.09	574	547
Fewer than 20 a day	0.20	–0.17	171	194
20 or more a day	–0.25	–0.20	75	73
% of variance explained	*50%*	*56%*		

NS not significant – p>0.05

Table 11.15 Multiple regression analysis for body weight for boys and girls

Variables in regression	Boys			Girls		
	Standardised regression coefficient	T-value	Significance of T-value	Standardised regression coefficient	T-value	Significance of T-value
Child's age	0.68	29.2	**p<0.01**	0.75	34.0	**p<0.01**
Child's birth weight	0.25	10.7	**p<0.01**	0.22	10.1	**p<0.01**
Whether mother had qualifications at or above GCE 'A' level:						
yes = 1; no = 0		1.1	NS	0.06	2.5	**p<0.05**
Whether parents receiving benefits:						
yes = 1; no = 0		–0.4	NS	–0.04	–1.9	**p<0.05**
Whether child lived in Scotland or Northern England:						
yes = 1; no = 0		0.9	NS		0.0	NS
Whether mother smokes:						
yes = 1; no = 0		1.7	NS		–0.9	NS
Whether head of household working:						
yes = 1; no = 0		0.6	NS		0.5	NS
Whether child in lone parent family:						
yes = 1; no = 0		1.0	NS		1.2	NS
Whether head of household in non-manual occupation:						
yes = 1; no = 0		1.4		NS	–1.0	NS
% of variance explained		*54%*			*60%*	

NS not significant – p>0.05

Table 11.16   Analysis of variance for standing height for boys and girls

Characteristic	Adjusted deviations from grand mean and significance of F ratios for height for:		No of cases	
	Boys	Girls	Boys	Girls
Grand mean (cm)	94.99	93.95		
Covariate – age	**p<0.01**	**p<0.01**		
Correlation coefficient	0.870	0.879		
Region	NS	NS		
Scotland	−0.21	0.66	*61*	*85*
Northern	−0.04	−0.03	*191*	*183*
Central, South West & Wales	0.07	0.05	*283*	*262*
London & South East	0.00	−0.28	*248*	*226*
Social class of HOH	**p<0.05**	NS		
Non-manual	0.36	0.00	*358*	*365*
Manual	−0.31	0.00	*425*	*391*
Employment status of HOH	NS	NS		
Working	0.14	−0.13	*589*	*560*
Unemployed	−0.88	0.51	*73*	*80*
Economically inactive	−0.13	0.27	*121*	*116*
Receipt of benefits	NS	NS		
Receiving	−0.06	−0.46	*238*	*245*
Not receiving	0.03	0.22	*545*	*511*
Family type	NS	NS		
Married couple with:				
one child	0.08	0.12	*153*	*168*
two or more children	−0.06	−0.07	*497*	*459*
Lone parent with:				
one child	0.09	0.17	*53*	*48*
two or more children	0.18	0.04	*80*	*81*
Mother's qualification level	NS	NS		
GCE 'A' level & above	0.15	0.30	*217*	*224*
Below GCE 'A' level	−0.07	0.00	*389*	*373*
None	−0.04	−0.42	*177*	*159*
Mother's smoking behaviour	NS	**p<0.05**		
Non-smoker	0.09	0.30	*547*	*506*
Fewer than 20 a day	0.04	−0.61	*164*	*179*
20 or more a day	−0.75	−0.61	*72*	*71*
% of variance explained	*77%*	*78%*		

NS not significant – p>0.05

Table 11.17   Multiple regression analysis for height for boys and girls

Variables in regression	Boys			Girls		
	Standardised regression coefficient	T-value	Significance of T-value	Standardised regression coefficient	T-value	Significance of T-value
Child's age	0.88	49.9	**p<0.01**	0.89	50.1	**p<0.01**
Mother's height	0.12	7.0	**p<0.01**	0.12	6.9	**p<0.01**
Father's height	0.13	7.4	**p<0.01**	0.11	6.0	**p<0.01**
Whether head of household working *yes=1; no=0*	0.04	2.2	**p<0.05**		−0.3	NS
Whether mother had qualifications at or above GCE 'A' level: *yes = 1; no = 0*		−0.3	NS		1.1	NS
Whether child lived in Scotland or Northern England: *yes = 1; no = 0*		−0.4	NS		0.3	NS
Whether parents receiving benefits: *yes = 1; no = 0*		−0.7	NS		−1.4	NS
Whether mother smokes: *yes = 1; no = 0*		−0.6	NS		−1.6	NS
Whether head of household in non-manual occupation: *yes = 1; no = 0*		0.3	NS		0.3	NS
% of variance explained	*80%*			*81%*		

NS not significant – p>0.05

Table 11.18 Analysis of variance for head circumference for boys and girls

Characteristic	Adjusted deviations from grand mean and significance of F ratios for height for:		No of cases	
	Boys	Girls	Boys	Girls
Grand mean (cm)	51.09	49.97		
Covariate – age	**p<0.01**	**p<0.01**		
Correlation coefficient	0.45	0.50		
Social class of HOH	NS	NS		
Non-manual	0.09	−0.04	380	388
Manual	−0.08	0.04	457	421
Mother's smoking behaviour	NS	**p<0.01**		
Non-smoker	0.08	0.15	587	544
Fewer than 20 a day	−0.16	−0.33	173	194
20 or more a day	−0.28	−0.27	77	71
% of variance explained	*21%*	*28%*		

NS not significant – p>0.05

Table 11.19 Analysis of variance for body mass index* for boys and girls

Characteristic	Adjusted deviations from grand mean and significance of F ratios for height for:		No of cases	
	Boys	Girls	Boys	Girls
Grand mean	16.35	16.06		
Covariate – age**	**p<0.01**	**p<0.01**		
Correlation coefficient	−0.25	−0.169		
Region	**p<0.01**	NS		
Scotland	0.03	−0.02	60	84
Northern	0.33	−0.02	177	178
Central, South West & Wales	−0.07	0.07	269	258
London & South East	−0.17	−0.06	239	220
Social class of HOH	NS	**p<0.05**		
Non-manual	0.01	−0.15	348	356
Manual	−0.01	0.14	397	384
Employment status of HOH	NS	NS		
Working	0.03	0.06	559	548
Unemployed	−0.15	0.08	70	79
Economically inactive	−0.07	−0.35	116	113
Receipt of benefits	NS	NS		
Receiving	0.05	−0.01	227	239
Not receiving	−0.02	0.00	518	501
Family type	NS	NS		
Married couple with:				
one child	−0.08	−0.06	140	167
two or more children	−0.01	−0.05	476	446
Lone parent with:				
one child	0.43	0.21	52	48
two or more children	−0.07	0.28	77	79
Mother's qualification level	NS	**p<0.05**		
GCE 'A' level & above	0.11	0.19	207	216
Below GCE 'A' level	−0.03	0.00	372	368
None	−0.07	0.25	166	156
Mother's smoking behaviour	NS	NS		
Non-smoker	−0.07	−0.02	520	495
Fewer than 20 a day	0.22	0.03	155	175
20 or more a day	0.05	0.04	70	70
% of variance explained	*10%*	*5%*		

NS not significant – p>0.05
  * For children aged under 2 years measurement of standing height has been used in calculating BMI.
** Age at time of measuring height of child.

259

Appendices

Appendix A

Fieldwork documents

Postal sift letter and postal sift form

Interviewer recall sift form

Multi-household selection sheet

Advance letter (A)

General purpose leaflet (B)

Interview questionnaire (C)

Prompt cards A to F

The correct position of the head when measuring height (Frankfort plane)

Home record diary (E)

Eating out diary (F)

Eating pattern check sheet (P)

Check list for weighing and recording (given to the informant) (R)

Interviewer check cards:
    Food description prompt card (K)
    Guide weights (L)
    Fats for spreading (M)
    Fats and oils for cooking (N)

Bowel movements card (Q)

Blood and anthropometry purpose leaflet (W)

Blood questionnaire (Z)

(Consent forms and results letters are reproduced in Appendix M)

Information for parents (about uses of blood sample) (Z1)

Dental recall form (T)

Postal sift letter and postal sift form

OPCS
OFFICE OF POPULATION CENSUSES & SURVEYS

Social Survey Division

St Catherine's House
10 Kingsway
London WC2B 6JP

Direct Dial   071-396
Switchboard   071-396 2200
        or   071-242 0262
GTN   3042

Fax   071-405 3C20

12 November 1992

our ref: N1340/W4/0

Dear Sir or Madam,

The Social Survey Division of the Office of Population Censuses and Surveys gathers information on different subjects in order to provide government departments with up-to-date information about people's views and living conditions. We have now been asked by the Department of Health and the Ministry of Agriculture, Fisheries and Food to find out about people's eating habits. To do this work properly we shall need to talk to representative samples of different kinds of people. Since we do not have information about the ages of individuals, we are asking for your help.

Your address is one of 28,000 chosen at random from a list of addresses in Great Britain. We would like you to help by filling in the form on the back of this letter, listing the sex and date of birth of everyone, including yourself, who usually lives in your household at the address shown on the label at the top of this letter. When you have completed the form I should like you to return it to us, as soon as possible, in the envelope provided (no stamp is needed).

As in all our surveys we rely on people's voluntary co-operation. Any information you give will be treated in strict confidence. The results will not be used in any way in which they can be associated with your name and address. No identifiable information will be passed to other government departments, local authorities, members of the public or the press.

Thank you for sparing the time to help us with this survey.

Yours faithfully,

Janet Gregory
Principal Social Survey Officer

If no-one lives permanently at the address on the label at the top of the letter, please tick one of the boxes below and return this form in the envelope provided.

Address is vacant. . . . . □ 1

Address is used for business purposes only. . . . . □ 2

Other address with no permanent residents (eg holiday home). . . . □ 3

Address is an institution (eg hotel, nursing home). . . . . . . □ 4

Please complete 1 and 2 below for everyone, including yourself, who usually lives in your household at the address shown on the label at the top of the letter.

Please include anyone who usually lives in your household but is temporarily away, for example, because they are in hospital, at school or on holiday. **Exclude** anyone who lives somewhere else permanently.

1. How many people are there in your household living at this address?

Total number of people in the household ──→ Number [ ]

2. For each person in the household, including yourself, please give their sex and date of birth

	Sex (please tick)		Date of birth (enter day, month and year)		
	Male	Female	Day	Month	Year
1					
2					
3					
4					
5					
6					
7					
8					
9					
10					

3. Is any part of the address shown on the label overleaf, *separately* occupied by persons not listed above?

Tick one box ──→ Yes [ ]   No [ ]

for office use only [ ]

Please return this form as soon as possible in the envelope provided.   Thank you for your help.

Interviewer recall sift form

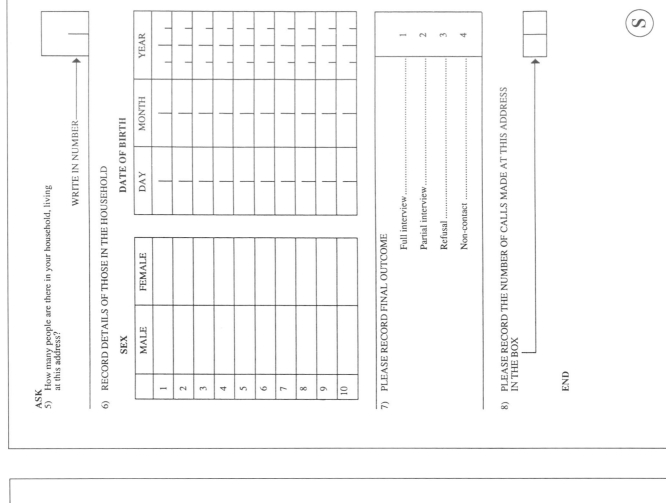

N1340/W4

INTERVIEWER POSTAL RECALL SIFT FORM

Serial no label

PLEASE COMPLETE THIS FORM FOR EACH ADDRESS ON YOUR LIST

RECORD
1) Is this address a . . . .

non-responder?	1
responding multi-household?	2

RECORD
2) Did you find the address?

Yes	1	
No	2	END

3) Was the whole address . . . .

RECORD

vacant/demolished?	1	END
business?	2	
no permanent residents?	3	
institution?	4	
eligible address?	5	Q4

4) Is this address occupied by more than one household?

Yes	1
No	2

IF YES
PLEASE COMPLETE A MULTI-HOUSEHOLD SELECTION SHEET AND SELECT HOUSEHOLD

WRITE IN HOUSEHOLD NUMBER SELECTED →

ADDRESS OF SELECTED HOUSEHOLD
(please describe as possible
including flat numbers etc)

POSTCODE

ASK
5) How many people are there in your household, living at this address?

WRITE IN NUMBER →

6) RECORD DETAILS OF THOSE IN THE HOUSEHOLD

	SEX		DATE OF BIRTH		
	MALE	FEMALE	DAY	MONTH	YEAR
1					
2					
3					
4					
5					
6					
7					
8					
9					
10					

7) PLEASE RECORD FINAL OUTCOME

Full interview	1
Partial interview	2
Refusal	3
Non-contact	4

8) PLEASE RECORD THE NUMBER OF CALLS MADE AT THIS ADDRESS IN THE BOX →

END

Ⓢ

Multi-household selection sheet

Interviewer name ....

N1340/W4 YOUNG CHILDREN'S DIETARY SURVEY

MULTI-HOUSEHOLD (A)
SELECTION SHEET

SERIAL NO. LABEL

TO BE RETURNED TO FIELD WITH
POSTAL SIFT FOLLOW-UP FORM

List of Households

H/hold No. (1)	DESCRIPTION OF HOUSEHOLDS eg location and surnames (2)	No. of h/hlds found at address (3)	Interview at household (4)	Outcome code (5)
1		1	1	
2		2	1	
3		3	1	
4		4	4	
5		5	1	
6		6	6	
7		7	4	
8		8	7	
9		9	8	
10		10	3	
11		11	8	
12		12	3	
13		13	5	
14		14	11	
15		15	3	

IF MORE THAN 15 HOUSEHOLDS PLEASE TURN OVER

Procedure

1. Note down the households on the table above. This must be done systematically. If numbered then list in numerical order, ie. flat 1,2,3, etc. or flat A,B,C, etc. Otherwise start at the lowest floor and work in a clockwise direction.

2. Ring the number of households found at column 3. Read column (4) to identify which household s selected for interview Ring the selected household number in column (1).

3. Attach this form to the corresponding postal sift follow-up form.

FOR USE ON THE YOUNG CHILDREN'S DIETARY SURVEY ONLY
NOTE: YOU ONLY SELECT ONE HOUSEHOLD

H/hold No. (1)	DESCRIPTION OF HOUSEHOLDS eg location and surnames (2)	No. of h/hlds found at address (3)	Interview at household (4)	Outcome code (5)
16		16	1	
17		17	12	
18		18	14	
19		19	1	
20		20	2	
21		21	19	
22		22	11	
23		23	17	
24		24	12	
25		25	18	
26		26	18	
27		27	8	
28		28	12	
29		29	15	
30		30	7	

ENGLAND, WALES AND SCOTLAND

If more than 30 Households
Ring Sampling
extensions:- 2352
             2276
Answer Phone 071 831 7738

SCOTLAND ONLY

Where a multi-occupancy indicator count is shown on the address list and the number of households found at the address is 5 more or less than the indicator
Ring Sampling
Extensions:- 2352
             2276
Answer Phone 071 831 7738

A/W4

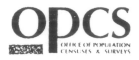

Social Survey Division

St Catherine's House
10 Kingsway
London WC2B 6JP

Direct Dial	071 - 396 2079
Switchboard	071 - 396 2200
or	071 - 242 0262
GTN	3042

| Fax | 071 - 405 3020 |

Our reference:
1340/W4

Date as postmark

Dear Householder

Young Children's Dietary Survey

I am writing to tell you about a survey that this Office will shortly be carrying out for the Ministry of Agriculture, Fisheries and Food and the Department of Health. The main aim of the survey is to find out, in detail, about the eating habits of young children and relate this to characteristics such as their age, sex, height and weight. The results of the survey will provide a better understanding of the relationship between diet and health.

The sample for this survey was selected from addresses on the Postcode Address File. The Postcode Address File is compiled by the Post Office and lists all addresses to which mail is sent. To visit all the addresses selected would take too long and cost far too much money and many of the households visited would not contain a young child. I therefore wrote in November to all the selected addresses asking for information on the age and sex of all people living there; some addresses where there is more than one household were visited by one of our interviewers. I am now writing again to all those households where there is a child aged under 5 years; yours is one of these addresses.

One of our interviewers will be calling on you in the next few weeks; he or she will show you their authorisation card and will tell you much more about the survey. Any information that you or any member of your household gives will be kept in strict confidence. Access to the completed questionnaires is restricted to Social Survey Division of OPCS and the Ministry of Agriculture, Fisheries and Food (MAFF). However the names and addresses of co-operating households will not be released to MAFF, to any other government department, to local authorities, members of the public or to the press. The survey results will not be presented in a form which can be associated with names and addresses.

I do hope that you will be able to help us with this survey; the results will be of great value both to MAFF and the Department of Health and I am sure that your household would find it interesting to take part. If you have any questions in advance of our interviewer calling please contact me at the address and telephone number shown at the top of this letter.

Thanking you in anticipation of your kind co-operation.

Yours faithfully

Janet Gregory

Janet Gregory
Principal Social Survey Officer

HA2 2 1/93

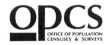
OFFICE OF POPULATION
CENSUSES & SURVEYS

The Young Children's Dietary Survey

This survey is being carried out by the Social Survey Division of the Office of Population Censuses and Surveys, for the Ministry of Agriculture, Fisheries and Food and the Departments of Health (in England, Wales and Scotland). This leaflet tells you more about why the survey is being done.

1. What is it about?

Over the past twenty years or so there has been a considerable increase in the range of foods available in the shops, and for many people, including children, this has meant changes in the kinds of foods they eat. We have been asked to carry out a large national survey to find out, in detail, about the eating habits of young children in Great Britain. The survey also collects information about the children themselves, not only their age and sex, but also some physical measurements, such as their height and weight. They are also asked to give a small sample of blood. This information, together with information about the foods they eat, will provide a better understanding about the relationship between diet and health, particularly at an early age. All the physical measurements are taken by our interviewers who have been carefully trained, and we employ qualified people who are particularly skilled in taking blood from small children to take this sample for us.

* * * * * * *

2. Why have we come to your household?

To visit every household in the country would take too long and cost far too much money.

Therefore we selected a sample of addresses from the Postcode Address File. The Postcode Address File is compiled by the Post Office and lists all the addresses to which mail is sent. We sent a letter to each selected address asking for details of the age and sex of everybody living there. We chose those addresses in a way that gave everyone the same chance of being selected. From the replies we were able to tell which households contained a child under 5, and from those we selected a sample to be interviewed. Your household is one of those chosen to be interviewed.

Some people think either that they and their family are not typical enough to be of any help in the survey or that they are very different from other people and they would distort the findings. The important thing to remember is that the community consists of a great many different types of people and families and we need to represent them all in our sample survey. It will therefore be appreciated if everyone we approach agrees to take part.

* * * * * * *

3. Is the survey confidential?

Yes We take very great care to protect the confidentiality of the information we are given. Access to the completed questionnaires and diaries is restricted to the Social Survey Division of OPCS and the Ministry of Agriculture, Fisheries and Foods (MAFF). However, the names and addresses of co-operating households will not be released to MAFF, to any other government department, to local authorities, members of the public or the press. The survey results will not be presented in a form which can be associated with names and addresses.

* * * * * * *

4. Is the survey compulsory?

In all our surveys we rely on voluntary co-operation, which is essential if our work is to be successful.

In appreciation of the help given a postal order payment of £10 is made to the child's parent, provided the food diary has been kept for the full four days.

* * * * * * *

We hope this leaflet answers some of the questions you might have, and shows the importance of the survey. The interviewer will leave another leaflet with you which tells you more about the measurements we are making and the blood sample.

Your co-operation is very much appreciated.

Social Survey Division
Office of Population Censuses and
 Surveys
St Catherine's House
10 Kingsway
London WC2B 6JP

telephone 071 - 242 0262 ext 2079

N1340 Young children's dietary survey.   HA2/5 4/92

Interview questionnaire (C)

Left panel

IN CONFIDENCE

1340/W4 : YOUNG CHILDREN'S DIETARY SURVEY

C

Serial no. label

Interviewer name ....

Authorisation no. ....

	Day	Month	Year
Date of Interview			9 3

	Hours	Mins
Enter start time - 24 hr clock		

INTERVIEWER CODE

(a) Who was interviewed as informant

Code one only

Child's mother (female parent- figure) 1

Child's father (male parent- figure) 2

Child's 'mother' and 'father' jointly 3

Enter per. no of informant(s)

1

Right panel

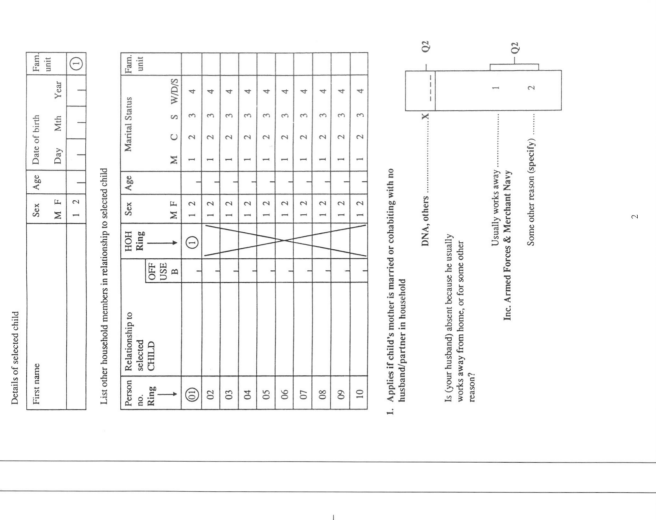

Details of selected child

First name	Sex	Age	Date of birth			Fam. unit
	M F		Day	Mth	Year	
	1 2					①

List other household members in relationship to selected child

Person no. Ring →	Relationship to selected CHILD	OFF USE B	HOH Ring →	Sex M F	Age	Marital Status				Fam. unit
						M	C	S	W/D/S	
⓪①			①	1 2		1	2	3	4	
02				1 2		1	2	3	4	
03				1 2		1	2	3	4	
04				1 2		1	2	3	4	
05				1 2		1	2	3	4	
06				1 2		1	2	3	4	
07				1 2		1	2	3	4	
08				1 2		1	2	3	4	
09				1 2		1	2	3	4	
10				1 2		1	2	3	4	

1. Applies if child's mother is married or cohabiting with no husband/partner in household

DNA, others .... X → Q2

Is (your husband) absent because he usually works away from home, or for some other reason?

Usually works away ....
Inc. Armed Forces & Merchant Navy 1

Some other reason (specify) .... 2 → Q2

2

Interview questionnaire (C) - continued

PRESENT ACCOMMODATION

Ring codes at Q2 and Q3

2. Type of accommodation occupied by **this household:**

Code one from observation, if in doubt ask informant

whole house, bungalow	1	— Q4
purpose-built flat or maisonette in block	2	— Q3
part of the house/converted flat or maisonette/ rooms in house	3	
dwelling with business premises	4	— Q4
caravan/houseboat	5	
Other (specify)	6	

3. To households coded 2 - 4

What is the floor level of the main living part of the accommodation?

Basement/semi-basement	1
Ground floor/street level	2
1st floor	3
2nd floor	4
3th floor	5
4th to 9th floor	6
10th floor or higher	7

4. Ask or record

Is there a garden or other area attached to your accommodation where.......... (CHILD) could play outside?

Yes	1
No	2

3

5. Do you have a kitchen, that is a separate room in which you cook?

Yes	1	(a)
No	2	(b)

(a) Do you share the kitchen with any other household?

Yes	1	— Q6
No	2	

(b) Are you able to cook a hot meal in this accommodation?

Yes, hot meal	1
No	2
Spontaneous: Hot drink only	3

6. Does your household have any of the following items in your (part of the) accommodation?

INCLUDE: **Items stored and under repair**

	Yes	No
Refrigerator?	1	2
Deep freezer or fridge freezer? ...	1	2
Microwave oven?	1	2

7. Is there a car or van **normally** available for use by you or any members of your household?

Yes	1	(a)
No	2	— Q8

INCLUDE: Any provided by employers if normally available for private use by informant or members of the household. EXCLUDE: Vehicles used solely for the carriage of goods.

(a) Is there one or more than one?

1	1	
2	2	— Q8
3 or more	3	

4

Interview questionnaire (C) - *continued*

EATING HABITS: Introduce

8. Do you find .... (CHILD) particularly easy, about average or particularly difficult to feed for a child of his/her age?

[*]

Easy	1	(a)
Average	2	Q9
Difficult	3	(a)

If easy or difficult

(a) In what way is (he/she) (easy/difficult) to feed?

9. How would you describe the variety of foods that .... (CHILD) generally eats? Does he/she

[*] Running prompt

eat most things	1
eat a reasonable variety of things..........	2
or is he/she a fussy or faddy eater? ...	3

10. Does .... (CHILD) have

[*] Running prompt

a good appetite..........	1
an average appetite..........	2
or a poor appetite	3
for a child of his/her age?	

11. Do you ever eat any food from .... (CHILD'S) plate to encourage him/her to eat it?

Yes..........	1	(a)
No	2	Q12

(a) How often do you do this? Is it

Running prompt

most mealtimes	1
some mealtimes	2
or very occasionally?..........	3

12. And does .... (CHILD) ever eat any food from your (or anyone else's) plate?

Yes..........	1	(a)
No..........	2	Q13

(a) How often does this happen? Is it

Running prompt

most mealtimes..........	1
some mealtimes	2
or very occasionally?..........	3

13. Are there any foods that .... (CHILD) does not eat because he/she does not like them?

Yes..........	1	Specify
No..........	2	Q14

IF YES SPECIFY WHICH FOODS

Interview questionnaire (C) - *continued*

14. Do avoid giving ....(CHILD) particular foods or drinks because he/she is allergic to them?

Yes............ 1   (a) - (c)

No 2   Q15

If yes

(a) Which foods do you avoid?

Specify

.... (b)

(b) What form does the allergy take?

Specify

.... (c)

(c) Has .... (CHILD'S) allergy been diagnosed by a doctor?

Yes............ 1

No 2

15. (Apart from these) Are there any (other) foods you do not give .... (CHILD) for health, religious or any other reasons?

Yes............ 1   (a)

No 2   Q16

(a) If yes specify which foods and give reasons

FOOD	REASON
....	....
....	....
....	....
....	....
....	....

---

16. I'd like to ask you about what your child usually has to eat at different times of the day, but first I'd like to find out what times he/she gets up, has breakfast, has lunch and so on.

At what time approximately does ....(CHILD) usually ....(EVENT)

Prompt each event for time on weekdays, on Saturdays and on Sundays. Record approx. times in the grid.

Event	Weekdays	Saturdays	Sundays
gets up on............at:	....	....	....
has breakfast on ....at:	....	....	....
has lunch on ....at:	....	....	....
has tea on ....at:	....	....	....
goes to bed on ....at:	....	....	....

17. I'd now like to know, in general terms, what ....(CHILD) usually has to eat and drink at these different times. For example, at breakfast, does he/she have cereal, or toast, or a cooked breakfast? Some children don't eat breakfast, so if ....(CHILD) does not have anything at a particular time, please tell me.

What does he/she usually have to eat and drink, if anything ....

Prompt each event for what eaten on weekdays, on Saturdays and on Sundays. Record brief description in grid.

Event	Weekdays	Saturdays	Sundays
in bed or before breakfast on	Nil............ x	Nil............ x	Nil............ x

Interview questionnaire (C) - *continued*

Event	Weekdays	Saturdays	Sundays
for breakfast on	Nil x	Nil x	Nil x
during the morning on..........	Nil x	Nil x	Nil x
for lunch on	Nil x	Nil x	Nil x
during the afternoon on	Nil x	Nil x	Nil x
for tea on..........	Nil x	Nil x	Nil x
between tea and bed-time on	Nil x	Nil x	Nil x
in bed or during the night on	Nil x	Nil x	Nil x

DRINKING

18. Does . . . . . (CHILD) usually drink from

a feeder beaker/beaker with spout	1	⎤ Q19
a plastic cup or beaker	2	
Running prompt an ordinary cup, mug or glass	3	⎦
a bottle	4	Q20
or from something else? (specify)	5	Q19

19. (May I check) Does . . . . . (CHILD) have a bottle at all these days, even just to go to bed with?

Include ALL drinks given in a bottle Yes, has a bottle	1	Q20
No, never has a bottle	2	Q21

20. On average, how many bottles does . . . . . (CHILD) have a day?

Fewer than 1 a day	00
Include ALL drinks given in a bottle 1 a day	01
2 a day	02
Prompt as necessary 3 a day	03
4 a day	04
More than 4 a day (specify)	–

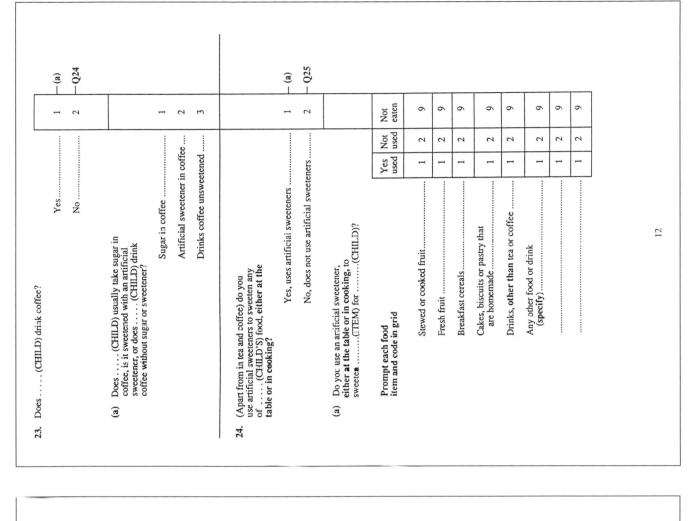

21. Does . . . . . (CHILD) drink tea?

Yes . . . . 1 —— (a)

No . . . . 2 —— Q22

   (a) Does . . . . . (CHILD) usually take sugar in tea, is it sweetened with an artificial sweetener, or does . . . . . (CHILD) drink tea without sugar or sweetener?

Sugar in tea 1

Artificial sweetener in tea 2

Drinks tea unsweetened 3

22. (May I check) does your child drink herbal teas **or** herbal infant drinks?

Yes, drinks herbal teas **or** herbal infant drinks . . . . 1 —— (a)(b)

No, drinks neither . . . . 2 —— Q23

   (a) <u>On average,</u> how often does . . . . . (CHILD) drink herbal tea or have a herbal infant drink?

| Show card A |

More than once a day 1

Once a day 2

Most days 3

At least once a week 4

At least once a month 5

Less than once a month 6

   (b) What brands of herbal tea or herbal infant drink are you giving your child at the moment?

| Record full brand name **and flavour** of all herbal teas/herbal infant drinks being given |

1. . . . .

2. . . . .

3. . . . .

Write in number of brands ⟶ |. . . . . .|

11

23. Does . . . . . (CHILD) drink coffee?

Yes . . . . 1 —— (a)

No . . . . 2 —— Q24

   (a) Does . . . . . (CHILD) usually take sugar in coffee, is it sweetened with an artificial sweetener, or does . . . . (CHILD) drink coffee without sugar or sweetener?

Sugar in coffee 1

Artificial sweetener in coffee 2

Drinks coffee unsweetened 3

24. (Apart from in tea and coffee) do you use artificial sweeteners to sweeten any of . . . . . (CHILD'S) food, **either at the table or in cooking?**

Yes, uses artificial sweeteners . . . . 1 —— (a)

No, does not use artificial sweeteners . . . . 2 —— Q25

   (a) Do you use an artificial sweetener, either **at the table or in cooking,** to sweeten . . . .(ITEM) for . . . .(CHILD)?

Prompt each food item and code in grid

	Yes used	Not used	Not eaten
Stewed or cooked fruit	1	2	9
Fresh fruit	1	2	9
Breakfast cereals	1	2	9
Cakes, biscuits or pastry that are homemade	1	2	9
Drinks, **other than tea or coffee**	1	2	9
Any other food or drink (specify)	1	2	9
. . . .	1	2	9
. . . .	1	2	9

12

Interview questionnaire (C) - *continued*

25. Applies if any artificial sweetener used
for child: Code 1 AT Q24 (any food)
Code 2 AT Q23(a) (in coffee)
Code 2 AT Q21(a) (in tea)

DNA, no artificial sweeteners used X

— Q26

What brands of artificial sweetener are you using to sweeten
.....(CHILD'S) food and drinks at the moment?

**Record full name and type - tablet, liquid, granulated,
of all artificial sweeteners being used for child**

1. ....

2. ....

3. ....

Write in number of brands ⟶

26. Do you usually add salt to ..... (CHILD'S) food during cooking?

Yes, includes sea salt 1

Yes, uses 'Lo Salt'/salt alternative
(<u>not</u> sea salt).............................. 2

No, does not use salt in cooking 3

Other (specify) 4

....

27. At the table, do you add salt to ..... (CHILD'S) food:

usually 1

Running   occasionally 2
prompt
rarely............................ 3

or never? 4

If uses 'Lo salt' or salt alternative (<u>not</u> sea salt) at table
ring code **1 - 3** <u>and</u> ring code ⟶   1

13

---

28. I would now like to ask you about some foods your child may eat.
Can you tell me about how often, on average, ... (CHILD) eats these foods.
Please choose your answer from this card.

| Hand informant Card A | Prompt each food listed below and code in grid. For 'seasonal foods' eg ice cream, prompt if necessary "......... *at this time of year*". |

	More than once a day	Once a day	Most days	At least once a week	At least once a month	Less than once a month	Never
Breakfast cereals	1	2	3	4	5	6	7
Cakes	1	2	3	4	5	6	7
Biscuits - any	1	2	3	4	5	6	7
Chocolate - confectionery	1	2	3	4	5	6	7
Other sweets	1	2	3	4	5	6	7
Ice cream or ice lollies	1	2	3	4	5	6	7
Yogurt (flavoured or plain but not fromage frais)	1	2	3	4	5	6	7
Cheese or cheese spread (not fromage frais)	1	2	3	4	5	6	7
Milk (dairy)	1	2	3	4	5	6	7
Eggs (include in home cooking)	1	2	3	4	5	6	7
Blackcurrant only drinks	1	2	3	4	5	6	7
Fruit juice (not squash)	1	2	3	4	5	6	7
Fizzy drinks (not mineral water)	1	2	3	4	5	6	7
Fish or shellfish, including fish fingers	1	2	3	4	5	6	7
Sausages - British type	1	2	3	4	5	6	7
Liver - not products	1	2	3	4	5	6	7
Beef, eg as a roast, steak or mince, in stews etc	1	2	3	4	5	6	7
Lamb, eg as a roast or chops, in stews etc	1	2	3	4	5	6	7
Pork, eg as a roast or chops, in stews etc	1	2	3	4	5	6	7
Chicken and poultry, eg as a roast, in casseroles	1	2	3	4	5	6	7

14

Interview questionnaire (C) - continued

28. (cont).

	More than once a day	Once a day	Most days	At least once a week	At least once a month	Less than once a month	Never
Baked beans - canned	1	2	3	4	5	6	7
Peas, in any form	1	2	3	4	5	6	7
Leafy green vegetables eg. spring greens, sprouts, broccoli	1	2	3	4	5	6	7
Chips	1	2	3	4	5	6	7
Other potatoes	1	2	3	4	5	6	7
Fresh fruit (any)	1	2	3	4	5	6	7

29. And how often, on average, does . . . . (CHILD) eat each of these foods?

Show Card A Prompt each food listed and code in grid.
For 'seasonal foods' prompt if necessary *"at this time of year"*.

	More than once a day	Once a day	Most days	At least once a week	At least once a month	Less than once a month	Never	(a) Skin eaten? Yes	(a) Skin eaten? No
Raw carrots	1	2	3	4	5	6	7	1	2
Cooked carrots	1	2	3	4	5	6	7	1	2
Other root vegetables, apart from carrots and potatoes e.g. parsnips, turnips, swedes	1	2	3	4	5	6	7	1	2
Button or baby mushrooms	1	2	3	4	5	6	7	1	2
Other mushrooms	1	2	3	4	5	6	7	1	2
Apples (fresh)	1	2	3	4	5	6	7	1	2
Pears (fresh)	1	2	3	4	5	6	7	1	2
Soft fruit (e.g. peaches, nectarines, grapes)	1	2	3	4	5	6	7	1	2
Citrus fruits (e.g. orange, tangerines, satsumas)	1	2	3	4	5	6	7	1	2
Fresh tomatoes	1	2	3	4	5	6	7	1	2
Cucumber	1	2	3	4	5	6	7	1	2

If child eats any of above ask for each food eaten

(a) Can you tell me whether . . . . . (CHILD) usually eats the skin on . . . . . (ITEM)

15

---

30. Applies if child **ever** eats potatoes **or** chips (see Q28)

DNA, **never** eats potatoes or chips . . . . 1 — Q31

Does your child eat the skin on . . . . . (TYPE OF POTATO) always, sometimes or never?

Prompt each type of potato listed below and code in grid.

	Eaten with skin left on Always	Sometimes	Never	Never eaten
Baked/jacket potatoes (cooked without fat)	1	2	3	4
Boiled new potatoes	1	2	3	4
Boiled old potatoes	1	2	3	4
Roast potatoes (in fat)	1	2	3	4
Fried potatoes or chips	1	2	3	4

16

Interview questionnaire (C) - continued

31. A lot of shops and supermarkets are selling foods which are labelled as 'organic' or 'organically grown', what do you understand by the term 'organic' or organically grown?

[*]

32. Do you buy any 'organic' foods for your child?

Yes .... 1 — (a)

No .... 2 — Q33

(a) Do you buy organic ..... (ITEM) for your child always, sometimes or never?

Prompt each food listed below and code in grid.

Buys for child	Always	Sometimes	Never
Organic fruit	1	2	3
Organic vegetables incl dried beans or lentils	1	2	3
Organic cereal products, rice, muesli, pasta etc	1	2	3
Meat	1	2	3
Anything else (specify)	1	2	3

17

33. Do you grow any of your own fruit and vegetables, either in your garden or on an allotment?

Include : salad vegetables

Exclude : herbs

Yes .... 1 — (a)(b)

No .... 2 — Q34

(a) Do you grow them without using pesticides?

Yes, all 1

Yes, some 2

No, none 3

(b) Do you grow them without using artificial fertilizers?

Yes, all 1

Yes, some 2

No, none 3

34. Does .....(CHILD) ever put soil into his/her mouth or eat soil these days?

Yes 1

No 2

35. Thinking about any food you have in the house today, which of the following items do you have here today?

Prompt each type of food listed below and code in grid.

	Has in house	Does not have in house
A breakfast cereal	1	2
Bread, or bread rolls	1	2
Milk, or liquid or powdered baby milk	1	2
A tin of baked beans or spaghetti	1	2
Eggs	1	2
Biscuits, of any kind	1	2
Potatoes	1	2
Chocolate, of any kind	1	2
Other sweets	1	2

18

36. Thinking now about different foods that come in cans.
How long, on average, would you keep ....(ITEM) in an opened can before eating/drinking it/them?

Show Card B

Prompt each type of food and code in grid below

	Code from Card B					Spontaneous only	
	More than a week	4 or 5 days	2 or 3 days	1 day	Use on same day	Never stored in open can	Not eaten/ drunk
Canned soft drinks eg cola, lemonade	1	2	3	4	5	6	7
Canned fruit juice	1	2	3	4	5	6	7
Baked beans	1	2	3	4	5	6	7
Spaghetti	1	2	3	4	5	6	7
Canned soup	1	2	3	4	5	6	7
Corned beef	1	2	3	4	5	6	7
Canned fish, eg, sardines, tuna	1	2	3	4	5	6	7

19

---

37. At present are you giving........(CHILD) fluoride tablets or drops?

Yes 1
No 2

38. And at present (apart from fluoride tablets/drops) are you giving ....(CHILD) any extra vitamins or minerals, as tablets, pills, powders, syrups or drops?

Yes 1
No 2

39. Applies if taking fluoride tablets/drops and/or supplements.

DNA .... X → Q40
(Qns 37 &38 coded No)

For each type taken record full description from bottle, including brand name and product licence number; record dose given to the child; how often taken, and form.

WRITE IN BLOCK CAPITALS   INCLUDE FLUORIDE

SUPPLEMENT 1

Full name , incl brand:
                                    Office use only

Dose: no. of tablets, drops, 5ml spoons:
                                    Office use only

Frequency: no. of times and period
eg 3 x day
                                    Office use only

Form: ring code   Drops 1
                   Pills/tablets 2
                   Liquid/syrup 3
                   Powder 4

Product licence number (if any)

PL:

SUPPLEMENT 2

Full name , incl brand:
                                    Office use only

Dose: no. of tablets, drops, 5ml spoons:
                                    Office use only

Frequency: no. of times and period
eg 3 x day
                                    Office use only

Form: ring code   Drops 1
                   Pills/tablets 2
                   Liquid/syrup 3
                   Powder 4

Product licence number (if any)

PL:

20

277

Interview questionnaire (C) - *continued*

Q39. (cont.)

SUPPLEMENT 3	**SUPPLEMENT 4**
Full name , incl brand: *Office use only* [ ]	Full name , incl brand: *Office use only* [ ]
Dose: no. of tablets, drops, 5ml spoons: *Office use only* [ ]	Dose: no. of tablets, drops, 5ml spoons: *Office use only* [ ]
Frequency: no. of times and period eg 3 x day *Office use only* [ ]	Frequency: no. of times and period eg 3 x day *Office use only* [ ]
Form: ring code Drops .... 1 Pills/tablets .... 2 Liquid/syrup .... 3 Powder 4	Form: ring code Drops .... 1 Pills/tablets .... 2 Liquid/syrup .... 3 Powder 4
Product licence number (if any) PL: [ ] / [ ]	Product licence number (if any) PL: [ ] / [ ]

SUPPLEMENT 5	**SUPPLEMENT 6**
Full name , incl brand: *Office use only* [ ]	Full name , incl brand: *Office use only* [ ]
Dose: no. of tablets, drops, 5ml spoons: *Office use only* [ ]	Dose: no. of tablets, drops, 5ml spoons: *Office use only* [ ]
Frequency: no. of times and period eg 3 x day *Office use only* [ ]	Frequency: no. of times and period eg 3 x day *Office use only* [ ]
Form: ring code Drops .... 1 Pills/tablets .... 2 Liquid/syrup .... 3 Powder 4	Form: ring code Drops .... 1 Pills/tablets .... 2 Liquid/syrup .... 3 Powder 4
Product licence number (if any) PL: [ ] / [ ]	Product licence number (if any) PL: [ ] / [ ]

21

CHILD'S MEDICAL HISTORY

40. **Code or ask:**

Is informant child's <u>natural</u> mother?

Yes 1   → Q41
No 2   → (a)

(a) Code or ask:

Is child's natural mother in the household?

Yes 1   ⎤
No 2   ⎦ → Q41

41. Thinking back to when . . . . . (CHILD) was born, was he/she born prematurely or early?

Don't know 9   → Q42
Yes/ yes - qualified answer 1   → (a)
No 2   → Q42

(a) How many weeks premature (early) was he/she?

[*]   Less than 1 week 00

Other: **specify no. of weeks** ⟶ [   ]

42. How much did (s)he weigh at birth?

[   ] Pounds   [   ] ounces

OR

[   ] Grams

Don't know/can't remember 1   ⎱ see Q43

22

Interview questionnaire (C) - *continued*

43. Applies if informant is child's natural mother, (Qn 40 coded 1)

DNA, informant is **not** child's natural mother X   Q44

Can I just check, how many children have <u>you</u> had, I mean all those who are living now (no matter what age) plus any who have died since birth including ..... (CHILD)?

> **Exclude stillborn, step, adopted and foster children**

Record number ⟶ ____

DNA, only one child X   Q44

(a) **If more than one ask**
Was ..... (CHILD) your first child, your second (or which)?

Record birth order number ⟶ ____   Q44

44. Has ..... (CHILD) ever had an accident which resulted in a hospital admission?

Yes 1
No 2

45. Has ..... (CHILD) ever had an operation?

Yes 1
No 2

46. Has ..... (CHILD) ever stayed in hospital as an inpatient, overnight or longer?

Yes 1
No 2

> **Exclude period after birth unless baby stayed in hospital after mother had left**

47. We would like to know about bowel movements of young children (as this is linked to their diets and health). How many times did ..... (CHILD) open his/her bowels yesterday?

Don't know 09   Q48
None 00   Q49
Write in number of times ⟶ ____   Q48

23

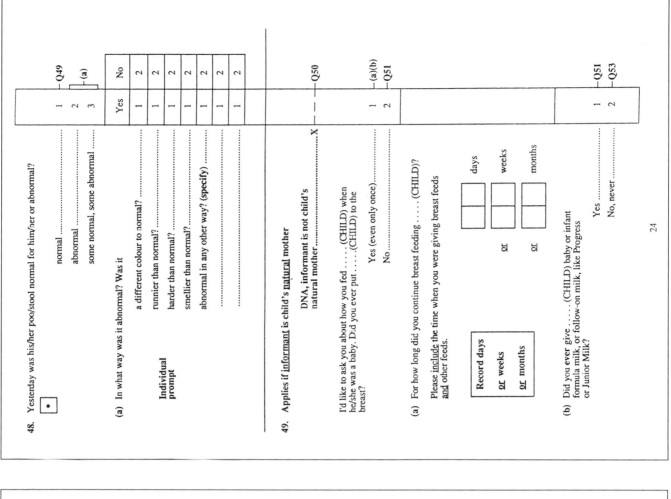

48. Yesterday was his/her poo/stool normal for him/her or abnormal?

[*]

normal 1   Q49
abnormal 2   (a)
some normal, some abnormal 3

(a) In what way was it abnormal? Was it

	Yes	No
a different colour to normal?	1	2
runnier than normal?	1	2
harder than normal?	1	2
smellier than normal?	1	2
abnormal in any other way? **(specify)**	1	2
	1	2
	1	2

Individual prompt

49. Applies if informant is child's <u>natural mother</u>

DNA, informant is not child's natural mother X   Q50

I'd like to ask you about how you fed ..... (CHILD) when he/she was a baby. Did you ever put ..... (CHILD) to the breast?

Yes (even only once) 1   (a)(b)
No 2   Q51

(a) For how long did you continue breast feeding ..... (CHILD)?

Please <u>include</u> the time when you were giving breast feeds <u>and</u> other feeds.

[ ] days
or [ ] weeks
or [ ] months

> **Record days or weeks or months**

(b) Did you **ever** give ..... (CHILD) baby or infant formula milk, or follow-on milk, like Progress or Junior Milk?

Yes 1   Q51
No, never 2   Q53

24

Interview questionnaire (C) - *continued*

50. Can I check, when ..... (CHILD) was a baby did (s)he ever have baby or infant formula milk, or follow-on milk like Progress or Junior Milk (not liquid cow's milk)?

Yes	1	— Q51
No, never	2	⌐ Q53
Don't know	3	⌐

51. At present is ..... (CHILD), having any baby or infant formula milk, or follow-on milk like Progress or Junior Milk, even just at bedtime?

Exclude liquid cow's milk

Yes	1	— Q53
No	2	— Q52

52. How old was ..... (CHILD) when he/she stopped having any baby, infant, formula or follow-on milk, even at bedtime?

Exclude liquid cow's milk

under 1 month	00
1 month - under 2 months	01
2 months - under 3 months	02
3 months - under 6 months	03
6 months - under 9 months	04
9 months - under 1 year	05
1 year - under 1½ years	06
1½ years - under 2 years	07
2 years - under 2½ years	08
2½ years - under 3 years	09
3 years or older	10

Prompt as necessary

---

53. Nowadays, does ..... (CHILD) have cow's milk as a drink?

Yes	1	(b)
No	2	(a)

(a) Has he/she ever had cow's milk as a drink?

Yes	1	(b)
No, never	2	Q54

(b) How old was ..... (CHILD) when he/she started having cow's milk as a drink?

Code in grid at bottom of page

54. What kind of milk does ..... (CHILD) usually have as a drink these days?

Prompt as necessary

Whole milk	01	Q55
Semi-skimmed milk	02	
Skimmed milk	03	(a)
Powdered baby milk	04	
Does not drink milk	05	Q55
Other (specify)	06	

(a) How old was ..... (CHILD) when he/she first had ..... (TYPE OF MILK) as a drink?

Prompt as necessary

	Q53(b) Cow's milk	Q54(a) Semi-skimmed	Q54(a) Skimmed
under 3 months	01	01	01
3 months - under 6 months	02	02	02
6 months - under 9 months	03	03	03
9 months - under 1 year	04	04	04
1 year - under 1½ years	05	05	05
1½ years - under 2 years	06	06	06
2 years - under 2½ years	07	07	07
2½ years - under 3 years	08	08	08
3 years - under 3½ years	09	09	09
3½ years - under 4 years	10	10	10
4 years or over	11	11	11
Don't know/can't remember	12	12	12

Interview questionnaire (C) - continued

55. Apart from as a drink, what kinds of milk do you give.......(CHILD) on cereal, in puddings etc?

Prompt as necessary

Code all that apply

Whole milk	01
Semi-skimmed milk.........	02
Skimmed milk	03
Powdered baby milk	04
Doesn't have any milk	05
Other (specify)	06

---

56. 'MOTHER'S' EMPLOYMENT

DNA, no mother/female parent-figure in household	1	Q68

Did you do any paid work last week - that is in the seven days ending last Sunday - either as an employee or self-employed?

Yes	1	Q57
No	2	Q58

57. Were you working full or part time?

Full time = more than 30 hrs
Part time = 30 hrs or less

Full time.........	1	Q62
Part time.........	2	

58. Even though you were not working did you have a job that you were away from last week?

Yes, is on maternity leave............	1	Q62
Yes, has a job and is not on maternity leave	3	Q62
No............	2	Q59

59. Last week were you:

Individual prompt

Code first that applies

waiting to take up a job that you had already obtained?......	1	Q60
looking for work?	2	
intending to look for work but prevented by temporary sickness or injury? (Check: 28 days or less)	3	
going to school or college full time? ...... (aged 16 - 49 only)	4	
permanently unable to work because of long-term sickness or disability? ...... (aged 16 - 59 only)	5	Q61
retired (only if stopped work after 50)	6	
looking after the home or family?	7	
Or were you doing something else? (specify)	8	

60. Apart from the job you are waiting to take up have you ever had a paid job or done any paid work?

Yes	1	Q62
No........	2	

61. May I just check, have you ever had a paid job or done any paid work?

Yes	1	Q62
No........	2	Q68

Interview questionnaire (C) - *continued*

62. 'MOTHER'S' MAIN LIFE JOB

- has only ever had one job: record details of job
- has had more than one job: record details of main job
- has never worked, but waiting to take up new job: record details of new job

Job title:

Describe fully work done:

SOC

IND

Industry:

Full time	1	(a)
Part time	2	(b)

| Employee | 1 |
| Self-employed | 2 |

(a) If employee: ask or record

Manager	1	(i)
Foreman/supervisor	2
Other employee	3

(i) How many employees work(ed) in the establishment?

1 - 24	1	see Q63
25 - 499	2
500 or more	3

(b) If self-employed:

Do (did) you employ other people?

Yes, **Probe**: 1-24	1
25 or more	2
No employees	3

29

---

63. Applies if 'mother' currently working or has job which she is away from, NOT on maternity leave.
Q56 coded 1 or Q58 coded 3

DNA, mother not currently working or has job but is on maternity leave .... 1 → Q68

Thinking now about your current job,
on which days of the week do you usually work?

| Varies .... | 1 | (a) |
| Does not vary .... | 2 |

(a) **Record days and hours worked: if varies, record days and hours worked last week**

DAY	Works?		Times worked: (Code all that apply)			
	Yes	No	Morning 06.00 - 12.59	Afternoon 13.00 - 17.59	Evening 18.00 - 23.59	Night 0.00 - 05.59
Monday	1	2	1	2	3	4
Tuesday	1	2	1	2	3	4
Wednesday	1	2	1	2	3	4
Thursday	1	2	1	2	3	4
Friday	1	2	1	2	3	4
Saturday	1	2	1	2	3	4
Sunday	1	2	1	2	3	4

64. How many hours a week do you usually work leaving out meal breaks?

If varies: record hours worked last week

Number of hours ————→ |...|.....|

65. Do you go out to work or work at home?

Goes out to work	1
Works at home	2
Varies on different days	3

30

Interview questionnaire (C) - *continued*

66. When you are working is ..... (CHILD) usually looked after at home or away from home?

Looked after at home	1
Looked after away from home	2
Varies	3

If sometimes at home, sometimes away, record place child spends most time while mother working

67. At present who looks after ..... (CHILD) while you are working?

	Q67 All	Q67(a) Main
Child's 'mother', at home	01	01
Child's 'mother', takes child to work with her	02	02
Child's 'father'	03	03
Child's grandparent	04	04
Child's brother/sister	05	05
Other relative of child in household	06	06
Other relative of child outside household	07	07
Friend/neighbour	08	08
Nanny	09	09
Paid childminder	10	10
Nurseryschool/class	11	11
School	12	12
Day Nursery or Creche	13	13
Play group	14	14
Other (specify)	15	15

Code all that apply

Only one ..... X — — — Q68

(a) Applies if more than one person looks after child

Who mainly looks after ..... (CHILD) while you are working? ——→ Code in column above

31

68. TO ALL

Show Card C

At present, is .... (CHILD) going to any of these regularly each week?

None attended .... 9 — see Q69

Code those attended in grid below; INCLUDE any mentioned at Q67

For each attended ask (a) - (d) and code in grid below

(a) On how many days a week does .... (CHILD) usually go to the .... (PLACE/PERSON)?

(b) Does he/she usually go there:

Running prompt — all day / mornings or afternoons only / or some other time?

(c) Does he/she usually have a meal while he/she is there?

(d) Does he/she usually have any drinks or snacks while he/she is there?

	Q68 Yes / No	Q68(a) No. of days/week child attends	Q68(b) Hours attended? all day	mornings or afternoons only	other	Q68(c) Meals? Yes / No	Q68(d) Snacks? Yes / No
Play group/Play school	1 2		1	2	3	1 2	1 2
Mother and toddler group	1 2		1	2	3	1 2	1 2
Nursery school/class	1 2		1	2	3	1 2	1 2
Day nursery or creche	1 2		1	2	3	1 2	1 2
Primary/Infants school	1 2		1	2	3	1 2	1 2
Childminder	1 2		1	2	3	1 2	1 2
Other children's group or childcare (specify)	1 2		1	2	3	1 2	1 2
	1 2		1	2	3	1 2	1 2
	1 2		1	2	3	1 2	1 2

32

Interview questionnaire (C) - continued

69. 'FATHER'S' EMPLOYMENT (male parent-figure)
If no 'father' in household, ask about HOH

Enter per. no. from h'hold box →

DNA, no 'father' and 'mother' is HOH .. 1 — Q75 mother

Did (your husband/HOH) do any paid work last week, that is in the seven days ending last Sunday, either as an employee or self-employed?

Yes .... 1 — Q74
No .... 2 — Q70

70. Even though (he) was not working, did (he) have a job that he was away from last week?

Yes .... 1 — Q74
No .... 2 — Q71

71. Last week was (he):

Individual prompt

waiting to take up a job that (he) had already obtained? ..... 1 — Q72
looking for work? 2
intending to look for work but prevented by temporary sickness or injury? (Check: 28 days or less) 3
going to school or college full time? (aged 16-49 only) 4

Code first that applies

permanently unable to work because of long-term sickness or disability? 5
retired? (men 16-64; women 16-59 only) 6
(for women, only if stopped work after age 50) looking after the home or family? 7
or was (he) doing something else? (specify) 8
} — Q73

72. Apart from the job (he) is waiting to take up, has (he) ever had a paid job or done any paid work?

Yes .... 1 — Q74
No 2

73. May I just check, has (he) ever had a paid job, or done any paid work?

Yes .... 1 — Q74
No .... 2 — Q75

33

---

74. 'FATHER'S'/HOH's CURRENT JOB

- has one job at present: record details of job
- has more than one job at present: record details of main job
- is not currently working: record details of last job
- is waiting to take up job: record details of 'new job'

Job title:

Describe fully work done:

SOC

IND

Industry:

Full time 1
Part time 2

Employee .... 1 — (a)
Self-employed .... 2 — (b)

(a) If employee: ask or record

Manager 1
Foreman/supervisor ..... 2 — (i)
Other employee 3

(i) How many employees work(ed) in the establishment?

1 - 24 .... 1 — Q75
25 - 499 2
500 or more 3

(b) If self-employed:

Does (did) (he) employ other people?

Yes, **Probe:** 1-24 ...... 1 — Q75
25 or more 2
No employees 3

34

Interview questionnaire (C) - *continued*

75. 'PARENTS' EDUCATION

Ask Qns 75 and 76 about 'mother' and 'father' if present in household

	Mother figure	Father figure
Enter per no.		
DNA, no 'mother'	X	
DNA, no 'father'	-----X	-----X	— Q76

How old were you (was your husband) when you (he) finished your (his) continuous full-time education?

	Mother figure	Father figure
Not yet finished	1	1
14 or under	2	2
15	3	3
16	4	4
17	5	5
18	6	6
19 or over	7	7
No formal education	8	8

---

76. Please look at this card and tell me whether you (your husband) have (has) any of the qualifications listed. Start at the top of the list and tell me the first one you come to that you have/he has passed

Show Card D

	Mother figure	Father figure
Degree (or degree level qualification)	1	1
Teaching qualification	2	2
HNC/HND, BEC/TEC Higher, BTEC Higher		
City and Guilds Full Technological Certificate		
Nursing qualifications (SRN, SCM, RGN, RM RHV, Midwife)		
'A' levels/SCE higher	3	3
ONC/OND/BEC/TEC not higher		
City and Guilds Advanced/Final		
Code first that applies		
'O' level passes (Grades A-C if after 1975)	4	4
GCSE (Grades A-C)		
CSE (Grade 1)		
SCE Ordinary (Bands A-C)		
Standard Grade (Levels 1-3)		
SLC Lower		
SUPE Lower or Ordinary		
School Certificate or Matric		
City and Guilds Craft/Ordinary level		
CSE Grades 2-5	5	5
GCE 'O' level (Grades D & E if after 1975)		
GCSE (Grades D, E, F, G)		
SCE Ordinary (Bands D & E)		
Standard Grade (Level 4, 5)		
Clerical or commercial qualifications		
Apprenticeship		
CSE ungraded	6	6
Other qualifications (**specify**)	7	7
No qualifications	8	8

Interview questionnaire (C) - *continued*

77. Do you (does your husband) smoke cigarettes at all?

	Mother figure	Father figure
Yes	1	1
No	2	2

Applies if mother/father smoke

(a) About how many cigarettes a day do you (does he) usually smoke?

	Mother figure	Father figure
Less than 1	00	00
No. smoked a day ——→	...	...
Don't know	99	99

78. **'MOTHER'S' PLACE OF BIRTH - female parent figure**

	Mother figure	Father figure
DNA, no 'mother'	X → Q80	

In which country were you born?

England	1
Scotland	2
Wales	3
N Ireland	4
Outside UK	5

79. To which of the groups listed as this card do you consider you belong?

Show Card E

*

White	1	
Black - Caribbean	2	} Q80
Black - African	3	
Black - Other	4	(a)
Indian	5	
Pakistani	6	} Q80
Bangladeshi	7	
Chinese	8	
None of these (include mixed race)	9	(a)

(a) How would you describe the racial or ethnic group to which you belong?

*

---

80. Does your household own or rent this house or flat?

Owns - with mortgage/loan	01
- outright	02
Rents - local authority/new town	03
- housing association	04
- privately unfurnished	05
- privately furnished	06
- from employer	07
- other with payment	08
Rent free	09

Prompt as necessary

81. Can I just check are you (or your husband) currently receiving Family Credit?

Yes	1
No	2

82. And have you (or your husband) drawn Income Support at any time in the last 14 days?

Yes	1
No	2

83. Could you please look at this card and tell me which group represents the <u>gross</u> income of the whole household?

Please include income from all sources before any compulsory deductions such as income tax, national insurance and superannuation contributions.

Show Card F

Group number	
Don't know	88
Refused	99

Remind informant who is included in the household

84. Enter finish time for questionnaire

24 hr. clock

Hours	Mins.

Interview questionnaire (C) - *continued*

CHILD'S ANTHROPOMETRIC MEASUREMENTS

The measurements of height, and supine length for children under age 2, mid-upper arm circumference, head circumference and weight may be made in any order, and at any visit <u>except blood taking</u>.

If no measurements made ring code
and specify reasons

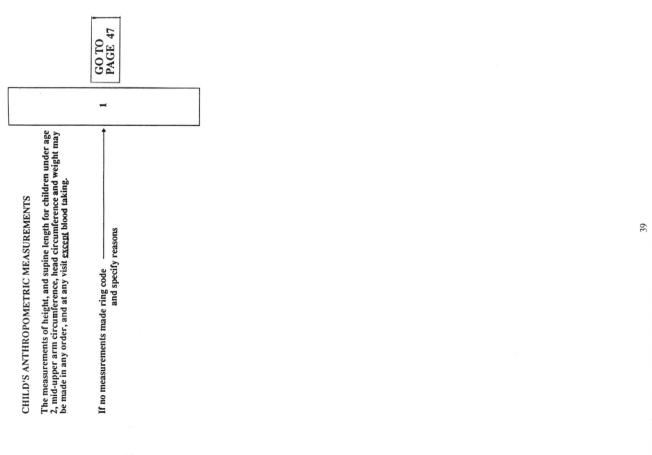

1	GO TO PAGE 47

M1. Child's weight (kilograms) ⟶ _____ . _____ (a)

(a) Date measured ⟶ Day | Mth | Yr → 9 3 (c)

(b) If refused, ring code and specify reasons ⟶ 1 next measure-ment

(c) Ring code if scales placed on:

    Code all that apply

    Uneven floor 1   (d)
    Carpet 2

(d) Ring code to show whether measurement made at:

    1st attempt.............. 1   (e)
    2nd attempt............. 2
    Other (specify number) ....

(e) Specify any special circumstances that might have affected weight

    Code all that apply

    No special circumstances 9   next measure-ment
    Wearing dry terry nappy 1
    Wearing dry disposable nappy 2
    Other (specify) 3

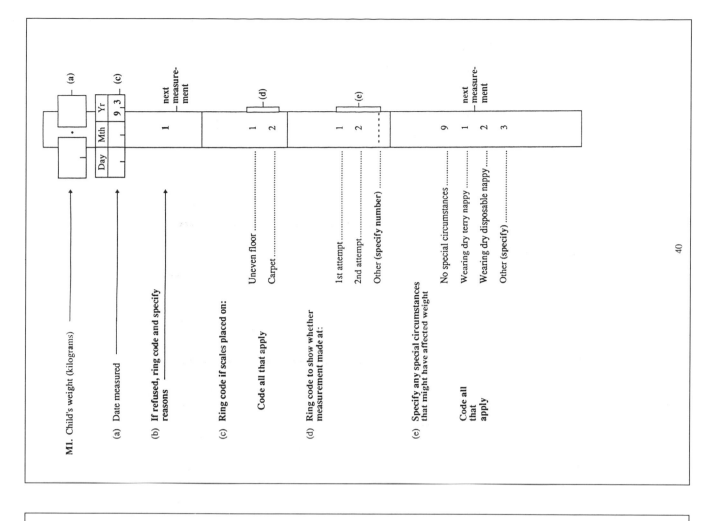

Interview questionnaire (C) - *continued*

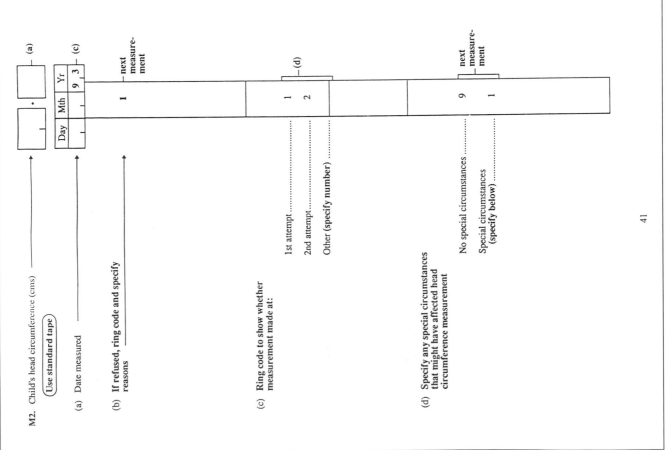

M2. Child's head circumference (cms) ──────────── (a)

[Use standard tape]

(a) Date measured ────────────── Day | Mth | Yr
9 | 3 (c)

(b) **If refused, ring code and specify reasons** ────────── 1 ── next measure-ment

(c) **Ring code to show whether measurement made at:**

1st attempt................. 1
2nd attempt................ 2
Other (specify number) .... (d)

(d) **Specify any special circumstances that might have affected head circumference measurement**

No special circumstances .... 9 ── next measure-ment
Special circumstances
(specify below) 1

41

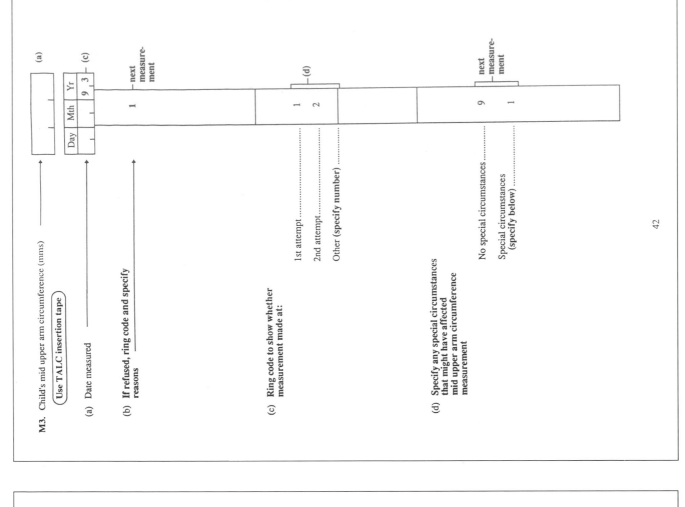

M3. Child's mid upper arm circumference (mms) ──────────── (a)

[Use TALC insertion tape]

(a) Date measured ────────────── Day | Mth | Yr
9 | 3 (c)

(b) **If refused, ring code and specify reasons** ────────── 1 ── next measure-ment

(c) **Ring code to show whether measurement made at:**

1st attempt................. 1
2nd attempt................ 2
Other (specify number) .... (d)

(d) **Specify any special circumstances that might have affected mid upper arm circumference measurement**

No special circumstances .... 9 ── next measure-ment
Special circumstances
(specify below) 1

42

Interview questionnaire (C) - continued

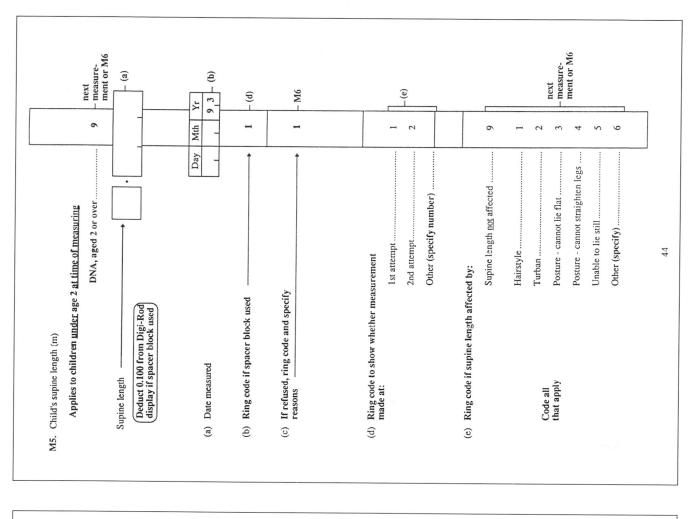

M5. Child's supine length (m)

Applies to children <u>under age 2 at time of measuring</u>

DNA, aged 2 or over .... 9 → next measurement or M6

(a)

Supine length →

Deduct 0.100 from Digi-Rod display if spacer block used

(a) Date measured

Day	Mth	Yr
		9 3

(b)

(b) Ring code if spacer block used — 1 (d)

(c) If refused, ring code and specify reasons — 1 → M6

(d) Ring code to show whether measurement made at:

1st attempt 1

2nd attempt 2

Other (specify number) .... (e)

(e) Ring code if supine length affected by:

Supine length <u>not</u> affected .... 9 → next measurement or M6

Hairstyle 1

Turban 2

Posture - cannot lie flat 3

Posture - cannot straighten legs 4

Unable to lie still 5

Other (specify) 6

Code all that apply

44

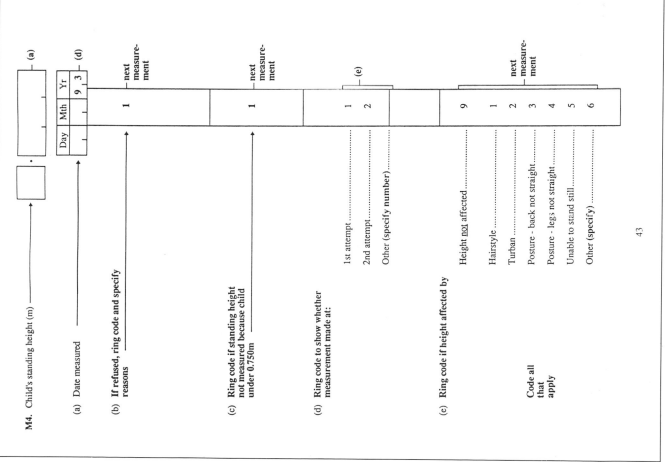

M4. Child's standing height (m) →

(a)

(a) Date measured

Day	Mth	Yr
		9 3

(d)

(b) If refused, ring code and specify reasons — 1 → next measurement

(c) Ring code if standing height not measured because child under 0.750m — 1 → next measurement

(d) Ring code to show whether measurement made at:

1st attempt 1

2nd attempt 2

Other (specify number) .... (e)

(e) Ring code if height affected by:

Height <u>not</u> affected .... 9 → next measurement

Hairstyle 1

Turban 2

Posture - back not straight 3

Posture - legs not straight 4

Unable to stand still 5

Other (specify) 6

Code all that apply

43

289

Interview questionnaire (C) - *continued*

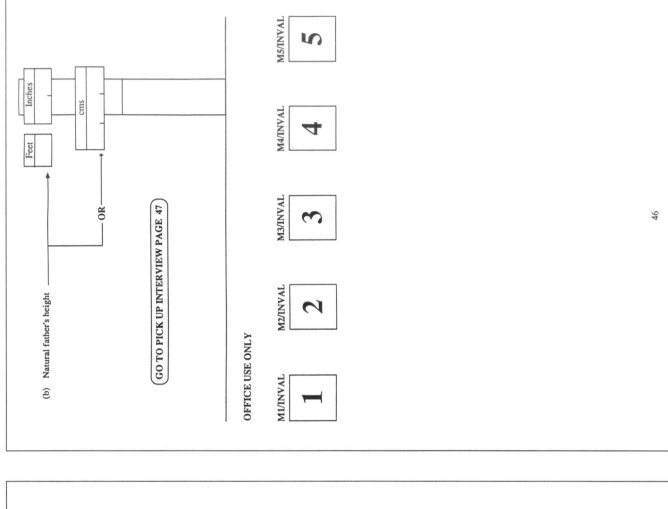

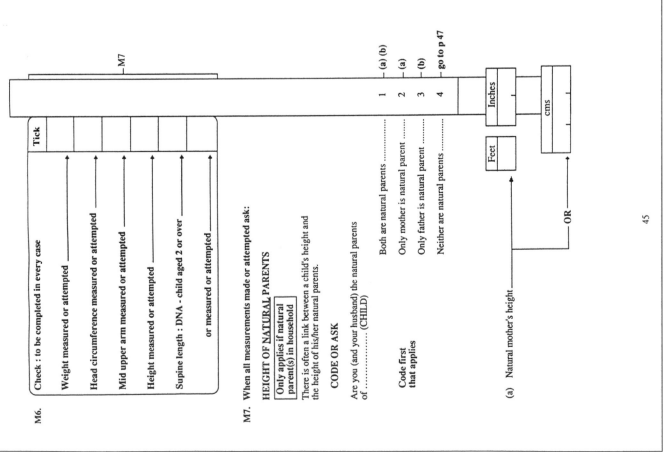

M6. Check : to be completed in every case

	Tick
Weight measured or attempted	
Head circumference measured or attempted	
Mid upper arm measured or attempted	
Height measured or attempted	
Supine length : DNA - child aged 2 or over	
or measured or attempted	

M7

M7. When all measurements made or attempted ask:

HEIGHT OF NATURAL PARENTS

Only applies if natural parent(s) in household

There is often a link between a child's height and the height of his/her natural parents.

CODE OR ASK

Are you (and your husband) the natural parents of .... (CHILD)

Code first
that applies

Both are natural parents .... 1 (a) (b)

Only mother is natural parent .... 2 (a)

Only father is natural parent .... 3 (b)

Neither are natural parents .... 4 go to p 47

(a) Natural mother's height

Feet | Inches

OR

cms

45

(b) Natural father's height

Feet | Inches

OR

cms

GO TO PICK UP INTERVIEW PAGE 47

OFFICE USE ONLY

M1/INVAL	M2/INVAL	M3/INVAL	M4/INVAL	M5/INVAL
1	2	3	4	5

46

Interview questionnaire (C) - *continued*

FOLLOW-UP QUESTIONNAIRE TO BE ASKED AT PICK-UP CALL

F1. Interviewer code

Dietary record refused	1	(a)
Partial dietary record	2	
4 day dietary record	3	F2

(a) Specify reasons dietary record refused/partial dietary record

F2. Applies if partial or 4 day dietary record obtained

DNA, no dietary record ...... X ----- F23

Interviewer code

Bowel movements card fully/partially completed	1	F3
No bowel movements card	2	(a)

(a) Specify reasons why no bowel movements card

GO TO F3

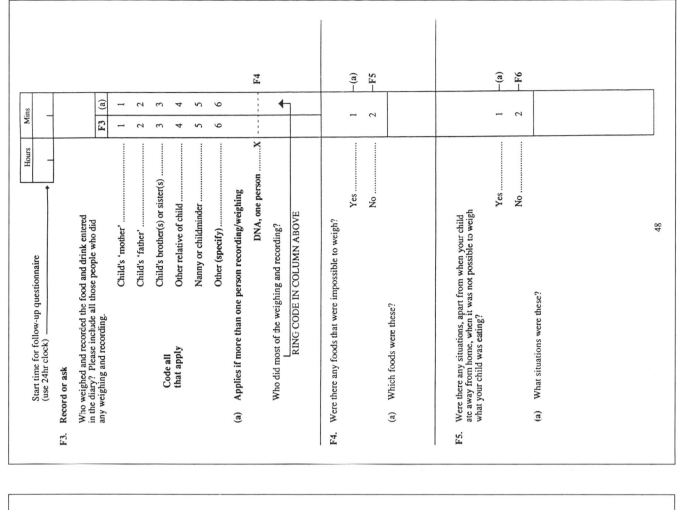

Start time for follow-up questionnaire (use 24hr clock)

Hours	Mins

F3. Record or ask

Who weighed and recorded the food and drink entered in the diary? Please include all those people who did any weighing and recording.

	F3	(a)
Child's 'mother'	1	1
Child's 'father'	2	2
Child's brother(s) or sister(s)	3	3
Other relative of child	4	4
Nanny or childminder	5	5
Other (specify)	6	6

Code all that apply

DNA, one person ...... X ----- F4

(a) Applies if more than one person recording/weighing

Who did most of the weighing and recording?

RING CODE IN COLUMN ABOVE

F4. Were there any foods that were impossible to weigh?

Yes	1	(a)
No	2	F5

(a) Which foods were these?

F5. Were there any situations, apart from when your child ate away from home, when it was not possible to weigh what your child was eating?

Yes	1	(a)
No	2	F6

(a) What situations were these?

Interview questionnaire (C) - *continued*

F6. Were there any occasions when you forgot to weigh and record any food or drink that your child had?

Yes .... 1 — (a) (b) (c)
No .... 2 — F7

(a) How often did this happen?

Several times a day 1
About once a day 2
Once or twice during the 4 days 3
Other (specify) 4
....

(b) What sorts of foods or drink did you forget to weigh?

(c) What did you do if you forgot to weigh something?

Prompt as necessary

Code all that apply

Missed it out completely 1
Put it in the diary with no weight 2
Weighed a similar item and entered this weight in the diary instead 3
Noted it down in the eating out diary 4
Other (specify) 5
....

F7. Do you consider your child to be a messy eater?

Yes .... 1 — (a)
No .... 2 — F9

(a) Did this cause you any problems with keeping the diary?

Yes .... 1 — (i)
No .... 2 — F8

(i) What sorts of problems did you have?

[*]

49

F8. If your child made a mess with their food did you manage to scrape it up and reweigh it as leftovers:

always 1
most of the time 2
only sometimes 3
or never? 4

Running prompt

F9. If your child ever left any of the food he/she was served, did you remember to weigh the leftovers and write the weight of them down in the diary:

Never any leftovers = code 1

always 1
most of the time 2
only sometimes 3
or never? 4

Running prompt

F10. If any food was wasted or eaten by someone else and therefore could not be reweighed as leftovers, did you remember to write this down in the diary:

Never wasted or eaten by somebody else = code 1

always 1
most of the time 2
only sometimes 3
or never? 4

Running prompt

50

Interview questionnaire (C) - continued

F11. During the (4) days that you were weighing and recording your child's food do you think you offered your child more, less or about the same amount of ....(ITEM) as usual?

Prompt each item listed below and code in the grid

	DNA, never eats item	Foods offered to your child		
		More	Less	Same
Biscuits	9	1	2	3
Sweets	9	1	2	3
Crisps	9	1	2	3
Drinks	9	1	2	3
Snacks	9	1	2	3

F12. On the whole, do you think that you offered your child:

Running prompt bigger	1
smaller	2
or the same size portions as usual while you were keeping the diary?	3

F13. During the (4) days do you think your child ate out of the home including at friends or nursery:

Running prompt more often..........................	1
less often	2
or about the same as usual?	3

F14. While you were weighing and keeping the diary, did you give your child food that was easier to weigh than you would normally give him/her?

Yes, easier to weigh	1
No, same as usual	2

51

F15. Do you think you changed your child's normal diet in any other way during the time you were weighing his/her food?

Yes..........	1	(a)
No	2	**F16**

(a) In what way did you change your child's normal diet?

[*]

F16. Do you think you weighed and recorded the food more accurately at:

Running prompt the beginning of the diary,..........	1	
or towards the end of the diary	2	
or was there no difference over the (4) days?	3	

F17. Did you always weigh each item or did you sometimes copy down the weight from a previous occasion, for example, the weights of biscuits, drinks or any other item your child has regularly?

Weighed every item..........	1	**F18**
Sometimes copied down weights..........	2	(a)

(a) Which items were weights copied over from?

52

293

Interview questionnaire (C) - *continued*

F18. Ask or record

Did the eating out diary have to be left with
someone else, for example a childminder or
playgroup worker, for them to record food
and drink eaten by your child?

Yes............... 1 —(a)

No .... 2 —F19

(a) Were there any problems in keeping the
eating out diary when your child was with
someone else?

Yes............... 1 —(i)

No .... 2 —F19

(i) What were these problems?

[*]

F19. Did you have any other problems with the weighing
and recording of what your child had to eat and drink
during the (4 day) period?

Yes............... 1 —(a)

No .... 2 —F20

(a) What were these problems?

[*]

F20. (During the past few days/while you were keeping the
diary) has ....(CHILD) been unwell at all;
has he/she:

	Yes	No
been teething?	1	2
Individual had any diarrhoea?	1	2
prompt been sick or vomited?	1	2
been unwell in any other way (specify)	1	2
....	1	2
....	1	2

DNA, not unwell during diary days....... 1 —F21

(a) Applies if <u>any</u> F20 coded 'yes'

On which day did he/she have (................ PROBLEM)

	Day 1	Day 2	Day 3	Day 4
DNA, not unwell this day	9	9	9	9
DNA, no diary this day	8	8	8	8
teething	1	1	1	1
diarrhoea	2	2	2	2
vomiting	3	3	3	3
other (specify)	4	4	4	4
....	5	5	5	5
....	6	6	6	6

(b) Ask for each day on which
child was unwell

Did being unwell affect his/her
eating habits on this day?

	Day 1	Day 2	Day 3	Day 4
Yes, eating affected........	1	1	1	1
No, eating not affected......	2	2	2	2

(RECORD COMMENTS AND PROBE
AMBIGUITIES)

Interview questionnaire (C) - continued

F21. Have there been any (other) unusual circumstances which have affected ....(CHILD'S) eating habits (during the past few days/while you were keeping the diary)?

Yes.................. 1 — (a)

No.................. 2 — F22

(a) What has been different about ....(CHILD'S) eating habits over these days?

[*]

F22. Is there anything you would like to say about the diary you kept for your child?

Yes (specify)...... 1

No.................. 2 ──────────────► F23

Finish time for follow-up questionnaire
(use 24hr clock)

Hours	Mins

55

F23. Applies to all

If kept diary ask: Since you started keeping the diary, that is, since last ...., has .... (CHILD) been taking any medicines, tablets or pills that have been prescribed for him/her by a doctor?

If no diary ask: At present, is .... (CHILD) taking any medicines, tablets or pills that have been prescribed for him/her by a doctor?

Yes, taking prescribed medicines .... 1 — (a)

No prescribed medicines .... 2 — F24

Include prescribed creams, drops, injections, inhalers etc.

For each prescribed medicine ask (a)
(a) What is it? Has it a brand name?

Ask to see all containers for prescribed medicines being taken (during recording period/now). Record the full names of each prescribed medicine in the grid below.

PLEASE USE BLOCK CAPITALS

PRESCRIBED MEDICINE 1	PRESCRIBED MEDICINE 2
Full name:	Full name:
Brand name:	Brand name:
Strength: *Office use only*	Strength: *Office use only*
Product licence no:	Product licence no:
P/L	P/L

56

Interview questionnaire (C) - *continued*

PRESCRIBED MEDICINE 3

Full name:

Brand name:

Office use only

Strength:

Product licence no:

P/L

PRESCRIBED MEDICINE 4

Full name:

Brand name:

Office use only

Strength:

Product licence no:

P/L

PRESCRIBED MEDICINE 5

Full name:

Brand name:

Office use only

Strength:

Product licence no:

P/L

PRESCRIBED MEDICINE 6

Full name:

Brand name:

Office use only

Strength:

Product licence no:

P/L

PRESCRIBED MEDICINE 7

Full name:

Brand name:

Office use only

Strength:

Product licence no:

P/L

PRESCRIBED MEDICINE 8

Full name:

Brand name:

Office use only

Strength:

Product licence no:

P/L

F24. INTERVIEWER'S ASSESSMENT SHEET

To be completed in every case where diary kept.

DNA, no diary X

F25

Please record your own assessment of the quality of weighing and recording in the home record and eating out diary. Note any circumstances that you think might have affected eating habits or the quality of the diaries

Prompt cards A TO F

CARD A

N1340

1. More than once a day
2. Once a day
3. Most days
4. At least once a week, but not most days
5. At least once a month, but less often than once a week
6. Less than once a month
7. Never

CARD B

N1340

1. More than a week
2. No more than 4 or 5 days
3. No more than 2 or 3 days
4. No more than 1 day
5. Use on same day

Interview questionnaire (C) - *continued*

F25. INTERVIEWER'S PROGRESS CHECK

	Tick if full or partial	Ring if DNA or refused
Collect: home record diary, with any wrappers (E)	- - - - -	X
eating out diary, with any wrappers (F)	- - - - -	X
bowel movements chart	- - - - -	X
Collect scales (and box) and bowl	- - - - -	X
Complete incentive payment letter and form (**if 4 day diary**) (Y)	- - - - -	X
Complete measurements of child	- - - - -	X
Collect: measuring equipment:		
Scales	- - - - -	X
TALC tape and pen	- - - - -	X
Tape	- - - - -	X
Digi-rod and block	- - - - -	X
Record measurement of parents' height	- - - - -	X

F26. To be completed after asking dental recall questions at final call

Copy code from Q1 on dental recall sheet

Yes, to interview and examination	1
Yes, to interview only	2
Yes, other/conditional	3
No	4
Dental recall qns not asked	5 — (a)

(a) Specify reasons why dental recall qns not asked

59

The correct position of the head when measuring height (Frankfort plane)

Prompt cards A to F - *continued*

CARD C

N1340

1. Playgroup or play school

2. Mother and toddler group

3. Nursery school or nursery class

4. Day nursery or creche

5. Primary or infants school

6. Childminder

7. Other children's group or childcare

N1340   CARD E

1. White

2. Black-Caribbean

3. Black-African

4. Black-Other

5. Indian

6. Pakistani

7. Bangladeshi

8. Chinese

9. None of these

N1340   CARD D

Degree (or degree level qualification)

Teaching qualification
HNC/HND, BEC/TEC Higher, BTEC Higher
City and Guilds Full Technological Certificate
Nursing qualifications (SRN, SCM, RGN, RM,
RHV, Midwife)

'A' levels/SCE higher
ONC/OND/BEC/TEC not higher
City and Guilds Advanced/Final level

'O' level passes (Grade A-C if after 1975)
GCSE (grades A-C)
CSE Grade 1
SCE Ordinary (Bands A-C)
Standard Grade (Level 1-3)
SLC Lower
SUPE Lower or Ordinary
School Certificate or Matric
City and Guilds Craft/Ordinary level

CSE Grades 2-5
GCSE 'O' level (Grades D&E if after 1975)
GCSE (Grades D,E,F,G)
SCE Ordinary (Bands D&E)
Standard Grade (Level 4,5)
Clerical or commercial qualifications
Apprenticeships

CSE ungraded

Other qualifications (specify)

No qualifications

N1340   CARD F

GROSS HOUSEHOLD INCOME

per week	Group	per year
less than £40	01	less than £2,000
£40 - less £80	02	£2,000 - less £4,000
£80 - less £120	03	£4,000 - less £6,000
£120 - less £160	04	£6,000 - less £8,000
£160 - less £200	05	£8,000 - less £10,000
£200 - less £240	06	£10,000 - less £12,000
£240 - less £280	07	£12,000 - less £14,000
£280 - less £350	08	£14,000 - less £18,000
£350 - less £400	09	£18,000 - less £20,000
£400 - less £500	10	£20,000 - less £25,000
£500 - less £600	11	£25,000 - less £30,000
£600 or more	12	£30,000 or more

(E)

CONFIDENTIAL
N1340/W4 NATIONAL DIET AND NUTRITION SURVEY;
CHILDREN AGED 1½ - 4½ YEARS

Serial no. label

Interviewer number

Sex

Boy   Girl

Date of Birth

HOME RECORD BOOK

Please record all food and drink as shown inside. Thank you

The interviewer will call again on:

Day	Date	Time

Office of Population Censuses and Surveys
Social Survey Division
St Catherines House
10 Kingsway, London WC2B 6JP

Home Record Book

These instructions tell you how you to describe the food and drink items you weigh. You should also read the instructions at the front of the eating out diary.

Please read through all these notes carefully before starting the 4 days of weighing and recording. The interviewer will go over the main points with you, and can help with any difficulties you might have. The check list card is a quick reminder of how to use the scales and record food items.

DESCRIBING FOOD AND DRINK: as full a description of each food and drink, together with its brand name is needed.

Column A: Write down the time the food will be eaten, indicating whether the time was a.m. or p.m. Each plate entry should have a time written in this column. If you are preparing food for your child to take out of the home for lunch tomorrow, record the information on tomorrow's sheet.

Column B: Tick the first box if the food is being eaten at home; tick the second box if the food was eaten away from home.

Column C: Tick the first box if you are the child's mother or father recording the food and drink; tick the second box if you are someone else, eg the nanny, childminder, child's grandmother recording the food or drink.

Column D: Write down the brand or product name of the food. Please give as much information as possible. Describe each item ON A SEPARATE LINE. Fresh meat, fresh fish, fresh fruit and vegetables, doorstep milk, unwrapped bread and cakes and other fresh foods which are not pre-packed (cheese, cooked meats and pasta which are not pre-packed) do not need brand or product names. In these cases no information is required, so leave the space in this column blank. Do NOT write in the name of the shop where the item was bought. However, remember to record 'own brand' names in this column, eg Sainsbury's (baked beans).

Column E: Write down the description of the food. Please give as much information as possible - type of food, name, and how it was cooked. If the food was fried or roasted, please write down the type of fat or oil it was cooked in. If the food includes homemade pastry please write down the type of fat used to make the pastry. If the food was a bought dessert, for example, a yoghurt or fromage frais, write down what flavour it was and whether it was low fat, diet/ reduced sugar or not. If you need to, you may use more than one line, but please put EACH SEPARATE ITEM ON A SEPARATE LINE. If the item was a cooked dish made from several items, for example, Shepherd's pie, weigh the whole portion and describe it as Sheperd's pie in the diary. Do not try to weigh the potato and meat parts separately. Write down the recipe used to make the dish on the back of the previous page.

Column F: If the food item is fresh fruit or fresh vegetables please tick a box in this column against the item to show whether it was homegrown or not. By homegrown, we mean grown IN YOUR OWN GARDEN OR ALLOTMENT.

Column G: Write in the weight of the food or drink.

Column H: We need to know the weight of any leftovers, including any inedible parts, such as fruit stones or peel. You should weigh the plate with the leftovers on it and write the weight in column H next to the weight you wrote down for the empty plate. Make sure to put a tick next to each item of food left.

Column J: If something is spilt or eaten by someone other than the child and therefore not reweighed as leftovers, tick the box in column J. Write in the space along side the item about how much of the original item you think was lost: for example "about ½ spilt". If it was a plateful of different foods that were spilt and you cannot estimate how much of each individual item was lost then bracket together all the items that were lost and estimate how much of the original plateful was lost.

For foods that already come in containers like yoghurt or trifles you can weigh the full container and then weigh the container again when your child has eaten the food. Or, if you prefer, you can tip out the food into a bowl which you have just weighed.

To weigh bread and butter or anything else you spread on bread, start by weighing the plate as usual. Press the button again to set the scale back to zero and weigh the bread. Press the button again to set the scale back to zero then remove the bread and quickly spread the butter. Put the bread back on the scales and it will show the weight of the butter or margarine you have just spread. Now set the scale back to zero and then remove the bread again to quickly spread the jam or marmalade. Put the bread back on the scale and it will show the weight of the jam you have put on. If the scales switch off before you have buttered your bread, or spread the filling, do not worry. Switch the scales on again and record the total weight of plate, bread, butter etc. However, please make a note against the entry to show what happened, for example, 'total weight of plate, one slice of toast, butter, marmalade'.

Children have a lot of drinks during the day. We need to know about ALL of them. If your child has a drink of squash, please weigh the concentrate and water separately and give a full description of the squash in column E. The 'Check List For Weighing' card has a step-by-step guide to weighing squash to help you.

Home record diary (E) - example page

A COMPLETED PAGE IN THE HOME RECORD BOOK SHOULD LOOK LIKE THIS

Serial Number

Day ... Friday ... day   Date 0 3 0 7 9 2

TICK A BOX TO SHOW WHICH DAY THIS IS
DAY 1 2 ✓ 3 4

OFF. USE DAY OR WEEK 1   TICK A BOX TO SHOW WHETHER CHILD IS WELL OR UNWELL TODAY
Wel ✓ Unwell 2

Please use a separate line for each item eaten: write in weight of plate; leave a line between different 'plate' entries

A Time eaten am/pm	B TICK A BOX Food eaten at home / away	C TICK A BOX Weighed by mother / other	D Brand name of each item, in full (except for fresh produce)	E Full description of each item including: - whether fresh, frozen, dried, canned - what flavour, whether sweetened - how cooked, what type of fat food fried in	F If fresh fruit or veg, was it home grown? TICK BOX Yes / No	G Weight served gms	H Weight of plate & leftovers TICK ITEMS LEFT OVER	OFFICE USE ONLY Est weight? Tick if YES	Brand	Food	J If any of this item was spilt or eaten by someone else and therefore not reweighed as leftovers TICK BOX: and estimate how much of the original item was lost. Give details of any other problems → Yes
8.05am	✓ 1	✓ 1		Bowl	1 / 2	400	442				1
			Kelloggs	Coco - pops	1 / 2	57	✓				1
			Unigate	Whole milk, pasteurised, Silver top	1 / 2	63	✓				1
			Silver-Spoon	Sugar (granulated)	1 / 2	6	✓				1
					1 / 2						1
8.05am	✓ 1	✓ 1		Glass	1 / 2	220					1
			Tesco	Orange juice, unsweetened longlife	1 / 2	64					1
				diluted with tap water	1 / 2	30					1
					1 / 2						1
11am	✓ 1	✓ 1		Plate	1 / 2	176					1
			Champion	Sliced softgrain bread, 2 slices toasted	1 / 2	76					¹/₂ slice of toast fed to the dog ✓ 1
			Flora	Margarine	1 / 2	8					✓ 1
				Marmite	1 / 2	8					✓ 1
					1 / 2						1

CHECK LIST

EACH PAGE SHOULD HAVE:
day and date;
whether child was well or unwell that day.

WHEN RECORDING:
ALL food should be weighed on a plate and all drinks weighed in a container.

Weigh the plate or container first.

Foods that come in pots or containers and are eaten from them, such as yoghurt, should be weighed before and after contents are eaten.

Start each new food item on a separate line: you can use more than one line to write the description of a food.

Leave a line before starting a new plate or container.

REMEMBER:
Record ALL drinks, including tap water.

Record ALL vitamin and mineral supplements, including fluoride supplements.

Record ALL condiments (eg tomato sauce) used at the table.

Show, by a tick in column F, whether fresh fruit and vegetables were home grown.

Weigh all leftovers on the plate or in the container, and tick those foods which have been left in column H.

Show in column J, whether any of the original item was lost or spilt and could not be reweighed. Estimate the proportion of food or drink lost.

VA43/06 1/93

301

Home record diary (E) - recording sheet

PLEASE START A NEW PAGE FOR EACH DAY EVEN IF ONLY SOME OF THIS PAGE IS USED

Day .... day   Date _____

Serial Number _____

OFF. USE	TICK A BOX TO SHOW WHETHER
DAY OF WEEK	CHILD IS WELL OR UNWELL TODAY
	Well [1] Unwell [2]

TICK A BOX TO SHOW WHICH DAY THIS IS
DAY   1 [1]   2 [2]   3 [3]   4 [4]

Please use a separate line for each item eaten: write in weight of plate; leave a line between different 'plate' entries

A	B		C		D	E	F		G	H		OFFICE USE ONLY			J
Time eaten am/pm	TICK A BOX Food eaten at		TICK A BOX Weighed by		Brand name of each item, in full (except for fresh produce)	Full description of each item including: - whether fresh, frozen, dried, canned - what flavour, whether sweetened - how cooked, what type of fat food fried in	If fresh fruit or veg, was it home grown? TICK BOX		Weight served gms	Weight of plate & leftovers		Est weight? Tick If YES	Brand	Food	If any of this item was spilt or eaten by someone else and therefore not reweighed as leftovers TICK BOX - and estimate how much of the original item was lost. Give details of any other problems.
	home	away	mother	other			Yes	No		TICK ITEM					Yes
	[1]	[2]	[1]	[2]			[1]	[2]							[ ]
	[1]	[2]	[1]	[2]			[1]	[2]							[ ]
	[1]	[2]	[1]	[2]			[1]	[2]							[ ]
	[1]	[2]	[1]	[2]			[1]	[2]							[ ]
	[1]	[2]	[1]	[2]			[1]	[2]							[ ]
	[1]	[2]	[1]	[2]			[1]	[2]							[ ]
	[1]	[2]	[1]	[2]			[1]	[2]							[ ]
	[1]	[2]	[1]	[2]			[1]	[2]							[ ]
	[1]	[2]	[1]	[2]			[1]	[2]							[ ]
	[1]	[2]	[1]	[2]			[1]	[2]							[ ]
	[1]	[2]	[1]	[2]			[1]	[2]							[ ]
	[1]	[2]	[1]	[2]			[1]	[2]							[ ]
	[1]	[2]	[1]	[2]			[1]	[2]							[ ]
	[1]	[2]	[1]	[2]			[1]	[2]							[ ]
	[1]	[2]	[1]	[2]			[1]	[2]							[ ]

VA43/3a 1/93

N1340/W4

(F)

Serial no. label

Eating Out Diary

Mothers/carers:- Please use this notebook to write down any food or drink the child has while away from home, even if the food was brought from home.

Carers:- Please hand this notebook back to the mother each day.

OPCS
St Catherine's House
10 Kingsway
London WC2B 6JP

VA43/5 1/93

When out of the home:
Write down <u>everything</u> the child eats and drinks in this eating out diary. EVEN if the food has been made (and weighed) at home to eat out.

Write down:
- the day and date on each page you use;

- the time and place where the food or drink was eaten or drunk;

- the brand name of each item of food and drink (where possible);

- a full description of the food and drink including, if it was bought, the price and place of purchase.

Make a note of any food or drink left over. If none of a particular item is eaten, please note this down. For example, if a child had a cheese and tomato sandwich but all the tomato is left, write this down.

The pocket book has a ruler printed on every page. Use this to help describe the size of the portion. For example, if the child has a piece of chocolate sponge pudding, measure it, noting its size: 6cm square and 4cm deep.

Example page:

Time eaten am/pm	Place where item was eaten	Brand name, in full, unless fresh produce.	Description, including price, where it was bought, and quantity.	Any leftovers?
2pm	Nan's House	Walkers Crisps	125g packet of ready salted crisps	No
3pm	Nan's House	Robinson's	Apple & blackcurrant juice drink (individual carton)	No
4pm	Car		Apple	Yes left core

cm 1 2 3 4 5 6 7 8 9 10 11 12 13 14 15 16 17 18 19

Please start a new page for each day even if only some of this page is used

Serial Number

Day ....

Date ....

VA43/5

Time eaten am/pm	Place where item was eaten	Brand name, in full, unless fresh produce.	Description, including price, where it was bought, and quantity.	Any leftovers?

cm 1 2 3 4 5 6 7 8 9 10 11 12 13 14 15 16 17 18 19

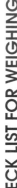

(R)

CHECK LIST FOR WEIGHING

Turn scales on and wait until 'O' is displayed. The scales are now ready for use.

Weigh your plate or other container and record weight in diary.

Leave plate or container on scales and press button to set scales back to 'O'.

Put first food item on plate or in container on scales and record weight.

Leave plate or container on scales, and press button again to set scale back to 'O'.

Repeat the same procedure for all other food items.

Remove plate or container from scales.

Press button twice to switch off scales.

Example:

Weighing a drink of orange squash;
- turn on scales: wait till 'O' appears;
- weigh cup or glass; record weight;
- press button to zero scales;
- add orange squash concentrate;
- record weight and description of squash;
- press button to zero scales;
- add water;
- record weight and description of water (ie tap water);
- remove cup of squash;
- press button twice to turn off scales.

Note: You can remove the cup or plate from the scales to add water or any other item as long as you zero the scales **before** you remove it. The scales will display a negative number until you return the cup or plate to the scales.

HA003092

(P)

N1340/W4 YOUNG CHILDREN'S DIETARY SURVEY

Serial number label

EATING PATTERN CHECK SHEET

Complete one sheet for each dietary record. Ring code to show number of items eaten each day.

Day	Drinks		Crisps & savoury snacks		Biscuits & sweets		Supplements, inc fluoride		Tick here if note in diary
	At home	Out	At home	Out	At home	Out	At home	Out	
.....day	1 5	1 5	1 5	1 5	1 5	1 5	1	1	
	2 6	2 6	2 6	2 6	2 6	2 6	2	2	
	3 7	3 7	3 7	3 7	3 7	3 7	3	3	
	4 8	4 8	4 8	4 8	4 8	4 8	4	4	
.....day	1 5	1 5	1 5	1 5	1 5	1 5	1	1	
	2 6	2 6	2 6	2 6	2 6	2 6	2	2	
	3 7	3 7	3 7	3 7	3 7	3 7	3	3	
	4 8	4 8	4 8	4 8	4 8	4 8	4	4	
.....day	1 5	1 5	1 5	1 5	1 5	1 5	1	1	
	2 6	2 6	2 6	2 6	2 6	2 6	2	2	
	3 7	3 7	3 7	3 7	3 7	3 7	3	3	
	4 8	4 8	4 8	4 8	4 8	4 8	4	4	
.....day	1 5	1 5	1 5	1 5	1 5	1 5	1	1	
	2 6	2 6	2 6	2 6	2 6	2 6	2	2	
	3 7	3 7	3 7	3 7	3 7	3 7	3	3	
	4 8	4 8	4 8	4 8	4 8	4 8	4	4	

HA24/41/93

Check list for weighing and recording (R) - *continued*

CHECK LIST FOR RECORDING IN THE DIARY

EACH PAGE SHOULD HAVE:
day and date;

whether child was well or unwell that day.

WHEN RECORDING:
ALL food should be weighed on a plate and all drinks weighed in a container.

Weigh the plate or container first.

Enter the time, am or pm, against each plate or container entry.

Foods that come in pots or containers and are eaten from them, such as yoghurt, should be weighed before and after contents are eaten.

Start each new food item on a separate line; you can use more than one line to write the description of c food.

Leave a line before starting a new plate or container.

REMEMBER:
Record **ALL** drinks, including tap water.

Record **ALL** vitamin or mineral supplements, including fluoride supplements.

Record **ALL** medicines.

Record **ALL** condiments (eg tomato sauce) used at the table.

Show, by a tick in column F, whether fresh fruit and vegetab es were home grown.

Weigh all leftovers on the plate or in the container, and tick those foods which have been left in column H.

Show in column J whether any of the original item was lost cr spilt and could not be reweighed. Estimate the proportion of food lost.

305

(K)

FOOD DESCRIPTION PROMPT CARD

N1340

Bought Form

Fresh
Frozen; chilled
Canned; bottled
Dried; dehydrated
Ready-meal
Smoked; not smoked

Cooking Method

Uncooked; raw
Rehydrated; reconstituted
Boiled; stewed; casseroled
Poached, in milk or water
Steamed
Baked - no added fat ?
Grilled - added fat ?
Deep fried ⎤ what fat ?
Shallow fried ⎦
Roasted - added fat
Microwaved - with fat = fried; grilled with fat
Microwaved - with little water = boiled

Leftovers

Meat: fat, bones, skin
Fish: bones, skin
Fruit: skin, peel, stones, pips

Coatings

Flour
Batter: egg, flour and milk
Crumbs: and eggs?

Brand Codes

Herbal teas; infant herbal drinks
Mineral waters; soft drinks
Artificial sweeteners

Meat Preparation

Fat trimmed before eating or cooking
Fat skimmed from meat dishes
Lean and fat eaten, or only

Gravy and sauces

Thickened: with flour, cornflour, Bisto, Gravy
    Granules
Skimmed; fat skimmed or no added fat
Casseroles: thickened; skimmed with
    vegetables/potatoes

Pastry

One or two crusts
Type of pastry: shortcrust; flaky
Type of flour: white; wholemeal
Type of fat

Soft drinks

Juice; juice drink
Pasteurised; UHT
Sweetened; unsweetened
Canned; bottled; cartons
Decaffeinated; not decaffeinated
Carbonates: Cola; lemonade; other
Diet; not diet
Fortified; not fortified

Water - code brand

Bottled; not bottled

Artificial Sweeteners - code brand

Record and code separately

Fats and oils

Blended vegetable oil: home fried or takeaway
Butter; salted or unsalted
Dripping
Lard
Margarine, NOT polyunsaturated
Polyunsaturated margarine or oil

Dairy Products

Low fat; full fat
Milk: skimmed; semi-skimmed; whole; UHT
Yogurt: very low fat; low fat; creamy; UHT;
    sweetened with sugar; artificial sweetener;
    unsweetened; fortified; not fortified
Cheese: low fat; full fat; made with sunflower oil

Vegetables

Homegrown; not homegrown
Carrots: old; new
Potatoes: old; new

Chips

Old/new potatoes; fresh/frozen
Cut: crinkle, straight, fine, thick
Oven ready; fried
Fat used

Fruit

Canned in syrup; canned in juice
Fruit only; fruit and juice/syrup
Sweetened with sugar, artificial
    sweetener, or unsweetened
Homegrown; not homegrown

HA1/23/92

N 1340 YOUNG CHILDREN'S DIETARY SURVEY (L)

GUIDE WEIGHTS - typical portion sizes for children aged 1½ to 4½ years

Note: these weights are a guide; reported weights outside these ranges may be correct, but should have a note to explain the circumstances. You should only use this sheet in the early days of the fieldwork. After the first two weeks of fieldwork you should rely on your own experience.

Approximate conversion (grams ➤ pounds/ounces)

454 gms = 1lb
228 gms = 8oz
114 gms = 4oz
60 gms = 2oz
30 gms = 1oz

FOOD	WEIGHT(g)
Ready Brek (dry)	20
Rice Krispies	20
Shreddies	25
Weetabix (one)	20
White bread (one slice)	30
White bread without crust (one slice)	21 - 12
Fat spread on a slice of bread	4
Cheddar cheese	20
Spaghetti canned in tomato sauce	40 - 200
Baked beans canned in tomato sauce	50 - 150
Fish finger (one)	20 - 25
Sausage (large)	60
Sausage (small/chipolata)	35
Chicken meat	30
Ham	20
Carrots boiled	20 - 80
Peas boiled	10 - 50
Potatoes mashed/boiled	40 - 120
Chips	40 - 120
Yoghurt	100 - 150
Fromage Frais	40 - 100
Apple (one)	80 - 160
Digestive biscuit (large)	17
Digestive biscuit (small)	13
Semi-sweet biscuit, e.g. Marie	7
Cream sandwich biscuit, e.g custard cream	12
Short sweet biscuit, e.g. cookies, crunch	10
Pink wafer biscuit	7
Children's milk chocolate bar, e.g. Wildlife	20
Square of chocolate (one)	7
Finger of Fudge bar	30
Treat sized bars	15 - 20
Crisps, one packet	25 - 30
Cornsnacks, one packet	20 - 25
Drinks	
Carton of drink	50 - 200 / 200 - 250
Squash concentrate	30

N1340 Young Children's Dietary Survey (M)

Fats for SPREADING - alphabetical list

FAT	DESCRIPTION	% FAT
Anchor Half Fat Spread	low fat spread, **not** polyunsaturated	40%
Anchor Low Fat Spread	low fat spread, **not** polyunsaturated	40%
Asda Golden Soft	low fat spread, **not** polyunsaturated	40%
Asda Sunflower Low Fat Spread	low fat spread, polyunsaturated	40%
Banquet soft margarine	soft margarine, **not** polyunsaturated, **not** low fat	
Beef fat	SPECIFY: flag entry	
Blue Band sunflower margarine	soft margarine, polyunsaturated, **not** low fat	
Blue Leaf soft margarine	soft margarine, **not** polyunsaturated, **not** low fat	
Butter, concentrated	SPECIFY: flag entry	
Butter, salted or slightly salted	butter; salted, slightly salted	
Butter, unsalted	butter; unsalted	
Butter, spreadable	butter; salted, slightly salted	
Clover	reduced fat spread, **not** polyunsaturated	70 - 80%
Clover, lightly salted	reduced fat spread, **not** polyunsaturated	70 - 80%
Clover Extra Lite	low fat spread, **not** polyunsaturated	40%
Co-op Good Life Low Fat Sunflower Spread	low fat spread, polyunsaturated	40%
Co-op Red Seal Soft Spread	reduced fat spread, **not** polyunsaturated, **not** olive oil	60%
Dairy Crest Willow	reduced fat spread, **not** polyunsaturated	70 - 80%
Delight	low fat spread, **not** polyunsaturated	40%
Delight Extra Low	very low fat spread, **not** polyunsaturated	20 - 25%
Echo hard margarine	hard, block margarine	
Encore Sol	soft margarine, polyunsaturated, **not** low fat	40%
Encore Sol Light	low fat spread, polyunsaturated	
Encore Supersoft Luxury margarine	soft margarine, **not** polyunsaturated, **not** low fat	
Flora	soft margarine, polyunsaturated, **not** low fat	40%
Flora Extra Light	low fat spread, polyunsaturated	
Flora reduced salt	soft margarine, polyunsaturated, **not** low fat	
Gold (St Ivel)	low fat spread, **not** polyunsaturated	40%
Gold Lowest (St Ivel)	very low fat spread, **not** polyunsaturated	20 - 25%
Gold for cooking	reduced fat spread, **not** polyunsaturated, **not** olive oil	60%
Golden Crown (Golden Churn)	reduced fat spread, **not** polyunsaturated,	70 - 80%
Golden Crown Light	reduced fat spread, **not** polyunsaturated, **not** olive oil	60%
Golden Olive	low fat spread, with olive oil	40%
Golden Vale	reduced fat spread, **not** polyunsaturated	70 - 80%
Granose	soft margarine, polyunsaturated, **not** low fat	
Half Fat Anchor	low fat spread, **not** polyunsaturated	40%
Half fat butters - own brand	low fat spread, **not** polyunsaturated	40%
Hard margarine - own brand	hard, block margarine	
"I can't believe it's not butter"	reduced fat spread, polyunsaturated	70 - 80%

Interviewer check card: Fats for spreading (M) - *continued*

Kerrygold Light	low fat spread, **not** polyunsaturated	40%
Kraft Special Soft	reduced fat spread, **not** polyunsaturated	70 - 80%
Krona (gold/silver label)	reduced fat spread, **not** polyunsaturated	70 - 80%
Krona Spreadable	reduced fat spread, **not** polyunsaturated, **not** olive oil	60%
Latta	low fat spread, polyunsaturated	40%
Marks and Spencer		
English Churn	reduced fat spread, **not** polyunsaturated	70 - 80%
Sunglow	low fat spread, **not** polyunsaturated	40%
Sunflower Lite	low fat spread, polyunsaturated	40%
Meadowcup	reduced fat spread, **not** polyunsaturated	70 - 80%
Mello	reduced fat spread, **not** polyunsaturated, **not** olive oil	60%
Olive Gold (Sainsbury)	reduced fat spread, with olive oil	60%
Olivio	reduced fat spread, with olive oil	60%
Outline	very low fat spread, **not** polyunsaturated	20 - 25%
Safeway		
Golden Low Fat Spread	low fat spread, **not** polyunsaturated	40%
Low Fat Sunflower Spread	low fat spread, **not** polyunsaturated	40%
Meadow	reduced fat spread, **not** polyunsaturated	70 - 80%
Olive	reduced fat spread with olive oil	60%
Soft margarine	soft margarine, **not** polyunsaturated, **not** low fat	
Reduced Fat Soft Spread	reduced fat spread, **not** polyunsaturated, **not** olive oil	60%
Very Low Fat Spread (Simplesse)	very, very low fat spread	5%
Sainsbury		
County Spread	reduced fat spread, **not** polyunsaturated	70 - 80%
County Light	low fat spread, **not** polyunsaturated	40%
Half Fat Spread	low fat spread, **not** polyunsaturated	40%
Olive Gold	reduced fat spread, with olive oil	60%
Luxury Soft margarine	soft margarine, **not** polyunsaturated, **not** low fat	
Soft Spread	reduced fat spread, **not** polyunsaturated, **not** olive oil	60%
Sunflower Low Fat Spread	low fat spread, polyunsaturated	40%
Sunflower Very Low Fat Spread	very low fat spread, polyunsaturated	20 - 25%
Shape Sunflower Spread	low fat spread, polyunsaturated	40%
Slimmers Gold Sunflower Low Fat Spread	low fat spread, polyunsaturated	40%
Somerfield Supersoft Margarine	soft margarine, **not** polyunsaturated, **not** low fat	
Soya margarine - own brands	soft margarine, polyunsaturated, **not** low fat	
Spreadable butter	butter, salted, slightly salted	
St Ivel Gold	low fat spread, **not** polyunsaturated	40%
St Ivel Gold Lowest	very low fat spread, **not** polyunsaturated	20 - 25%
Stork	hard, block margarine	
Stork Light Blend	reduced fat spread, **not** polyunsaturated, **not** olive oil	60%
Stork SB	soft margarine, **not** polyunsaturated, **not** low fat	
Summer County reduced fat spread	reduced fat spread, **not** polyunsaturated	60%
Sunflower margarine - own brands	soft margarine, polyunsaturated, **not** low fat	
Sunflower low fat spread	low fat spread, polyunsaturated	40%
Sunflower very low fat spread	very low fat spread, polyunsaturated	20 - 25%

Tesco		
Golden Blend	reduced fat spread, **not** polyunsaturated	70 - 80%
Half Fat Sunflower spread	low fat spread, polyunsaturated	40%
Healthy Eating Very Low Fat Spread	very low fat spread, **not** polyunsaturated	20 - 25%
Healthy Eating Lowest Ever 5% Fat Spread	very, very low fat spread	5%
Soft Spread	reduced fat spread, **not** polyunsaturated	70 - 80%
Tomor hard margarine	hard, block margarine	
Vitalite	reduced fat spread, polyunsaturated, **not** olive oil	70 - 80%
Vitalite Light	reduced fat spread, polyunsaturated, **not** olive oil	60%
Vitaquelle	soft margarine, polyunsaturated, **not** low fat	
Weight Watchers	low fat spread, **not** polyunsaturated	40%
Willow (Dairy Crest)	reduced fat spread, **not** polyunsaturated	70 - 80%

HA/1/11/92

Interviewer check card: Fats and oils for cooking (N)

(N)

N1340 Toddlers' Dietary Survey

Fats and oils for COOKING - alphabetical list

FAT	DESCRIPTION
Anchor Half Fat	SPECIFY: flag entry
Anchor Low Fat Spread	SPECIFY: flag entry
Banquet soft margarine	margarine, **not** polyunsaturated
Beef fat	dripping
Blended vegetable oil	blended vegetable oil
Blue Band sunflower margarine	polyunsaturated margarine
Butter, concentrated	SPECIFY: flag entry
Butter, salted or slightly salted	butter
Butter, unsalted	butter
Butter, spreadable	butter
Clover	SPECIFY: flag entry
Clover, lightly salted	SPECIFY: flag entry
Clover Extra Lite	SPECIFY: flag entry
Cookeen compound cooking fat	SPECIFY: flag entry
Corn oil	polyunsaturated oil
Country Fare solid oil	dripping
Dairy Crest Willow	SPECIFY: flag entry
Delight	SPECIFY: flag entry
Delight Extra Low	SPECIFY: flag entry
Echo hard margarine	margarine, **not** polyunsaturated
Encore Sol	polyunsaturated margarine
Encore Sol Light	SPECIFY: flag entry
Encore Supersoft margarine	margarine, **not** polyunsaturated
Flora	polyunsaturated margarine
Flora Baking	polyunsaturated margarine
Flora Extra Light	SPECIFY: flag entry
Flora oil	polyunsaturated oil
Flora reduced salt	polyunsaturated margarine
Flora white	SPECIFY: flag entry
Gold (St Ivel)	SPECIFY: flag entry
Gold for cooking	SPECIFY: flag entry
Gold Lowest (St Ivel)	SPECIFY: flag entry
Golden Crown (Golden Churn)	SPECIFY: flag entry
Golden Crown Light	SPECIFY: flag entry
Golden Olive	SPECIFY: flag entry
Golden Vale	SPECIFY: flag entry
Granose	polyunsaturated margarine
Groundnut oil	polyunsaturated oil
Half Fat Anchor	SPECIFY: flag entry
"I can't believe it's not butter"	SPECIFY: flag entry
Kerrygold Light	SPECIFY: flag entry
Krisp and Dry oil (Spry)	blended vegetable oil
Krona (gold/silver label)	SPECIFY: flag entry
Krona Spreadable	SPECIFY: flag entry
Latta	SPECIFY: flag entry
Maize oil	polyunsaturated oil
Mazola	polyunsaturated oil
Meadowcup	SPECIFY: flag entry
Mello	SPECIFY: flag entry
Olive oil	SPECIFY: flag entry
Olivio	SPECIFY: flag entry
Outline	SPECIFY: flag entry
Own brands	
blended oil	blended vegetable oil
block margarine	margarine, **not** polyunsaturated
hard margarine	margarine, **not** polyunsaturated
soft margarine, **not** polyunsaturated	margarine, **not** polyunsaturated
soft margarine, polyunsaturated	polyunsaturated margarine
low fat spreads	SPECIFY: flag entry
reduced fat spreads	SPECIFY: flag entry
reduced fat spreads with olive oil	SPECIFY: flag entry
very low fat spreads	SPECIFY: flag entry
Palm oil	SPECIFY: flag entry
Peanut oil	polyunsaturated oil
Pork fat	lard
Pura Big Fry solid cooking oil	dripping
Pura solid vegetable oil	blended vegetable oil
Rapeseed oil	blended vegetable oil
Safflower oil	polyunsaturated oil
Sesame oil	polyunsaturated oil
Shape Sunflower Spread	SPECIFY: flag entry
Soya margarine - own brands	polyunsaturated margarine
Soya oil	polyunsaturated oil
St Ivel Gold	SPECIFY: flag entry
St Ivel Gold for cooking	SPECIFY: flag entry
St Ivel Gold Lowest	margarine, **not** polyunsaturated
Stork	SPECIFY: flag entry
Stork Light Blend	margarine, **not** polyunsaturated
Stork SB	polyunsaturated margarine
Summer County reduced fat spread	margarine, **not** polyunsaturated
Sunflower margarine - own brands	polyunsaturated margarine
Sunflower oil	polyunsaturated oil
Spry compound cooking fat	SPECIFY: flag entry
Tesco Healty Eating Lowest Ever 5% fat Spread	SPECIFY: flag entry
Tomor hard margarine	margarine, **not** polyunsaturated
Trex compound cooking fat	SPECIFY: flag entry
Vegetable oil - unspecified	blended vegetable oil
Very low fat spread - own brand	SPECIFY: flag entry
Vitalite	SPECIFY: flag entry
Vitalite Light	SPECIFY: flag entry
Vitaquelle	polyunsaturated margarine
Walnut Oil	polyunsaturated oil
Weight Watchers	SPECIFY: flag entry
White Cap	lard
Willow (Dairy Crest)	SPECIFY: flag entry

Bowel movements card (Q)

N1340 YOUNG CHILDREN'S DIETARY SURVEY

BOWEL MOVEMENTS

Serial number label

Please keep a record of the number of bowel movements your child has each day that you keep the food record diary.

On the first day that you keep a record of what your child eats write in the day in the 1st column, for example, Thursday.

When your child has a bowel movement that day circle the number 1 in the 2nd column. If your child is in nappies, and when you get him or her up in the morning he or she has a dirty nappy, count that as the first bowel movement. If your child has a second bowel movement that day circle number 2, and so on.

Keep a record for each of the four days, ending at midnight on the fourth day. If your child does not have a bowel movement on any day please circle the number 9 in the 3rd column.

Office use only

1

Day	Number of bowel movements			No bowel movements
.... day	1	2	3	4	9
	5	6	7	8	
.... day	1	2	3	4	9
	5	6	7	8	
.... day	1	2	3	4	9
	5	6	7	8	
.... day	1	2	3	4	9
	5	6	7	8	

The interviewer will collect this sheet when she collects the completed food diary.

Thank you for your help.

HA7/5 7/92

(Q)

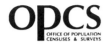

The Young Children's Dietary Survey

This survey is being carried out by the Social Survey Division of the Office of Population Censuses and Surveys, for the Ministry of Agriculture, Fisheries and Food and the Departments of Health (in England, Wales and Scotland). This leaflet tells you more about measurements we are making and the blood sample.

1. Height, weight and other measurements

Obviously what children eat affects their weight, so we are interested in the weight of the children in the survey. By itself though, weight is of limited use because taller children will probably weigh more anyway. Hence we need to know about weight in relation to size - not just height, but bone size and the amount of muscle and fat. A measurement of head circumference will give us some information on bone size and growth, and the arm circumference is a useful measure of body size.

* * * * * * *

2. Blood sample

We ask if you would agree to your child providing us with a sample of blood. This is a very important aspect of the survey as the analysis of all the blood samples will tell us a great deal about the health of the children in the survey and further information on their diet. You are, of course, free to choose not to consent to the blood sample being taken.

A small amount of blood (no more than 4ml) is taken from your child's arm using new, sterile equipment by a qualified person who is skilled in taking blood from small children. If you prefer your child to have a finger prick then we are happy to do so. The blood is sent to three medical laboratories, in Cambridge, at Hull University and at Great Ormond Street Children's Hospital in London, for a number of analyses, including measurements of ferritin, haemoglobin and vitamins. The sample is **not** used for viral analyses such as an AIDS test.

Haemoglobin is the red pigment in the blood which carries oxygen. A low level of haemoglobin in the blood is called anaemia. One reason for a low level of haemoglobin may be a shortage of iron. Ferritin is a measure of the body's iron stores.

* * * * * * *

With your consent we let your child's GP know that you have agreed to your child taking part in the survey and we will let you know the results of the haemoglobin analysis.

* * * * * * *

3. Are the measurements compulsory?

In all our surveys we rely on voluntary co-operation, which is essential if our work is to be successful. The measurements and the blood sample are a particularly important part of this survey, as from these results we can find out much more about the health of small children than would be possible with just the information about their diet.

* * * * * * *

We hope this leaflet answers some of the questions you might have and that it shows the importance of the survey.

Your co-operation is very much appreciated.

Social Survey Division
Office of Population Censuses and
 Surveys
St Catherine's House
10 Kingsway
London WC2B 6JP

telephone 071 - 242 0262 extension 2079

N1340 Young children's dietary survey.   HA3/1 3/93

Blood questionnaire (Z)

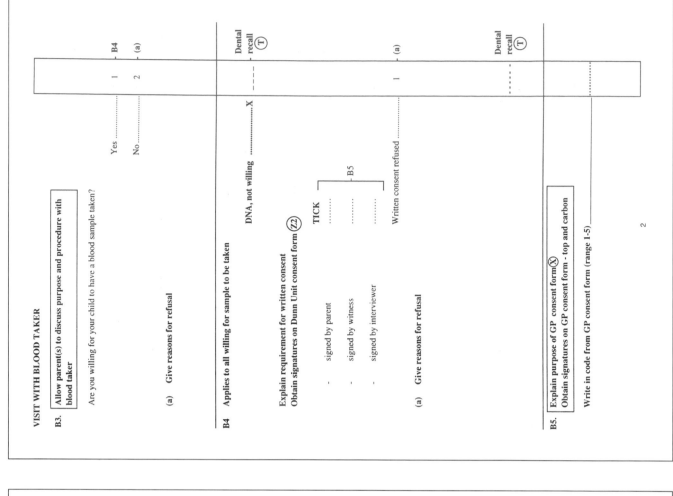

(Z)

N1340/W4: Young Children's Dietary Survey
BLOOD QUESTIONNAIRE

Serial number label

Explain purpose and outline procedure for taking blood sample

Hand 'Information Sheet for Parents' to parent(s) - (Z1)

Explain that parent(s) will have opportunity to discuss purpose with person taking blood

B1. May I make an appointment to call back with the person who would be taking the blood sample?

Yes, willing for sample to be taken	1	} B2
Yes, wishes to discuss further/think about it	2	
Yes, other conditional answer	3	(a)
No, outright refusal	4	
Blood not introduced, no blood taker available	5	Dental recall (T)

(a) Give reasons for refusal and specify conditional answers

B2. Applies to all "willing" or "conditional" - B1 coded 1, 2 or 3

DNA, outright refusal ..... X — Dental recall (T)

Leave 'Information Sheet' Z1 with parent(s) and make appointment to call with blood taker

Day: _____ day _____ th

Time: _____ am/pm

1

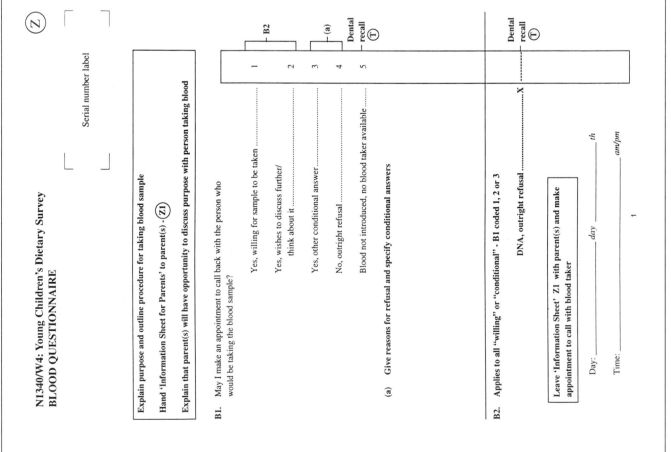

VISIT WITH BLOOD TAKER

B3. **Allow parent(s) to discuss purpose and procedure with blood taker**

Are you willing for your child to have a blood sample taken?

Yes	1	B4
No	2	(a)
DNA, not willing	X	Dental recall (T)

(a) Give reasons for refusal

B4 **Applies to all willing for sample to be taken**

Explain requirement for written consent
Obtain signatures on Dunn Unit consent form (Z2)

TICK
- signed by parent ....
- signed by witness .... } B5
- signed by interviewer ....

Written consent refused .... 1 — (a)
Dental recall (T)

(a) Give reasons for refusal

B5. **Explain purpose of GP consent form (X)**
Obtain signatures on GP consent form - top and carbon

Write in code from GP consent form (range 1-5)

2

Blood questionnaire (Z) - *continued*

B6. Outcome: ring code

Attempted, obtained blood 1
Attempted, did not obtain blood 2
Not attempted 3

B7 (a)

(a) **Specify reasons why blood sample not attempted**

B7. **Applies if blood sample obtained or attempted**

DNA, not attempted .... 1 | **Dental recall T**

Date sample obtained/last attempted:

Day	Month	Year
		9 | 3

B8

B8. Time sample obtained/last attempted: **(Use 24 hr clock)**

Hours	Mins

B9

B9. Number of attempts made to obtain sample:

1
2

B10. Site of attempt(s) to obtain sample:

Specified answers:

1st attempt site ....

2nd attempt site ....

	1st attempt	2nd attempt
Venepuncture - arm	1	1
Venepuncture - hand	2	2
Finger prick	3	3
Other (specify)	4	4

B11. Amount of blood obtained:

None 9
Less than 1 ml 8
Other (specify mls) ....

(Consult blood taker)

Blood questionnaire (Z) - *continued*

B12. **Were there any difficulties in attempting to obtain/obtaining the sample?**

Yes, difficulties..........	1
No, no difficulties..........	2

(a)
Check list

(a) Specify difficulties

GO TO CHECKLIST

Interviewer check list:

				TICK
*	Blood consent form 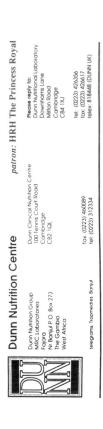 (Z2)	:	to blood taker	------
*	GP consent form (X)	:	top copy to blood taker	------
			carbon to HQ	
*	GOSH analysis card	:	complete with serial no.	------
			lable - to blood taker	
*	Set of serial no. labels	:	to blood taker	------

NOW GO TO DENTAL RECALL (T)

5

Information for parents (Z1)

Dunn Nutrition Centre   *patron*: **HRH The Princess Royal**

Dunn Nutrition Group
MRC Laboratories
Fajara
Nr Banjul P.O. Box 273
The Gambia
West Africa

telegrams Toomedies Banjul

fax (0223) 460089
tel (0223) 312334

Please reply to:
Dunn Clinical Nutrition Centre
100 Tennis Court Road
Cambridge
CB2 1QL

Dunn Nutritional Laboratory
Downhams Lane
Milton Road
Cambridge
CB4 1XJ

tel: (0223) 426356
fax: (0223) 426617
telex: 818448 (DUNN UK)

INFORMATION FOR PARENTS

The Departments of Health and the Ministry of Agriculture, Fisheries and Food have decided that there is a need to measure the amount and type of food young children are eating in Great Britain. The Social Survey Division of the Office of Population Censuses and Surveys is undertaking these measurements and will be inviting you to record the amount of food your child eats, as well as measuring your child's height and weight.

As part of the survey we would also like to take a small sample of blood from your child's arm.

The Medical Research Council's Dunn Nutrition Unit have been asked by the Departments of Health and the Ministry of Agriculture, Fisheries and Food to take responsibility for the arrangements associated with obtaining the blood samples. We are working closely with the Social Survey Division and we together with Great Ormond Street Hospital will be analysing the blood samples.

The blood will be taken by a suitably trained person who is qualified and skilled in taking blood from small children. He or she will be accompanied by the Social Survey interviewer and they will take time to put your child at ease. We are asking for a sample to be taken from the child's arm because this is less painful than a finger prick. If you would prefer your child to have a finger prick then we are happy to do so.

We would be grateful if you would agree to your child providing us with a sample of blood. This is a very important aspect of the survey as the analysis of all the blood samples will tell us a lot about the health of the children in the survey in relation to what they eat and their body measurements. You are, of course, free to choose not to consent to a blood sample being taken.

The blood sample will be sent to the medical laboratories for a number of analyses, including levels of haemoglobin, ferritin and vitamins; it will <u>not</u> be used to look for infections such as AIDS.

Haemoglobin is the red pigment in the blood which carries oxygen. A low level of haemoglobin in the blood is called anaemia. One reason for a low level of haemoglobin may be shortage of iron. Ferritin is a measure of the body's iron stores.

If any of these measurements are abnormal we will, if you agree, inform your general practitioner, who will be able to advise you about treatment.

Medical Research Council and the University of Cambridge

Dental recall form (T)

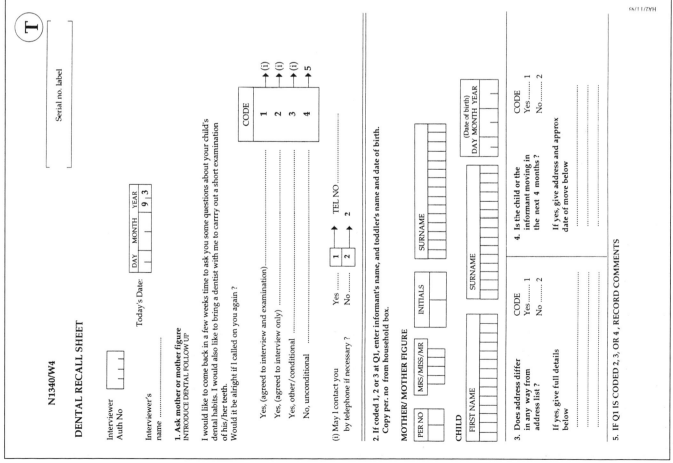

T

Serial no. label

N1340/W4

DENTAL RECALL SHEET

Interviewer
Auth No [ ]

Today's Date: | DAY | MONTH | YEAR |
| --- | --- | 9,3 |

Interviewer's
name ....

1. Ask mother or mother figure
INTRODUCE DENTAL FOLLOW UP

I would like to come back in a few weeks time to ask you some questions about your child's
dental habits. I would also like to bring a dentist with me to carrry out a short examination
of his/her teeth.
Would it be alright if l called on you again ?

	CODE	
Yes, (agreed to interview and examination)	1	(i)
Yes, (agreed to interview only)	2	(i)
Yes, other/conditional	3	(i)
No, unconditional	4	5

(i) May l contact you   Yes .... 1 → TEL NO ....
by telephone if necessary ?   No .... 2 → 2

2. If coded 1, 2 or 3 at Q1, enter informant's name, and toddler's name and date of birth.
Copy per. no from household box.

MOTHER/ MOTHER FIGURE

PER NO	MRS/MISS/MR	INITIALS	SURNAME

CHILD

FIRST NAME	SURNAME	(Date of birth) DAY MONTH YEAR

3. Does address differ   CODE
in any way from   Yes 1
address list ?   No 2

If yes, give full details
below

....

....

4. Is the child or the   CODE
informant moving in   Yes 1
the next 4 months ?   No 2

If yes, give address and approx
date of move below

....

....

5. IF Q1 IS CODED 2, 3, OR 4 , RECORD COMMENTS

HAZ/11/93

315

Appendix B

Survey letters to: Chief Constables of Police, Directors of Social Services, and Directors of Public Health

Letter to Chief Constables of Police

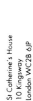

OPCS OFFICE OF POPULATION CENSUSES & SURVEYS

Social Survey Division

St Catherine's House
10 Kingsway
London WC2B 6JP

Direct Dial   0171 396
Switchboard 0171 - 396 2200
         or 0171 - 242 0262
GTN   3042

Fax   0171 405 3020
              0171 396 2383

our ref: N1340

Dear Chief Constable

National Diet and Nutrition Survey: Children aged 1½ to 4½ years

The Social Survey Division of the Office of Population Censuses and Surveys, which is the government's survey organisation, has been commissioned by the Ministry of Agriculture, Fisheries and Food and the Departments of Health (in England, Wales and Scotland) to carry out a survey to determine the diet and nutritional status of children aged 1½ to 4½ years living in private households in Great Britain.

Because of the age of the children and some of the procedures involved in this study I am writing to all Chief Constables and all Directors of Social Services in the areas where the survey is being carried out. The survey is taking place in 100 areas in Great Britain over a 12-month period starting in July 1992. Within the area for which you have responsibility, one of our interviewers will be working:

in ...... during the period from 5 October 1992 to 3 January 1993;

and in .... during the period from 4 January 1993 to 3 April 1993;

The survey aims to obtain information from the parents of about 1500 children, about 15 in each area. The sample of addresses for the survey has been selected at random from the Post Office's Postcode Address File. Before the start of fieldwork each sampled address will be sent a letter explaining briefly about the survey and that an interviewer from this Office will be calling in the following few weeks. When the interviewer calls at the home he or she will explain to the child's parents what the survey involves and will seek their voluntary co-operation.

317

If co-operation is obtained, the survey starts with a short personal interview to collect information about the child and their household and about their general eating habits and health. Mothers (or guardians) are then asked to keep a detailed diary for four days weighing and describing every item of food and drink that the child consumes over the period. A payment of £10 is made as a token of our appreciation. The interviewer will then seek the mother's co-operation in measuring the child's height and supine length, weight, head circumference and mid upper arm circumference. Parents will then be invited to consent to allowing a sample of blood to be taken from their child for analysis. If written witnessed consent is obtained the interviewer will recall at the address with a person qualified to take the blood sample. At the end of the survey parents will be invited to co-operate with a further study to find out about their child's dental habits and condition. This will involve a further short interview and a brief dental examination, carried out by a qualified community dentist in the child's home.

All the interviewers working on the study are employed by Social Survey Division; all have been trained and are experienced in carrying out surveys on a wide range of topics covering different groups in the population and additionally they will all receive five day's special training for this survey prior to the start of fieldwork. All our interviewers carry identification issued by this Office, and before starting work they will call at the main Police Station(s) covering the sample area to make themselves known to the local police. The usual procedure is for their name to be entered in the station 'Day Book'. As the names and addresses of people who take part in any of our surveys are confidential to this Division, we are unable to divulge these to the local police or other authorities.

The blood samples are being taken by persons qualified in taking blood, usually a phlebotomist from the local hospital. These personnel have been specially recruited for the study by the Medical Research Council's Dunn Nutrition Unit, which is based in Cambridge, and which has been contracted to carry out all the procedures associated with the blood sampling aspects of the survey. These personnel will also receive a specialised briefing before the start of fieldwork.

The survey protocol, and in particular the procedures associated with taking the blood sample have been approved by your Local Area National Health Service Ethical Committee. The British Medical Association and the British Paediatric Association have been informed of the survey.

2

I should stress that, as with all surveys undertaken by this Division, co-operation is voluntary, although we rely on people's willingness to take part in order to achieve results which will be representative of the whole population being studied. In the case of this study, written consent from the child's parent or guardian and verbal consent from the child are required for the blood sample; it will be made clear to parents that they are free to withdraw at any stage.

All the procedures associated with this survey of major importance have been thoroughly tested in feasibility and pilot studies. All the equipment and instruments being used are of the highest standard to meet the rigorous requirements for quality data demanded by the Ministry of Agriculture, Fisheries and Food and the Departments of Health. At the feasibility and pilot study stages, which were designed primarily to assess the acceptability of the procedures, our interviewers achieved high levels of co-operation from parents and children.

If you would like any further information about the survey, please contact me at the above address.

Yours faithfully

Jan Gregory
Principal Social Survey Officer - Project Manager

3

OPCS
OFFICE OF POPULATION
CENSUSES & SURVEYS

Social Survey Division

St Catherine's House
10 Kingsway
London WC2B 6JP

Direct Dial   0171 · 396
Switchboard   0171 · 396 2200
         or   0171 · 242 0262
GTN   3042

Fax   0171 · 405 3020
               0171 · 396 2383

our ref: N1340

Dear Director

National Diet and Nutrition Survey: Children aged 1½ to 4½ years

The Social Survey Division of the Office of Population Censuses and Surveys, which is the government's survey organisation, has been commissioned by the Ministry of Agriculture, Fisheries and Food and the Departments of Health (in England, Wales and Scotland) to carry out a survey to determine the diet and nutritional status of children aged 1½ to 4½ years living in private households in Great Britain.

Because of the age of the children and some of the procedures involved in this study I am writing to all Directors of Social Services and all Chief Constables in the areas where the survey is being carried out. The survey is taking place in 100 areas in Great Britain over a 12-month period starting in July 1992. Within the area for which you have responsibility, one of our interviewers will be working in .... during the period from 5 October 1992 to 3 January 1993.

The survey aims to obtain information from the parents of about 1500 children, about 15 in each area. The sample of addresses for the survey has been selected at random from the Post Office's Postcode Address File. Before the start of fieldwork each sampled address will be sent a letter explaining briefly about the survey and that an interviewer from this Office will be calling in the following few weeks. When the interviewer calls at the home he or she will explain to the child's parents what the survey involves and will seek their voluntary co-operation.

If co-operation is obtained, the survey starts with a short personal interview to collect information about the child and their household and about their general eating habits and health. Mothers (or guardians) are then asked to keep a detailed diary for four days weighing and describing every item of food and drink that the child consumes over the period. A payment of £10

1

is made as a token of our appreciation. The interviewer will then seek the mother's co-operation in measuring the child's height and supine length, weight, head circumference and mid upper arm circumference. Parents will then be invited to consent to allowing a sample of blood to be taken from their child for analysis. If written witnessed consent is obtained the interviewer will recall at the address with a person qualified to take the blood sample. At the end of the survey parents will be invited to co-operate with a further study to find out about their child's dental habits and condition. This will involve a further short interview and a brief dental examination, carried out by a qualified community dentist in the child's home.

All the interviewers working on the study are employed by Social Survey Division; all have been trained and are experienced in carrying out surveys on a wide range of topics covering different groups in the population and additionally they will all receive five day's special training for this survey prior to the start of fieldwork. All our interviewers carry identification issued by this Office, and before starting work they will call at the main Police Station(s) covering the sample area to make themselves known to the local police. The usual procedure is for their name to be entered in the station 'Day Book'. As the names and addresses of people who take part in any of our surveys are confidential to this Division, we are unable to divulge these to Social Services Departments, the local police or other authorities.

The blood samples are being taken by persons qualified in taking blood, usually a phlebotomist from the local hospital. These personnel have been specially recruited for the study by the Medical Research Council's Dunn Nutrition Unit, which is based in Cambridge, and which has been contracted to carry out all the procedures associated with the blood sampling aspects of the survey. These personnel will also receive a specialised briefing before the start of fieldwork.

The survey protocol, and in particular the procedures associated with taking the blood sample have been approved by your Local Area National Health Service Ethical Committee. The British Medical Association and the British Paediatric Association have been informed of the survey.

I should stress that, as with all surveys undertaken by this Division, co-operation is voluntary, although we rely on people's willingness to take part in order to achieve results which will be representative of the whole population being studied. In the case of this study, written consent from the child's parent or guardian and verbal consent from the child are required for the blood sample; it will be made clear to parents that they are free to withdraw at any stage.

All the procedures associated with this survey of major importance have been thoroughly tested in feasibility and pilot studies. All the equipment and instruments being used are of the

2

Dunn Nutrition Centre

Patron: **HRH The Princess Royal**

Dunn Nutrition Group
MRC Laboratories
Fajara
Mr Banjul P.O Box 273
The Gambia
West Africa

Telegrams Tropmedres Banjul

Dunn Clinical Nutrition Centre
Hills Road
Cambridge
CB2 2DH

tel: (0223) 415695
fax: (0223) 413763

Please reply to:
Dunn Nutritional Laboratory
Downhams Lane
Milton Road
Cambridge
CB4 1XJ

tel: (0223) 426356
fax: (0223) 426617

Dear

Re: National Diet and Nutrition Survey of Children aged 1.5 to 4.5 Years

The above study is being carried out in 100 randomly selected areas throughout the UK. The _____ area within your Health District has been chosen, and families are being approached to assist with the survey. A separate approach is being made to the Ethical Committee, to obtain approval.

I am enclosing a Protocol which sets out fully the details of the study, for your information. If you have any queries or require any further information relating to the study, please do not hesitate to let me know.

Yours sincerely,

Peter S.W. Davies   B.Sc, M.Phil, Ph.D
MRC Staff Scientist
Infant & Child Nutrition Group

Medical Research Council and the University of Cambridge

---

highest standard to meet the rigorous requirements for quality data demanded by the Ministry of Agriculture, Fisheries and Food and the Department's of Health. At the feasibility and pilot study stages, which were designed primarily to assess the acceptability of the procedures, our interviewers achieved high levels of co-operation from parents and children.

If you would like any further information about the survey, please contact me at the above address.

Yours faithfully

Jan Gregory
Principal Social Survey Officer - Project Manager

3

Appendix C

Sample design and response

1 Requirements of the sample

A representative sample of children aged 1½ to 4½ years living in private households in Great Britain was required.

In determining the sample size, account was taken of the need to achieve adequate numbers for analysis by sex within three age groups, 1½ to 2½, 2½ to 3½ and 3½ to 4½ years, and a requirement to achieve dietary records for approximately equal numbers of these six sex/age cohorts. No oversampling would be required as the sex and age groups are approximately equally distributed in the population. Account also needed to be taken of the resources required for the survey, particularly the high unit cost of using a weighed intake dietary methodology, and the relatively large number of calls that would need to be made to each participating household. Bearing these factors in mind, it was decided that about 1500 dietary records should be obtained.

It was recognised that the survey would be very onerous for the parents and carers of young children, involving their commitment over a period of time. It was therefore decided that only one eligible child per household should be included in the survey. Because there is likely to be considerable similarity between the diets of children of similar ages in the same household, by selecting only one child in a household a greater variety of diets would be covered in a sample of 1500. It was also thought likely that collecting dietary information from more than one child in the same household would produce less accurate data. For example, food weights might be duplicated across eligible children in the household, rather than each child's food being weighed individually.

2 Selection of eligible households

A number of sampling frames were evaluated, but none were found which contained only households with children aged 1½ to 4½ years. One of the sampling frames evaluated was the Department of Social Security's (DSS) Child Benefit Register. However this was found to have a number of deficiencies which made it unsuitable for use at the time as a sampling frame for this survey. In particular the selection of a suitable primary sampling unit was made difficult by the way in which addresses were held on the Register and the fact that not all the addresses had a postcode. DSS could not accurately estimate the number of deficient addresses and hence the potential sample bias could not be assessed. Thus the Postcode Address File (PAF) was used, with a sample of addresses being selected and households containing an eligible child being identified from response to a postal questionnaire.

To achieve 1500 four-day weighed intake records the sample size took account of:

(a) the proportion of households in Great Britain containing a child aged 1½ to 4½ years — estimated to be 8.9% from combined data from the General Household Surveys for 1988 and 1989[1,2];

(b) an assumed overall response rate of 70%; and

(c) the proportion of addresses on the PAF which are ineligible because they are not private households or do not exist because they have either been demolished, not yet built or are empty — about 12%.

It was estimated that a set sample of 28000 addresses would be required to achieve 1500 dietary records.

In selecting addresses a stratified multi-stage, random probability design was used. The stages in the selection of the sample were as follows:

(i) in order that addresses would be clustered giving areas of an economic size for interviewers to work, postal sectors, which are similar in size to wards, were selected as primary sampling units. All postal sectors in England, Wales and mainland Scotland[3] were stratified by region, then according to the proportion of heads of household in socio-economic groups (SEGs) 1 to 5 and 13, and by the proportion of females in private households who were aged 16 and over and economically active[4]. The regional stratification differentiated between metropolitan and non-metropolitan areas within standard regions, and the Scottish Highlands were defined as a separate stratum in order to ensure at least one selection from this area. One hundred postal sectors were systematically selected, with the chance of selection of each sector being proportional to its size, as given by the number of delivery points in the sector.

(ii) Because dietary habits may be seasonally related, fieldwork was required to cover a 12 month period. For organisational reasons it was decided to conduct the survey in four fieldwork waves of approximately 10 to 12 weeks each. The 100 postal sectors were systematically allocated to one of four waves of fieldwork, ensuring as far as possible a similar distribution of all regions in each wave.

As the proportion of children aged 1½ to 4½ years is known to vary by area, possibly affecting the number of achieved interviews per wave, an attempt was made to allocate areas to waves in a way which would minimise this variability. This was done by stratifying selected areas by the proportion of pensioners and the proportion of females in private households who were aged 16 and over and economically active[5].

Thus in each wave fieldwork took place in 25 postal sectors throughout Great Britain.

(iii) For each of the 25 postal sectors in each wave, 280 addresses were systematically selected with a random start from the small users' file of the PAF.

(iv) Approximately three months before the beginning of each wave of fieldwork, each selected address was sent a sift form which asked for details of the sex and date of birth of every person living in the household. In order to avoid any response bias the accompanying letter did not mention an interest in any specific age group or the subject matter of the survey. A reminder letter was sent two weeks and four weeks after the date of the original mailing to those who had not responded. Residual non-responding addresses were subsequently called on by an interviewer who attempted to collect the same information. Sift procedures were carried out as close as possible to the start of each wave of fieldwork to minimise the number of households which might move. The sift form and letter are reproduced in Appendix A.

Response to the postal and interviewer sift stages is shown at the end of this Appendix.

3 Multi-household addresses

Most addresses listed on the PAF contain only one private household; a few, such as institutions, contain no private households. In England and Wales about 3.5% are known to contain more than one household but there is no indication on the PAF of how many households are contained at any address. For Scotland the PAF contains a multi-household indicator which is used in the selection of households.

In order to identify concealed multi-household addresses in England and Wales a question was asked on the sift form[6]. All multi-household addresses were visited by interviewers who listed all households and selected one using a random number grid. Interviewers had four different multi-household selection grid sheets which were used consecutively to vary the chance of selection of a household relative to the number of households found at the address and these are reproduced in Appendix A.

This procedure gave each household an equal chance of selection at a multi-household address. However the probability of selecting one household at a multi-household address was dependent on the number of households identified at the address, whereas addresses containing only one household had a unitary probability of selection. Because the sift procedures meant that only one household was selected at a multi-household address there is a bias in the selection of households, but this is small as only a small proportion of addresses contain concealed multi-households.

As in the postal sift, details of the sex and date of birth of all members of the selected household were then recorded.

4 Ineligible addresses

Children living in non-private households, such as residential hospitals and care units, were not eligible for the survey. The small users' file of the PAF excludes any delivery point which receives more than 25 items of mail a day and hence excludes most large institutions and non-residential addresses; some small institutions may however be included on the small users' file. These were identified at the sift stage, and were excluded as ineligible.

5 Selection of eligible children

A child's eligibility (being aged between 1½ and 4½ years) was determined by taking the mid-point of the fieldwork wave as the reference point for defining eligible dates of birth.[7] Households containing an eligible child were identified from completed sift forms. If more than one eligible child was present in the household, all eligible children were listed and one selected at random.

Each wave of fieldwork covered a ten to twelve week period, and as the mid-point of the fieldwork period was taken as the reference date for defining eligibility, a few children in this survey were slightly older than 4½ years or slightly younger than 1½ years at the time of interview. However for analysis purposes children under 1½ years are included in the 1½ to 2½ years cohort, and children over 4½ years are included in the 3½ to 4½ years cohort.

Where a child was included in the interview sample but subsequently found to be ineligible, mainly because the date of birth had been recorded wrongly, no interview was carried out.

In a very small number of cases at the main interview stage the selected child was found to have a medical condition which affected his or her diet, or growth and development. Interviews were conducted as for other children, but details of the condition (anonymised) were referred to DH and advice taken as to whether it was appropriate to include such children in the analysis.

6 Response to the postal and interviewer sift stages

Figure 1 represents the various stages in the identification of households containing an eligible child. At the postal sift stage households containing an eligible child were identified from returns from single-household addresses; multi-household addresses, along with non-responding addresses were issued to interviewers. Response rates for the sift stages are based on the number of private households identified, known as the eligible sample.

Response to the postal sift stage was 74%; the same response rate was achieved for the interviewer follow up. Overall response was increased by about a quarter, from 74% to 93%, as a result of the interviewer follow up. Only 4% of residents refused to co-operate with the postal sift and interviewer follow up.
(Table 1)

Table 1 also shows the interviewer follow up boosted the number of households identified as containing an eligible child by 370; overall 8.3% of eligible addresses were found to contain a household with an eligible child. This is only slightly lower than the GHS and comparisons between this survey and the GHS (see *Chapter 3*) provide no evidence of any bias in the preschool children's survey sample.

Response rates to the sift stages were very similar by wave, although in Wave 1 (July to September 1992) there was a higher number of ineligible addresses than in the other waves, as Table 2 shows. This was due to a large number of derelict addresses being selected in one sector in that wave.

A total of 2101 households containing eligible children were identified by the sift stages. This number is referred to as the interview sample and is the base for response calculations given in Chapter 3.

Not all informants completed all elements of the survey and Chapter 3 discusses response to these different elements. The maximum response is defined as those agreeing to the initial questionnaire interview and Table 3 shows that this was achieved for 88% of the interview sample; only 7% of households refused to take part in any aspect of the survey.

The maximum response rate is almost constant across fieldwork waves, the varying numbers of co-operating cases reflecting variation in the number of eligible children identified in the different waves at the sift stages.

References and notes

1 Foster K, Wilmot A, Dobbs J. *1988 General Household Survey*. HMSO (London, 1990)
2 Breeze E, Trevor G, Wilmot A. *1989 General Household Survey*. HMSO (London, 1991)
3 Areas of Scotland excluded from the sample were: the Orkneys, Shetlands, Western Isles and other Scottish Islands. Also excluded from the sampling frame were the Channel Islands, Isle of Man and the Scilly Isles.
4 As 1991 Census data were not available when stratification took place, 1981 Census variables were used to stratify postal sectors.
5 1981 Census variables were used in the allocation of postal sectors to waves of fieldwork.
6 For the definition of household see Appendix S.
7 Eligible dates of birth were:

wave	fieldwork dates	mid-point	eligible dates of birth
1	28.06.92 to 03.10.92	15.08.92	15.02.88 to 14.02.91
2	05.10.92 to 03.01.93	18.11.92	18.05.88 to 17.05.91
3	04.01.93 to 03.04.93	17.02.93	17.08.88 to 16.08.91
4	05.04.93 to 04.07.93	19.05.93	19.11.88 to 18.11.91

Figure 1 Postal and interviewer follow up sift stages

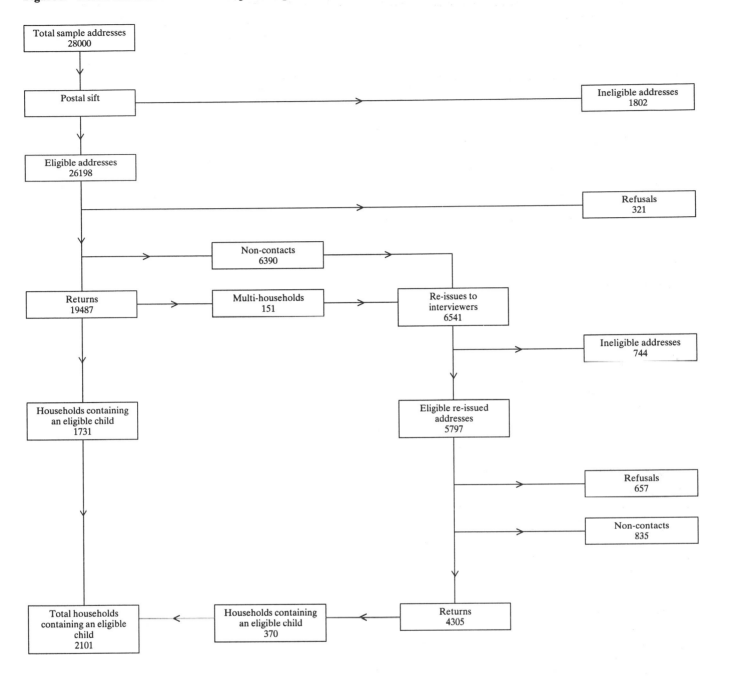

Table 1   Response to the postal sift and interviewer follow up of non-responders and multi-households

(i) Postal sift

	No.	%
Total sample addresses	**28000**	*100*
Ineligibles	1802	
Eligible addresses	**26198**	*100*
Refusals	321	*1*
Non-contacts (re-issued to interviewers)	6390	*24*
Returns: multi-household addresses (re-issued to interviewers)	151	*1*
Returns: single household addresses	19336	*74*
Single household addresses identified from returns to the postal sift containing an eligible child	**1731**	**6.6**

(ii) Interviewer follow up

	No.	%
Addresses issued to interviewers	**6541**	*100*
Ineligibles	744	
Eligible addresses	**5797**	*100*
Refusals	657	*11*
Non-contacts	835	*14*
Returns	4305	*74*

(iii) Overall response

	No.	%
Total sample addresses	**28000**	*100*
Ineligibles	2546	
Total eligible addresses	**25454**	*100*
Refusals	978	*4*
Non-contacts	835	*3*
Returns	23641	*93*
Total households identified from returns as containing an eligible child	**2101**	**8.3**

Table 2   Response rates for sift stages (combined) by fieldwork wave*

	Wave of fieldwork									
	Wave 1		Wave 2		Wave 3		Wave 4		Total	
	No.	%	No.	%	No.	%	No.	%	No.	%
Total sample addresses	**7000**	*100*	**7000**	*100*	**7000**	*100*	**7000**	*100*	**28000**	*100*
Ineligible addresses	834	*12*	575	*8*	505	*7*	632	*9*	2546	*9*
Eligible addresses sample	**6166**	*100*	**6425**	*100*	**6495**	*100*	**6368**	*100*	**25454**	*100*
Refusals	270	*4*	246	*4*	257	*4*	205	*3*	978	*4*
Non-contacts	206	*3*	223	*3*	194	*3*	212	*3*	835	*3*
Returns: of which	5690	*93*	5956	*93*	6044	*93*	5951	*94*	23641	*93*
addresses containing at least one eligible child	474	*7.7%*	544	*8.5%*	559	*8.6%*	524	*8.2%*	2101	*8.3%*

*Wave 1: July to September 1992.
 Wave 2: October to December 1992.
 Wave 3: January to March 1993.
 Wave 4: April to June 1993.

Table 3   Maximum response rate by fieldwork wave*

	Wave of fieldwork									
	Wave 1		Wave 2		Wave 3		Wave 4		Total	
	No.	%	No.	%	No.	%	No.	%	No.	%
Interview sample	**474**	*100*	**544**	*100*	**559**	*100*	**524**	*100*	**2101**	*100*
Non-contacts	1	*0*	6	*1*	5	*1*	–	*–*	12	*1*
Movers	14	*3*	25	*5*	13	*2*	24	*5*	76	*4*
Refusals	33	*7*	41	*7*	38	*7*	42	*8*	154	*7*
Response to questionnaire	426	*90*	472	*87*	503	*90*	458	*87*	1859	*88*

*Wave 1: July to September 1992.
 Wave 2: October to December 1992.
 Wave 3: January to March 1993.
 Wave 4: April to June 1993.

Appendix D

Sampling errors

This appendix examines the sources of error associated with survey estimates and presents sampling errors of survey estimates, referred to as standard errors, and design factors for a number of key variables shown in this Report. Note that tables showing standard errors in the analysis chapters of this Report have assumed a simple random sample design. In testing for the significance of the differences between two survey estimates, proportions or means, the sampling error calculated as for a simple random sample design was multiplied by an assumed design factor of 1.5 to allow for the complex sample design.

1.1 The accuracy of survey results

Survey results are subject to various sources of error. The total error in a survey estimate is the difference between the estimate derived from the data collected and the true value for the population. It can be thought of as being comprised of random and systematic errors, and each of these two main types of error can be subdivided into error from a number of different sources.

Random error

Random error is the part of the total error which would be expected to average zero if a number of repeats of the same survey were carried out based on different samples from the population.

An important component of random error is sampling error, which arises because the estimate is based on a survey rather than a census of the population. The results of this or any other survey would be expected to vary from the true population values. The amount of variation depends on both the size of the sample and the sample design.

Random error may also arise from other sources such as the informant's interpretation of the questions or from errors associated with taking measurements. As with all surveys carried out by Social Survey Division, considerable efforts were made on this survey to minimise these effects through interviewer and blood taker training and through pilot work; however it is likely some will still remain which is not possible to quantify.

Systematic error

Systematic error, or bias, applies to those sources of error which will not average to zero over repeats of the survey. The category includes, for example, bias due to omission of certain parts of the population from the sampling frame, and that due to interviewer or coder variation. Again a substantial effort is put into avoiding systematic errors, but it is likely some will still remain.

Non-response bias is another type of systematic error, of particular concern. It occurs if non-respondents to the survey or to particular elements of the survey differ in some respect from respondents, so that the responding sample is not representative of the total population. Non-response can be minimised by training interviewers in how to deal with potential refusals, and with strategies to minimise non-contacts. However a certain level of non-response is inevitable in any voluntary survey. The resulting bias, is however, dependent not only on the absolute level of non-response but on the extent to which non-respondents differ from respondents in terms of the measures which the survey aims to estimate.

Although informants were encouraged to take part in all elements of the survey, some refused certain components. Chapter 3 examined the characteristics of groups responding to the different parts of the total survey package. The age and sex profiles of the responding and diary samples were found to be virtually identical, and analysis of non-response to the postal sift and interviewer follow-up stages showed no evidence of response bias. However for the anthropometric measurements and blood analytes there is likely to be an age bias, as younger children tended to be more difficult to measure and were harder to obtain a blood sample from.

1.2 True standard errors for NDNS of children 1½ to 4½ years estimates

As described in Chapter 1 and Appendix C this survey used a multi-stage sample design which involved both clustering and stratification. In considering the reliability of estimates, standard errors calculated on the basis of a simple random sample design need to be adjusted for the effect of the complex sample design.

This dietary survey sample was clustered using postcode sectors as primary sampling units (PSUs). While clustering can increase standard errors, stratification tends to reduce them and is of most advantage where the stratification factor is of relevance to the survey subject matter. The stratifiers used on this survey were region, which differentiated between metropolitan and non-metropolitan areas within standard region, the proportion of heads of household in socio-economic groups 1 to 5 and 13, and the proportion of females in private households who were aged 16 and over and were economically active.

In a complex sample design the size of the standard error of any estimate depends on how the characteristic of interest is spread within and between PSUs and strata, and this is taken into account in the way data are grouped in order to calculate the standard error. The method described here is called *successive differencing* because it uses the differences between adjacent clusters (postal sectors) in the characteristic of interest[1]. The ordering of PSUs reflects the ranking of postal sectors on the stratifiers used in the sample design.

The formula used to estimate the true standard error for this survey's estimates is known as the ratio estimator, and is shown below. The method explicitly allows for the fact that the percentages and means are actually ratios of two survey estimates, both of which are subject to random error.

$$var(r) = \frac{1}{x^2}[var(y) + r^2 var(x) - 2r\,cov(yx)]$$

Var (r) is the estimate of the variance of the ratio, *r*, expressed in terms of *var(y)* and *var(x)* which are the estimated variances of *y* and *x*, and *cov(y,x)* which is their estimated covariance. The resulting estimate is only valid if the denominator is not too variable[2].

Tables 1 to 11 give true standard errors, taking account of the complex sample design used on this survey, for most of the key variables presented in this Report. The characteristic is the numerator, for example the average daily intake of iron, and the sample size the denominator in the ratio estimate.

For certain nutrients, blood analytes, and anthropometric measurements, estimates are shown by age and sex. Standard errors for estimates of other subgroups, such as social class and family type have not been presented because of the large number of possible estimates to be covered.

1.3 Estimating standard errors for other survey estimates

Although true standard errors can be calculated readily by computer, there are practical problems in presenting a large number of survey estimates. One solution is to calculate true standard errors for selected variables and, from these, identify design factors appropriate for the specific survey design and for different types of survey variable. The standard error of other survey measures can then be estimated using the appropriate design factor together with the sampling error assuming a simple random sample.

1.3.1 The Design Factor (deft)

The effect of a complex sample design can be quantified by comparing the observed variability in the sample with that which would be expected if the survey had used a simple random sample. The most commonly used statistic is the design factor (deft) which is calculated as a ratio of the true standard error for a survey estimate, allowing for the full complexity of the sample design, to the standard error assuming that the result has come from a simple random sample. The deft can be used as a multiplier to the standard error based on a simple random sample, $se(p)_{srs}$, to give the standard error of the complex design, $se(p)$, by using the following formula:

$$se(p) = deft \times se(p)_{srs}$$

Tables 1 to 11 show defts for certain Dietary Survey measures. The level of deft varies between survey variables reflecting the degree to which the characteristic is clustered within PSUs or is distributed between strata. For a single variable the level of the deft also varies according to the size of the subgroup on which the estimate is based, and on the distribution of the subgroup between PSUs and strata.

The deft values presented here for certain nutrients and main characteristics are for all children in the diary sample. Defts for blood analytes and anthropometric measurements are for children for whom these measures were obtained, and exclude cases where a quality control variable indicated that a particular measurement or result was unreliable (see *Chapters 10 and 11*). Defts are also presented for certain nutrients, anthropometric measurements and blood analytes by age and sex; these will, on average be higher than those for smaller subgroups. Their application to smaller subsamples will result in a more conservative test of significance.

Eighty per cent of the design factors presented in Tables 1 to 11 were less than 1.2. Design factors of this order are considered to be small and they indicate that the characteristic is not markedly clustered geographically. Higher defts were recorded for a number of the blood analytes. This may be explained in part by the lower response rate to this element of the survey and by possible differences between blood takers in their success in obtaining 4ml of blood.

For socio-demographic characteristics where geographic clus-

tering would be expected design factors above 1.2 were found for virtually all characteristics. *(Table 1)*

1.3.2 Testing differences between means and proportions

Standard errors can be used to test whether an observed difference between two proportions or means in the sample is likely to be entirely due to sampling error.

The formula for the standard error of a difference between percentages assuming a simple random sample is:

$$se(p_1 - p_2) = \sqrt{\left(\frac{p_1 q_1}{n_1} + \frac{p_2 q_2}{n_2}\right)}$$

where p_1 and p_2 are the observed percentages for the two subsamples, q_1 and q_2 are respectively $(100-p_1)$ and $(100-p_2)$, and n_1 and n_2 are the subsample sizes.

The equivalent formula for the standard error of the difference between the means for subgroups 1 and 2 is:

$$se(diff) = \sqrt{se_1^2 + se_2^2}$$

Allowance for the complex sample design is then made by multiplying the standard error for the difference, from the above formula, by the appropriate value of the deft.

In this report the calculation of the difference between proportions and means assumed a deft of 1.5 across all survey estimates. The calculation of complex sampling errors and design factors for key characteristics thus show this was a conservative estimate for most characteristics. Therefore there will be some differences in sample proportions and means which are not commented on in the text but which are significantly different at least at the $p < 0.05$ level.

Confidence intervals can be calculated around a survey estimate using the true standard error for that estimate. For example, the 95% confidence interval is calculated as 1.96 times the standard error, on either side of the estimated proportion or mean value. At the 95% confidence level, over many repeats of the survey under the same conditions, 95% of these confidence intervals would contain the population estimate. However, when assessing the results of a survey, it is usual to assume that there is only a 5% chance that the true population value will fall outside the 95% confidence interval calculated for the survey estimate.

References and notes

1   The calculation of true standard errors and design factors for this survey used the package EPSILON which was developed by Social Survey Division for samples drawn using multi-stage designs. For further details of the method of calculation see Butcher B and Elliot D. *A sampling errors manual*. OPCS (London, 1987) (NM13).
2   This variability can be measured by the co-efficient of variation of x, denoted by cv (x), which is the standard error of x expressed as a proportion of x:

$$cv(x) = \frac{se(x)}{x}$$

It has been suggested that the ratio estimator should not be used if cv (x) is greater than 0.2. The co-efficient of variation of x did not exceed 0.2 for any of the estimates presented in this Appendix.

Table 1 True standard errors and design factors for socio-demographic characteristics of the diary sample

Characteristic	%(p)	Standard error of p	Design factor
Age			
1½ to 2½ years	34.39	1.16	1.00
2½ to 3½ years	36.18	1.21	1.03
Boys 3½ to 4½ years	14.92	0.76	0.87
Girls 3½ to 4½ years	14.51	0.74	0.86
Whether child was reported as being unwell during four-day dietary recording period			
Unwell, eating affected	15.88	0.92	1.03
Unwell, eating not affected	11.34	0.89	1.14
Not unwell	72.78	1.29	1.19
Region			
Scotland	9.85	0.96	1.31
Northern	25.49	1.36	1.28
Central, South West and Wales	33.61	1.45	1.26
London and South East	31.04	1.38	1.22
Social class of head of household			
Non-manual	44.87	1.62	1.33
Manual	52.01	1.59	1.30
Employment status of head of household			
Working	74.57	1.61	1.52
Unemployed	9.97	0.80	1.09
Economically inactive	15.46	1.33	1.51
Whether child's parents receiving Income Support or Family Credit			
Receiving benefit(s)	31.90	1.83	1.61
Not receiving benefit(s)	68.10	1.83	1.61
Mother's highest educational qualification			
Above GCE 'A' level	18.24	1.39	1.47
GCE 'A' level or equivalents	10.94	0.88	1.15
GCE 'O' level or equivalents	35.29	1.35	1.16
CSE or equivalents	14.11	1.12	1.31
None	21.41	1.54	1.53
Family type			
Married or cohabiting couple with:			
one child	21.85	1.28	1.27
more than one child	60.36	1.64	1.37
Lone parent with:			
one child	7.22	0.72	1.13
more than one child	10.57	0.86	1.15
Sample size		*1675*	

Table 2 True standard errors and design factors for average daily intakes of energy and macronutrients

Macronutrients	Mean r	Standard error of r	Design factor
Energy (kcal)	1140	6.67	1.05
Energy (kJ)	4798	28.04	1.06
Total sugars (g)	87.07	0.92	1.27
Starch (g)	68.13	0.59	1.10
% energy from total carbohydrate	51.12	0.17	1.12
% energy from sugars	28.64	0.23	1.31
% energy from starch	22.47	0.17	1.26
Protein (g)	36.81	0.29	1.14
% energy from protein	12.98	0.06	1.04
Total fat (g)	45.69	0.33	1.03
Saturated fatty acids (g)	20.56	0.18	1.14
Cis monounsaturated fatty acids (g)	14.18	0.10	1.00
Cis n-3 polyunsaturated fatty acids (g)	0.87	0.01	1.09
Cis n-6 polyunsaturated fatty acids (g)	5.00	0.05	0.94
Trans fatty acids	2.20	0.02	1.05
Cholesterol (mg)	139	1.91	1.14
% energy from total fat	35.90	0.14	1.06
Sample size		*1675*	

Table 3 True standard errors and design factors for average daily intakes of selected vitamins from all sources

Vitamins	Mean r	Standard error of r	Design factor
Total carotene (µg)	872	21.69	1.16
Vitamin A (retinol equivalents) (µg)	578	21.30	1.01
Thiamin (mg)	0.81	0.01	1.06
Riboflavin (mg)	1.21	0.01	0.99
Niacin equivalents (mg)	16.32	0.14	1.16
Vitamin B_6 (mg)	1.24	0.01	1.17
Vitamin B_{12} (µg)	2.83	0.04	1.02
Folate (µg)	132	1.21	1.02
Vitamin C (mg)	51.76	1.49	1.44
Vitamin D (µg)	1.89	0.06	1.07
Vitamin E (mg)	4.42	0.05	0.93
Sample size		*1675*	

Table 4 True standard errors and design factors for average daily intakes of selected minerals from all sources

Minerals	Mean r	Standard error of r	Design factor
Iron (mg)	5.55	0.06	1.06
Calcium (mg)	638	6.08	0.98
Phosphorus (mg)	742	5.78	1.05
Magnesium (mg)	136	0.98	1.07
Sodium (mg)	1506	14.24	1.24
Potassium (mg)	1507	11.34	1.09
Sample size		*1675*	

Table 5 True standard errors and design factors for average daily intakes of energy and macronutrients by age and sex of child

Macronutrients	All aged 1½ – 2½ years			All aged 2½ – 3½ years			All aged 3½ – 4½ years Boys			All aged 3½ – 4½ years Girls		
	mean r	se of r	deft	mean r	se of r	deft	mean r	se of r	deft	mean r	se of r	deft
Energy (kcal)	1045	10.50	1.03	1160	9.43	0.96	1273	17.59	1.04	1183	18.16	1.16
Energy (kJ)	4393	44.05	1.03	4882	39.55	0.96	5355	74.00	1.05	4976	76.08	1.16
Carbohydrate (g)	139	1.51	0.98	159	1.43	0.95	177	2.71	1.06	162	2.30	1.08
Total sugars (g)	79.91	1.30	1.10	89.19	1.11	0.96	97.80	2.30	1.09	87.71	1.82	1.08
Starch (g)	58.75	0.77	0.93	69.91	0.90	1.04	79.38	1.24	0.88	74.34	1.35	1.06
% energy from total carbohydrate	49.92	0.29	1.05	51.53	0.25	1.03	52.32	0.42	1.14	51.71	0.42	1.11
% energy from sugars	28.69	0.35	1.12	28.82	0.30	1.07	28.77	0.53	1.10	27.92	0.46	1.09
% energy from starch	21.20	0.24	1.00	22.71	0.21	0.98	23.55	0.31	0.94	23.78	0.36	1.09
Protein (g)	35.40	0.47	1.11	36.76	0.38	0.90	39.37	0.68	1.04	37.66	0.77	1.14
% energy from protein	13.62	0.10	0.92	12.69	0.09	0.88	12.40	0.13	0.92	12.75	0.16	1.03
Total fat (g)	42.51	0.56	1.07	46.30	0.54	1.07	50.08	0.89	1.04	47.16	1.03	1.19
Saturated fatty acids (g)	19.74	0.30	1.12	20.76	0.27	1.07	21.90	0.42	1.03	20.65	0.49	1.17
Cis monounsaturated fatty acids (g)	13.02	0.17	1.05	14.39	0.18	1.06	15.72	0.29	1.01	14.81	0.34	1.18
Cis n-3 polyunsaturated fatty acids (g)	0.78	0.02	1.09	0.88	0.02	1.06	0.99	0.03	0.82	0.95	0.03	0.94
Cis n-6 polyunsaturated fatty acids (g)	4.29	0.07	0.93	5.14	0.09	1.03	5.85	0.14	0.99	5.50	0.16	1.08
Trans fatty acids (g)	2.03	0.03	0.91	2.23	0.05	1.26	2.4	0.07	1.10	2.26	0.07	1.21
Cholesterol (mg)	133	2.50	0.87	138	2.81	1.01	147	4.49	1.08	144	4.39	0.95
% energy from total fat	36.45	0.25	1.06	35.78	0.23	1.08	35.28	0.37	1.16	35.55	0.37	1.16
Sample size	576			606			250			243		

Table 6 True standard errors and design factors for average daily intakes of selected vitamins from all sources by age and sex of child

Vitamins	All aged 1½ – 2½ years			All aged 2½ – 3½ years			All aged 3½ – 4½ years Boys			All aged 3½ – 4½ years Girls		
	mean r	se of r	deft	mean r	se of r	deft	mean r	se of r	deft	mean r	se of r	deft
Total carotene (μg)	796	20.54	0.86	874	30.44	0.99	1029	70.28	1.06	884	48.56	0.93
Vitamin A (retinol equivalents) (μg)	589	48.07	1.03	579	26.74	0.87	568	29.68	1.07	561	48.75	1.07
Thiamin (mg)	0.76	0.01	1.03	0.81	0.01	0.90	0.89	0.02	0.96	0.86	0.02	1.02
Riboflavin (mg)	1.22	0.02	0.97	1.21	0.02	0.87	1.23	0.03	1.09	1.17	0.03	0.97
Niacin equivalents (mg)	14.94	0.20	1.10	16.40	0.18	0.90	18.22	0.30	0.91	17.46	0.35	0.98
Vitamin B$_6$ (mg)	1.14	0.02	1.14	1.25	0.02	0.96	1.36	0.03	0.97	1.31	0.04	1.05
Vitamin B$_{12}$ (μg)	2.88	0.09	0.97	2.80	0.05	0.81	2.81	0.09	1.02	2.80	0.11	1.11
Folate (μg)	120	1.64	0.91	134	2.07	1.02	145	3.20	1.00	140	2.82	0.90
Vitamin C (mg)	50.75	2.25	1.25	52.25	1.93	1.08	54.61	3.20	1.17	49.97	2.37	1.06
Vitamin D (μg)	1.85	0.11	1.12	1.85	0.08	0.88	2.09	0.14	0.98	1.92	0.14	1.06
Vitamin E (mg)	3.93	0.08	1.09	4.51	0.06	0.76	5.12	0.15	1.01	4.65	0.14	1.07
Sample size	576			606			250			243		

Table 7 True standard errors and design factors for average daily intakes of selected minerals from all sources by age and sex of child

Minerals	All aged 1½ – 2½ years			All aged 2½ – 3½ years			All aged 3½ – 4½ years Boys			All aged 3½ – 4½ years Girls		
	mean r	se of r	deft	mean r	se of r	deft	mean r	se of r	deft	mean r	se of r	deft
Iron (mg)	5.04	0.09	0.95	5.59	0.10	1.06	6.19	0.14	1.11	5.96	0.17	0.92
Calcium (mg)	664	11.43	1.01	635	9.80	0.93	625	15.32	1.07	595	14.90	1.09
Phosphorus (mg)	735	10.06	1.03	740	8.93	0.97	767	14.32	1.07	736	14.52	1.09
Magnesium (mg)	132	1.55	0.98	137	1.50	0.99	146	2.88	1.18	137	2.41	1.06
Sodium (mg)	1365	21.80	1.18	1528	21.00	1.12	1658	24.78	0.87	1632	32.11	1.00
Potassium (mg)	1476	19.31	1.09	1513	17.27	0.96	1573	30.66	1.15	1501	27.19	1.07
Sample size	576			606			250			243		

Table 8   True standard errors and design factors for anthropometric measurements

Body measurements	Mean r	Sample size	Standard error of r	Design factor
Weight (kg)	14.38	1707	0.06	1.04
Standing height (cm)	94.49	1606	0.19	1.02
Supine length (cm)	84.67	191	0.25	1.00
Body mass index	16.20	1549	0.05	1.26
Head circumference (cm)	50.53	1720	0.06	1.31
Mid upper-arm circumference (cm)	17.0	1719	0.05	1.31

Table 9   True standard errors and design factors for anthropometric measurements by age and sex of child

Age and sex of child	Body measurements	Mean r	Sample size	Standard error of r	Design factor
	Weight (kg)				
Boys 1½ to 2½ years		12.62	294	0.09	0.97
Girls 1½ to 2½ years		11.87	283	0.08	0.82
Boys 2½ to 3½ years		14.93	307	0.09	0.89
Girls 2½ to 3½ years		14.30	314	0.10	1.03
Boys 3½ to 4½ years		16.62	251	0.13	0.97
Girls 3½ to 4½ years		16.38	258	0.11	0.83
	Standing height (cm)				
Boys 1½ to 2½ years		86.94	252	0.24	0.98
Girls 1½ to 2½ years		85.30	236	0.25	0.90
Boys 2½ to 3½ years		95.55	305	0.20	0.87
Girls 2½ to 3½ years		94.69	304	0.24	0.97
Boys 3½ to 4½ years		102	255	0.29	1.02
Girls 3½ to 4½ years		101	254	0.25	0.93
	Body mass index				
Boys 1½ to 2½ years		16.79	240	0.09	0.97
Girls 1½ to 2½ years		16.38	229	0.09	0.93
Boys 2½ to 3½ years		16.36	289	0.08	0.99
Girls 2½ to 3½ years		15.92	297	0.09	1.08
Boys 3½ to 4½ years		15.94	244	0.09	0.94
Girls 3½ to 4½ years		15.89	250	0.09	1.05
	Head circumference (cm)				
Boys 1½ to 2½ years		50.11	298	0.10	1.05
Girls 1½ to 2½ years		48.82	285	0.09	0.91
Boys 2½ to 3½ years		51.30	316	0.11	1.05
Girls 2½ to 3½ years		50.16	309	0.10	1.12
Boys 3½ to 4½ years		51.94	257	0.09	1.04
Girls 3½ to 4½ years		50.99	255	0.12	1.26
	Mid upper-arm circumference (cm)				
Boys 1½ to 2½ years		16.5	293	0.07	1.02
Girls 1½ to 2½ years		16.2	286	0.08	1.02
Boys 2½ to 3½ years		17.0	314	0.07	0.91
Girls 2½ to 3½ years		17.0	312	0.07	0.99
Boys 3½ to 4½ years		17.5	256	0.10	0.98
Girls 3½ to 4½ years		17.6	258	0.08	0.95

Table 10   True standard errors and design factors for selected blood analytes

Blood analytes	Mean r	Sample size	Standard error of r	Design factor
Haemoglobin (g/dl)	12.16	951	0.04	1.29
Ferritin (µg/l)	23.49	930	0.66	1.08
ZPP (µmol/mol haem)	54.37	950	0.91	1.33
Vitamin B_{12} (pmol/l)	636	817	9.85	1.07
Plasma folate (nmol/l)	21.12	819	0.46	1.35
Plasma ascorbate (vitamin C) (µmol/l)	67.61	744	1.55	1.39
α-carotene (µmol/l)	0.10	807	0.004	1.38
Retinol (µmol/l)	1.02	816	0.01	1.33
Plasma total cholesterol (mmol/l)	4.28	683	0.03	1.07
HDL cholesterol (mmol/l)	1.14	683	0.02	1.60

Table 11 True standard errors and design factors for selected blood analytes by age and sex of child

Age and sex of child	Blood analytes	Mean r	Sample size	Standard error of r	Design factor
	Haemoglobin (g/dl)				
All 1½ to 2½ years		11.98	310	0.06	1.12
All 2½ to 3½ years		12.19	351	0.05	1.03
Boys 3½ to 4½ years		12.40	137	0.07	0.82
Girls 3½ to 4½ years		12.26	153	0.08	1.23
	Ferritin (µg/l)				
All 1½ to 2½ years		21.38	300	0.93	0.86
All 2½ to 3½ years		23.85	345	0.80	0.82
Boys 3½ to 4½ years		24.92	135	1.54	0.85
Girls 3½ to 4½ years		25.62	150	1.57	1.15
	ZZP (µmol/mol haem)				
All 1½ to 2½ years		58.43	309	1.63	1.08
All 2½ to 3½ years		53.76	351	1.10	1.09
Boys 3½ to 4½ years		50.68	137	1.55	0.92
Girls 3½ to 4½ years		50.87	153	0.94	1.04
	Vitamin B$_{12}$ (pmol/l)				
All 1½ to 2½ years		620	254	18.68	1.10
All 2½ to 3½ years		645	308	14.99	1.01
Boys 3½ to 4½ years		654	124	17.67	0.73
Girls 3½ to 4½ years		627	131	22.71	1.01
	Plasma folate (nmol/l)				
All 1½ to 2½ years		21.05	255	0.67	1.10
All 2½ to 3½ years		21.10	309	0.64	1.13
Boys 3½ to 4½ years		22.04	124	0.85	0.93
Girls 3½ to 4½ years		20.45	131	0.81	1.04
	Plasma ascorbate (vitamin C) (µmol/l)				
All 1½ to 2½ years		66.69	218	2.53	1.18
All 2½ to 3½ years		68.97	284	2.15	1.18
Boys 3½ to 4½ years		61.96	117	3.07	1.18
Girls 3½ to 4½ years		71.37	125	2.71	1.04
	α-carotene (µmol/l)				
All 1½ to 2½ years		0.11	238	0.01	1.03
All 2½ to 3½ years		0.10	310	0.01	1.34
Boys 3½ to 4½ years		0.10	124	0.01	0.99
Girls 3½ to 4½ years		0.10	135	0.01	0.82
	Retinol (µmol/l)				
All 1½ to 2½ years		1.03	242	0.02	1.08
All 2½ to 3½ years		1.02	313	0.02	0.96
Boys 3½ to 4½ years		0.98	125	0.02	1.09
Girls 3½ to 4½ years		1.02	136	0.03	1.26
	Plasma total cholesterol (mmol/l)				
All 1½ to 2½ years		4.26	195	0.06	1.09
All 2½ to 3½ years		4.29	256	0.05	1.04
Boys 3½ to 4½ years		4.23	111	0.07	1.16
Girls 3½ to 4½ years		4.32	121	0.07	1.03
	HDL cholesterol (mmol/l)				
All 1½ to 2½ years		1.13	195	0.02	1.18
All 2½ to 3½ years		1.16	256	0.02	1.16
Boys 3½ to 4½ years		1.17	111	0.03	1.07
Girls 3½ to 4½ years		1.09	121	0.03	1.21

Appendix E

The feasibility and pilot studies

The mainstage survey was preceded by a feasibility study, with fieldwork carried out in October and November 1989, and a pilot survey in 1991.

The feasibility study was designed to assess whether the proposed questionnaire and methods were feasible for use in a home-based national survey, and would provide reliable data on the diets of young children throughout the country. As part of the feasibility study, the methodology for collecting the dietary data by weighed intake record was validated by comparing the computed energy intake from the food intake with the energy expenditure measured at the same time as the food record was being kept, by the doubly-labelled water method. Blood sampling was not included in the feasibility study; blood-taking procedures and acceptability were tested by the 1991 pilot survey.

Feasibility study

Details of the design of the feasibility study and its main findings have been published elsewhere[1,2], and are summarised here. The study involved:

1. Short interviews with the parents, usually the mothers, of 96 children aged 1½ to 4½ years. The sample was not designed to be nationally representative. Instead, children from a range of different social and economic backgrounds were included in order to test the suitability of the methods and procedures for a national survey. Some cases were specifically included which it was considered might present particular difficulties: for example, where mothers were working, and where mothers had other young children.

2. A record for four days of weighed intake of all food and drink consumed by the child both in and out of the home.

3. Weight, supine length, mid upper-arm circumference, head circumference, waist circumference and hip circumference measurements for each child.

4. An assessment of total energy expenditure via the doubly-labelled water method. This involved the child drinking a dose of water labelled with a stable isotope and providing a urine sample daily for a total of 10 days.

5. A short interview with parents at the end of the survey to find out about any difficulties they had with the survey, especially in keeping the dietary record.

The study showed that the length of the interview was acceptable to parents and that the questionnaire successfully elicited the information required. Recommendations for some minor amendments are described in the study report[1].

Overall parents coped well with the food diary, the OPCS nutritionists and staff coding the diary data judging that over 70% of the dietary records were good or very good. The study identified a few problems with weighing food, in particular with squash type drinks and snack items such as biscuits, crisps and sweets, and with recording leftover items such as gravy, milk etc. These findings led to emphasis on these items at the main survey interviewer training sessions, and to some improvements in diary design to encourage recording of such items. The results of the doubly-labelled water procedure confirmed that the quality of record keeping was generally very high[2].

At the end of the four-day recording period, parents were asked whether they could have carried on keeping the dietary record for longer. It was considered likely that increasing the record-keeping period would lead to loss of response and accuracy.

The main difficulties with the anthropometric measurements were with supine length and waist and hip circumferences. Interviewers found it difficult to locate children's waists and hips with any degree of confidence and therefore these measurements were not included in the main survey. New, specially designed equipment for measuring height and supine length was tested in the pilot survey.

Pilot survey

A pilot exercise on a sample of 48 children was carried out in 1991. This incorporated many of the recommendations from the feasibility study with respect to the design of the questionnaire, dietary methodology and dietary recording documents as well as providing a further opportunity to test all aspects of the survey package.

Its main aims were to test:

— sampling procedures;
— the suitability of new dietary scales;
— the suitability of new equipment for measuring height and supine length;
— the procedures associated with obtaining a sample of blood.

Sample

It was recognised that obtaining a nationally representative sample of preschool children would not be easy because, for example, children of this age are not yet registered for attendance at school. Two options were considered. Use of the Postcode Address file (PAF) was assessed and found to be suitable. For the pilot survey 2,000 addresses, randomly selected from the PAF were sent a short postal questionnaire to identify eligible households. This method was selected for use at the main survey, and the details of the procedures involved are described in Appendix C.

An alternative method of selecting the samples was to use the National Register for Child Benefit held by the Department of Social Security. This would have similarities with the sampling method in the 1967/8 survey[3], which had used the national Welfare Food Scheme as a basis for selecting participant children. However preliminary investigation established that the use of the Child Benefit Register was not a practical possibility.

Blood taking

The pilot survey showed that taking blood was acceptable to most parents and to children: the mothers of 32 of the 48 children included in the survey agreed to a blood sample being taken although blood was only obtained from 24 children. While generally working satisfactorily, the pilot survey identified the need for blood takers to be briefed on the background to the survey, trained in the blood taking protocol, and recruited with sufficient availability to be able to visit households at a time convenient to parents.

The methodology adopted for the main survey, and tested in the pilot is described in Chapters 2 and 10 and Appendix L.

The MRC Dunn Nutrition Unit were responsible for obtaining ethical approval for the blood sampling procedures, for the recruitment and training of blood takers and for taking and analysing the blood samples. These aspects of the survey were contracted to the Dunn Nutrition Unit for the main stage of the survey.

Equipment

The new equipment was considered acceptable, and adopted for the main survey (see *Chapter 2* and *Appendix 0*).

References

1 White A J, Davies P S W. *Feasibility Study for the National Diet and Nutrition Survey of Children aged 1½ to 4½ years*. OPCS (London, 1994). (NM22)

2 Davies P S W, Coward W A, Gregory J, White A J, Mills A. Total energy expenditure and energy intake in the pre-school child: a comparison. *Brit J Nutr* 1994; **72(1):** 13–20.

3 Department of Health and Social Security. Report on Health and Social Subjects: 10. *A Nutrition Survey of Pre-School Children, 1967–68*. HMSO (London, 1975). See also *Appendix P*.

Appendix F

Dietary methodology: details of the recording and coding procedures

Chapter 2 outlined the weighing, recording, coding and editing procedures used on this survey. This Appendix gives further information on these procedures and the reasons why the weighed intake method was preferred to other dietary methodologies.

1 Choice of dietary methodology

A number of different methodologies can be used to collect data on food consumption. These include weighed intake records, duplicate diets, 24-hour recall methods and food frequency questionnaires. Recall methods and food frequency questionnaires may include methods to estimate the quantity of food items eaten by reference, for example, to food models or photographs, but generally they do not involve direct weighing.

Each method has advantages and disadvantages, and in deciding which to adopt a number of factors need to be considered. These include the aims of the study, the precision required for the results, the age and ability of the population, the likely effect of the methodology on the quality of the data, and on co-operation and response rates, and the resources available.

The weighed intake methodology is the preferred method for collecting quantitative information on food and drink consumption when estimates of nutrient and energy intakes are required for individuals, with sufficient precision to be related to health indices, such as nutritional status as measured by blood analytes. Distributions of nutrient and energy intakes for groups can also be calculated. The method avoids recall errors and, for foods eaten at home, minimises estimates of quantities consumed, if carried out properly[1,2].

Nevertheless the method has disadvantages; it requires a high level of motivation from subjects assisted by regular calls from interviewers. Precision scales must be provided. It is resource intensive and expensive, it requires an adequate level of comprehension by the subject, and, the most frequent criticism, it may cause changes in eating habits, or lead to under-recording. However, the feasibility study indicated that the method was feasible, and produced good quality information[3].

Weighed intake methods provide information on a subject's current intake, whereas recall methods and food frequency questionnaires, because they generally cover a longer reference period, may be more likely to reflect a subject's usual diet.

2 Recording in the 'home record' diary

Parents were asked to start a new diary page at the beginning of each day and record the day and date on every page used. Each food or group of foods was preceded by an entry for a container, such as a plate, bowl or cup, which was first weighed. The scales were then set to zero and the first food item put on the plate and weighed[4]; the scales were then 'zeroed' again and subsequent items added and weighed in the same way. Each food item was recorded in the diary on a separate line, with a full description including brand information, as shown on the example page of the 'home record' diary, reproduced in Appendix A.

Foods eaten straight from containers: for some food items like yogurt, which are usually eaten directly from the container, it was difficult or inappropriate to follow this recommended method for weighing and recording. Therefore, foods such as yogurts were initially weighed as a complete item, container plus contents, and then the container was reweighed empty or with any leftovers. Such entries were later re-written to the standard format by the interviewer or office coders.

Second helpings were weighed and recorded in the same way as the initial serving; the plate, with any items remaining was put on the scales and the scales zeroed. Each second serving of a food was then added to the plate and weighed and recorded separately. These items were then flagged for the attention of the nutritionists who combined the weights of first and second helpings giving an overall weight for each food item consumed.

Items too light to be weighed: for items which were too light to be weighed, for example a thin spreading of Marmite, a description of the quantity was recorded.

Leftovers were also recorded. At the end of each eating occasion the plate or container was reweighed with all the leftover items; the total weight was recorded in the leftover column next to the initial entry for the container with a tick in the leftovers column to indicate each food item that was left. Parents were encouraged also to record additional information on leftovers, for example, that half the mashed potato was left or all the serving of carrots. For foods which have inedible parts such as some meats, fish, fruit and nuts, the parent was asked to note whether the weight of leftovers included the weight of inedible parts, such as bones, peel or shells.

Spilt or dropped food. If any item was spilt or dropped after weighing, parents and carers were encouraged wherever possible to recover and reweigh it, for example by scraping food from the child's bib and reweighing it on the original plate together with any other leftovers. In some cases this was not possible, for example, because the spilt food was eaten by the dog, so an estimate was made of how much of the original item was lost, and recorded in the spillage column of the 'home record'.

Recipes for homemade dishes were recorded on the back of the recording sheets in the 'home record' diary. Informants were asked to give as much detail as possible about quantities of ingredients used, including liquids added during cooking, and the cooking method used.

3 Recording in the 'eating out' diary

Where items could not be weighed, generally because they were consumed away from home, a description of each item was required together with information on portion size, price, where it was bought and details of any leftovers. At the coding stage interviewers transcribed the entries from the eating out diary to the home record and split composite items such as sandwiches into their constituent parts (bread, spread and filling).

Strategies for obtaining information about items which had not been weighed

Weight information for foods eaten away from home which could not be weighed was collected in a variety of ways and added to the record. For items purchased from local shops or cafes, such as cakes, sandwiches and chips, interviewers used the information about price and place of purchase to buy a duplicate item which was either weighed directly or, if it was a composite item, split into its component parts and weighed. Interviewers were also asked to find out further details of foods purchased from takeaway outlets so that they could be correctly coded; for example the type of fat used for frying, and the type of spread used in sandwiches.

Where it was not possible to collect information on the weights of the components of a composite item, individual weights were estimated by the nutritionists. For prepackaged foods eaten outside the home, for example confectionery and soft drinks, weight information was obtained from the packaging. To encourage parents and carers to keep wrappers and cartons they were given small plastic bags which were then returned to the interviewer.

All estimated weights entered by the record keeper or interviewer were checked by the nutritionists to make sure they were consistent, for example that the weight recorded for a standard 'chocolate' bar corresponded with the weight on the packaging.

4 Children looked after by a childminder or other carer

If the child was looked after by a childminder or went to a nursery where food was served, the interviewer encouraged the parent to give the home record diary and a set of scales to the childminder or nursery teacher. If the parent agreed, and it could be arranged, the interviewer explained the weighing and recording procedure direct to the carer. In other cases the parent explained the procedure. Where carers were not able or willing to weigh the food the child ate, they were asked to record all details in the eating out diary, including a description of the amounts consumed and any leftovers.

5 Checks by the interviewer

Interviewers were required to call back on parents approximately 24 hours after placing the diary. Feasibility work had shown that this call was essential in giving encouragement to parents to continue keeping the record and to help with any problems they were having with the weighing or recording[3]. At this call interviewers checked in particular that weights were not being recorded cumulatively, that leftovers were being weighed and recorded correctly, that descriptions of foods consumed were sufficiently detailed, and that composite items were being split before weighing. To help interviewers spot cumulative weights they were provided with a list of typical portion weights for commonly consumed foods, such as breakfast cereals.

Depending on how much support parents appeared to need interviewers made extra calls throughout the recording period, checking for any obvious difficulties in recording and probing for more details of foods that were inadequately described. At these calls interviewers also checked for food items that the parents might have forgotten to record, for example, drinks during the night. In such cases a duplicate item was weighed, recorded in the diary and noted as an estimated weight.

6 Eating pattern check sheet

As part of the checking process interviewers completed an eating pattern check sheet for each child, summarising the number of sweets, savoury snacks, biscuits, drinks and dietary supplements taken each day. This check sheet was designed to alert the interviewer to marked changes in the dietary record from day to day, such as a decline over time in the number of snacks or drinks being recorded, which could then be checked at the next call. At each checking call interviewers took away completed diary pages to be coded; any additional information needed to code the food item could then be asked for at the next visit.

7 Coding

Interviewers were responsible for food and brand coding; this

ensured early identification of inadequate descriptions and gave them the opportunity to resolve queries quickly by calling back on informants.

A large amount of detail needed to be recorded in the dietary record to enable similar foods prepared and cooked by different methods to be coded correctly, as such foods will have different nutrient compositions. For example, the nutrient composition of crinkle cut chips made from new potatoes and fried in a polyunsaturated oil is different from the same chips fried in lard. Therefore, depending on the food item, information could be needed on cooking method, preparation and packaging as well as an exact description of the product before it could accurately be coded.

Food coding
The following information was required in order to code food items:

- the form in which the food was bought, for example, whether it was fresh, frozen or canned;

- whether the product was low fat and whether any fat had been trimmed or skimmed from meat or meat dishes;

- the cooking method, for example whether the food item had been baked, grilled or fried, and if fried, the type of fat used;

- whether a coating was used for fish and meat, and whether sauces and gravies were thickened;

- whether foods had been sweetened and, if so, whether sugar or an artificial sweetener had been used;

- details of the type of fat and flour used in home-baked items;

- whether products such as cheese, fish and meat were smoked or not.

MAFF compiled the nutrient databank, details of which are given in Appendix H, and associated food code list which contained over 3000 food codes. A page from the food code list is reproduced in Appendix G. Interviewers were provided with this list and an alphabetical index to help them find particular foods. The code list was regularly updated to take account of products, commonly eaten by young children, which came on the market during the fieldwork period. A separate list of raw foods not expected to occur in food diaries, for example raw chicken, was also provided.

A number of check lists were prepared for interviewers by OPCS and MAFF which helped interviewers correctly code particular food groups which required a lot of detail, for example for soft drinks, and for fats used for spreading where codes differed according to the fat content.

Composite and recipe items
Composite items which could be split into their constituent parts
Where foods could be split into their individual components they were weighed and recorded separately, for example, a drink of orange squash would be weighed and recorded as orange squash concentrate and water; a sandwich as bread, spread and filling(s).

If such composite items had not been split and weighed separately then the interviewer recorded an estimate of the quantity of each of the constituent parts; this could be a relatively standard amount, such as the number of slices of bread, or could involve a description of the quantity or relative proportions of each component, for example the quantity of each vegetable in a mixed salad. Using this information the OPCS nutritionists apportioned the total weight between the components of the dish.

Recipe items
Informants were asked to record recipes for most home-made

dishes, such as chicken casserole or apple crumble. Where such foods were included in the food code list, they were identified by 'R' preceding the code number which indicated that their nutrient values were based on standard recipe ingredients. Recipes were individually checked by the OPCS nutritionists and the type and proportions of ingredients used were compared with those of the standard recipe to which the food code referred. If the ingredients differed from the standard recipe in a way which was nutritionally significant the existing food code was not used and a new food code allocated to the item; the appropriate nutrients for the new recipe code were calculated by MAFF and added to the nutrient database.

Where recipe items were eaten away from the home, for example shepherd's pie eaten at a restaurant, and it was not possible to establish details of the ingredients, the standard food code for that item was used. However interviewers were encouraged to collect details of ingredients used in such recipes as this information enabled items to be coded appropriately. Codes were also included in the food code list for menu items purchased from national fast-food chains, for example, Mac-Donalds, where data on the nutritional content of the foods were available.

Brand information

Brand information was recorded for all pre-packaged foods. For some food items, for example, confectionery, biscuits and some breakfast cereals, the brand name was needed in order to code correctly the food item.

Artificial sweeteners, herbal teas and herbal infant drinks, soft drinks and mineral waters were the only food items to be brand coded. This was necessary to provide accurate information on non-nutrient components such as sweeteners.

References and notes

1 Fehily AM. Epidemiology for nutritionists: four survey methods. *Hum Nutr: Appl Nutr*. 1983; **37A**: 419–425.
2 Bingham SA. The dietary assessment of individuals; methods, accuracy, new techniques and recommendations. *Nutr Abstr Rev*. (Series A) 1987; **57**: 10; 705–742.
3 White A, Davies PSW. *Feasibility Study for the National Diet and Nutrition Survey of children aged 1½ to 4½ years*. OPCS (1994) (NM22).
4 The scales had a digital display and a tare facility, and were calibrated in one gram units up to one kilogram and in two gram units thereafter.

Appendix G

Example page from the food code list

If made with fresh or homefrozen potatoes code whether potatoes home grown or not.

D: Chips purchased from a Takeaway or Fast Food Outlet

1853	Chips, old potatoes, fresh, fried in blended vegetable oil, purchased from a takeaway shop
1850	Chips, old potatoes, fresh, fried in dripping
1851	Chips, old potatoes, fresh, fried in lard
1852	Chips, old potatoes, fresh, fried in polyunsaturated oil or margarine
1858	Chips, new potatoes, fresh, fried in blended vegetable oil, purchased from a takeaway shop
1855	Chips, new potatoes, fresh, fried in dripping
1856	Chips, new potatoes, fresh, fried in lard
1857	Chips, new potatoes, fresh, fried in polyunsaturated oil or margarine
1863	Crinkle cut frozen chips, fried in blended vegetable oil, purchased from a takeaway shop
1860	Crinkle cut frozen chips, fried in dripping
1861	Crinkle cut frozen chips, fried in lard
1862	Crinkle cut frozen chips, fried in polyunsaturated oil or margarine
1949	Fine cut frozen chips, fried in blended vegetable oil, purchased from a fast food outlet. NOT McDonalds
7865	Fine cut frozen chips, purchased from McDonalds only
1865	Fine cut frozen chips, fried in dripping
1866	Fine cut frozen chips, fried in lard
1867	Fine cut frozen chips, fried in polyunsaturated oil or margarine
8549	Steak cut/Thick cut frozen chips, fried in blended vegetable oil, purchased from a takeaway shop
1869	Steak cut/Thick cut frozen chips, fried in dripping
1870	Steak cut/Thick cut frozen chips, fried in lard
1871	Steak cut/Thick cut frozen chips, fried in polyunsaturated oil or margarine
1876	Straight cut frozen chips, fried in blended vegetable oil, purchased from a takeaway shop

Appendix H

The nutrient databank and details of nutrients measured

1 The nutrient databank

Intakes of nutrients were calculated from the records of food consumption using a specially adapted nutrient databank. The nutrient databank developed by MAFF for The Dietary and Nutritional Survey of British Adults[1] was revised for this survey of children aged 1½ to 4½ years. Some nutrients were added, some nutrient values were updated and many new codes were added to accommodate foods and drinks consumed by this age group. The databank now contains nutritional information on over 3500 foods and drinks, including manufactured products and recipe dishes, many soft drinks and children's vitamin and mineral supplements.

Each food on the databank has values assigned for 54 nutrients and energy. All the nutrients on the databank for the adults' survey are included, with a number of additions.

These are:

- manganese;
- non-starch polysaccharides (NSP) (Englyst fibre);
- individual sugars (glucose, fructose, sucrose, maltose, lactose, other sugars);
- total sugars split into:
    - i) non-milk extrinsic;
    - ii) intrinsic and milk sugars;
- individual carotenoids (α-carotene, ß-carotene, ß-cryptoxanthin) and
- haem and non-haem iron.

The nutrient values assigned to the foods on the databank are based on *McCance and Widdowson's The Composition of Foods*[2] and its supplements. The Ministry of Agriculture, Fisheries and Food has an ongoing programme of nutritional analysis of foods and a project was commissioned to analyse foods consumed by children of this age as identified in the feasibility study for the survey[3]. Data obtained from food manufacturers were also used, as was nutritional information given on labels. All data were carefully evaluated before being incorporated onto the databank.

In order to calculate the nutrient intakes from the consumption data it is important that there are no missing nutrient values on the databank. For some foods no reliable information was available for certain nutrients. Therefore it was sometimes necessary to estimate values for foods for which there were few available data, by referring to similar foods. For home-made dishes and manufactured products for which no data were available, nutrients were calculated from their constituents using a computer recipe program that allows adjustments to be made for weight and vitamin loss in cooking.

During the survey fieldwork period the range of foods included in the databank was extended as new products with different nutrient contents were consumed by the children, for example, fortified soft drinks.

Further details of MAFF's nutrient databank have been published[4].

1.1 Dietary supplements
Information was collected on brand name, type (tablets, drops or syrup), strength, and quantity of each supplement taken over the four-day recording period. Each supplement was given a code. Manufacturers' data were applied to each individual supplement taken by the children in the survey and the total nutrients provided by the supplements was calculated.

2 Details of nutrients measured and units

Nutrient	Units
water	(g)
sugars	(g) total sugars, expressed as monosaccharide
starch	(g) expressed as monosaccharide
dietary fibre	(g) expressed as modified Southgate method[5]
non-starch polysaccharides	(g) expressed as Englyst method[6]
energy (kJ)	(17 x protein) + (37 x fat) + (16 x carbohydrate) + (29 x alcohol)
energy (kcal)	(4 x protein) + (9 x fat) + (3.75 x carbohydrate) + (7 x alcohol)
protein	(g)
fat	(g)
carbohydrate	(g) sum of sugars plus starch, expressed as monosaccharide equivalent
alcohol	(g)
sodium	(mg)
potassium	(mg)
calcium	(mg)
magnesium	(mg)
phosphorus	(mg)
iron	(mg)
haem iron	(mg)
non-haem iron	(mg)
copper	(mg)
zinc	(mg)
chloride	(mg)
iodine	(μg)
manganese	(mg)
retinol	(μg) sum of trans retinol + (0.75 x *cis* retinol) + (0.9 x retinaldehyde) + (0.4 x dehydroretinol)
carotene	(μg) largely as ß-carotene
α-carotene	(μg)
ß-carotene	(μg)
ß-cryptoxanthin	(μg)
thiamin	(mg)
riboflavin	(mg)
niacin equivalent	(mg) niacin + (tryptophan ÷ 60)
vitamin B$_6$	(mg)
vitamin B$_{12}$	(μg)
folate	(μg)
pantothenic acid	(mg)
biotin	(μg)
vitamin C	(mg)
vitamin D	(μg)
vitamin E	(mg)
fatty acids	
saturated	(g)
cis monounsaturated	(g)
cis n-3 polyunsaturated	(g)

cis n-6 polyunsaturated	(g)
trans	(g)
cholesterol	(mg)
sugars	
glucose	(g)
sucrose	(g)
fructose	(g)
lactose	(g)
maltose	(g)
other sugars	(g)
non-milk extrinsic sugars	(g) includes all the sugars in fruit juices + table sugar + honey + sucrose, glucose and glucose syrups added to food + 50% of the sugars in canned, stewed, dried or preserved fruits[7].
intrinsic & milk sugars	(g) includes all sugars in fresh fruit and vegetables + 50% of the sugars in canned, stewed, dried or preserved fruits + lactose in milk

References

1 Gregory J, Foster K, Tyler H, Wiseman, M. *The Dietary and Nutritional Survey of British Adults.* HMSO (London, 1991).

2 Holland B, Welsh AA, Unwin ID, Buss DH, Paul AA and Southgate DAT. *McCance and Widdowson's The Composition of Foods.* 5th edition. HMSO (London, 1991).

3 White AJ, Davies PSW. *Feasibility Study for the National Diet and Nutrition Survey of Children aged 1½–4½ years* OPCS (London, 1994) (NM22).

4 Smithers G. MAFF's Nutrient Databank. *Nut & Fd Science* 1993; **2:** 16–18.

5 Southgate DAT. Dietary fibre analysis and food sources. *Am J Clin Nutr* 1978; **31:** Suppl. S107–S110.

6 Englyst HN Cummings JH. An improved method for the measurement of dietary fibre as the non-starch polysaccharides in plant foods. *J Assoc Off Anal Chem.* 1988; **71:** 808–814.

7 Buss DH, Lewis J and Smithers G. Non-milk extrinsic sugars. *J Hum Nut & Dietetics.* 1994; **7:** 87.

Appendix I

(i) Main and subsidiary food groups

Food types are in bold and consist of one or more food group.
Food groups are expressed as integers.
Food subgroups are integers with an alphabetical suffix.

1	**Pasta, rice and other miscellaneous cereals**
1A	– Pasta
1B	– Rice
1C	– Pizza
1R	– Other cereals
2	**White bread**
3	**Wholemeal bread**
4	**Other breads**
4A	– Soft grain bread
4R	– Other bread
5	**Wholegrain and high fibre breakfast cereals**
6	**Other breakfast cereals**
7	**Biscuits**
8	**Buns, cakes, pastries and fruit pies**
8A	– Fruit pies
8R	– Buns, cakes and pastries
9	**Puddings and ice cream**
9A	– Milk puddings
9B	– Ice cream
9D	– Sponge type puddings
9C	– Other puddings

1–9 Total cereals and cereal products

10	**Whole milk**
11	**Semi-skimmed milk**
12	**Skimmed milk**
13	**Other milk and cream**
13A	– Infant formula
13R	– Other milk and cream
14	**Cheese**
14A	– Cottage cheese
14R	– Other cheeses
15	**Yogurt and fromage frais**
15A	– Fromage frais
15R	– Yogurt

10–15 Total milk and milk products

16	**Eggs and egg dishes**
17	**Butter**
18	**'Polyunsaturated' margarine and oils**
18A	'Polyunsaturated' margarine
18B	'Polyunsaturated' oils
19	**Low fat spread**
19A	– 'Polyunsaturated' low fat spread
19R	– Low fat spread NOT polyunsaturated
20	**Block margarine**
21	**Other margarines, spreads and oils**
21A	– Soft margarine (not polyunsaturated)
21B	– 'Polyunsaturated' reduced fat spread
21C	– Reduced fat spread (not polyunsaturated)
21R	– Cooking fats and oils (not polyunsaturated)

17–21 Total fats

22	**Bacon and ham**
23	**Beef, veal and dishes**
24	**Lamb and dishes**
25	**Pork and dishes**
26	**Coated chicken and turkey**
27	**Chicken and turkey dishes**
28	**Liver and dishes, liver paté and liver sausage**
29	**Burgers and kebabs**
30	**Sausages**
31	**Meat pies and pastries (incl. chicken pies)**
32	**Other meat and meat products (incl. game and offal; excl. liver)**

22–32 Total meat and meat products

33	**White fish, coated or fried (including fish fingers)**
34	**Other white fish, shellfish and fish dishes**
34B	– Shellfish
34A	– Other white fish and fish dishes
35	– Oily fish (incl. canned)

33–35 Total fish and fish dishes

36	**Salad and raw vegetables**
36A	– Carrots (raw)
36B	– Other salad and raw vegetables
36C	– Tomatoes (raw)
37	**Vegetables (not raw)**
37A	– Peas
37B	– Runner beans
37C	– Baked beans
37D	– Leafy green vegetables (incl. broccoli)
37E	– Carrots (not raw)
37F	– Fresh tomatoes (not raw)
37R	– Other vegetables
38	**Fried or roast potatoes (incl. chips)**
38A	– Potato chips
38B	– Other fried or roast potatoes
38R	– Other potato products
39	**Other potatoes**
42	**Savoury snacks**

36–39 & 42 Total vegetables

40	**Fruit and nuts**
40A	– Apples and pears
40B	– Oranges, tangerines, etc
40C	– Bananas
40D	– Canned fruit in juice
40E	– Canned fruit in syrup
40F	– Nuts, fruit and nut mixes
40R	– Other fruit

40 Total fruit and nuts

41	**Sugar, preserves and sweet spreads**
41A	– Sugar
41B	– Preserves
41R	– Sweet spreads, fillings and icing
43	**Sugar confectionery**

(ii) Examples of foods in food groups

FOOD GROUP		
1	Pasta, rice and other miscellaneous cereals	includes boiled/fried rice, pasta - all types (dried, fresh and canned), Yorkshire pudding, dumplings, pizza.
2	White bread	includes sliced, unsliced, french stick, milk loaf, slimmers' type, white pitta bread and white chapatis, white rolls.
3	Wholemeal bread	includes sliced, unsliced, wholemeal chapatis and pitta breads, wholemeal rolls.
4	Other breads	includes brown bread, granary, soft grain bread, high fibre white, rye, crumpets, muffins, pikelets, brown and granary rolls.
5	Wholegrain and high fibre breakfast cereals	includes All Bran, Branflakes, Shredded Wheat, muesli, porridge, Weetabix.
6	Other breakfast cereals	includes cornflakes, Rice Krispies, Special K, Sugar Puffs, Smacks.
7	Biscuits	all types, including sweet and savoury.
8	Buns, cakes, pastries and fruit pies	includes danish pastry, Chelsea bun, doughnut, Eccles cake, frangipane tart, jam tart, scones (sweet and savoury), sponge cake, fruit cake, meringue, fruit pies (all types).
9	Puddings and ice cream	includes instant whip, fruit crumble, Arctic roll, batter pudding, custard/blancmange, rice pudding, trifle, mousse, cheesecake, cream desserts, jelly, fruit fool, sponge pudding, milk pudding, sorbets, ice cream.
10	Whole milk	all types including pasteurised, UHT, sterilised, Channel Island.
11	Semi-skimmed milk	all types including pasteurised, UHT, flavoured, canned, milk with added vitamins.
12	Skimmed milk	all types including pasteurised, UHT, sterilised, canned, milk with added vitamins.
13	Other milk and cream	includes condensed, evaporated, dried milk, infant formula, goats' milk, sheep's milk, soya milk, milk shakes and all creams.
14	Cheese	all types including hard and soft cheese, cream cheese, processed cheese, cottage and curd cheese, low fat cheeses.
15	Yogurt and fromage frais	includes low fat, thick and creamy, soya yogurt, frozen yogurt, 'diet' yogurt and fromage frais, goats' and sheep's milk yogurt, yogurt drink.
16	Eggs and egg dishes	includes boiled, fried, poached, scrambled, omelette (sweet and savoury), souffle, quiche and flans, scotch egg.
17	Butter	includes butter ghee.
18	'Polyunsaturated' margarines and oils	margarines and oils that can make a claim to be high in polyunsaturated fatty acids.
19	Low fat spread	spreads containing 40% or less fat (includes polyunsaturated and non-polyunsaturated).
20	Block margarine	
21	Other margarines, spreads and oils	includes soft margarines (not polyunsaturated) and reduced fat spreads (polyunsaturated and non-polyunsaturated).
22	Bacon and ham	includes bacon joints and rashers, gammon joints/steaks, ham (all types).
23	Beef, veal and dishes	includes beef (and veal) joints, steaks, minced beef, stewing steak, beef stew and casserole, meat balls, lasagne, chilli con carne, beef curry dishes, bolognaise sauce.
24	Lamb and dishes	includes lamb joints, chops, cutlets, lamb curry dishes, Irish stew, lamb stew and casserole.
25	Pork and dishes	includes joints, chops, steaks, belly rashers, pork stew and casserole, sweet and sour pork, spare ribs.
26	Coated chicken and turkey	includes chicken and turkey drumsticks, chicken pieces, nuggetts, fingers, burgers etc. coated in egg and crumb, Kentucky Fried Chicken.
27	Chicken and turkey dishes	includes roast chicken and turkey, barbecued, fried (no coating), pieces, curry, stew and casserole, chow mein, in sauce, spread, chicken/turkey roll.

28	Liver and dishes, liver paté and liver sausage	includes all types of liver (fried, stewed, grilled), liver sausage casserole, liver sausage, liver paté.	

28 Liver and dishes, liver paté and liver sausage — includes all types of liver (fried, stewed, grilled), liver sausage casserole, liver sausage, liver paté.

29 Burgers and kebabs — includes beefburger, hamburger, cheeseburger (with or without roll), doner/shish/kofte kebab (with pitta bread and salad).

30 Sausages — includes beef, pork, turkey, polony, sausage in batter, saveloy, frankfurter, peperoni.

31 Meat pies and pastries — includes chicken/turkey pie, vol-au-vent, beef pie, steak and kidney pie, pork pie, veal and ham pie, pasty, sausage roll, meat samosa.

32 Other meat and meat products — includes game (eg duck, grouse, hare, pheasant), rabbit, offal (not liver), faggots, black pudding, meat paste, tongue, luncheon meat, corned beef salami, meat loaf, chop suey.

33 White fish coated or fried including fish fingers — includes cod, haddock, hake, plaice etc, coated in egg and crumb, batter or flour and any fried fish without coating; coated fried cartilaginous fish (eg dogfish, skate), scampi, fillet-o-fish, fish cakes, fish fingers, cod roe fried, prawn balls.

34 Other white fish, shellfish and fish dishes — includes cod, haddock, hake, plaice etc, (poached, grilled, smoked, dried), shellfish, curried fish, fish paste, fish in sauce, fish pie, kedgeree.

35 Oily fish — includes herrings, kippers, mackerel, sprats, eels, herring roe (baked, fried, grilled), salmon, tuna, sardines, taramasalata, mackerel paté.

36 Salad and raw vegetables — includes raw leafy green vegetables (eg endive, lettuce, chicory), other raw vegetables (eg cabbage, carrots, tomatoes, radish, spring onion), coleslaw, purchased prepared salad.

37 Vegetables (not raw) — includes beans/pulses, baked beans, cooked vegetables, vegetable stew and casserole, vegetable curry dishes, tofu, ratatouille, vegetable lasagne and cauliflower cheese, vegieburgers.

38 Fried or roast potatoes incl. chips — chips (fresh and frozen), oven chips, potato waffles, hash browns, roast, sautéed, croquettes.

39 Other potatoes — includes boiled, mashed, jacket, potato salad, canned potato, potato-based curry, instant potato.

40 Fruit and nuts — includes fruit cooked (with and without sugar), raw, canned, dried, fruit pie filling (not fruit pie); nuts incl. almonds, hazelnuts, mixed nuts, peanuts, peanut butter, bombay mix, seeds (eg sunflower, sesame).

41 Sugars, preserves and sweet spreads — includes sugar (white and brown), glucose liquid/powder, black molasses, treacle, syrup, honey, jam, marmalade (incl. low sugar varieties), glacé cherries, mixed peel, marzipan, chocolate spread, icing, ice cream sauce.

42 Savoury snacks — includes crisps, other potato and cereal products (eg puffs, rings), Twiglets.

43 Confectionery—sugar — includes boiled sweets, gums, pastilles, fudge, chews, mints, rock, liquorice, toffee, popcorn.

44 Confectionery—chocolate — includes chocolate bars, filled bars, assortments.

45 Fruit juice — includes single fruit and mixed fruit 100% juices; canned, bottled, carton; carbonated, still, freshly squeezed; includes vegetable juice.

46 Soft drinks, including diet or low calorie — includes carbonated soft drinks (eg lemonade, coca cola), fruit squash, cordial, fruit drink (concentrated or ready to drink), Ribena, rosehip syrup, mineral water, tonic water.

47 Spirits and liqueurs — includes cream liqueurs, Pernod, Southern Comfort, 70% proof spirits, Pimms.

48 Wine — includes white, red, rosé, sparkling, champagne, port, sherry.

49 Beer/cider/perry — includes beer and lager (both non-premium and premium and low alcohol versions), stout, strong ale (bottled, draught and canned), cider and low alcohol cider, Babycham, perry.

50 Miscellaneous — includes sauces, ketchup, condiments, chutney, pickle, gravy, mayonnaise, soup, beverages (not tea or coffee) and herbal tea.

51 Tea, coffee and water — instant and leaf/bean, also lemon tea, vending machine tea and coffee; tap water.

52 Commercial infant and toddler foods and drinks — includes instant and ready to eat foods and drinks specifically manufactured for the infant and young child.

53 Vitamin and mineral supplements — includes vitamin and mineral preparations in tablet, liquid or syrup form; cod liver oil; fluoride supplements.

54 Artificial sweeteners — includes granulated table top sweeteners; liquid, tablet or mini cube sweeteners.

Appendix J

Number and pattern of recording days and the effect of weighting

1 Number of days

The number of days over which to collect the dietary record and hence energy and nutrient intakes for an individual are an important consideration. Ideally sufficient numbers of days are required to give reliable information on usual food consumption and hence nutrient intakes, but previous studies have shown that the number of days to achieve a given reliability of classification of individuals into quantiles of the distribution for different nutrients varies [1,2,3]. In addition, consideration has to be given to the likelihood of poor compliance, the possible interference with eating habits and the cost if the recording period is lengthy.

It is generally accepted that for free-living subjects seven days is sufficiently long to obtain representative assessments of daily energy, protein, fat and carbohydrate intakes[2]. However in planning this survey it was recognised that it might not be feasible to collect information on food consumption for all seven days of the week. It was therefore necessary to investigate whether fewer days would provide adequate estimates of intake and if particular days or types of day, that is weekend days and weekdays, were significantly different from each other, in order to arrive at informed decisions on how many and on which days recording should take place.

A four-day period was chosen for the feasibility study, comprising two weekdays and the weekend, as this was felt to be long enough to include most of the range of foods that pre-school children eat, but not to be so long as to affect adversely the quality of response[4]. For some children, day of the week probably does make a difference to what they eat; for example, mothers may work on one day but not on another which might mean that the child is fed differently on working and non-working days. However, as this will vary between mothers, overall the picture is likely to be reasonably representative.

The mothers who took part in the feasibility study were asked whether they would have been prepared to complete the dietary record for seven days; 61% said they could have carried on keeping the dietary record for longer but of these 44% qualified their answer saying that although they could have gone on longer they were glad they did not have to do so. Many mentioned that they would have had difficulty maintaining motivation and some said they thought the accuracy would have declined had they gone on longer; 39% thought four days was the maximum they could have managed. The feasibility report concluded that four days was likely to be the maximum period acceptable to respondents if a high level of co-operation was to be obtained[4].

This decision was supported by the fact that in the feasibility study estimates of energy expenditure using doubly-labelled water showed a high level of agreement for the three one-year age cohorts when compared with energy intake estimated from the four-day weighed intake record (*Appendix E*).

Energy and nutrient intake data from the feasibility study were analysed and the standard deviation ratio (SDR) for each of a number of nutrients was calculated by MAFF to predict the effect of the number of diary days on the precision of the main survey's estimates for each nutrient of interest. The SDR is the ratio of the standard deviation over individuals' average intake levels (*inter* individual) to the average of each individual's standard deviation over separate days (*intra* individual):

$$SDR = SD_{inter} / SD_{intra}$$

The observed Standard Deviation Ratios (SDR) for the selected nutrients, energy (kcal), carbohydrate, starch, sugar, protein, total fat, total saturated fatty acids, percentage energy from fat, ratio of polyunsaturated to saturated fatty acids (P:S), iron, and zinc, ranged from 0.74 to 1.04 and were typically around 0.8 to 0.9 (*Table 1*). For some nutrients the distribution of intake is skewed, and a logarithmic transformation was used. The same analysis was therefore applied to the natural logarithms of the nutrient intakes. The results are set out in Table 2; with the exception of energy and percentage energy from fat, taking logarithms made little difference to the SDR. MAFF used theoretical probability distributions to demonstrate that values of SDR in the region of 0.8 to 0.9 were likely to provide sufficient precision for the main survey's estimates for each nutrient. *(Tables 1 and 2)*

The analysis demonstrated that if the feasibility study statistics continued to hold true for the main survey, at least 90% of individuals would be successfully classified with 95% confidence at the upper or lower decile with a group size of 250 children. When terciles were examined, the success rate for classification decreased to around 65% to 75% of individuals correctly classified in their own tercile. However where it is necessary to distinguish the highest, or indeed the lowest, tercile from the other two, rather than model all three simultaneously, there is about 85% correct classification.

2 Days of the week

The significance of differences between each individual's intake by days of the week and by type, that is weekend days and weekdays, was assessed both by a non-parametric sign test and by Student's t-test. The sign test was used in order to test the hypothesis that the number of children whose consumption increases is equal to the number whose consumption decreases. Student's t-test allowed examination of the actual difference in intake for each child; it was used to test the hypothesis that the true mean difference is zero. The latter test is more powerful, but strictly depends on assumptions of Normality for its validity.

Statistical significance (probability level) for the non-parametric sign test and the Student's t-test along with 95% confidence intervals (CI) of the differences found in the mean nutrient intake for selected nutrients for all the subjects between Monday and Friday, between Saturday and Sunday, and between weekdays and weekend days are shown in Table 3. The confidence intervals are in terms of percentage deviance from the unweighted average intake levels for the nutrients. *(Table 3)*

There were statistically significant differences using the sign test between weekdays and weekend days for starch. The t-test revealed significantly different intakes of total energy, carbohydrate, starch, sugar, and iron on weekdays and weekend days. The sign test showed a significant difference in the intake of protein between Saturday and Sunday.

The sample was not nationally representative nor was it controlled for the representation of social class or other factors that might be thought to affect dietary behaviour. However, it was necessarily assumed that a sample of 1500 children in the main survey would exhibit similar behaviour.

In any dietary record with fewer than seven days there is a need to consider the choice of diary recording days. Investigation of differences in average nutrient intake for certain nutrients on different days of the week revealed significant differences between weekdays and weekend days. Although the p-values quoted for both the non-parametric sign test and the t-test are not expected to be in complete agreement, they do tend to agree on the highly significant differences. While protein was the only nutrient for which there was a significant difference in intakes between Saturdays and Sundays according to the sign test, this was not strictly confirmed by the t-test (p=0.07). However, owing to the relatively small number of cases in the feasibility study, the t-test can only return significant results (p<0.05) for differences of 14% or more. Since the greater size of the mainstage survey means that smaller real differences, around 10%, are detectable, this was taken as sufficient evidence of the likelihood of actual differences between the two weekend days.

3 Weighting the dietary data and the effect when estimating the food consumption and nutrient intake

In order to produce information on food consumption and nutrient intakes which would allow comparisons to be made with other dietary survey data, which are conventionally expressed as seven-day intakes, the food consumption data was weighted to provide an estimate of the total amount consumed over a seven-day period. Thus the total consumption of each item of food and drink recorded for the two weekdays was multiplied by $5 \div 2$ and then added to the total consumption of the item recorded for Saturday and Sunday. The weighting applied to the data assumes that the consumption pattern on the three non-recording weekdays will be the same as on the two recording weekdays; information for the two weekend days is not subject to any reweighting. While the analysis of nutrients described above provides reasonable confidence that the intake of nutrients for the sample does not differ significantly between weekdays, there are possible effects of weighting on the amounts of foods consumed.

In Chapter 4 the proportion of the sample of children consuming a food represents consumers over a four-day period and is likely to be lower than the proportion of those children who would be consumers of this food over a seven-day period. For most staple foods eaten daily the effect of weighting on the amounts of food consumed and hence the intakes of nutrients is negligible but for foods eaten infrequently, for example less than twice a week (foods such as liver and oily fish), the effect of weighting on the measures of mean and median for consumers is difficult to predict. Any effect would be at the individual level rather than at the population level.

For example, if a child's regular eating pattern includes consumption of fish on only one weekday, and that weekday happens to be one of the two recorded weekdays, then the amount consumed by that individual child will be overesti-

mated as a result of weighting the mean of the two weekdays up to five days. The estimated consumption of fish for this individual child would be 2.5 times the 'true' amount for five weekdays and similarly for the seven days if no fish was eaten on Saturday and Sunday. For example, 50g fish for one day becomes 125g for the five weekdays and hence for the weighted estimate for seven days.

However there is also a chance that the child will not eat fish on either of the two recording days which would lead to an underestimation of fish consumption for that child since weighting can only be applied to the foods consumed on the recording days. Clearly for such infrequently eaten foods the estimate of the amount eaten for an individual child based on four days recorded intake reweighted is unreliable. But estimates for population groups of the mean and median amounts of an infrequently eaten food remain unbiased after weighting, given that each child has an equal chance of being a consumer or non-consumer over the recording period. Even without reweighting there is an underestimation of the number of consumers and thereby an overestimation of the mean for consumers.

Weighting has also been observed to affect the nutrient intake at the individual level where an infrequently eaten food is also a food with a high level of a particular nutrient. For example liver has a high level of retinol and iron (lamb's liver, fried contains $22680\mu g$ retinol/100g and 10mg iron/100g[5]) and, as a result, where liver has been eaten on a recorded weekday and reweighted the estimation of retinol and iron for that individual will be high. The effect of this on the mean and median intakes of these nutrients at the population level should be negligible. However there is an effect at the extreme end of the range of intakes where an estimated high intake of a nutrient might appear to be an outlier. The results of nutrient intakes are presented in this report as reweighted daily estimates of population mean, median, lower and upper 2.5 percentiles and standard error of the mean. Any effect at individual level at the extremes of intakes will only be apparent when considering the full range of intakes, for example minimum and maximum, and then only for a limited number of foods and nutrients.

References

1 Marr JW, Heady JA. Within-and between-person variation in dietary surveys: Number of days needed to classify individuals. *Hum Nut: App Nut.* 1986; **40A:** 347–364

2 Levine JA, Morgan MY. Assessment of dietary intake in man: a review of available methods. *Journal of Nutritional Medicine.* 1991; **2:** 65-81.

3 James WPT, Bingham SA, Cole TJ. Epidemiological assessment of dietary intake. *Nutrition and Cancer.* 1981; 2: **4:** 203–212.

4 White A, Davies PSW. *Feasibility Study for the National Diet and Nutrition Survey of Children aged 1½ to 4½ years.* OPCS (1994) (NM22).

5 Holland B, Welsh AA, Unwin ID, Buss DH, Paul AA and Southgate DAT. *McCance and Widdowson's The Composition of Foods.* 5th edition. HMSO (London, 1991).

Table 1 Inter-SD and intra-SD and SDR for nutrients

Direct values: intake or attribute	Mean daily intake $n=93$	Inter-SD $n=93$	Intra-SD* $n=93$	SDR**
Energy (kcal)	1140	209	261	0.80
Sugar (g)	98.3	24.0	28.6	0.84
Fat (g)	43.9	11.1	15.0	0.74
% energy from fat	31.9	4.8	6.0	0.80
P:S ratio	0.38	0.16	0.2	0.81
Iron (mg)	5.4	1.80	1.7	1.04
Zinc (mg)	4.2	1.30	1.5	0.87

*Intra-SD values are the means of unbiased estimates of individuals'
standard deviations over four days of recorded intake.
**SDR = Standard Deviation Ratio = Inter-SD ÷ Intra-SD
These estimates of SDR are slightly biased. The unbiased estimates
are very similar.

Table 2 Inter-SD and intra-SD and SDR for natural log nutrients

Natural logs: intake or attribute	Mean daily intake $n=93$	Inter-SD $n=93$	Intra-SD* $n=93;$	SDR**
Log energy	7.0	0.18	0.24	0.74
Log sugar	4.5	0.26	0.30	0.87
Log fat	3.7	0.28	0.38	0.74
Log % energy from fat	3.4	0.18	0.21	0.87
Log P:S ratio	−1.13	0.41	0.52	0.79
Log iron	1.6	0.33	0.32	1.02
Log zinc	1.3	0.33	0.38	0.87

*Intra-SD values are the means of unbiased estimates of individuals'
standard deviations over four days of recorded intake.
**SDR=Standard Deviation Ratio = Inter-SD ÷ Intra-SD
These estimates of SDR are slightly biased. The unbiased estimates
are very similar.

Table 3 Differences between days

	Sign test	Student's t-statistic	
	p-value	p-value	95% confidence interval % of joint mean
Energy (kcal)			
Monday v Friday	0.22	0.35	(−4, 11)
Saturday v Sunday	0.40	0.40	(−11, 4)
Weekend day v Weekday	0.30	**0.02**	**(3, 12)**
Total fat (g)			
Monday v Friday	0.46	0.92	(−10, 11)
Saturday v Sunday	0.83	1.00	(-10, 10)
Weekend day v Weekday	0.53	0.11	(−1, 13)
Saturated fat (g)			
Monday v Friday	0.81	0.72	(−3, 12)
Saturday v Sunday	0.67	0.95	(−10, 12)
Weekend day v Weekday	1.00	0.22	(−9, 13)
Carbohydrate (g)			
Monday v Friday	1.00	0.17	(−2, 13)
Saturday v Sunday	0.20	0.30	(−12, 4)
Weekend day v Weekday	0.06	**<0.01**	**(5, 15)**
Starch (g)			
Monday v Friday	0.22	0.14	(−3, 18)
Saturday v Sunday	0.09	0.07	(−21, 1)
Weekend day v Weekday	**<0.01**	**<0.01**	**(6, 18)**
Sugar (g)			
Monday v Friday	1.00	0.33	(−5, 14)
Saturday v Sunday	0.83	1.00	(−9, 9)
Weekend day v Weekday	0.06	**<0.01**	**(3, 15)**
Protein (g)			
Monday v Friday	0.81	0.25	(−4, 16)
Saturday v Sunday	0.02	0.07	(−15, 1)
Weekend day v Weekday	0.68	0.60	(−5, 8)
Iron (mg)			
Monday v Friday	0.46	0.09	(−2, 23)
Saturday v Sunday	0.83	0.69	(−11, 8)
Weekend day v Weekday	0.06	0.02	**(2, 15)**

Appendix K

Blood analytes in order of priority for analysis

Analyte	No of cases with reported results	Unit of measurement	Conversion from SI units (factor)	Resulting metric units
Haematology				
Haemoglobin concentration	951	g/dl	*	*
Mean corpuscular volume	951	fl	*	*
Haematocrit	951	l/l	*	*
Mean cell haemoglobin	951	pg	*	*
Mean cell haemoglobin concentration	951	g/dl	*	*
Ferritin	930	μg/l	*	*
Zinc protoporphyrin	950	μmol/mol haem	**	**
Water soluble vitamins and plasma zinc				
Plasma folate	819	nmol/l	× 0.441	μg/l
Vitamin B$_{12}$	817	pmol/l	× 1.357	ng/l
The erythrocyte glutathione reductase activation coefficient	828	ratio	***	***
Plasma zinc	602	μmol/l	× 0.065	mg/l
Fat soluble vitamins and carotenoids				
Plasma retinol	816	μmol/l	× 0.286	mg/l
α-carotene	807	μmol/l	× 0.537	mg/l
ß-carotene	812	μmol/l	× 0.537	mg/l
α-cryptoxanthin	811	μmol/l	× 0.552	mg/l
ß-cryptoxanthin	813	μmol/l	× 0.552	mg/l
Lycopene	807	μmol/l	× 0.537	mg/l
Lutein	812	μmol/l	× 0.569	mg/l
Plasma 25-hydroxyvitamin D	737	nmol/l	× 0.400	mg/l
α-tocopherol	816	μmol/l	× 0.552	mg/l
γ-tocopherol	816	μmol/l	× 0.417	mg/l
Blood lipids				
Plasma triglycerides	682	mmol/l	****	****
Plasma total cholesterol	683	mmol/l	× 0.387	g/l
High density lipoprotein cholesterol	683	mmol/l	× 0.387	g/l
Acute phase proteins				
Caeruloplasmin	763	g/l	*	*
α$_1$-antichymotrypsin	763	g/l	*	*
Albumin	754	g/l	*	*
Red cell folate	743	nmol/l	× 0.441	μg/l
Plasma ascorbate	744	μmol/l	× 0.176	mg/l
Immunoglobulins				
IgA	105	g/l	*	*
IgG	106	g/l	*	*
IgM	99	g/l	*	*

* Analyte measured in metric units.

** The metabolite ratio μmol/mol haem is the expression of choice. Porphyrin concentration units found in the literature include:
> μg ZPP/dl whole blood
> μg ZPP/dl RBC
> μg ZPP/g haemoglobin.

Direct, retrospective conversion to the ratio is not possible without haemoglobin concentration having been obtained at the time of the ZPP assay. Where this is available, the conversion becomes, for example:
> (μg ZPP * 64,500) : (g Hb * 562.27 * 4)
> = (μg ZPP/g haemoglobin) * 28.68
> = μmol ZPP/mol haem.

*** Analyte measured as a ratio.

**** Triglycerides are measured as glycerol; the molecular weight of a triglyceride molecule varies with different fatty acid constituents; conversion from SI to metric units is not appropriate.

Appendix L

The blood sample: further information on stages up to and including local laboratory processing of the collected samples

Chapter 2 gave details of the purpose of taking the blood samples and of the blood sampling procedures up to the stage at which the blood sample was taken, including the training of the phlebotomists, the consent procedures that preceded taking the sample, and the system for reporting results to parents and children's General Practitioners.

This Appendix gives further information on these, including details on the recruitment of the phlebotomists and also describes the stages in the local laboratory processing of the collected samples. It includes tables giving information on the outcomes of the attempts to take blood, for example the number of attempts made and the volume of blood obtained. Copies of the various consent forms and letters for reporting results to parents and GPs that were used on the survey will be found in Appendix M.

The final stage processing of the blood samples, methods of analysis and the laboratory quality control procedures are described in Appendix N.

1 Recruitment of the phlebotomists

Attempts were made to recruit a phlebotomist in each of the survey areas. The first approach was usually made to the head of the haematology laboratory in the hospital closest to the survey area. Details of the survey were discussed with the head laboratory manager and written information provided about the survey background and the requirements. The laboratory manager was usually then able to recommend a potentially suitable phlebotomist.

Any potential phlebotomist needed to have current experience in venepuncture procedures in children under 5 years of age and be reasonably available for variable appointment times made by the interviewer. The majority of phlebotomists recruited to the survey were already working part time, usually in the morning, and consequently the majority of blood samples were obtained in the early afternoon.

A written reference was obtained from each phlebotomist's manager or head of department. In a few areas where it was not possible to recruit a local phlebotomist, local hospital doctors or general practitioners took the blood samples.

2 The recruitment of a local processor of the blood sample

Some local processing of the blood sample (described in detail below) was required. In many cases the phlebotomist undertook this work at his or her hospital but if the recruited phlebotomist did not have the appropriate experience in laboratory-based procedures another member of the laboratory staff undertook the local processing requirements. In a few cases processing of the sample took place at a hospital laboratory other than that normally employing the phlebotomist.

3 The equipment provided

Each phlebotomist was sent all the equipment that would be required, except needles and syringes. These they were asked to provide themselves to ensure that they would be familiar and confident with the equipment being used. The equipment sent to each phlebotomist consisted of:

- 1ml ethylenediamine tetra-acetic acid (EDTA) containers
- 5ml lithium heparin containers
- padded protective bags ('Jiffy' bags) pre-addressed to the Department of Haematology, Hospital for Sick Children, Great Ormond Street, London, and stamped.
- plastic or cardboard protective containers for EDTA containers
- sharps disposal bin
- plastic sample rack
- sticky tape and tissues
- subject record card
- re-freezable ice brick.

Each local processor was sent a number of 2ml containers for the storage of processed blood and small polythene resealable bags. The containers had red, blue, green or neutral caps for the different aliquots of the whole blood sample. The green-capped contained 0.15ml (10% w/v) metaphosphoric acid to stabilise vitamin C in a plasma sample; the blue-capped contained 1.35ml (1% w/v) ascorbic acid (pH 4.6) to stabilise red cell folate and the red and neutral-capped contained no stabiliser. Both the blue and green-capped containers were kept frozen until a blood sample was being processed.

4 The venepuncture procedure

Approval for venepuncture as part of the survey protocol had been obtained from each Local NHS Ethics Committee.

Once witnessed, written consent to the blood sample being taken had been obtained, the OPCS interviewer arranged a suitable appointment time to call with the phlebotomist at the child's home[1]. In making an appointment, as well as the convenience to the family and the availability of the phlebotomist, the following constraints needed to be taken into account:

- The blood sample had to be taken in the child's home.
- Sufficient time had to be allowed to put the child and family at ease prior to and following the venepuncture.
- The blood sample had to be delivered to the local laboratory within 4 hours, and in sufficient time for the initial local processing to be done that day.
- A portion (1ml) of the sample needed to be posted to Great Ormond Street Hospital, before the last postal collection that day.

Although consent to the blood sample being taken had been given, if in the professional opinion of the phlebotomist the child or family was overtly distressed venepuncture was not attempted. Consent by the child or parent could be withdrawn at any time.

Parents were offered the choice of venepuncture or a finger prick and the interviewer explained that venepuncture was less painful. If a finger prick was still requested up to 1ml of blood could be taken. Only 7% of the attempts to obtain a blood sample used fingerprick.

The venepuncture procedures adopted in this survey were designed to produce minimal anxiety, trauma and pain to the child. Only skilled phlebotomists were recruited and venepuncture procedures were monitored. Some NHS Local Ethics Committees approved the protocol only if it included the use of local anaesthetic cream prior to venepuncture. Emla cream is a preparation of lignocaine for surface anaesthesia. It was applied over both ante-cubital fossae for at least one hour before venepuncture. Although effective in reducing the pain of needle insertion, there were concerns that the prolonged wait before anaesthesia was induced, might engender anxiety. There were also concerns that this ointment might cause contamination of the blood sample especially with zinc, although subsequent laboratory tests did not confirm this.

The protocol, as approved by the local NHS Ethics Committees, allowed only two attempts to obtain blood. Even if a parent encouraged the phlebotomists to try again, which sometimes occurred, no further attempts could be made. In 90% of cases only one attempt to obtain blood was made — although it should be noted that not all of these resulted in blood being obtained. Blood taken by venepuncture was taken only from the ante-cubital fossa or the back of the hand[2].

The blood was divided as follows:

- 1ml of whole blood was placed in the 1ml EDTA container, gently mixed by inversion and labelled with the child's serial number. The container was placed in the plastic or cardboard protective container. This container was placed in the pre-stamped and addressed 'Jiffy' bag with a card showing the child's date of birth, sex and serial number. The bag was sealed and posted to the Department of Haematology, Hospital for Sick Children, Great Ormond Street, that day, before the last postal collection.
- Any remaining blood was placed in the 5ml lithium heparin container, labelled with the child's serial number and placed next to the plastic ice brick in a small opaque bag. The lithium heparin container was kept cool and in the dark prior to processing in the laboratory.

A report form was completed by the phlebotomist following a visit to a child. This recorded:

- the child's serial number;
- the date and time venepuncture or finger prick was attempted;
- the child's date of birth and sex;
- the site of the first and second attempt (if any), that is, ante-cubital fossa or hand;
- a brief description of why venepuncture or finger prick was not attempted, if this was the case;
- the total volume of blood taken, recorded to nearest half ml;
- a record of whether a sample was sent to the Hospital for Sick Children, London;

and after local processing at the laboratory:

- a record of containers used in processing, B(lue), G(reen), N(eutral), R(ed);
- the time the containers were put in the freezer;
- comments, that is any information that may be relevant;
- laboratory comments.

If the phlebotomist was not carrying out the processing, liaison with the laboratory was necessary to complete the last four points.

Tables 1 to 5 give information on attempts made to obtain blood, the site of venepuncture attempts, the volume of blood obtained and the proportion of cases where some difficulty in obtaining or attempting to obtain a sample was recorded by the interviewer or phlebotomist on the survey questionnaire.

(Tables 1 to 5)

In the laboratory one of two procedures was adopted depending on how much blood was obtained from the child.

If 4ml of blood had been obtained, the blood in the lithium heparin container was mixed thoroughly by inversion; 0.15ml was removed and added to the blue capped-container and mixed by inversion. This container was labelled with the child's serial number and placed into a small polythene bag. This sample was used for red cell folate analysis.

The lithium heparin container was then centrifuged for 15 minutes at 3,000 RPM at 4°C; 0.15ml of plasma was removed placed into the green- capped container and mixed in a vortex mixer. This container was also labelled with the child's serial number and placed into a small polythene bag for later vitamin C analysis.

Using a clean plastic Pasteur pipette the remaining plasma from the lithium heparin container was placed in the neutral-capped container, serial-number labelled, and put into another small polythene bag.

The remaining red blood cells were washed by adding approximately a dual volume of saline to the lithium heparin tube using a clean plastic Pasteur pipette. The red blood cells were mixed with the saline by inversion, re-centrifuged as above and the layer of saline was discarded by pipette. The cells were washed twice in this way.

Using a clean wide-tipped plastic Pasteur pipette the cells were removed and placed in the red-capped container; this was labelled with the serial number and placed into a further small polythene bag.

The four bags of containers were placed into a larger polythene bag in a freezer at −40°C or below.

If between 1ml and 2.5ml of blood was obtained, only plasma and washed red cells were stored. The blue-capped (red cell folate analysis) and the green-capped (vitamin C analysis) containers were not used because these analyses had lower priority.

Samples were stored locally usually until the end of fieldwork in each area when samples were transferred to the Dunn Nutrition Unit, Cambridge, with the completed data forms.

The samples arrived on dry ice at times pre-arranged between the Dunn Nutrition Unit and the local laboratory. On arrival the samples were kept on dry ice while sorted into colour/analyte categories and serial number order. Each serial number was recorded and compared with details from the phlebotomists' data forms to ensure that all samples had been received by the Dunn Nutrition Unit and that the local processing was in agreement with laboratory documentation.

The samples were then filed in a colour-coded system for storage in a −80°C freezer. Green, blue, red and neutral-capped containers were filed in separate freezer containers. As areas did not complete their contribution to the survey in numerical order freezer filing was random in relation to the area code element of the serial number, but was ordered with regards to the children within each area. Samples from the individual fieldwork waves of the survey were also numerically identified.

Notes

1 If the child's parents wished to discuss some aspect of the blood sample with the phlebotomist before deciding whether to consent to the procedure, the appointment for the interviewer and phlebotomist to call had to be made before obtaining consent, but no attempt was made to take a sample from the child until the consent forms were signed and witnessed. This sometimes meant a further appointment had to be made after the discussion between the child's parents and the phlebotomist (see also *Chapter 2, section 2.7.3*). Copies of the various consent forms used in the survey are included in Appendix M.

2 A consideration of the ethical aspects of taking blood from preschool children for survey purposes has been submitted for publication. It includes an analysis of the responses of parents and of children to the request for a blood sample and to the procedure of venepuncture. These data were collected as a separate study, by postal questionnaire after the main study fieldwork had been completed. Davies PSW, Collins DL, Clarke P C. *Reactions to Venepuncture in Children aged 1½ to 4½ years.* In preparation.

Table 1 Proportion of children from whom a second attempt to obtain a blood sample was made by age and sex of child*

Age and sex of child	% where a second attempt made	All children from whom attempted to obtain a blood sample = 100%
All aged 1½ – 2½ years	15	378
All aged 2½ – 3½ years	8	400
All aged 3½ – 4½ years	8	324
All boys	10	555
All girls	10	547
All children	10	1102

* Maximum of 2 attempts allowed.

Table 2 Site of first and second attempt to obtain blood*

Site of attempt to obtain blood	1st attempt	2nd attempt	All attempts
	%	%	%
By venepuncture:			
from ante-cubital fossa	83	60	81
from hand	12	13	12
By fingerprick	5	23	7
Not recorded	0	3	7
Total attempts to obtain blood = 100%	1102	116	1218

* Maximum of 2 attempts allowed.

Table 3 Site of attempts to obtain a blood sample by age and sex of child*

Site of attempt to obtain blood	Age of child			Sex of child		All children
	1½ – 2½ years	2½ – 3½ years	3½ – 4½ years	Boys	Girls	
	%	%	%	%	%	%
By venepuncture:						
from ante-cubital fossa	78	83	83	82	79	81
from hand	12	11	11	11	12	12
By fingerprick	10	5	5	6	8	7
Not recorded	1	1	1	1	0	1
Total attempts to obtain blood sample = 100%	436	433	349	613	605	1218

* Maximum of 2 attempts allowed.

Table 4 Volume of blood obtained from children from whom attempted to obtain a blood sample by age and sex of child*

Volume of blood obtained	Age of child			Sex of child		All children
	1½ – 2½ years	2½ – 3½ years	3½ – 4½ years	Boys	Girls	
	%	%	%	%	%	%
None	11	9	7	9	9	9
Less than 1ml	8	4	6	7	6	6
1ml – less than 2ml	13	6	5	7	9	8
2ml – less than 3ml	6	6	4	5	6	6
3ml – less than 4ml	8	10	6	8	8	8
4ml	54	64	71	63	62	62
All children from whom attempted to obtain blood sample = 100%	378	400	324	555	547	1102

* Maximum of 4ml allowed.

Table 5 Proportion of children where difficulties in obtaining or attempting to obtain a blood sample were reported*

Age and sex of child	% where difficulties reported	All children from whom attempted to obtain a blood sample = 100%
All aged 1½ – 2½ years	34	378
All aged 2½ – 3½ years	27	400
All aged 3½ – 4½ years	24	324
All boys	27	555
All girls	30	547
All children	29	1102

* Difficulties reported by the interviewer or blood taker.

Appendix M

(i) Letters to parents and General Practitioners reporting normal and abnormal blood results

Dunn Nutrition Centre *Patron:* **HRH The Princess Royal**

Dunn Nutrition Group
MRC Laboratories
Fajara
Nr Banjul P.O. Box 273
The Gambia
West Africa

Dunn Clinical Nutrition Centre
Hills Road
Cambridge
CB2 2DH

tel: (0223) 415695
fax: (0223) 413763

Telegrams Tropmedres, Banjul

Please reply to:
Dunn Nutritional Laboratory
Downhams Lane
Milton Road
Cambridge
CB4 1XJ

tel: (0223) 426356
fax: (0223) 426617

Dear Parents or Guardians,

You will doubtless remember taking part recently in the National Diet and Nutrition Survey of children aged 1.5 to 4.5 years, being carried out by Social Survey Division of the Office of Population Censuses and Surveys for the Departments of Health and the Ministry of Agriculture, Fisheries and Food.

As part of the survey you were kind enough to consent to a sample of blood being taken from your child for analysis. We said that we would be letting you and if you agreed, your child's GP, know the results of the measurement of haemoglobin.

Your childs haemoglobin result was   g/dl. We would normally expect the result to be over 11g/dl.

Thank you for helping with the survey.

Yours faithfully,

Peter S.W. Davies B.Sc, M.Phil, Ph.D
MRC Staff Scientist
Infant & Child Nutrition Group

Medical Research Council and the University of Cambridge

Dunn Nutrition Centre *Patron:* **HRH The Princess Royal**

Dunn Nutrition Group
MRC Laboratories
Fajara
Nr Banjul P.O. Box 273
The Gambia
West Africa

Dunn Clinical Nutrition Centre
100 Tennis Court Road
Cambridge
CB2 1QL

fax: (0223) 460089
tel: (0223) 312314

Telegrams Tropmedres, Banjul

Please reply to:
Dunn Nutritional Laboratory
Downhams Lane
Milton Road
Cambridge
CB4 1XJ

tel: (0223) 426356
fax: (0223) 426617
telex: 818448 (DUNN UK)

INFORMATION FOR PARENTS

The Departments of Health and the Ministry of Agriculture, Fisheries and Food have decided that there is a need to measure the amount and type of food young children are eating in Great Britain. The Social Survey Division of the Office of Population Censuses and Surveys is undertaking these measurements and will be inviting you to record the amount of food your child eats, as well as measuring your child's height and weight.

As part of the survey we would also like to take a small sample of blood from your child's arm.

The Medical Research Council's Dunn Nutrition Unit have been asked by the Departments of Health and the Ministry of Agriculture, Fisheries and Food to take responsibility for the arrangements associated with obtaining the blood samples. We are working closely with the Social Survey Division and we together with Great Ormond Street Hospital will be analysing the blood samples.

The blood will be taken by a suitably trained person who is qualified and skilled in taking blood from small children. He or she will be accompanied by the Social Survey interviewer and they will take time to put your child at ease. We are asking for a sample to be taken from the child's arm because this is less painful than a finger prick. If you would prefer your child to have a finger prick then we are happy to do so.

We would be grateful if you would agree to your child providing us with a sample of blood. This is a very important aspect of the survey as the analysis of all the blood samples will tell us a lot about the health of the children in the survey in relation to what they eat and their body measurements. You are, of course, free to choose not to consent to a blood sample being taken.

The blood sample will be sent to the medical laboratories for a number of analyses, including levels of haemoglobin, ferritin and vitamins; it will not be used to look for infections such as AIDS.

Haemoglobin is the red pigment in the blood which carries oxygen. A low level of haemoglobin in the blood is called anaemia. One reason for a low level of haemoglobin may be shortage of iron. Ferritin is a measure of the body's iron stores.

If any of these measurements are abnormal we will, if you agree, inform your general practitioner, who will be able to advise you about treatment.

Medical Research Council and the University of Cambridge

Patron: **HRH The Princess Royal**

Dunn Nutrition Centre

Dunn Nutrition Group
MRC Laboratories
Fajara
Nr Banjul P.O. Box 273
The Gambia
West Africa

telegrams: Tropmedres, Banjul

tel: (0223) 415695
fax: (0223) 413763

Dunn Clinical Nutrition Centre
Hills Road
Cambridge
CB2 2DH

Please reply to:
Dunn Nutritional Laboratory
Downhams Lane
Milton Road
Cambridge
CB4 1XJ

tel: (0223) 426356
fax: (0223) 426617

Dear Parents or Guardians,

You will doubtless remember taking part recently in the National Diet and Nutrition Survey of children aged 1.5 to 4.5 years being carried out by the Social Survey Division of the Office of Population Censuses and Surveys for the Departments of Health and the Ministry of Agriculture, Fisheries and Food.

As part of the survey you were kind enough to consent to a sample of blood being taken from your child for analysis. We offered to report to parents or guardians any abnormal result for Haemoglobin (g/dl), Zinc Protoporphyrin (µmol/mol haem), Ferritin (µg/l), Vitamin A and Vitamin D. In the case of your child we found the following result:

which falls outside the expected range for a child of this age. Such a value is often associated with anaemia.

It is likely that your child's GP could find out the cause of this, and I suggest that you arrange for «child» to see him or her at your convenience. As you agreed at the time, I am writing to your child's GP to let him/her know of this result.

Thank you for helping with the survey.

Yours faithfully,

Peter S.W. Davies   B.Sc. M.Phil, Ph.D
MRC Staff Scientist
Infant & Child Nutrition Group

Alternative versions of the letter opposite were sent to parents whose children had no GP, and to parents who had not consented to their child's GP being informed of any abnormal blood result.

If no GP, the penultimate paragraph read:

It is likely that a family doctor (GP) could find out the cause of this, and I suggest that you arrange for your child to see one at your convenience, taking this letter with you. Your local Post Office should have a list of family doctors in your area, or the Child Health Clinic may be able to advise you.

If GP consent refused, the penultimate paragraph read:

It is likely that your child's GP could find out the cause of this, and I suggest that you arrange for (child) to see him or her at your convenience, taking this letter with you.

356

Medical Research Council and the University of Cambridge

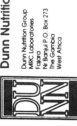

Dunn Nutrition Centre   *Patron:* **HRH The Princess Royal**

Dunn Nutrition Group   Dunn Clinical Nutrition Centre   **Please reply to:**
MRC Laboratories   Hills Road   Dunn Nutritional Laboratory
Fajara   Cambridge   Downhams Lane
Nr Banjul P.O. Box 273   CB2 2DH   Milton Road
The Gambia   Cambridge
West Africa   CB4 1XJ

Telegrams: Tropmedres, Banjul   tel: (0223) 415695   tel: (0223) 426356
                                   fax: (0223) 413763   fax: (0223) 426617

Dear Parents or Guardians,

You will doubtless remember taking part recently in the National Diet and Nutrition Survey of Children aged 1.5 to 4.5 years being carried out by the Social Survey Division of the Office of Population Censuses and Surveys for the Departments of Health and the Ministry of Agriculture, Fisheries and Food.

As part of the survey you were kind enough to consent to a sample of blood being taken from your child for analysis. We said that we would be letting you, and if you agreed, your child's GP, know the result of the measurement of haemoglobin.

Unfortunately in _____ case we were not able to measure the amount of haemoglobin. This was due to _____. The fact that we were unable to analyse this sample does not indicate that there was any abnormality.

This is of course regretful, but in a large study such as the National Diet and Nutrition Survey a few problems are bound to occur. Nevertheless, the other information you provided has been extremely useful to us.

Thank you for helping with the survey.

Yours faithfully,

Peter S.W. Davies   B.Sc, M.Phil, Ph.D
MRC Staff Scientist
Infant & Child Nutrition Group

Dunn Nutrition Centre   *Patron:* **HRH The Princess Royal**

Dunn Nutrition Group   Dunn Clinical Nutrition Centre   **Please reply to:**
MRC Laboratories   Hills Road   Dunn Nutritional Laboratory
Fajara   Cambridge   Downhams Lane
Nr Banjul P.O. Box 273   CB2 2DH   Milton Road
The Gambia   Cambridge
West Africa   CB4 1XJ

Telegrams: Tropmedres, Banjul   tel: (0223) 415695   tel: (0223) 426356
                                   fax: (0223) 413763   fax: (0223) 426617

Dear

Re:

The parent or guardian of the above named child who is one of your patients agreed to co-operate in a survey being carried out by the Social Survey Division of the Office of Population Censuses and Surveys for the Ministry of Agriculture Fisheries and Food and the Departments of Health.

As part of this National Diet and Nutrition Survey of children aged 1.5 to 4.5 years a venous blood sample was obtained to assess iron status and a wide range of micronutrient levels. It is our policy to report to General Practitioners and to parents the results of the measurement of haemoglobin. In the above named patient measurement of haemoglobin was _____ g/dl.

I hope this information may be of use to you.

Yours sincerely,

Peter S.W. Davies   B.Sc, M.Phil, Ph.D
MRC Staff Scientist
Infant & Child Nutrition Group

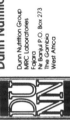

Dunn Nutrition Centre　　　　*Patron:* **HRH The Princess Royal**

Dunn Nutrition Group
MRC Laboratories
Fajara
Nr Banjul P.O. Box 273
The Gambia
West Africa

telegrams: Tropmedres, Banjul

Dunn Clinical Nutrition Centre
Hills Road
Cambridge
CB2 2DH

tel: (0223) 415695
fax: (0223) 413763

Please reply to:
Dunn Nutritional Laboratory
Downhams Lane
Milton Road
Cambridge
CB4 1XJ

tel: (0229) 426356
fax: (0223) 426617

Dear

Re:

The parent or guardian of the above named child who is one of your patients agreed to co-operate in a survey being carried out by the Social Survey Division of the Office of Population Censuses and Surveys for the Ministry of Agriculture Fisheries and Food and the Departments of Health.

As part of this National Diet and Nutrition Survey of children aged **1.5 to 4.5 years** a venous blood sample was obtained to assess iron status and a wide range of micronutrient levels. It is our policy to report to General Practitioners and to parents the results of the measurement of haemoglobin. In the above named patient measurement of haemoglobin was　　　　g/dl.

I hope this information may be of use to you.

Yours sincerely,

Peter S.W. Davies　B.Sc, M.Phil, Ph.D
MRC Staff Scientist
Infant & Child Nutrition Group

Dunn Nutrition Centre　　　　*Patron:* **HRH The Princess Royal**

Dunn Nutrition Group
MRC Laboratories
Fajara
Nr Banjul P.O. Box 273
The Gambia
West Africa

telegrams: Tropmedres, Banjul

Dunn Clinical Nutrition Centre
Hills Road
Cambridge
CB2 2DH

tel: (0223) 415695
fax: (0223) 413763

Please reply to:
Dunn Nutritional Laboratory
Downhams Lane
Milton Road
Cambridge
CB4 1XJ

tel: (0223) 426356
fax: (0223) 426617

Dear

Re:

The parent or guardian of the above named child who is one of your patients agreed to co-operate in a survey being carried out by the Social Survey Division of the Office of Population Censuses and Surveys for the Departments of Health and the Ministry of Agriculture Fisheries and Food.

As part of this National Diet and Nutrition Survey of children aged 1.5 to 4.5 years a venous blood sample was obtained to assess iron status and a wide range of micronutrient levels. It is our policy to report to GP's and parents any abnormal value for haemoglobin (g/dl), ferritin (µg/l), zinc protoporphyrin (µmol/mol Haem), vitamin A and vitamin D. In the above named patient we found the following result:

which falls outside the normal range for a child of this age. The child's parents/guardians have been informed and advised to arrange for the child to see you.

Yours sincerely,

Peter S.W. Davies　B.Sc, M.Phil, Ph.D
MRC Staff Scientist
Infant & Child Nutrition Group

Medical Research Council and the University of Cambridge

(ii) Copies of consent forms

N1340 Young Children's Dietary Survey - GP consent form

Serial number label

Today's date: [9 | 3]

Name of child: ....
first name   surname

Child's date of birth

Sex of child: Boy / Girl
delete as appropriae

Address: ....

Name of child's GP: Dr ....

Address: ....
....

I consent to:

(i)   The Social Survey Division of the Office of Population Censuses and Surveys informing the Medical Research Council's Dunn Nutrition Unit of the above information.

Signature of parent/guardian: ....

(ii)   The Medical Research Council's Dunn Nutrition Unit writing to my child's GP informing him/her of my participation in this survey.

Signature of parent/guardian: ....

(iii) I consent to the Dunn Nutrition Unit notifying my child's GP of the results of the haemoglobin analysis, and, if any result is abnormal, to the Dunn Nutrition Unit notifying my child's GP of all the results of the blood analyses carried out on the sample provided.

Signature of parent/guardian: ....

INTERVIEWER USE ONLY	ring code
Full consent given	1
No GP	2
Consent (i) refused	3
Consent (ii) refused	4
Consent (iii) refused	5

Dunn Nutrition Centre
patron: HRH The Princess Royal

Dunn Nutrition Group
MRC Laboratories
Fajara
Nr Banjul P.O. Box 273
The Gambia
West Africa

Dunn Clinical Nutrition Centre
100 Tennis Court Road
Cambridge
CB2 1QL

tel: (0223) 462099
fax: (0223) 312434

tel: (0223) 426356
fax: (0223) 426617
Telex: 818448 (DUNN UK)

Teagram, incamesh, Banjul

YOUNG CHILDRENS DIETARY SURVEY

Consent for a Minor to take part in research.
(Ages under 16)

NAME OF CHILD: ....

DATE OF BIRTH: ....

I, ...

acting as the parent/guardian of the above-named child give my consent to his/her taking part in the research project named above, and providing a blood sample.

- I understand that the research is designed to add to medical knowledge, and will add to medical knowledge which will help other children.

- I have read the note of explanation about the study.   Yes/No
  This is attached and I have had time to consider it.

- I have had the study explained to me by ....   Yes/No

- I have been told that I may withdraw my consent at any stage without giving a   Yes/No
  reason, and without prejudice to the treatment of my child.

Signed: ....

I also consent to the blood sample taken being analysed for haematological status, vitamins, trace elements, fat, albumin and markers of immune function. The sample **will not** be tested for HIV (i.e. AIDS tests).

Signed: ....

I also consent to any remaining blood being stored and that it may be analysed in other ways.

Signed: ....

Witness: I confirm that the parent/guardian

....   I confirm that the parent/guardian of

.... has given consent to the study freely and readily.

Signed: ....
(A witness should not be a member of the project team)

I confirm that I have explained to the parent/guardian the nature of this study, and have given adequate time to answer any questions concerning it.

Signed: ....
(Senior investigator or member of the project team acting on their behalf)
(Survey interviewer)

Medical Research Council and the University of Cambridge

359

Appendix N

Methods of blood analysis and quality control

1.0 Haematology

1.1 Blood counts including haemoglobin
Blood counts were performed using a Coulter S Plus Junior, a Coulter Max M or Coulter T660. Both these counters employ impedance counting methodology and haemoglobins were measured using a cyanmethaemoglobin colorimetric technique at 540nm. Samples were analysed on the day of receipt, that is within 24 hours of taking blood, in almost all cases.

The machine was controlled daily using Coulter 4C commercial control material. Instrument drift was controlled by running mean analysis (Bull Algorithm) on all samples. External quality control consisted of the UK National External Quality Assessment Scheme (NEQAS) and the Addenbrooke's External Quality Assessment Scheme (EQAS). Quality control data for haemoglobin are shown in Table 1.

1.2 Zinc protoporphyrin (ZPP)
ZPP estimation used the Helena Protofluor. One drop of EDTA whole blood mixed with two drops of Protofluor reagent on a coverslip was exposed to light at 415nm. Excited zinc protoporphyrin emits light at 595nm which is filtered and focused on to a photomultiplier tube. A current, level in response to the light reaching it, is proportional to the ZPP/haem ratio. In the five seconds after measurement, the average of 1000 light level readings gives a value for ZPP/mol haem.

The machine was controlled on a daily basis using Helena Protofluor high and low level controls. No other control material was available. Quality control data are shown in Table 2.

Concerns have been expressed, particularly in North America, about the precision of the Helena Protofluor method of mea-suring protoporphyrin levels. Quality control materials, provided by the manufacturer, may not always give long-term consistency of results. Daily calibration was particularly important.

1.3 Plasma ferritin
EDTA samples were centrifuged after blood counts and ZPP estimations had been performed. Plasma was removed and stored at –40°C until assayed. The assay, with Becton-Dickinson monoclonal antibody-coated tubes, used an immunoradiometric (IRMA) assay ('sandwich technique') where excess amounts of antibodies are used to form a complex with the analyte.

The Becton-Dickinson ferritin monoclonal antibody solid phase system contains a monoclonal antibody immobilised on the surface of a plastic tube and radioactive monoclonal antibody directed against ferritin. This procedure is not subject to loss of precision of the assay at high values, samples with high ferritin values will not give false values in the normal ranges, and levels of up to 2000μg/l may be measured without dilution.

Radioactivity in the samples was measured using LKB-Wallac 1261 Multigamma counter and data reduction performance by means of Riacalc software.

Internal quality control used Becton-Dickinson Riatrac three level control material, and external quality control was by means of UK NEQAS for haematinic assays run by haematology department, North Manchester General Hospital NHS Trust. Quality control data are shown in Table 3.

2.0 Fat soluble vitamins

2.1 Retinol, tocopherols, lutein/zeaxanthin, lycopene, cryptoxanthins, α-carotene and β-carotene in plasma
The assay was based on the procedure described by Thurnham et al, 1988[1]. The measurement of lutein (representing lutein plus zeaxanthin) has also been added to that of the other carotenoids.

Plasma proteins are precipitated using ethyl alcohol to release the nutrients into the aqueous alcoholic solution from which they are then extracted into heptane. A portion of the heptane extract is evaporated to dryness and reconstituted with mobile phase prior to injection on to a 100 x 4.6mm, 3μm Spherisorb ODS-2 column for separation and quantification. A guard column is not used and the column is protected by a 0.5μm pore size, stainless steel frit. Flow rate is approximately 0.8ml/min and run time is approximately 10 minutes.

The nutrients were measured in 0.1ml aliquots of plasma and other reagents were scaled down accordingly except heptane. The mobile phase was methanol, acetonitrile and chloroform (47:47:6,v/v/v) in which was dissolved 25mg/l butylated hydroxytoluene. The standardisation of the individual nutrients is described in the paper except for lutein for which a mM extinction coefficient of 145.1 (445nm, in ethyl alcohol) was used to obtain the response factor.

Extinction coefficients are used to calculate the concentration of the individual standards. Response factors are obtained from the areas of the standards after adjusting for purity. Standardisation is checked after any modification in the chromatography, for example new batch of solvents, new column, new bulb etc.

Plasma samples were analysed for retinol, γ- and α-tocopherol, α- and ß-carotene, lutein, lycopene, α- (pre) and ß-cryptoxanthin by high pressure liquid chromatography (HPLC) on a 4.6 x 100mm, 3μm ODS-2 Spherisorb column after heptane extraction. Absorbance was measured at 450nm to quantify carotenoids, 325nm for retinol and 292nm for the tocopherols (Thurnham et al[1]). External quality assurance (EQA) for most of these components was by participating in the National Institute of Standards Scheme organised in Washington DC. Internal quality assurance (IQA) was obtained using in-house serum samples stored at -40°C (Thurnham and Flora[2]). QC data collected in the four three-month fieldwork periods (waves) are shown in Table 4.

The retinol assay gave good agreement in both EQA and IQA throughout the survey.

Quality control data for α- and ß-carotenes, and for the tocopherols showed a small fall in mean results between Waves 1 and 2 in both EQA and IQA. The results of quality control assays throughout all four waves, using both external and internal quality assessments were scrutinised. There was a minor degree of downward drift in the results from internal quality control materials from Wave 2 through to Wave 4. It was decided retrospectively that the IQA materials, being three years old, were deteriorating during the period of the survey. This had not been identified during the survey since the marker substance used to assess the quality of the IQA material was retinol and this showed no such loss. EQA results for these three waves were consistently satisfactory. It was concluded that all results of assays of the samples from the survey should be accepted as reliable.

For lutein, lycopene and the cryptoxanthins the results of assays of quality control materials showed a larger fall between Waves 1 and 2 than described for the other analytes above. In subsequent waves the mean IQA results were more consistent and comparison of results with the EQA showed acceptable limits of variation (fewer laboratories are available for comparison so the EQA results provide more limited information). To adjust for the likelihood that assay results from Wave 1 of lutein, lycopene and the cryptoxanthins may have been somewhat too high, when compared with Waves 2, 3 and 4, the sample results from Wave 1 were adjusted on the basis of factors developed to take account of both IQA and EQA results. Thus for Wave 1 only, lutein was multiplied by 0.785, lycopene by 1.18 and the cryptoxanthins by 0.56.

2.2 25-hydroxyvitamin D in plasma
The assay employed a kit produced by INCSTAR Corpn, Minnesota USA: '25-hydroxyvitamin D ^{125}I RIA Kit', based on the method of Hollis and Napoli[3]. An antibody to 25-hydroxyvitamin D has been generated in rabbits by the vitamin D analog: the 23, 24, 25, 26, 27-pentanor-C(22)-carboxylic acid of vitamin D, chemically coupled with bovine serum albumin. Following extraction of human plasma samples with acetonitrile, the extracted 25-hydroxyvitamin D is mixed with ^{125}I-labelled tracer vitamin D, and then interacts with the specific rabbit antibody. The ligand-antibody complex is mixed with a second antibody to give a precipitate, which is collected by centrifugation and counted in a gamma-counter. This assay is a newly-marketed modification of the [3]H-25-hydroxyvitamin D RIA Kit from the same manufacturer. Because of the high degree of specificity introduced by the rabbit antibody, pre-purification of the acetonitrile extract is not necessary.

Quality control included the manufacturer's quality control serum with an assigned 25-hydroxyvitamin D value, and a pool of normal human heparinised plasma obtained from Dunn laboratory staff, stored in small aliquots at -80°C.

Coefficients of variation (CV) of assays of control materials over approximately a 12-month assay period using both in-house (plasma stored at -80°C) and commercial quality control materials (kit and Lyphochek controls) ranged between 11% and 13%, intra-assay CV's were 7%. Both were comparable with the manufacturer's values. Average values obtained for each are shown in Table 5. Towards the end of Wave 4, BioRad control gave a concentration value of 27.39 ng/ml over five runs compared to assigned value with Incstar kit of 26ng/ml (range 18–34).

3.0 Water soluble vitamins

3.1 Erythrocyte glutathione reductase for riboflavin status, in red blood cells
This assay was adapted from the manual technique developed by Glatzle and colleagues[4] for use with a 'Cobas Bio' centrifugal analyser[5]. The initial reactivation of the unsaturated apoenzyme in the sample is carried out for a relatively long period (30 minutes at 37°C), in order to ensure full reactivation of apoenzyme with only a low final concentration of flavin adenine dinucleotide (FAD) (1.5μM). This is necessary in order to eliminate activation coefficients (ratios) less than 1.0, which can be caused by partial enzyme inhibition by FAD or its breakdown products, if the amount of FAD used is too high.

After collection and centrifugation of the heparinised blood sample and removal of plasma at the local laboratory, the red cells were washed with saline to remove adherent plasma and the buffy coat layer. Following transport to Dunn Nutrition Laboratory, Cambridge, on dry ice, and storage at -80°C, batches of samples were thawed, diluted in buffer, centrifuged, and the extracts were incubated with and without FAD (30 minutes at 37°C). Addition of assay reagents (oxidised glutathione and reduced pyridine nucleotide coenzyme) took place in the centrifugal analyser, and was followed by a 5 minute measurement of the reaction rate at 340nm, 37°C. The ratio of FAD—stimulated to unstimulated activity, known as 'EGRAC' (erythrocyte glutathione reductase activation coefficient)—measures riboflavin status.

Quality control samples comprised pools of red cell haemolysates with low and high values of the activation coefficient, prepared from samples from United Kingdom and Gambian subjects, stored in aliquots at -80°C, and thawed on the day of analysis. Mean values for these analyses for each wave are shown in Table 6.

3.2 Folates in red blood cells
A number of studies have shown that there is adequate stability of red cell folate at 4°C provided the samples are subsequently extracted in the presence of ascorbate.

The assay used the BioRad (California, USA) Quantaphase Folate radioassay kit, in which a sample of heparinised whole blood, diluted 1:10 in 1% w/v ascorbic acid pH 4.6 is mixed with an equal volume of human serum albumin ('red cell folate diluent'). After storage at -80°C, blood is assayed by a competitive protein-binding assay, using microbeads that have been coupled to a specific folate binder. Labelled folate, to be displaced by the unlabelled folate of the sample-extracts, is ^{125}I-labelled pteroyl glutamic acid and the calibration standards (0-45nM) comprise unlabelled pteroyl glutamic acid in a human serum albumin solution. In order to eliminate all unwanted folate-binding by components of the sample, and also to ensure equivalent activities by the different forms of folate that are present in blood and in the assay, there is an initial heating step in the presence of buffer and of dithiothreitol, and the assay is then performed at pH 9.1. The concentration of folate in the packed red cells was calculated from the haematocrit, measured at the Great Ormond Street Laboratory with a correction for plasma folate.

In order to assess quality control, lyophilised samples of Bio-Rad Lyphochek Whole Blood, with assigned values for red cell folate (2 levels), were reconstituted in 1% ascorbate pH 4.5 and were stored in small aliquots at -80°C; a fresh sample was thawed for each assay. The mean values for these analyses are shown in Table 6.

3.3 Plasma folate and vitamin B_{12}

Plasma folate and vitamin B_{12} measurements were carried out using BioRad kit. The assay of plasma folate and vitamin B_{12} are performed simultaneously. The principle involved is competitive binding. In the case of the vitamin B_{12} assay, both B_{12} in the sample (or standard/control) and ^{57}Co labelled vitamin B_{12} are competing for the same binder, porcine intrinsic factor. The more B_{12} present in the sample, the less ^{57}Co labelled B_{12} will bind to the intrinsic factor.

For folate assay, the principle is the same as the B_{12} assay, but the binder is a purified folate binder from bovine milk and the tracer is ^{125}I labelled folate.

As the two assays use different radioisotopes, they may be performed together, but counted independently on the gamma counter.

Internal quality control was performed using Becton-Dickinson Riatrac three level control materials, and external quality control was by UK NEQAS for haematinic assays run by haematology department, North Manchester General Hospital NHS Trust. These samples are distributed monthly. Quality control data are shown in Table 7.

3.4 Vitamin C in plasma

The assay was based on the procedure described by Vuilleumier and Keck[6] in 1989. Conversion of ascorbic acid to de hydroascorbic acid by a specific enzyme, ascorbate oxidase, obtainable from Sigma, London, is followed by coupling of the resulting dehydroascorbate with ortho-phenylene diamine, to give a fluorescent quinoxaline. The formation of this quinoxaline is linearly related to the amount of vitamin C in the sample, over the range, $0–10\mu g/ml$ ($0-57\mu M$) which is a typical range for vitamin C in plasma, after dilution 1:2 with 10% metaphosphoric acid. The assay was performed on a Roche 'Cobas Bio' centrifugal analyser with fluorescence attachment.

It is well documented that levels of vitamin C in whole blood deteriorate rapidly unless stabilised. Nevertheless, it has been shown (M Levine, personal communication) that if normal heparinised blood is stored at 4°C in the dark, no deterioration in its vitamin C content is demonstrable for up to 29 hours. In another study by Galan et al[7] 17 heparinised blood samples were stored for 8 hours at 4°C in the dark and subsamples were analysed every 2 hours. There was no evidence of any downward trend in content and only a 3% random fluctuation around the mean. Therefore, unless the blood sample is unusual, for example haemolysed or containing a large amount of pro-oxidant, the evidence available supports storage for 5 to 8 hours with probably negligible loss and for 24 hours with not more than 10% loss. For this reason blood samples collected in this survey were kept next to an ice brick and in the dark prior to stabilization.

Each set of assays was calibrated with freshly prepared vitamin C standards which comprised heparinised plasma, with vitamin C added to give three known concentrations, and stored at -80°C in metaphosphoric acid. The mean values of these analyses are shown in Table 8. Preliminary trial runs verified the stability of vitamin C under the collection, stabilisation and storage conditions used (see *Appendix L*), and the validity of the fluorometric assay procedure, by cross-correlation with HPLC-based assays, and by experiments on whole blood with added vitamin C at known concentrations.

3.5 Vitamin B_6

Several vitamin B_6 related analytes have been used as status indices, none of which when used alone, are currently considered reliable and accurate. None of them have generally agreed limits of normality, in relation to the risk of deficiency for young children. Pilot studies, using a commercial kit for the measurement of pyridoxal phosphate concentrations in plasma samples revealed that inter-run reproducibility was poor, and that the method was designed for the specific use of EDTA-anticoagulated blood samples, which were not readily available in this survey. For these reasons it was concluded that results obtained by this method could not be guaranteed as accurate or easy to interpret. Consequently vitamin B_6 was not measured in this survey.

4.0 Zinc in plasma

Standardised precautions were taken to minimise the possibility of zinc contamination (acid-washed glassware; single use of trace element-free plastic containers, zinc-free gloves, Elgastat deionised water etc). Haemolysed samples were discarded.

The assay employed a kit produced by Wako Chemicals GmbH, Neuss, Germany. Zinc in the sample (plasma deproteinised with trichloroacetic acid) is chelated by the reagent '5-Br-PAPS' (2 – (5 – bromo – 2 – pyridylazo) – 5 – (N – propyl – N – sulfopropylamino) – phenol). The colour produced by this complex is directly proportional to the amount of zinc in the plasma sample, and has been shown, both by the manufacturer and Dunn Nutrition Laboratory, to correlate closely with results obtained by the more conventional flame atomic absorption spectrometry procedure.

Quality controls comprised a reconstituted lyophilized human serum sample, with an assigned zinc value (Versieck, Belgium: $9.6\mu g/g$ ($147nM/g$) freeze-dried material), and two controls (BioRad Lyphochek Unassayed Chemistry Human Serum), reconstituted and stored in small aliquots at -80°C. The mean values of these analyses are shown in Table 9.

5.0 Acute phase proteins

5.1 α_1-Antichymotrypsin

This assay was as in the Dakopatt's brochure which is based on the procedure described by Calvin and Price, 1986[8]. Serum/plasma is diluted 1:41 times with dilution buffer. Standards are prepared from Calibrator Human Serum Standard (Code no X908) to cover the range 0.2–2.39g/l. Antisera (Dako Ltd) are diluted 1:5.5 (v/v) in dilution buffers. Diluted serum ($80\mu l$) is incubated with $10\mu l$ water at 37°C for 20 seconds. The reaction is started by adding $50\mu l$ diluted α_1-antichymotrypsin antiserum. Formation of the immunoprecipitate is monitored at 340nm over 10 minutes at 37°C. Calibration uses a standard curve measured for each new preparation of antibody. The measurement is carried out in a Cobas Fara. The reaction buffer consists of 7% (w/v) polyethylene glycol (PEG) 6000 in 0.1M-phosphate buffer (pH 7.4) containing sodium azide (1.0g/l sodium phosphate buffer). The dilution buffer is the same as the reaction buffer but without PEG. Quality control data are shown in Table 10.

The assay was calibrated at the start of each new preparation of antibody and in addition each plate of 30 samples contained one or two 'in-house' QC samples. (Serotech HPSO1, Seronorm Protein Standard).

5.2 Caeruloplasmin

Caeruloplasmin was measured as described for α_1-antichymotrypsin. The method is that outlined in the Dakopatt's brochure. (TA900601).

Serum/plasma is diluted 1:41 with dilution buffer. Standards (Calibrator code no X908) are diluted with dilution buffer to cover the range of concentrations 0.06–1.3g/l. The anti-caeruloplasmin antibody is diluted 1:6 with the same diluent, then diluted 1:5 with reaction buffer containing 7% (w/v) PEG. Diluted serum ($80\mu l$) is incubated at 37°C with $10\mu l$ water for 20 seconds. The reaction is then started by the addition of $250\mu l$ diluted antiserum. The formation of the immunoprecipitate is followed over 4 minutes at 340nm and 37°C. Calibration is by reference to the standard curve prepared freshly from each new preparation of antibody.

Caeruloplasmin was measured using immunoprecipitation on a Cobas-Fara (Roche Diagnostics). IQA samples (Serotec and Seronorm) were used with each batch analysed. No EQA samples were used. Data for the two IQA samples for each wave of fieldwork are shown in Table 10.

5.3 Albumin
Albumin was measured as described for α_1-antichymotrypsin using the procedure described by Dakopatt for the Cobas-Fara centrifugal analyser. Serum/plasma is diluted 1:164 with dilution buffer and a range of standards from 22 to 45g/l is prepared from the calibrator reference serum (X908). Antiserum is diluted 1:33 with dilution buffer then diluted 1:5.5 with reaction buffer containing 5% (w/v) PEG.

Diluted serum (5μl) is incubated with 30ml water at 37°C for 20 seconds. The reaction is then started by adding 250μl diluted albumin antiserum. The formation of the immunoprecipitate is monitored at 340nm for 5 minutes at 37°C. The readings are calibrated by reference to the standard curve prepared freshly for each new preparation of antibody. Quality control data are shown in Table 10.

Mean results for α_1-antichymotrypsin and albumin for the children's samples in Wave 3 were high by comparison with the other waves. However there was no evidence of the same trend in the IQA or caeruloplasmin results suggesting that neither methodological bias nor sample drying was responsible. Likewise caeruloplasmin results in Wave 1 were higher than those in other waves but this was not observed in the IQA data.

6.0 Immunoglobulins

The principle of measuring all three immunoglobulins A,G and M is the same as that described for α_1-antichymotrypsin.

Serum was diluted 1:41 with the dilution buffer. Standards were prepared from Calibrator Human Serum Standard (Code no. X908) to cover the appropriate ranges.

IgA standard range 0.5g/l to 11g/l
IgG standard range 2.2g/l to 49g/l
IgM standard range 0.2g/l to 0.5g/l

Antisera (Dako Ltd) were diluted in the dilution buffer as follows:

IgA (Q 332) 1:6.6 volumes with dilution buffer
IgG (Q 331) 1:6.6 volumes with dilution buffer
IgM (Q 333) 1:3.67 volumes with dilution buffer

Each antisera was then diluted 1:5 with reaction buffer (5% PEG).

IgA   Diluted serum/standard (15μl) was incubated at 37°C on the Cobas with 75μl water for 20 seconds. The reaction was started by addition of 250μl diluted IgA antisera. The formation of the immunoprecipitate was monitored at 30nm for 10 minutes at 37°C. Readings were calibrated by reference to a standard curve prepared freshly for each new preparation of antiserum.

IgG   Diluted serum or standard (5μl) was incubated on the Cobas at 37°C with 80μl water, otherwise reaction conditions were the same as for IgA.

IgM   Diluted serum or standard (80μl) was incubated on the Cobas at 37°C with 10μl water otherwise reaction conditions were the same as those for IgA.

Immunoglobulin measurements for IgA, IgG and IgM were done on approximately 100 samples (25 from each three month period of fieldwork; *Table 11*) using immunoprecipitation techniques (Dakopatt). Samples from the different waves were measured in discrete batches. IQA results were similar which suggests that there were no differences between batches.

7.0 Lipids

The majority of samples were taken between 9am and 5pm from survey participants who were not fasting. An aliquot of 500μl was set aside for assays of lipid and zinc. The assays were carried out on a Roche 'Cobas Bio' centrifugal analyser using Roche kits.

Each assay was calibrated using a reconstituted lyophilised Roche lipid Control Serum and Boehringer Manheim Precinorm L. Lyophilised sera were reconstituted, bulked and divided into small aliquots prior to storage at -85°C. A sufficient number of aliquots for a day's assays were defrosted and assayed simultaneously and in the same manner as the survey samples. Waves 1 and 2 were analysed together; Waves 3 and 4 were analysed as each became available.

Instrument precision tests were made prior to each batch of analyses. Coefficients of variation were only accepted if they were below 1% and generally were between 0.3% to 0.5%.

7.1 Triglycerides in plasma
This is an enzymatic colorimetric test with glycerol phosphate oxidase and 4-aminophenazone. Plasma triglycerides are converted to glycerol by lipoprotein lipase. The glycerol in turn is converted to glycerol-3-phosphate by glycerol kinase and thence converted to dehydroxyacetone phosphate and hydrogen peroxide which, in the presence of peroxidase, effects the oxidative coupling of 4-chlorophenol and 4-aminophenazone to form a red coloured quinoneimine derivative. The colour intensity is proportional to the triglycerides concentration and is determined at a wavelength of 520nm. The level of triglycerides may be difficult to interpret when the subject is non-fasting as in this survey. This analysis required 4μl of plasma.

Quality control sera were included with each batch of samples. BCL 'Precinorm' was the material of choice.

Quality control data for trigylcerides are shown in Table 12. No trend was noted in the 32 batches analysed.

7.2 Total cholesterol
This is an enzymatic colorimetric test with cholesterol esterase, cholesterol oxidase and a peroxidase catalysed indicator reaction. Cholesterol ester is converted to cholesterol by cholesterol esterase and thence to Δ^4-cholesten-3-one and H_2O_2 by cholesterol oxidase. The liberated hydrogen peroxide in the presence of peroxidase effects the oxidative coupling of phenol and 4-aminoantipyrine to form a red coloured quinoneimine derivative. The colour intensity is directly related to the cholesterol concentration and is determined at a wavelength of 500nm. This analysis required 4μl of plasma.

Quality control sera were included with each batch of samples. BCL 'Precinorm' was the material of choice.

Quality control data for total cholesterol are shown in Table 12. No trend was noted in the 32 batches analysed.

7.3 HDL Cholesterol
Low density and very low density lipoproteins are precipitated using a phosphotungstate/magnesium chloride reagent. After centrifugation at 4000rpm for 10 minutes, the high density lipoproteins remain in the supernatant. The HDL cholesterol can then be assayed enzymatically using the cholesterol oxidase/4-amino-antipyrine method. This analysis required 100μl of plasma.

Quality control sera were included with each batch of samples. BCL 'Precinorm' was the material of choice.

Quality control data for HDL cholesterol are shown in Table 12. No trend was noted in the 32 batches analysed.

Expert review of laboratory procedures

The Department of Health commissioned an expert independent review of several of the laboratory procedures. We are grateful to Dr Elaine Gunter, Chief of the Laboratory of the National Health and Examination Survey (NHANES) in the United States of America for giving an expert opinion. NHANES is the third national survey conducted by the National Center for Health Statistics of the Centers of Disease Control of the US Departments of Health and Human Services in Atlanta, USA.

Dr Gunter visited the MRC Dunn Nutrition laboratories on 2 March 1993. She received written accounts and a presentation of methodologies, in particular, the specimen collection and processing and the methods for analysis of vitamins A and D, lipids, acute phase proteins, vitamin C, red cell folate, plasma zinc, and riboflavin. Although Dr Gunter did not visit the Hospital for Sick Children in London, she commented on written accounts of the haematology, protoporphyrin, ferritin, plasma folate and vitamin B_{12} assays.

The consultation has led to useful collaboration between Dr Gunter's laboratory and the MRC Dunn Nutrition laboratory concerning the laboratory procedures for this survey. A few modifications of technique were adopted for the analysis of blood samples following discussion with Dr Gunter. Dr Gunter records at the time of the review "I was very favourably impressed with the laboratory progress to date at the MRC Dunn Nutrition Unit".

Following the visit from Dr Gunter, it was decided not to attempt assay of vitamin B_6 in the samples. Further enquiries were made about the reliability of the Helena protofluor instrument for measuring zinc erythrocyte protoporphyrin since manufacture of this machine has now ceased (see *section 1.2* above).

References

1 Thurnham DI, Smith E, Flora PS. Concurrent liquid-chromatographic assay of retinol, α-tocopherol, β-carotene, α-carotene, lycopene and β-cryptoxanthin in plasma, with tocopherol acetate as internal standard. *Clin Chem.* 1988; **34**: 377-81.

2 Thurnham DI, Flora PS. Stability of individual carotenoids, retinol and tocopherol in stored plasma, *Clin Chem.* 1988; **34**: 1947.

3 Hollis BW, Napoli JL. Improved radioimmunoassay for vitamin D and its use in assessing vitamin D status. *Clin Chem.* 1985; **35**: 1815-9.

4 Glatzle D, Korner WF, Christeller S, Wiss O. Method for the detection of a biochemical riboflavin deficiency. Stimulation of $NADPH_2$ - dependent glutathione reductase from human erythrocytes by FAD *in vitro*. Investigations on the vitamin B_2 status in healthy people and geriatric patients. *Internat J Vit Nutr Res.* 1970 **40**: 166-83.

5 Powers H J, Bates C J, Prentice AM, Lamb WH, Jepson M, Bowman H. The relative effectiveness of iron and iron with riboflavin in correcting a microcytic anaemia in men and children in rural Gambia. *Hum Nutr: Clin Nutr.* 1983; **37C**: 413-25.

6 Vuilleumier J P, Keck E. Fluorometric assay of vitamin C in biological materials using a centrifugal analyser with fluorescence attachment. *J Micronutrient Anal* 1989; **5**: 25-34.

7 Galan P, Hercberg S, Keller H E, Bellio J P, Bourgeois C F, Fourlon CH. Plasma ascorbic acid determination: is it necessary to centrifuge and to stabilize blood samples immediately in the field? *Internat J Vit Nutr Res.* 1988; **58**: 473-474.

8 Calvin J, Price CP. Measurement of serum $α_1$-antichymotrypsin by immunoturbidimetry. *Ann Clin Biochem.* 1986; **23**: 206-209.

Acknowledgements

We wish to acknowledge the following who were involved in the analyses. Dr D I Thurnham and Mr L Edmund at the University of Ulster, Coleraine, for the analysis of fat soluble vitamins. The following staff at the Dunn Nutrition Unit, Cambridge: Dr A Prentice and Ms J Abbotts for vitamin D analysis, Mr B Baker for the assessment of lipids, Ms V Christeanssen for analysis of water-soluble vitamins and Mrs J Day for preparation of biochemical samples. Mr S Early and Ms D Muggleston for the haematological analyses at the Hospital for Sick Children, Great Ormond Street. We wish specifically to acknowledge the major contribution by Dr C Bates in all the analyses and all aspects of the biochemical assessment in this survey.

We are also indebted to personnel at the following hospitals for their assistance in local sample processing and storage.

Aberdeen Royal Hospitals NHS Trust; Arrowe Park Hospital NHS Trust (Liverpool); Blackburn Royal Infirmary; Bradford Hospitals NHS Trust; Bridgend District NHS Trust; Burnley General Health Care NHS Trust; Burton Hospitals NHS Trust; Carlisle Hospital NHS Trust; Coventry and Warwickshire Hospital Walsgrave NHS Trust; Derby City General Hospital NHS Trust; Dumfries and Galloway Royal Infirmary Acute and Maternity Services NHS Trust; Falkirk and District Royal Infirmary NHS Trust; Freeman Group of Hospitals NHS Trust (Newcastle); Friarage Hospital NHS Trust (Northallerton); Glenfield Hospital NHS Trust (Leicester); Good Hope Hospital NHS Trust (Sutton Coldfield); Grimsby General Hospital NHS Trust; Havering Hospital Trust (Romford); Homerton Hospital (London); Kent and Sussex Weald; Kettering General Hospital NHS Trust; Kidderminster Healthcare NHS Trust; Kings College Healthcare; Kingston General Hospital NHS Trust (London); Law Hospital NHS Trust (Motherwell); Luton and Dunstable Hospital NHS Trust; Maidstone Hospital NHS Trust; Maidstone Priority Care NHS Trust; Mansfield Hospital NHS Trust; Norfolk and Norwich Healthcare NHS Trust; Northampton General Hospital NHS Trust; Northern General Hospital NHS Trust (Sheffield); Northwick Park and St Marks NHS Trust (London); Oxford Radcliffe Hospital NHS Trust; Pontefract Hospitals NHS Trust; Queen Alexandra Hospital (Portsmouth); Raigmore Hospital NHS Trust (Inverness); Rotherham General Hospital NHS Trust; Royal Alexandra Hospital NHS Trust (Paisley); Royal Cornwall Hospitals NHS Trust; Royal Gwent Hospital; Glanhafren Trust; Royal Manchester Children's Hospital NHS Trust; Royal Oldham Hospital NHS Trust; Royal Preston Hospital NHS Trust; Royal Sussex County Hospital NHS Trust; Royal United NHS Trust (Bath); Royal West Sussex Trust (Chichester); Salisbury District Hospital NHS Trust; Selly Oak Hospital; Southend Healthcare Trust; Southmead Health Services NHS Trust; St Georges Hospital NHS Trust (London); St Lukes Hospital NHS Trust (Guilford); St Peters NHS Trust; St Richards Hospital; Stepping Hill Healthcare Trust (Stockport); University Hospital of Wales; Victoria (Kirkcaldy) Hospital NHS Trust; Warwick Hosptial NHS Trust; West Cumbria Health Care NHS Trust (Whitehaven); West Middlesex University Hospital NHS Trust; West Morland Hospitals NHS Trust; Whiston Hospital (Prescot); Withybush General Hospital NHS Trust (Haverfordwest); Wycombe General Hospital NHS Trust; York Hill NHS Trust (Glasgow).

Table 1   Quality control data for blood counts and haemoglobin

Instrument	Test	Result	DI	Median*	SD	CV%	N	
Coulter Max M	Haemoglobin concentration (g/l)							
	Sample 1	127	0.45	126	2.22	1.8	916	All
			0.68	126	1.48	1.2	171	Group
	Sample 2	123	0.45	122	2.22	1.8	915	All
			0.68	122	1.48	1.2	171	Group
Coulter Max M	Haematocrit (l/l)							
	Sample 1	0.378	−0.19	0.380	0.0104	2.7	883	All
			−0.27	0.380	0.0074	1.9	171	Group
	Sample 2	0.367	0.09	0.366	0.0111	3.0	882	All
			0.17	0.366	0.0059	1.6	171	Group
Coulter Max M	Mean Corpuscular Volume (fl)							
	Sample 1	90.1	−0.58	91.0	1.56	1.7	874	All
			−1.01	91.0	0.89	1.0	169	Group
	Sample 2	91.8	−0.28	92.3	1.78	1.9	873	All
			−0.67	92.4	0.89	1.0	169	Group
Coulter Max M	Mean Cell Haemoglobin (pg)							
	Sample 1	30.3	0.38	30.1	0.52	1.7	851	All
			0.38	30.1	0.52	1.7	154	Group
	Sample 2	30.7	−0.17	30.8	0.59	1.9	849	All
			0.00	30.7	0.59	1.9	154	Group
Coulter Max M	Mean Cell Haemoglobin Concentration (g/dl)							
	Sample 1	33.7	0.85	33.0	0.82	2.5	850	All
			1.04	33.0	0.67	2.0	154	Group
	Sample 2	33.3	0.21	33.2	0.96	2.9	848	All
			0.30	33.2	0.67	2.0	154	Group

Sample 1 = Partially fixed human whole blood
Sample 2 = Partially fixed human whole blood
DI = Deviation Index = (result − median)/SD

*Quality control values are expressed as medians in line with standard practice in clinical haematological laboratories.

Table 2   Quality control data for zinc protoporphyrin (µmol/mol haem)*

Precision data**			Internal quality control			
			Target	Lab value	Dev Index	
Mean	51.25	Internal	77.7	78	0.1	
SD	2	QC	77.7	74		−0.5
CV%	3.9	Sample	77.7	81	0.4	
N	20					

* Sample Quality Assessment not available
**That is values obtained from repeated analysis (20 times) of the same sample.

Table 3   Quality control data for plasma ferritin (µg/l)

Precision data*			Internal quality control		
			Target	Lab value	Dev Index
Mean	16.5	Low level QC	11.4	10.9	−0.4
SD	1.1			9.5	−1.7
CV%	6.7	Medium level QC	61.2	71.3	1.7
N	20			78.1	1.7
		High level QC	449	439	−0.2
				397	−0.12

External Quality Assessment

	Method mean	Lab value	Dev index
Sample 1	45.1	48	0.32
Sample 2	8.3	7	−0.77

*That is values obtained from repeated analysis (20 times) of the same sample.

Table 4 Quality control data for fat soluble vitamins, lutein and lycopene

Analyte and Wave*	High level quality control				Low level quality control			
	Mean	SD	CV	N	Mean	SD	CV	N
Retinol (μmol/l)								
1	1.46	0.111	8	23	0.73	0.066	9	19
2	1.45	0.090	6	6	0.71	0.063	9	6
3	1.47	0.120	8	5	0.70	0.008	1	4
4	1.47	0.077	5	8	0.76	0.113	15	5
β–carotene (μmol/l)								
1	0.974	0.131	13	23	0.330	0.038	11	19
2	0.809	0.233	27	6	0.314	0.031	10	6
3	0.685	0.102	15	5	0.295	0.096	30	4
4	0.783	0.128	16	8	0.289	0.028	10	5
α–carotene (μmol/l)								
1	0.309	0.037	12	23	0.050	0.008	16	19
2	0.249	0.064	25	6	0.046	0.006	13	6
3	0.234	0.031	13	5	0.030	0.008	28	4
4	0.273	0.023	9	8	0.040	0.010	28	5
Cryptoxanthins (μmol/l)								
1	0.369	0.033	9	23	0.191	0.022	11	19
2	0.319	0.020	6	6	0.178	0.007	4	6
3	0.286	0.029	10	5	0.136	0.020	14	4
4	0.267	0.023	9	8	0.145	0.018	12	5
Lutein (μmol/l)								
1	0.274	0.013	8	23	0.242	0.013	5	19
2	0.254	0.017	7	6	0.221	0.018	8	6
3	0.227	0.018	8	5	0.220	0.040	18	4
4	0.212	0.018	9	8	0.192	0.012	6	5
Lycopene (μmol/l)								
1	0.782	0.064	8	23	0.617	0.099	16	19
2	0.696	0.149	21	6	0.547	0.209	38	6
3	0.445	0.049	11	5	0.416	0.136	33	4
4	0.546	0.102	19	8	0.474	0.045	9	5
Tocopherols (μmol/l)								
1	20.26	0.69	4	23	13.59	0.520	4	19
2	18.04	2.25	12	6	11.78	0.612	5	6
3	17.48	1.45	8	5	10.88	1.460	13	4
4	17.41	1.43	8	8	11.77	1.770	15	5

*Fieldwork periods:
 Wave 1 – July to September 1992
 Wave 2 – October to December 1992
 Wave 3 – January to March 1993
 Wave 4 – April to June 1993

Table 5 Quality control data for 25-hydroxyvitamin D (nmol/l)

Wave*	Kit control				In-house control				Lyphochek control			
	Mean	SD	CV	N	Mean	SD	CV	N	Mean	SD	CV	N
1	32.02	1.93	6.0	16	47.10	5.60	11.9	32	79.17	10.10	12.7	15
2	34.57	2.85	8.2	23	54.72	5.12	9.4	46	83.62	7.95	9.5	22
3	38.95	3.50	9.0	21	56.62	7.10	12.5	42	85.62	9.77	11.4	20
4	37.27	3.17	8.5	26	58.35	8.10	14.2	52	86.00	9.12	10.6	25

*Fieldwork periods:
 Wave 1 – July to September 1992
 Wave 2 – October to December 1992
 Wave 3 – January to March 1993
 Wave 4 – April to June 1993

Table 6   Quality control data for the erythrocyte glutathione reductase activation coefficient and red cell folate

Analyte and Wave*	Low level QC				High level QC			
	Mean	SD	CV	N	Mean	SD	CV	N
The erythrocyte glutathione reductase activation coefficient (ratio)								
1	1.30	0.05	3.8	12	1.80	0.10	5.4	12
2	1.40	0.10	7.1	1	1.87	0.15	7.9	1
3	1.43	0.02	1.1	12	1.88	0.06	3.1	12
4	1.42	0.12	8.4	12	1.89	0.07	4.0	12
Red cell folate (nmol/l)								
1	118	2	1.6	6	1256	52	4.1	6
2	111	23	20.2	7	1010	349	34.5	7
3	139	10	7.3	7	1340	420	31.3	7
4	153	3	2.0	7	1587	103	6.5	7

*Fieldwork periods:
 Wave 1 – July to September 1992
 Wave 2 – October to December 1992
 Wave 3 – January to March 1993
 Wave 4 – April to June 1993

Table 7   Quality control data for plasma folate and vitamin B_{12}

Precision data*			Internal Quality Control		
			Target	Lab value	Dev Index
Vitamin B_{12}					
Mean	168	Level 1	163	190	1.7
SD	14			171	0.5
CV%	8.3	Level 2	398	412	0.4
N	20			420	0.6
		Level 3	940	998	0.6
				1005	0.7
Plasma folate					
Mean	4.93	Level 1	1.6	1.5	−0.6
SD	0.23			1.3	−1.9
CV%	4.6	Level 2	4	3.9	−0.3
N	20			3.6	−1.0
		Level 3	11.4	13	1.4
				1.5	0.1

External Quality Assessment

	Method mean	Lab value	Dev Index
Vitamin B_{12}			
Sample 1	251	327	1.37
Sample 2	385	485	1.3
Plasma folate			
Sample 1	8.1	7.3	−0.49
Sample 2	9.1	8.5	−0.33

*That is values obtained from repeated analysis (20 times) of the same sample.

Table 8   Quality control data for plasma ascorbate (vitamin C) (μmol/l)

Wave*	Low level QC				Medium level QC				High level QC			
	Mean	SD	CV (%)	N	Mean	SD	CV (%)	N	Mean	SD	CV (%)	N
1	4.5	1.7	37.0	6	33.4	2.4	6.8	6	68.6	3.8	5.4	6
2	5.1	0.8	15.0	5	34.5	2.6	7.2	5	72.2	3.0	4.0	5
3	5.3	1.3	24.0	6	31.2	3.7	11.8	6	72.8	1.0	1.3	6
4	6.8	0.6	8.0	5	29.5	2.2	7.2	5	67.7	2.0	2.9	5

*Fieldwork periods:
 Wave 1 – July to September 1992
 Wave 2 – October to December 1992
 Wave 3 – January to March 1993
 Wave 4 – April to June 1993

Table 9 Quality control data for plasma zinc (µmol/l)

Wave*	Versieck control				BioRad control 1				BioRad control 2			
	Mean	SD	CV (%)	N	Mean	SD	CV (%)	N	Mean	SD	CV (%)	N
1	8.6	1.0	12.1	3	12.2	1.4	11.1	3	14.2	1.3	9.2	3
2	6.9	0.4	5.7	4	10.6	0.2	2.2	4	12.7	0.5	3.7	4
3	10.0	2.0	20.0	4	13.8	2.6	19.1	4	15.2	0.9	5.8	4
4	9.1	0.2	2.2	3	14.3	0.8	5.7	3	12.5	3.6	28.4	3

*Fieldwork periods:
Wave 1 – July to September 1992
Wave 2 – October to December 1992
Wave 3 – January to March 1993
Wave 4 – April to June 1993

Table 10 Quality control data for acute phase proteins (g/l)

Analyte and Wave*	IQA 1**				IQA 2***			
	Mean	SD	CV	N	Mean	SD	CV	N
α_1–antichymotrypsin (g/l)								
1	0.233	0.007	3	7	0.696	0.048	7	7
2	0.244	0.005	2	7	0.680	0.024	3	6
3	0.236	0.005	2	8	0.633	0.018	3	8
4	0.240	0.000	0	8	0.633	0.034	5	8
Caerulopasmin (g/l)								
1	0.220	0.005	2	6	0.450	0.020	5	6
2	0.210	0.012	6	7	0.420	0.015	3	7
3	0.190	0.010	6	6	0.370	0.010	3	6
4	0.200	0.010	5	8	0.390	0.020	6	8
Albumin (g/l)								
1	26.55	1.78	7	6	53.90	3.46	6	6
2	26.70	0.64	2	7	49.66	2.26	5	5
3	30.34	1.76	6	8	55.09	4.76	9	8
4	29.19	0.41	1	8	54.97	0.71	1	8

*   Fieldwork periods:
   Wave 1 – July to September 1992
   Wave 2 – October to December 1992
   Wave 3 – January to March 1993
   Wave 4 – April to June 1993
** Internal Quality Assurance: control material with a low assigned value.
***Internal Quality Assurance: control material with a high assigned value.

369

Table 11 Quality control data for immunoglobulins (g/l)

Wave*	Children's samples		IQA 1**	IQA 2***
	Mean	N	Mean	Mean
IgA (g/l)				
1	0.949	27	1.53	3.85
2	0.777	23	1.49	3.85
3	1.094	24	1.49	3.72
4	0.885	27	1.50	3.87
IgG (g/l)				
1	9.84	27	8.77	17.07
2	8.20	23	8.61	16.80
3	10.13	26	8.48	17.56
4	8.77	27	8.57	17.10
IgM (g/l)				
1	0.96	27	0.61	1.61
2	0.79	23	0.63	1.67
3	0.98	26	0.63	1.67
4	0.80	27	0.63	1.70

*   Fieldwork periods:
     Wave 1 – July to September 1992
     Wave 2 – October to December 1992
     Wave 3 – January to March 1993
     Wave 4 – April to June 1993
**   Internal Quality Assurance: control material with a low assigned
     value
***Internal Quality Assurance: control material with a high assigned
     value

Table 12 Quality control data for blood lipids (mmol/l)

Wave*	Triglycerides				Plasma total cholesterol				HDL cholesterol			
	Mean	SD	CV (%)	N	Mean	SD	CV (%)	N	Mean	SD	CV (%)	N
1 and 2	1.629	0.021	1.289	32	4.546	0.045	0.990	32	0.974	0.034	3.491	32
3	1.674	0.031	1.852	32	4.653	0.076	1.633	32	0.970	0.026	2.680	32
4	1.713	0.032	1.868	32	4.588	0.078	1.700	32	0.992	0.019	1.915	32

*Fieldwork periods:
 Waves 1 and 2 – July to December 1992
 Wave 3 – January to March 1993
 Wave 4 – April to June 1993

Appendix O

Protocols for making the anthropometric measurements

Measurements taken were height, weight, mid upper-arm circumference, head circumference, and for children under two years, supine length. Weight was recorded to the nearest 100 grams, height and length, mid upper-arm and head circumferences to the nearest millimetre.

As gaining the co-operation of young children in taking measurements can be difficult and more than one attempt is often needed, it was decided that measurements could be taken by the interviewer at any point after the initial interview, and that a particular time of day would not be specified.

If interviewers were unhappy with the accuracy of any measurement they could repeat it until they were satisfied with its accuracy. However only one accurate measurement was required; feasibility work suggested that repeating a measurement to validate its accuracy might affect co-operation as some children would not tolerate re-measuring[1]. Interviewers recorded the number of attempts made to obtain each measurement along with any special circumstances which might have affected its accuracy. Measurements which were likely to have been inaccurate, or unreliable due to special circumstances have been excluded from the analyses. The numbers of children who co-operated with each of measurements are shown in Table 11.1, Chapter 11.

The date the measurement was taken and details of reasons for refusal of any measurement were also recorded on the questionnaire.

Interviewers were encouraged to explain to the child what they were doing, for example that they wanted the child to stand up straight or be a statue, and with young or fractious children they tried to get parents and any brothers and sisters to assist.

Interviewers were trained in accurate measurement techniques at the residential briefings. They practised the techniques on each other and on young children recruited from local playgroups. However it was not possible to assess intra-observer variation because it was not feasible to recruit the same children for each briefing, and the children would not tolerate repeated measurements by all interviewers.

1 Stature (height)

Height was measured using a portable, telescopic stadiometer, with a digital display[2].

The child was undressed to vest and pants and any nappy removed. Socks were also removed as these made it difficult to see whether the feet remained flat on the floor. Parents were asked not to put their child's hair in elaborate non-permanent styles, such as buns, as this would make measurement difficult and inaccurate.

Careful positioning of the child is crucial to obtaining an accurate measurement and the assistance of the parent was encouraged. The stadiometer was placed on a hard, level surface, switched on and the headplate extended above the height of the child. The child stood on the baseplate with his or her back to the rod. The interviewer then checked that the child's feet were together and flat on the ground, the legs and back were straight and that arms were at the sides. The headplate was then gently lowered until it was a little above the child's head. The head was positioned in the Frankfort plane (Fig 1) and

gentle traction was applied to the head to extend the child to maximum height.

Figure 1 **The correct position of the head when measuring height**

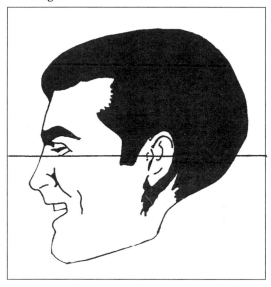

To achieve the correct Frankfort position the bottom of the orbital (eye) socket should be in line with the external auditory meatus, the protruding flap of firm skin on the front edge of the ear above the ear lobe. *(Fig 1)*

After gentle traction had been applied the headplate was lowered onto the child's head, checking that the child's feet were still flat on the baseplate. Once satisfied that the maximum height had been achieved the interviewer pressed the 'hold' button on the stadiometer freezing the measurement; the headplate was then raised above the child, allowing him or her to move away safely, and the measurement was recorded. *(Fig 2)*

The interviewer recorded on the questionnaire any difficulties in making the measurements and any other relevant information, for example posture problems, or known growth deficiency.

Supine length

This was attempted for all children who were under 2 years of age on the day of measuring.

The child was undressed as for the measurement of standing height. The stadiometer was switched on, extended and laid on an even, preferably uncarpeted floor, ideally with the baseplate against a wall or other solid vertical surface.

The child lay with his or her back on the floor and feet against the baseplate. The child's heels were placed together and the interviewer checked that the back and shoulders were on the floor and arms to the sides. The child's head was positioned facing forward with eyes looking up and in the Frankfort plane. Gentle traction was applied as for the measurement of height to stretch the child to the maximum length. The headplate was then moved onto the child's head. Once the interviewer was satisfied with the position of the child the measurement was recorded. *(Fig 3)*

Weight

Weight was taken using Soehnle Quantratronic scales calibrated in 100 gram units. The scales were checked for accuracy before being issued to interviewers and the batteries regularly changed.

The scales were placed on a hard, level surface. If only a carpeted surface was available then this was noted on the questionnaire.

The child was undressed to vest and pants and any nappy removed. If this was not possible the additional clothing or nappy being worn was recorded on the questionnaire. The scales were switched on, and when the display showed zero, the child was asked to stand on the scales with feet together, heels on the back edge, arms loosely at the sides, head facing forward and to remain still. The measurement was recorded on the questionnaire.   *(Fig 4)*

Mid upper-arm circumference

The measurement was made in two stages. With the left arm bare and at 90° across the body the mid point of the upper arm was located. Using a conventional tape the distance between the inferior border of the acromion and the tip of the olecranon process was measured, and the mid-point marked on the child's arm with a dermatological pen. To measure the circumference at the mid-point the child's arm was positioned loosely at the side. Using an insertion tape of non-stretchable material[3]

the circumference was measured, ensuring that the tape was horizontal, in contact with the arm around the entire circumference, and without pressure to compress the tissue. The measurement was recorded on the questionnaire.   *(Fig 5)*

Head circumference

This measurement was made with the child seated. An insertion tape was passed around the child's head, over the hair, just above the brow ridges and its position adjusted to the maximum circumference. Checking that the tape was horizontal, in contact with the child's head throughout its length, and under tension the reading was taken to the nearest millimetre.*(Fig 6)*

References and notes

1 White AJ, Davies PSW. *Feasibility study for the National Diet and Nutrition Survey of children aged 1½ to 4½ years.* OPCS (1994) (NM22).
2 The stadiometer was modified, to OPCS' specification from a Rabone building surveyor's measuring device by Glentworth Fabrications Ltd, Molly Millar's Bridge, Molly Millar's Lane, Wokingham, Berkshire, UK.
3 The insertion tape used to take mid upper-arm circumference was made by Teaching Aids at Low Cost (TALC) and is commonly used by field workers in developing countries to measure the head circumference of children. Tapes are available from TALC PO Box 49, St Albans, Herts, AL1 4AX.

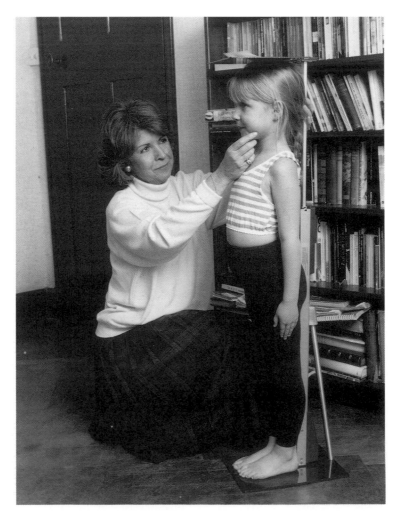

Figure 2   Measurement of standing height

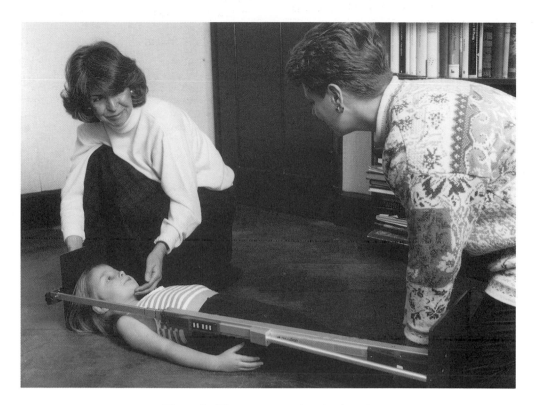

Figure 3   Measurement of supine length

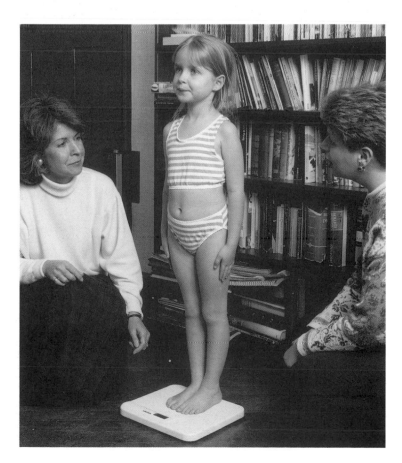

Figure 4   Measurement of weight

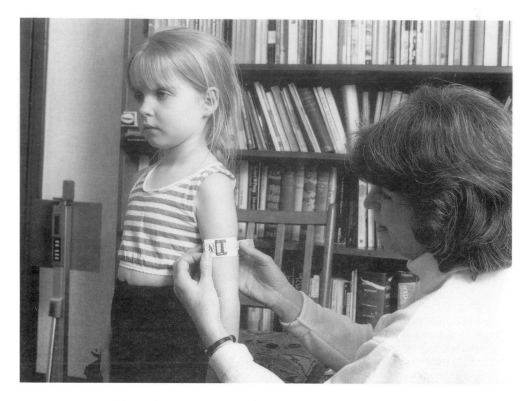

Figure 5   Measurement of mid upper-arm circumference

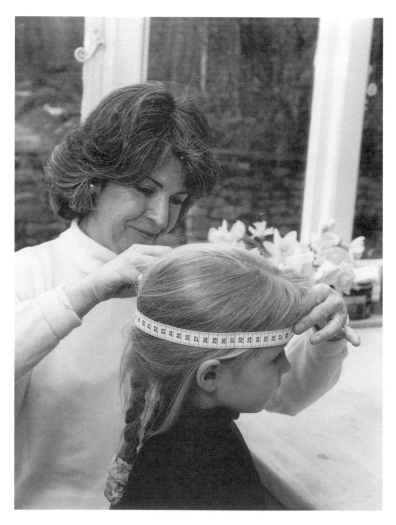

Figure 6   Measurement of head circumference

Appendix P

The 1967-68 survey of pre-school children[1]

In developing the protocol for the National Diet and Nutrition Survey of children aged 1½ – 4½ years, account was taken of an earlier Government survey carried out in 1967–68. This Appendix gives a brief account of the methodology and some of the main findings from this earlier survey. It is provided to allow the reader more convenient comparison with the current survey since the Government report published in 1975 may not be readily accessible.

1 The sample

Children in this survey were aged between 6 months and 4½ years. All of the children were living at home which excluded children in care. Children attending nursery or other day schools were also excluded, which particularly affected the group aged 3 to 4½ years. The selection of children was stratified to select children from different family sizes: families with one or two children, families with three children or families with four or more children. The sample was chosen using lists for Welfare Milk allocation with additional information on family size provided from health visitors' lists of children under their responsibility. There were compromises in choosing a sample on the basis of family size, especially in London where, for administrative reasons, it was not possible to use Welfare Milk records for sampling.

The sample was selected from 39 areas, in 38 Local Authorities in Great Britain. These 39 areas were regarded as corporately representative of the country, and comprised 4 areas in Scotland, 2 in Wales and 33 in England. Dates of fieldwork were October 1967 to September 1968.

The set sample size was 2,085 and from these an interview was obtained for 1,938 children; 63.4% of the sample participated fully in the survey.

2 Information collected for the survey

This included:

- social and demographic data
- height and weight of child
- heights of both parents
- weighed record of all food and drink consumed during seven consecutive days
- medical examination (only a proportion were invited to be examined)
- questionnaire about matters of dental interest (for example the use of dummies and infant feeders)
- dental examination (children aged 1½ to 4½ years only)

3 Characteristics of the sample

- Dietary records were obtained for 1321 children.
- The age distribution and social class distributions for fully co-operating children were as follows:

Age	
6 months – 1½ years:	201 children
1½ – 2½ years:	394 children
2½ – 3½ years:	407 children
3½ – 4½ years:	319 children

Social class	
I and II:	18%
III (non manual):	9%
III (manual):	48%
IV and V:	22%
Others:	3%

- School-leaving age of mother: 75.7% had completed their education by the age of 15 years.
- Child in a single parent family: 3.3%

4 Nutrient and dietary data

The food energy and nutrient intakes are shown in Table 1.

Milk provided the principal (23% of total) source of energy in the youngest group. It provided 15% of energy in the older groups, more protein than any other single food at all ages and it was the chief source of fat at all ages. It also provided more riboflavin and calcium than did any other individual food. In the older age groups, cakes and biscuits provided more fat than did milk. Carbohydrates provided 50% of the energy at all ages.

5 Children's heights and weights

The heights of 1627 children were measured at the time of the survey, and weight was recorded for 1688 children.

The weight of children was measured using apparatus designed to look, to the child, like a swing-seat suspended by ropes from a spring dial weighing machine. The clothes the child was wearing when weighed were subsequently weighed separately on the scales used for the dietary recording and the appropriate deduction made.

All children were measured in the supine position and the standing height of both parents was also measured. The equipment comprised a stainless steel footplate, containing an ordinary steel tape. Attached to the cowling of the steel tape was a flat flange - the head plate. Interviewers were instructed that no measurement of supine length was preferable to an unreliable measurement if the child was fractious or uncooperative.

Measurements of weight and height were adjusted by standardising to the mid-point of the age range by reference to normal rates of growth (Tanner, Whitehouse and Takaishi, 1966[2]).

The age-adjusted mean heights and weights of children by age group are shown in Table 2.

References

1 Department of Health and Social Security. Report on Health and Social Subjects: 10. *A Nutrition Survey of Pre-School Children in 1967–68*. HMSO (London, 1975).
2 Tanner JM, Whitehouse RH, and Takaishi M. Standards from birth to maturity for height, weight, height velocity and weight velocity; British children, 1965. *Arch. Dis. Childh.* 1966; **41:** 454–471; 613–635.

Table 1 Mean daily intakes of food energy and nutrients, including intakes from dietary supplements; Department Health and Social Security Survey of Nutrition of Pre-School Children 1967–8*

Nutrient	Age group		
	1½ – 2½ years	2½ – 3½ years	3½ – 4½ years
Energy (kcals)	1262	1401	1468
(MJ)	5.3	5.9	6.1
Total protein (g)	38.0	40.7	41.6
Precentage energy from protein	12.1	11.7	11.4
Fat (g)	54.4	59.7	61.9
Percentage energy from fat	38.8	38.4	37.9
Total carbohydrate (g)	164	186	197
Percentage energy from carbohydrate	48.7	49.8	50.3
Vitamin A (μg)	750	670	720
Thiamin (mg)	0.62	0.67	0.70
Riboflavin (mg)	1.07	1.07	1.08
Nicotinic acid (mg)	6.5	7.3	7.9
Vitamin B_6 (mg)	0.65	0.70	0.73
Vitamin C (mg)	40	37	38
Vitamin D (μg)	2.9	2.0	1.8
Calcium (mg)	691	658	661
Iron (mg)	6.6	6.8	7.1

* Department of Health and Social Security. Report on Health and Social Subjects: 10. *A Nutrition Survey of Pre-School Children 1967–8* HMSO (London, 1975).

Table 2 Mean heights and weights of pre-school children by age and sex; Department of Health and Social Security. Survey of Nutrition of Pre-School Children 1967–8*

Age and sex of child	Height			Weight		
	Mean (cm)	SD	No of children	Mean (kg)	SD	No of children
Boys aged:						
1½ – 2½ years	85.9	4.08	186	12.9	1.5	200
2½ – 3½ years	94.3	5.35	188	14.7	1.8	195
3½ – 4½ years	101.7	5.04	164	16.5	2.0	167
Girls aged:						
1½ – 2½ years	84.9	3.83	181	12.2	1.5	194
2½ – 3½ years	92.8	4.89	194	13.9	1.8	200
3½ – 4½ years	100.4	4.72	142	16.0	1.9	147

* Department of Health and Social Security. Report on Health and Social Subjects: 10. *A Nutrition Survey of Pre-School Children 1967–1968*. HMSO (London, 1975).

Appendix Q

The dental survey of children aged 1½ to 4½ years[1]: summary of main findings

Introduction

This dental survey is the first in many years to investigate the dental health of a nationally representative sample of British preschool children. It was carried out as the final component of the National Diet and Nutrition Survey (NDNS) of children aged 1½ to 4½ years[2].

The dental survey comprised a dental examination by a dentist seconded from the Community Dental Services of the National Health Service, and a dental interview. The examination included assessments for caries, trauma, or accidental damage, to the incisors and erosion of the upper incisors. The interview collected information on a range of topics including visits to the dentist, teething experiences, toothbrushing habits and the use of bottles, dinky feeders and dummies. Data relating to social and economic characteristics of children and their households were collected by questionnaire interview on the diet and nutrition survey and linked to the dental data. Some diet and nutrition survey data about dietary habits have also been linked to the dental data enabling investigation of a wide range of possible relationships between dietary behaviour and dental health. *(Chapter 1)*

The sample for the diet and nutrition survey and hence the dental survey was selected using a multi-stage random probability design. A total of 1658 children participated in the dental survey, representing 89% of those who took part in the diet and nutrition survey and 79% of those originally selected as eligible for the diet and nutrition survey (the eligible sample). For some children consent was given to the dental interview but not to the examination and for some children partial rather than complete examinations were carried out. A total of 1532 children had a complete examination for the caries component of the dental examination, 73% of the eligible sample. *(Chapter 2)*

Comparison of the characteristics of the responding sample with those of the total population and other large surveys showed very good agreement, confirming that the sample is representative of the population of children aged 1½ to 4½ years in private households in Britain. *(Chapter 2)*.

Dental decay among children aged 1½ to 4½ years *(Chapter 3)*

Overall, 17% of 1½ to 4½ year olds had some experience of dental decay. The proportion of children affected increased with age; 4% of 1½ to 2½ year olds, 14% of 2½ to 3½ year olds and 30% of those aged 3½ to 4½ years had some experience of dental decay. There was no variation in decay experience by sex. Most of children's decay experience was untreated or active decay. Only 2% of 1½ to 4½ year olds had filled teeth and 2% had teeth missing due to decay.

Overall, children aged 1½ to 2½ years had an average of 0.1 teeth with decay experience, those aged 2½ to 3½ years had 0.5 teeth affected and an average of 1.3 teeth showed decay experience among those in the oldest age cohort.

A higher proportion of children in households where the head was in a manual social class group, as defined by occupation, had experience of dental decay than was found among those from non-manual backgrounds. Decay experience was also related to the highest educational qualifications of children's mothers with those whose mothers had no educational qualifi-

cations having highest experience of dental decay and those whose mothers had GCE 'A' levels or above having lowest decay experience.

Decay experience varied noticeably among children from different parts of Britain; Scottish children and those in the North of England had more decay than those in other parts of England and Wales. Half of the 3½ to 4½ year olds in Scotland and 43% of those in the Northern region of England had some experience of dental decay compared with less than a quarter of those in the rest of England and Wales.

Children living in lone parent families, in households where the head was unemployed or economically inactive and in households where at least one adult was receiving Income Support or Family Credit were significantly more likely to have each type of dental decay than other children.

Dental care and advice *(Chapter 4)*

Prior to the survey, a quarter of 1½ to 2½ year olds, half the children aged 2½ to 3½ years and three quarters of those aged 3½ to 4½ years had been examined by a dentist.

Parents were asked whether they had received advice about what their child should be eating and drinking to look after their teeth, about cleaning their child's teeth and about giving or not giving their child fluoride drops or tablets; 60% had received advice on at least one of these issues and dentists and dental ancillaries were the main source of advice. Parents of children in Scotland were far more likely than those in other parts of Great Britain to have been advised to give their child fluoride drops or tablets; 65% of Scottish parents had received this advice compared with 24% of those in London and the South East, 18% in the Northern region and 12% in the Central and South West regions of England and Wales.

At the time of interview 98% of 1½ to 4½ year olds had started having their teeth brushed, either by an adult or themselves. For half the children in the survey toothbrushing started before the age of one year.

Most children sometimes brushed their own teeth and sometimes had their teeth brushed by an adult, however 10% of children had always brushed their own teeth. Over half the children in the survey (55%) had their teeth brushed (by self or other) more than once a day and one third had their teeth brushed once a day; 12% had their teeth brushed less than once a day.

Almost all children in the survey used fluoride toothpaste; about a third of children used toothpastes with low fluoride concentrations (below 600 parts per million). Eighteen per cent of children had used fluoride drops or tablets. The use of fluoride drops or tablets was more widespread in Scotland (over 50%) than elsewhere (less than 25%).

For many aspects of dental care, habits varied significantly for children with different social class backgrounds. Children from households with a non-manual head tended to have started toothbrushing at a younger age than those from manual backgrounds and they also brushed their teeth more frequently and were more likely to have been examined by a dentist prior to the survey.

The use of bottles, dinky feeders and dummies and the consumption of foods and drinks containing sugars *(Chapter 5)*

Overall, 87% of children had used bottles at some time; 49% of those aged 1½ to 2½ years and 8% of those aged 3½ to 4½ years were reported to be current bottle users. Thirty one per cent of 1½ to 2½ year olds were using bottles every night as were 6% of those in the oldest age cohort. Over half the children using bottles at night usually had milk in them (56%) while a quarter (24%) usually had a drink containing non-milk extrinsic sugars including squashes, carbonated drinks and flavoured milks[3].

Eighteen per cent of children had ever used a dinky feeder[4] and only 2% were said to be current users. Dinky feeders were mainly used during the day and drinks containing non-milk extrinsic sugars were most commonly consumed from them.

Just over half the children in the survey (53%) had ever used a dummy; only 5% of children had ever had a sweetened dummy.

The use of bottles, dinky feeders and dummies was more widespread among children from manual than from non-manual backgrounds.

Just under a third of children (31%) were reported to have a drink in bed every night and almost half (48%) sometimes had a drink in bed. When drinking in bed, 12% of children usually had a drink containing non-milk extrinsic sugars; two thirds of these children had a drink every night.

Five per cent of children were reported ever to have something to eat in bed or during the night.

Overall 43% of children had sugar confectionery and 24% had carbonated drinks on at least most days of the week, at the time of the survey (data from the dietary survey interview); for both the proportions consuming with this frequency increased with age. Children from manual backgrounds were much more likely to be frequent consumers of sugar confectionery and carbonated drinks than were those from non-manual households.

Dental care, dietary behaviour and dental decay *(Chapter 6)*

The younger children were when they started having their teeth brushed or brushing their own teeth and the more frequently the teeth were brushed, the lower the proportion having tooth decay. For example, 12% of those whose teeth were brushed (by self or other) before the age of one year had experience of caries compared with 34% of those who did not start toothbrushing until after the age of 2 years. Decay prevalence was higher among children who always brushed their own teeth than among those where an adult sometimes or always brushed their teeth for them.

Children who had never used a bottle, dinky feeder or dummy had considerably less experience of dental decay than those who had (13% compared with 32%).

A higher proportion of those aged 1½ to 2½ and 2½ to 3½ years who had a drink in bed every night had decay experience than of those who had a drink in bed only sometimes or never. Among all children who consumed drinks in bed every night, 29% of those who had a drink containing non-milk extrinsic sugars had experience of decay compared with 11% of those who had milk.

For children of all ages the frequency of consumption of sugar confectionery and of carbonated drinks reported in the dietary interview at the time of the survey was related to dental decay; for example, 40% of 3½ to 4½ year olds who had sugar confectionery most days or more often had experience of caries compared with 22% of those who consumed sugar confectionery less frequently.

Trauma to the incisors and erosion of the upper incisors *(Chapter 7)*

The incisors of 15% of children aged 1½ to 4½ years had experienced trauma (accidental damage); there was little variation by age or sex. Most of the trauma affected teeth on the upper jaw, only 2% of children had experienced trauma to the lower incisors. Fractures were the most common type of trauma recorded; 59% of children with some dental trauma had a tooth which was fractured only as far as the enamel while 14% and 2% had teeth which were fractured into the dentine and dental pulp respectively. Eight per cent of children with some experience of trauma had lost a tooth through accidental damage.

Dental erosion has been defined as the loss of dental hard tissue by a chemical process that does not involve bacteria[5]. The main causes of dental erosion are thought to be dietary habits such as the consumption of demineralizing acidic foods. An attempt to assess the national prevalence of erosion has been undertaken only once before this survey; on the 1993 survey of children's dental health in the United Kingdom[6]. This survey used the same methodology as the 1993 children's dental health survey to investigate erosion. The upper incisors were examined on both the buccal (front) and palatal (back) surfaces and for each surface an assessment was made as to whether there was erosion into the enamel, erosion into the dentine or erosion into the dental pulp. Erosion, especially into the enamel only, can be difficult to identify and different dentists may have made different assessments[7].

Erosion into the dentine or pulp affected the buccal surfaces of the teeth of 2% of children and the palatal surfaces of 8%. The prevalence of erosion increased with age, with 3% of children aged 1½ to 2½ years found to have some palatal erosion into the dentine or pulp compared with 13% of those aged 3½ to 4½ years.

For neither trauma nor erosion were differences identified by social class. Erosion was not found to be related to dental care or dietary behaviour.

References and notes

1 Hinds K, Gregory J. National Diet and Nutrition Survey: children aged 1½ to 4½ years. Volume 2: *Report of the dental survey.* HMSO (London, 1995).

2 This survey of the diet and nutrition of British children aged 1½ to 4½ years forms part of the National Diet and Nutrition Survey programme, which was set up jointly by the Ministry of Agriculture Fisheries and Food and the Department of Health to assess the dietary practices and nutritional status of different age groups within the British population. The dental component of this survey was commissioned from OPCS by the Department of Health. It is intended that dental surveys will also be linked to further surveys in the NDNS programme; these will focus on people aged 65 years and over, school children aged 5 to 15 years and adults aged 16 to 64 years.

3 Drinks containing non-milk extrinsic sugars included: fruit squash with sugar, blackcurrant drink (not diet), fruit juice or syrup, carbonated drinks (including low calorie carbonated drinks), hot chocolate, Ovaltine, Horlicks, flavoured milk, tea and coffee with sugar. A definition of non-milk extrinsic sugars is given in the Glossary to this report, Appendix G.

4 The term dinky feeder used in this report refers to the small comforter a child can be given, with a reservoir for small quantities of liquid behind the teat.

5 Pindborg J J (1970). *Pathology of Dental Hard Tissues* Copenhagen: Munksgaarrd, pp 312–321.

6 O'Brien M. *Children's Dental Health in the United Kingdom 1993* HMSO (London, 1994).

7 Further discussion of the methodology for the erosion examination is found in Chapter 7 of the Dental Report and Appendix F of the report of the 1993 survey of school children's dental health[6].

Appendix R

Units of measurement used in the Report

Units of energy

kcal   kilocalorie, 1000 calories. A unit used to measure the energy value of food.

kJ   kiloJoule, 1000 Joules. A unit used to measure the energy value of food.
1 kilocalorie = 4.18 kiloJoules

mJ   megaJoule, 1 million Joules

Units of length

cm   centimetre, one-hundredth of 1 metre

m   metre, 100 centimetres

mm   millimetre, one-thousandth of 1 metre

Units of volume

dl   decilitre, one-tenth of 1 litre

fl   femtolitre, 1 litre x 10^{-15}

l   litre, 1000 millilitres

l/l   litre per litre (ratio)

ml   millilitre, 10^{-3} litre, one-thousandth of 1 litre

Units of weight

g   gram

kg   kilogram, 1000 grams

mg   milligram, 10^{-3} grams, one-thousandth of 1 gram

mmol   millimol; the atomic or molecular weight of an element or compound in grams x 10^{-3}

μg   microgram, 10^{-6} grams, one-millionth of 1 gram

μmol   micromol; the atomic or molecular weight of an element or compound in grams x 10^{-6}

ng   nanogram, 10^{-9} grams, one-thousand-millionth of 1 gram

nmol   nanomol, the atomic or molecular weight of an element or compound in grams x 10^{-9}

pg   picogram, 10^{-12} grams, one-million-millionth of 1 gram

pmol   picomol, the atomic or molecular weight of an element or compound in grams x 10^{-12}

Appendix S

Glossary of abbreviations, terms and survey definitions

Benefits (receiving)	Receipt of Income Support or Family Credit by the child's mother or her husband/partner.
Biological parent	The term used to describe those who are biologically the parents of the child, that is, *not* adoptive, step or foster parents or cohabiting partners not genetically related to the child.
BMI	see *Body Mass Index*
Body Mass Index	A measure of body fatness which standardises weight for height: calculated as [weight (kg)/height (m)^2]. Also known as the Quetelet Index.
COMA	The Committee on Medical Aspects of Food Policy
CSE	Certificate of Secondary Education
cum %	Cumulative percentage (of a distribution)
CV	Coefficient of variation
Deft	Design factor; see *Notes* and *Appendix D*
DH	The Department of Health
DI	Deviation index: (result—mean) ÷ standard deviation (see *Appendix N*)
Diary sample	Children for whom a four-day dietary record, covering two weekdays and both weekend days, was obtained.
dna	Does not apply
DRV	Dietary Reference Value. The term used to cover *LRNI, EAR, RNI* and safe intake. (See Department of Health. Report on Health and Social Subjects: 41. *Dietary Reference Values for Food Energy and Nutrients for the United Kingdom*. HMSO (London, 1991))
DSS	The Department of Social Security
EAR	The Estimated Average Requirement of a group of people for energy or protein or a vitamin or a mineral. About half will usually need more than the EAR, and half less.
Economically inactive	Those neither working nor *unemployed*; includes students, the retired and individuals who were looking after the home or family.
Economic status	Whether at the time of interview the individual was *working, unemployed* or *economically inactive.*
EGRAC	The erythrocyte glutathione reductase activation coefficient
Emla cream	A topical local anaesthetic cream applied to the arm of some children at the site of the venepuncture.
EQA(S)	External quality assurance (scheme)
Extrinsic sugars	Any sugar which is not contained within the cell walls of a food. Examples are the sugars in honey, table sugar and lactose in milk and milk products.
Family	A unit within a *household* defined by their relationship to each other. A family unit can consist of: – married or cohabiting couple on their own;

	– a married or cohabiting couple/lone parent and their never married children; provided these children have no children of their own; – one person on their own.
Frankfort plane	The desired position for the child's head when measuring standing height and *supine length*. The position is achieved for standing height, when the line between the external auditory meatus and the lower border of the orbit is horizontal. In measuring *supine length* this line should be vertical.
GCE	General Certificate of Education
GHS	The General Household Survey; a continuous, multipurpose household survey, carried out by the Social Survey Division of OPCS on behalf of a number of government departments.
GP	General Practitioner
HDL cholesterol	High density lipoprotein cholesterol
Head of household	The head of household is defined as follows: (i) in a household containing only a husband, wife and children under age 16 years (and boarders), the **husband** is always the head of household (ii) in a cohabiting household the **male partner** is always the head of household (iii) when the household comprises other relatives and/or unrelated persons the **owner**, or **the person legally responsible** for the accommodation, is always the head of the household In cases where more than one person has equal claim, the following rules apply: (i) where they are of the same sex the oldest is always the head of household (ii) where they are of different sex the male is always the head of household
Highest educational qualification level	Based on the highest educational qualification obtained by the child's mother, grouped as follows:

Above GCE 'A' level
Degree (or degree level qualification)
Teaching qualification
HNC/HND, BEC/TEC Higher, BTEC Higher
City and Guilds Full Technological Certificate
Nursing qualifications (SRN, SCM, RGN, RM, RHV, Midwife)

GCE 'A' level and equivalent
GCE 'A' level/SCE higher
ONC/OND/BEC/TEC *not* higher

GCE 'O' level and equivalent
GCE 'O' level passes (Grades A-C if after 1975)
CSE (Grades A-C)
CSE (Grade 1)
SCE Ordinary (Bands A-C)
Standard Grade (Levels 1-3)
SLC Lower
SUPE Lower or Ordinary School Certificate or Matriculation
City and Guilds Craft/Ordinary Level

CSE and equivalent
CSE Grades 2-5, and ungraded
GCE 'O' Level (Grades D and E if after 1975)
GCSE (Grades D-G)
SCE Ordinary (Bands D and E)
Standard Grade (Levels 4 and 5)
Clerical or commercial qualifications
Apprenticeship
Other qualifications

None
No educational qualifications

The qualification levels do not in all cases correspond to those used in statistics published by the Department for Education

Household	The standard definition used in most surveys carried out by OPCS Social Survey Division, and comparable with the 1991 Census definition of a household was used in this survey. A household is defined as a single person or group of people who have the accommodation as their only or main residence and who either share one main meal a day or share the living accommodation. (See E McCrossan *A Handbook for interviewers*. HMSO: London 1985)
IgA, IgG, IgM	Three immunoglobulins—plasma antibodies—measured in the blood samples from some children

Intrinsic sugars	Any sugar which is contained within the cell wall of a food
IQA	Internal quality assurance (see also *EQAS, NEQAS*)
LRNI	The Lower Reference Nutrient Intake for protein or a vitamin or a mineral. An amount of the nutrient that is enough for only the few people in the group who have low needs.
MAFF	The Ministry of Agriculture, Fisheries and Food
Manual social class	Children living in households where the head of household was in an occupation ascribed to *Social Classes III manual, IV or V.*
Marital status	Informants were categorised according to their perception of marital status. Married and cohabiting took priority over other categories. Cohabiting includes anyone living with their partner (of the other gender) as a couple.
MCH	Mean cell haemoglobin
MCHC	Mean cell haemoglobin concentration
MCV	Mean corpuscular volume
Median	see *Quantiles*
MRC	The Medical Research Council
MUAC	Mid upper-arm circumference
NDNS	The National Diet and Nutrition Survey
NA	Not answered
NEQAS	The National External Quality Assurance Scheme
Non-manual social classes	Children living in households where the head of household was in an occupation ascribed to *Social Classes I, II or III non-manual.*
Non-milk extrinsic sugars	Extrinsic sugars, except lactose in milk and milk products
NSP	Non-starch polysaccharides. A precisely measurable component of foods. The best measure of 'dietary fibre'.
OPCS	The Office of Population Censuses and Surveys
PAF	Postcode Address File; the sampling frame for the survey
Percentiles	see *Quantiles*
Plasma 25-hydroxyvitamin D	Plasma vitamin D
Plasma ascorbate	Plasma vitamin C
PSU	Primary Sampling Unit; for this survey, postcode sectors
PUFA	Polyunsaturated fatty acid
QA (QC)	Quality assurance/Quality control
Quantiles	The quantiles of a distribution divide it into equal parts. The *median* of a distribution divides it into two equal parts, such that half the cases in the distribution fall, or have a value, above the median, and the other half fall, or have a value below the median.
Quetelet Index	see *Body Mass Index*

Region	Based on the Standard regions and grouped as follows:

Region — Based on the Standard regions and grouped as follows:

Scotland

Northern
    North
    Yorkshire and Humberside
    North West

Central, South West and Wales
    East Midlands
    West Midlands
    East Anglia
    South West
    Wales

London and South East
    London
    South East

The regions of England are as constituted after local government reorganisation on 1 April 1974. The regions as defined in terms of counties are listed in Chapter 3.

Responding sample — Informants who co-operated with any part of the survey

RNI — The Reference Nutrient Intake for protein or a vitamin or a mineral. An amount of the nutrient that is enough, or more than enough, for about 97% of the people in a group. If average intake of a group is at the RNI, then the risk of deficiency in the group is small.

se — Standard error of estimate; see *Notes and Appendix D* for method of calculation

sd — Standard deviation

SDR — Standard deviation ratio: the ratio of inter and intra individual standard deviations (*see Appendix J*)

SI units — *Système Internationale d'Unitès* (International System of Units)

Social Class — Based on the Registrar General's *Standard Occupational Classification,* Volume 3. HMSO (London, 1991). Social class was ascribed on the basis of the occupation of the head of household. The classification used in the tables is as follows:

Descriptive description	Social class
Non-manual	
Professional and intermediate	I and II
Skilled occupuations, non manual	III non-manual
Manual	
Skilled occupations, manual	III manual
Partly-skilled and unskilled occupations	IV and V

Social class was not determined for those whose head of household had never worked, was a full-time student, was in the Armed Forces or whose occupation was inadequately described. If the head of household was male, social class was determined on the basis of their present (main) occupation; if they were currently unemployed on the basis of the last occupation and if they were waiting to take up a new job, on the basis of that new occupation. If the head of household was female, social class was determined on the basis of what the informant regarded as her 'main' life occupation.

Supine length — Body length measured with the child lying down, face upward

Unemployed — Those actively seeking work, those intending to look for work but prevented by sickness (28 days or fewer) and those waiting to take up a job already obtained.

Working — In paid work, as an employee or self employed, at any time in the 7 days prior to the interview or not working in the 7 days prior to interview but with a job to return to, including, for women, being on maternity leave.

ZPP — Zinc protoporphyrin

Index

References are to table numbers; Appendix tables are referenced by letter, for example, D1 - Appendix D, Table 1. *References to figures are shown in italics.*